ATLAS OF ELECTROENCEPHALOGRAPHY

Second edition

Volume 1

Volume 1

Second edition

ATLAS OF ELECTROENCEPHALOGRAPHY

Philippe Gélisse and Arielle Crespel

Awake and sleep EEG
Activation procedures and Artifacts

John Libbey EUROTEXT

ISBN: 9-782-742-01507-8

Published by
Éditions John Libbey Eurotext
127, avenue de la République,
92120 Montrouge, France
Tél.: 01.46.73.06.60
Fax: 01.40.84.09.99
contact@jle.com
http://www.jle.com

John Libbey Eurotext
34 Anyard Road, Cobham
Surrey KT11 2LA
United Kingdom

PREFACE

More than ten years have elapsed since Arielle Crespel and Philippe Gélisse published the first edition of their EEG Atlas. It has been widely distributed, both in its French and in its English editions, and has remained a standard in many EEG labs around the world, as a practical guide and help for all those involved, especially EEG technicians and young neurophysiologists. This modern standard has gone out of print, and there was pressure, from many sides, for a second, updated edition. Here it is.

The authors rely on their extensive experience with the daily use of the EEG in clinical practice, in the setting of a reference, very active EEG lab, where the procedure is used for diagnostic and monitoring purposes in all its indications. There is a beginning, in the practice of EEG, that is often neglected: the good practices in the recording procedure, the detection of the numerous normal variants. All this is treated, in-depth, in the first volume of the 2nd edition of this atlas. There is of course a focus on epilepsy and the numerous pitfalls in its diagnosis, first and foremost because epilepsy is nowadays the main indication of EEG.

The authors have chosen not to insist on the special procedures used in highly specialized settings, such as intracranial recordings, or fusion procedures. This English-language edition complies with the international recording speed standard at 30 mm/sec. It covers both childhood and adult features, because there are indeed only slight age-related differences in the practical management of the EEG techniques. The high quality of iconography and accompanying legends will, I hope, ensure that a high level of technicity and reliability of the EEG – still often considered to be more "art" than "science" – will prevail among the new generations who lay their hands on this precious, useful, energy- and cost-effective procedure.

Pierre Genton, MD, Marseille, France

THE AUTHORS

Philippe Gélisse, M.D.

Neurologist and epileptologist, Dr Gélisse works in the Medical and Surgical Epilepsy Unit in Montpellier. His main research topics are juvenile myoclonic epilepsy, benign epilepsy with centro-temporal spikes, psychosis and epilepsy, and antiepileptic drug pharmacology. Dr Gélisse has published articles in international journals and has contributed chapters for books on these topics.

Arielle Crespel, M.D., PhD.

Dr Crespel is a neurologist and epileptologist in the Medical and Surgical Epilepsy Unit in Montpellier. This unit is designed for the management of children and adults with resistant epilepsy. Her main research topics are sleep and epilepsy, the physiopathology of medial temporal lobe epilepsies, and antiepileptic drug pharmacology. Dr Crespel has published articles in international journals and has contributed chapters for books on these topics.

CHAPITRE I

Normal awake electroencephalogram and unusual EEG patterns

CHAPITRE II

Activation procedures

CHAPITRE

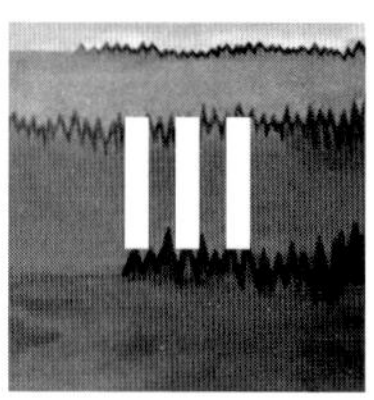

EEG and sleep

CHAPITRE

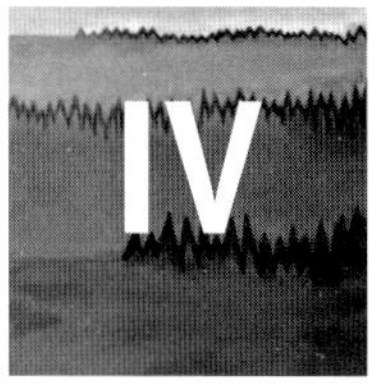

Artifacts

INTRODUCTION

The philosophy of our approach to EEG analysis

As neurologists in charge of the Epilepsy Unit at the University Hospital in Montpellier (France), our aim is to improve the knowledge of EEG analysis for junior collaborators, neurologists, neuropediatricians and EEG technologists. EEG analysis could be compared to a child who is growing up as, in both cases, maturing is a long process. For EEG analysis, the stages are as follows:

- stage I: nothing makes any sense,
- stage II: you think you understand but you see abnormalities everywhere,
- stage III: you gain more hindsight. You recognize a spike but wonder if it is actually significant,
- stage IV: you are finally able to form your own opinion, even if it is different from your teacher's. This last stage is the sign you have matured. You have acquired enough experience to have your own opinion and to discuss an EEG.

Although the valuable help of your teacher is undoubtedly a prerequisite to start out in EEG analysis, it is basically up to you to do the work. The more EEGs you interpret, the more questions you ask yourself, the more you will learn. When in doubt, having the curiosity to open a book or ask a colleague for his advice will greatly benefit your learning process.

When analyzing an EEG, you must ask yourself what the referring physician is expecting form the test, and how your analysis can help the patient. If I were the prescribing doctor and I received this clinical report, how would it be useful for me? The writing up of an EEG report corresponds to a formal and orderly process. In the first part, the recordings must be described (background activity, hyperventilation, intermittent photic stimulation, physiological sleep patterns, abnormalities...) then a conclusion must be given. Are the abnormalities significant? Is the pattern pathological? Your opinion must be clearly expressed, and therefore you must accept that you will sometimes be mistaken. It is also important to state that the EEG is normal whenever the case. Above all, avoid hastily jumping to conclusions or giving your opinion about patient management before seeing the patient or discussing the case with the prescribing doctor.

The EEG is a tool used to confirm clinical hypotheses. A patient should never be diagnosed as "epileptic" based merely on observation of spikes or similar abnormalities but in absence of any semiological evidence. In epileptology, it is preferable to claim the presence of too few rather than too many abnormalities. If the patient does actually have epilepsy, the clinical diagnosis will eventually make itself known. Indeed, the consequences of such a diagnosis for the patient are too serious to risk diagnosis of epilepsy due to misinterpretation. When in doubt, it is recommended to be cautious before attributing pathological significance to findings. Complementary recordings should be performed, including sleep recordings in particular. Needless to say, this critical attitude does not apply to all fields in neurology. For instance, encephalitis or acute focal dysfunction call for immediate intervention, which is why brain imaging has currently replaced EEGs as the firstline investigation in these emergency situations.

In the first volume of this collection, we will describe the normal awake and sleep EEGs, the activation procedures, the unusual rhythms, and the artifacts required to establish whether an activity is physiological or pathological. Pathological EEGs will be dealt with mainly in upcoming volumes. With this atlas, our aim is to provide a useful tool which we would have liked to have when we were learning how to analyze EEGs and when we started teaching EEG analysis ourselves. Each chapter begins with a review of the technical features and a description of the physiological EEG patterns. After that, these patterns are illustrated with full-size EEG plates. We hope this atlas will thus be useful for the electroencephalographer who is having trouble analyzing a tracing. We have intentionally left the original plates without any notes so that this book can be used for self-study. The comments on the plates can be used by the reader as a key to visual analysis.

Arielle Crespel **Philippe Gélisse**

EEG RECORDINGS

Digitalized electroencephalography has been used for more than two decades now. This technological advance has given EEG recordings of brain activity a new lease on life. Indeed, the standard 10-20 recording has now become a routine procedure, and the fact that the signals can be reformatted is undoubtedly a major breakthrough. The scope of analysis is broadened by the possibility to analyze an event in playback with different montages, modify voltage and speed, or use filters. With breakthroughs in neuroimaging (brain CT scans and MRIs), EEGs have found a new place and better indications. We are now using supplementary electrodes, sleep recordings, polygraphy, and video EEGs for many indications in neurology. Epileptology is the main indication for EEGs and, in this field, EEGs have led to major therapeutical breakthroughs as well as accurate classification of epileptic syndromes on the basis of clinical and electroencephalographic criteria. In this chapter, we will present the 10-20 montage system, recording methods, and an orderly approach to visual analysis.

The 10-20 montage system (see figures)

Routine 10-20 montage includes a minimum of 21 electrodes: Fp2, F4, C4, P4, 02, F8, T4, T6, Fpz, Fz, Cz, Pz, Oz, Fp1, F3, C3, P3, 01, F7, T3, T5. "Fp" stands for frontal-polar, "F" for frontal, "C" for central, "P" for parietal, "O" for occipital, and "T" for temporal. By convention, even numbers refer to the electrodes on the right side, odd numbers refer to the electrodes on the left side, and the letter "z" indicates a midline placement. The suprasylvian line runs along electrodes Fp2, F4, C4, P4 on the right and Fp1, F3, C3, and P3 on the left, while Fz, Cz, and Pz form the midline. F8 and F7 are the anterior temporal electrodes, also called inferior frontal because they are anatomically located at the frontal-temporal boundary. T4 and T3 are the midtemporal electrodes, and T6 and T5 posterior temporal. Lastly, O2 and O1 are the right and left occipital electrodes. The international 10-20 montage system enables consistent and anatomic placement of electrodes.

Specific measurements are taken between constant anatomical landmarks to determine the placement of electrodes. First, the distance from the nasion (bridge of nose) to the inion (external occipital protuberance) is measured. Then the first points are marked at an interval which is 10% of the nasion to inion line. The Fpz position is 10% above the bridge of the nose. The Oz position is 10% above the external occipital protuberance. Three other measurements are taken between Fpz and Oz at intervals corresponding to 20% of the nasion to inion line to mark Fz, Cz, and Pz.

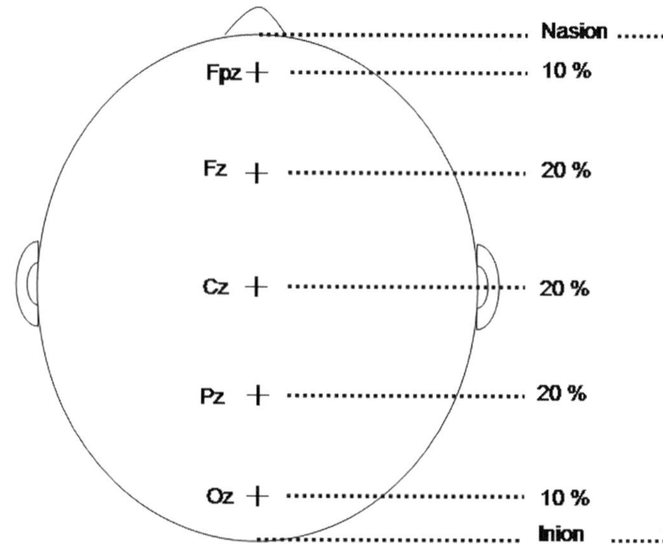

Then the second line is measured between the two preauricular points across Cz, the midline point at the top of the skull. As with the previous line, a point is marked at an interval corresponding to a 10% distance of the preauricular-to-preauricular line, and then the following points are determined at 20% intervals. Cz is then marked at the intersection of these two lines. Hence, T4, C4, C3, and T3 are marked.

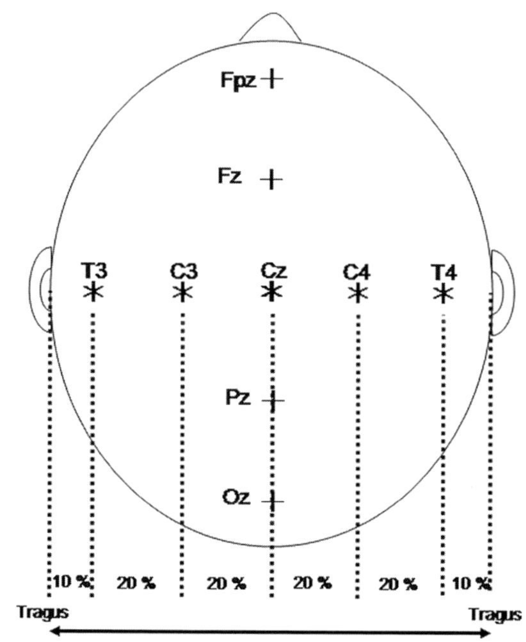

Then the circumference of the head is measured starting from the point at a 10% interval from the nasion (Fpz), through a 10% interval from the right preauricular point (T4), a 10% interval from the inion (Oz), and ending at a 10% interval from the left preauricular point (T3). Five percent of the circumference on each side of the Fpz position is measured to mark the Fp2 and Fp1 points. Then, starting from these frontal-polar points, F8, T4, T6, O2, T5, T3, and F7 are marked at 10% intervals of the circumference. T4 and T3 are thereby determined by the intersection of two measurements.

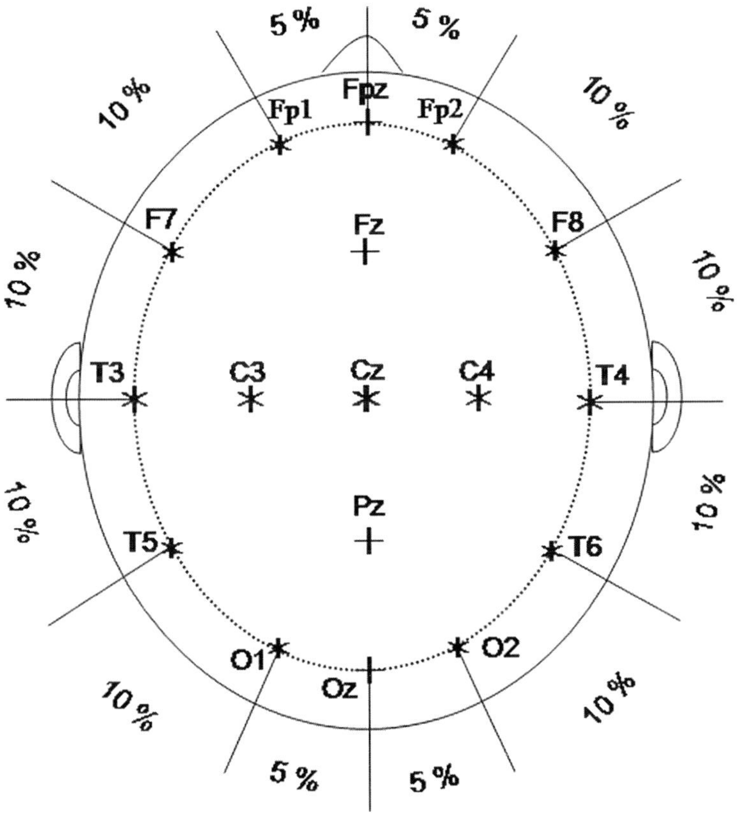

Then the longitudinal distance is measured (front to back), on the right between Fp2 and O2 through the first coordinate of C4, and on the left between Fp1 and O1 through the first coordinate of C3. For each of these measurements, the midline corresponds respectively to the final coordinates of C4 and C3. The first coordinate of F4 is midway between Fp2 and C4. Likewise, the first coordinate of F3 is midway between Fp1 and C3. Lastly, the first coordinate of P4 is midway between C4 and O2 and the first coordinate of P3 is midway between C3 and O1.

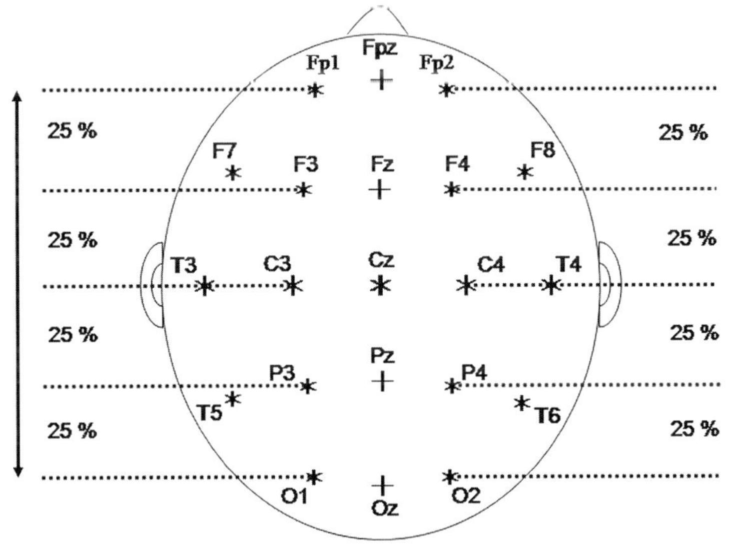

Measurements from F7 to F8 (left-right) through Fz and from T5 to T6 through Pz define the transverse coordinates. Toward the front, F4 is midway between F8 and Fz, and F3 is midway between F7 and Fz. Toward the back, P4 is midway between T6 and Pz, and P3 is midway between T5 and Pz. Hence all the 21 electrodes are marked.

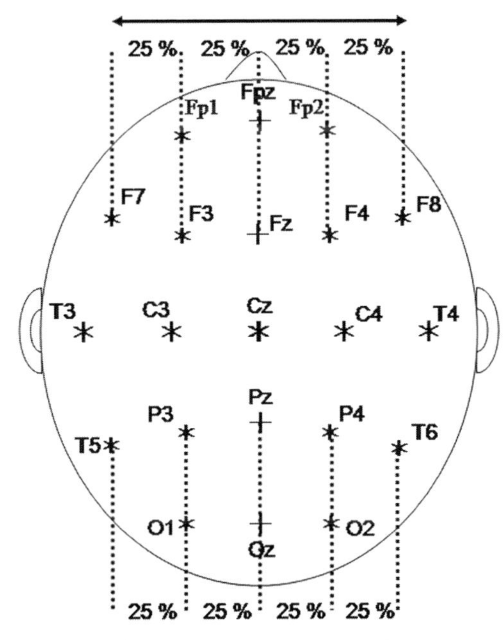

Additional electrodes and polygraphy

In certain situations, supplementary electrodes can be added to the 10-20 system. For instance, as the temporal derivation is too high with this system, its anterior part explores the lower part of the frontal lobe. To increase spatial resolution of the temporal lobe, it is recommended to add a lower temporal line. Three additional electrodes can be added to the 10-20 montage for this purpose. The lower temporal line is measured from the external auditory canal to the lateral canthus of the eye and divided by three. T1 and T2 are marked at one-third from the external auditory canal and TA1-TA2 (TA: temporal-anterior) are marked at one-third from the lateral canthus of the eye. The electrodes are placed one centimeter above these points. T1-T2 are the zygomatic electrodes and TA1-TA2 are the anterior lower temporal electrodes. Lastly, TP1-TP2 (TP: temporal-posterior) can be placed over the mastoid regions.

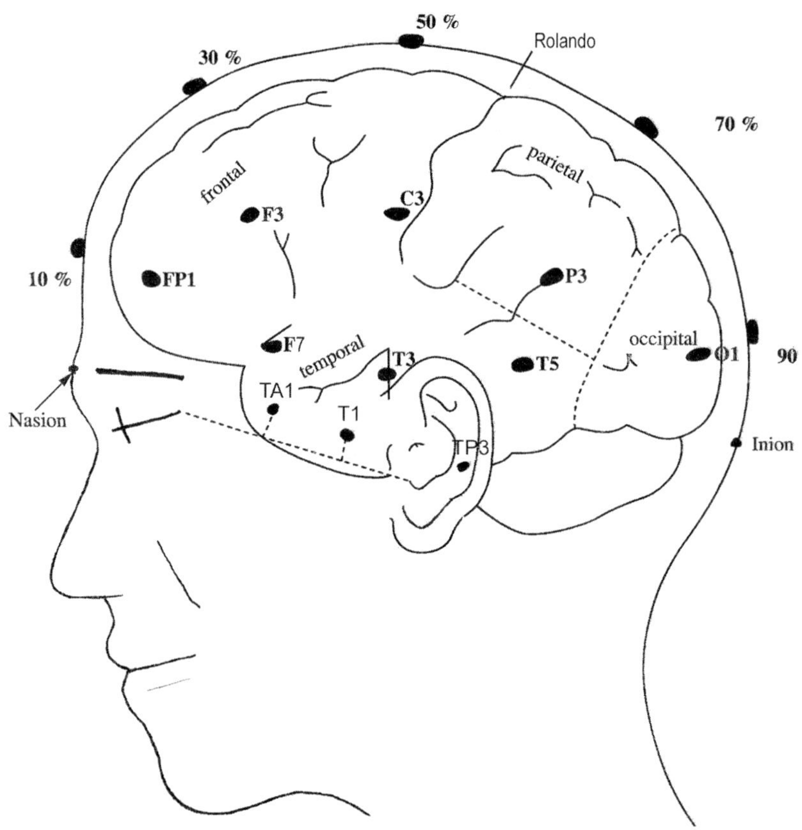

An ECG (electrocardiogram) is performed routinely with all EEGs. For infants, a recording of muscle activity (electromyogram) is routinely performed and respiration is routinely monitored. EMGs and breathing may also be used in other clinical situations.

Recording methods

In France, the standard EEG recording speed is 15 mm/s. In most countries, the standard speed in 30 mm/s. Due to digitalization, speed can be modified during subsequent reformatting to facilitate interpretation of faster or slower brain activity. Standard voltage is 7 or 10 µV/mm. In case of very low voltage or very high voltage signals, the amplifier's sensitivity setting can be increased or decreased. It is recommended to visualize the recording prior to using any filters, after which fast muscle activity can be attenuated at frequencies higher than 100, 75, or 35 Hz. A 50 Hz or 60 Hz filter setting can be used to attenuate noise which may interfere under certain circumstances (e.g. in case of strong electric fields).

In France, EEG activity is recorded with a high-pass filter of 0.53 Hz (0.35 with 30 mm/s). Lastly, it is important, prior to initialization, to verify that input impedance is not higher than 10 kOhms in order to obtain good quality EEG recordings.

Routine laboratory recordings are traditionally performed with clip electrodes underneath an elastic cap specifically designed for the 10-20 system. Each recording lasts 20 minutes and includes two hyperventilations and one intermittent photic stimulation (IPS). A polygraphic recording (EMG, respiration) or a video recording may be added. The procedure is performed on a patient lying down on a bed to allow deep relaxation and sleep if needed.

For recordings which last several hours, an elastic cap fitted with embedded electrodes is used for better comfort and optimized quality. Additional electrodes, polygraphy or video may also be added. For polysomnography, or recordings lasting 24 hours or more, the electrodes are glued directly onto the scalp.

Spatial analysis

With digital technology, calibration only needs to be performed once, and recalibrations of the initial recording can be obtained with different montages. A longitudinal montage is used to study brain wave activity "backward", anterior to posterior of the vertex, the right and left suprasylvian regions, the right and left infrasylvian regions.

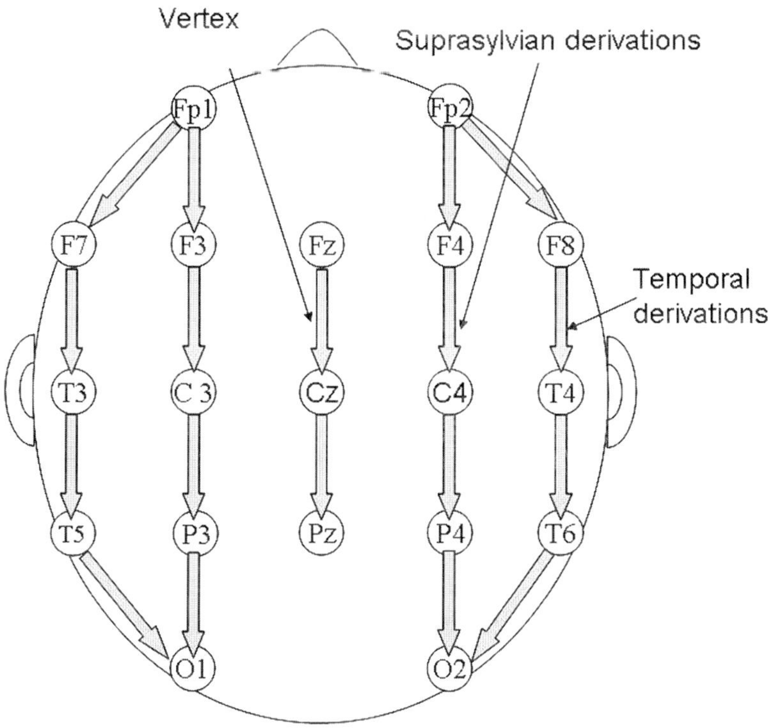

For the transverse montage, brain wave activity is read from one side to the other.

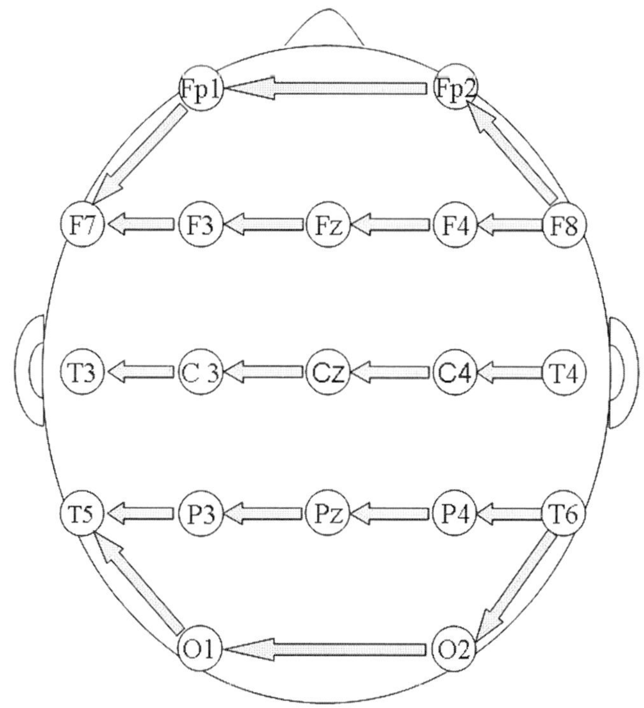

Furthermore, a montage can be calibrated from a given reference, or from the average of several or all of the electrodes (average reference montage). With each new montage, brain wave activity is reformatted, and the input voltage can be modified. Of course, other derivations can be selected for additional montages.

GLOSSARY

General terms

After-discharge: describes a persistent pattern following stimulus cessation. This is the case for example with persistent spike-wave discharge after cessation of intermittent photic stimulation.

Background activity: refers to the referential EEG rhythm corresponding to the patient's age and state of consciousness. When awake, background activity is posterior and can be observed when the eyes are closed. In adults, background activity is in the alpha frequency range.

Burst: a group of waves which appear abruptly and are clearly distinguished from background activity. A burst can be either physiological or pathological. When a burst lasts over a prolonged period, it can be called a **discharge**.

Cycles per second (c/s): indicates the number of elements observed within one second. Equivalent term for Hertz (Hz).

Discharge: a burst which lasts several seconds. Although discharges may be non-pathological, as rhythmic midtemporal discharge for instance, this term is most often used to describe epileptic events.

Epoch: the period of time corresponding to one 30-cm page of EEG recording. It is calculated according to recording speed. At 15 mm/s, an epoch lasts 20 seconds and at 30 mm/s, an epoch lasts 10 seconds.

Focus: the region displaying a given pathological activity.

Frequency: the number of cycles per second.

Harmonic: this term is used to describe a rhythm which is half the basic frequency (subharmonic) or twice the basic frequency (fast alpha variant).

Ictal: Ictal activity corresponds to an epileptic seizure, whether it is clinical or subclinical. It is opposed to **interictal** activity, a non-seizure related activity which is usually brief. **Post-ictal** activity corresponds to activities recorded during the regressive phase of the seizure.

Paroxysm: an abrupt phenomenon that can clearly be distinguished from background activity.

Pattern: corresponds to any characteristic EEG activity.

Phase reversal: in bipolar montages, simultaneous deflections in opposite directions caused by a wave in two linked derivations with the electrode common to both derivations. This opposition indicates that the electrode is near the generator source.

Reactivity: a modification of rhythms observed in response to sensory (visual, auditory, somato-sensory...), motor, behavioral, or pharmacological stimulation.

Sinusoidal: applied to EEG waves resembling sine waves. The alpha rhythm is a characteristic example.

Slowing: refers to a pattern characterized by slow waves. Slowing may be local or diffuse. Slowing can either be physiological, as with hyperventilation, or pathological

Description of EEG activities

• Description of elementary paroxysmal activities

Wave: any change of the potential difference between pairs of electrodes forming a single EEG element. According to duration, the waves are said to be slow (> 200 ms) or sharp (70 to 200 ms).

Spike: an EEG transient (20 to 70 ms). Spikes are usually diphasic, i.e. composed of a negative and a positive deflection.

Spike-wave complex: a spike followed by a wave with the same polarity. Depending on the number of cycles per second, they are referred to as slow spike-waves (2.5 c/s or less), or spike-waves (3 c/s or faster).

Polyspike complex: a sequence of two or more spikes.

Polyspike-wave complex: a sequence of two or more spikes followed immediately by one or more slow waves with the same polarity.

Sharp wave: a wave of great amplitude lasting between 70 and 200 ms, to be distinguished from spikes which are of shorter duration. When it starts with a nearly vertical slope, it is called a steep wave front.

Triphasic wave: a slow wave with three components alternating about the baseline. Duration of the second wave, which resembles a sharp wave, is the longest. This repetitive, rhythmic activity (every 1 to 3 c/s) is observed in particular in metabolic encephalopathies.

Slow complexes: a sequence of two or more slow waves, generally of higher amplitude. This type of activity is generally periodic, and may be found for instance in encephalitis

• Description with regard to amplitude

Low voltage: activity less than 20 µV. If voltage is less than 10 µV, it is referred to as very-low-voltage activity.

High voltage: activity more than 50 µV.

• Description with regard to distribution

Focal activity: activity involving a very limited area of the brain.

Localized activity: activity involving several neighboring electrodes (covers a larger area than focal activity).

Lateralized activity: activity involving all of the electrodes on one side of the head.

Diffuse activity: activity overlapping the two hemispheres, whether synchronous or not.

Generalized activity: all of the electrodes on both hemispheres are involved, most often synchronous.

Multifocal activity: presence of several independent intra and/or interhemispheric foci.

Asymmetrical activity: difference between the two hemispheres (the opposite of **symmetrical activity**). Forms, amplitude and frequency can be asymmetrical.

• Description with regard to timing

Synchronous activity: two events occurring simultaneously as opposed to an **asynchronous activity**.

Bilateral activity: activity occurring on both hemispheres (but not necessarily at the same time). An activity can be both bilateral and synchronous (bisynchronous), for instance with 3 c/s spike-waves in childhood absence epilepsy.

• Description with regard to frequency

Delta frequency: under 4 c/s.

Theta frequency range: from 4 c/s to under 8 c/s.

Alpha frequency range: from 8 c/s to under 13 c/s.

Beta frequency: over 13 c/s.

• Description with regard to regularity

Monomorphic activity: mainly a morphologically rhythmic repetitive pattern with regular amplitude and frequency.

Polymorphic activity: with variations of waveform amplitude, frequency and morphology.

• Description with regard to repetition

Rhythmic activity: regular activity with similar duration of both waves and intervals between the waves (no separate elements). Epileptic seizures are an example of this kind of activity.

Arhythmic activity: activity occurring irregularly with inconstant intervals between individual waveforms.

Periodic activity: activity with regular intervals of longer duration than the individual waves. These intervals last between one and several seconds. They are referred to as short periodic activities under or equal to 4 seconds (periodic complexes in Creutzfeldt-Jakob disease) or as long periodic activities over 4 seconds. Long periodic activity is seen in SSPE (sub-acute sclerosing panencephalitis).

Pseudoperiodic activity: intervals between individual waves are slightly irregular.

Technical terminology

Derivation: a difference of potential between a pair of electrodes. An EEG montage is composed of the combination of simultaneously recorded derivations. Montages can be longitudinal, transverse, or referential.

Electrode impedance: For EEGs, electrode impedance corresponds to its resistance. It is calculated in kiloOhms. For quality EEG recordings, it should remain below 5 kΩ.

Low-frequency filter/high-pass filter/time constant: a filter that allows higher frequencies to pass through the amplifier. For a speed of 15 mm/s, the most commonly used low-frequency filter setting is 0.53 Hz.

High-frequency filter/low-pass filter: a filter that attenuates all frequencies above the selected frequency. Commonly referred to as the EEG filter, it can attenuate rapid activities such as muscle activities (a 70-Hz filter attenuates all frequencies above 70 Hz).

Selective/Single-band filter/ Notch filter: a filter which attenuates only one frequency band, for example a 50-Hz filter to attenuate the noise from mains electrical input (60 Hz in some countries).

Ground electrode: Referential electrode, i.e. an electrode which is neutral for the amplifiers, so that extraneous signals, whose source may be the patient or surrounding metal objects from the electromagnetic field, and which may act as an antenna and interfere with the recording, can be attenuated.

Reference electrode: the electrode the least likely to pick up the same EEG activity recorded by an exploring electrode, and which the signal of the other electrodes can be compared to.

Sensitivity: the input voltage necessary to cause a 1 mm deflection. EEG recordings are usually carried out with a sensitivity of 7 μV/mm at 30 mm/s.

Normal awake electroencephalogram and unusual EEG patterns

CHAPITRE I

BACKGROUND OR FUNDAMENTAL ACTIVITY

• Frequency

An individualized background activity appears in the posterior regions when the patient's eyes are closed. The normal range for the frequency of the alpha rhythm in adults between 15 and 65 years old is 8 to 12 Hz. The alpha rhythm consists of sinusoidal wave forms. In children and in the elderly, background activity may be slower. In children, frequency increases with maturation, whereas wave amplitude decreases. There is no predominant alpha rhythm under age 3 years. The frequency is approximately 5 Hz at 6 months, 6 to 7 Hz from 9 to 18 months and 7 to 8 Hz by age 2 years. It increases to 9 Hz by age 7 years. In young adults, it is commonly 10-11 Hz. However, around age 60 years, background activity usually decreases to about 9 Hz and it is estimated at 8 Hz for hundred-year-olds. An alpha rhythm slower than 8 Hz should raise the suspicion of an abnormality in a healthy elderly person.

• Amplitude

From a physiological point of view, the amplitude of the alpha rhythm is slightly asymmetrical, with a higher amplitude on the non-dominant side.

If the amplitude is high enough (in children, adolescents and young adults, or in some adults), there may be single alpha waves with "sharp" peaks in the sinusoidal alpha rhythm without any pathological significance. Conversely, low amplitude of the alpha rhythm can be found in some individuals due to anxiety, also commonly in alcoholics, but mostly as a nonpathological individual trait. Moreover, the amplitude of the alpha rhythm tends to decrease with age and low amplitude is more frequent in elderly persons with posterior-to-anterior spread of background activity.

Lastly, certain drugs (antiepileptic, antihistaminic, neuroleptic, psychotropic drugs...), can modify brain activity and provoke predominantly "sharp" or irregular patterns.

• Reactivity of the alpha rhythm

Reactivity upon eye opening and closing must be tested. Normally, the alpha rhythm is present when eyes are closed and blocked when the person is asked to open his eyes. Concentrated mental effort also blocks the alpha rhythm. This is referred to as reactivity. Reactivity is a sign that the person's activity is well-organized. It is important to test eye reactivity several times during a recording session. Likewise, posterior slow waves of youth block with eye opening.

• Alpha variants

The alpha rhythm can sometimes become fragmented at a slower frequency of 4 to 6 Hz. It becomes monomorphic with rhythmic notched theta waves. This is referred to as the slow alpha variant pattern or the subharmonic alpha pattern. This pattern can either be symmetrical or alternate between the two hemispheres. It can be the predominant background activity or it can be mixed with the regular alpha activity. Although slow alpha variants are sometimes unilateral, they share the same topographic distribution and reactivity to eye opening with the alpha rhythm. Lastly, they can be blocked by intermittent photic stimulation (IPS) at half the frequency of the alpha rhythm that appears elsewhere in the record and display a subharmonic pattern.

Even more rarely, the background activity can be twice the frequency of the restful alpha rhythm, ranging from 16 to 20 Hz, which constituted the fast alpha variants. They share the same topographic distribution and reactivity to eye opening with the alpha rhythm. They can be mixed with the alpha activity. These harmonic patterns can be activated by IPS.

• Paradoxical alpha

Paradoxical alpha rhythm occurs with open eyes in drowsy subjects who awaken. Paradoxical alpha represents an alerting response and does not correspond to an abnormal response.

• Posterior slow waves of youth

In children of 3 to 10 years of age, posterior slow waves may be intermixed with the alpha rhythm, sometimes resembling spike-waves, which can be very misleading. As with the alpha rhythm, posterior slow waves are blocked in children when eyes are open. They are also activated by hyperventilation. Pathological posterior slow waves differ from the latter in that the activity is more monomorphic, waveforms are often larger and eye reactivity is not as constant.

OTHER RHYTHMS

• Mu Rhythm

Gastaut *et al.* (1952) were the first to describe in detail the features of mu rhythm. This rhythm is physiological and can be detected from infancy on (Gelisse & Crespel, 2006). Its incidence is estimated to be 10% of the population (Niedermeyer & Koshino, 1975). Mu rhythms are essentially seen during resting wakefulness but can also be observed in REM sleep (Duntley *et al.*, 2001; Gelisse & Crespel, 2014). It commonly occurs in the central region at 7 to 11 Hz, and does not block with eye opening. It is easier to identify when eyes are open, due to the blocked alpha rhythm. Mu waves occur in small bursts and have a characteristic low-frequency arch-like or comb-like shape. Although sometimes present bilaterally, mu rhythm is most often asymmetrical and asynchronous. Mu rhythm blocks unilaterally upon contraction of the contra-lateral hand, or upon movement of the contra-lateral foot if the rhythm is near the vertex (Cz), or sometimes with the thought of movement of the contra-lateral limb. With skull defects, in particular after neurosurgery, the amplitude can be higher and the rhythm present on only one side (on the operated side). The reactivity is less constant.

• Beta rhythms

The frequency of beta rhythms is above 13 Hz, with low amplitude waves and the same frequency on both sides of the anterior regions. They can be detected during wakefulness, are usually enhanced during drowsiness, and decrease in deeper sleep stages. They tend to reappear in REM sleep. The incidence of beta rhythms increases with age. In adults, beta rhythms are physiological and more or less persistent. In elderly people, there is no clear correlation between beta activity of high amplitude and cognitive decline. On the contrary, it has been suggested that a decrease in beta activity may indicate a loss of intellectual capacities (Williamson *et al.*, 1990). Beta rhythms may become very pronounced in patients on benzodiazepines or barbiturates.

• Lambda waves

These sharp waves occur in the occipital regions in wakefulness, particularly when individuals are visually scanning a picture in a well-illuminated room. The amplitude is commonly low (< 50 μV). Lambda waves are often bilateral. According to some authors, a marked asymmetry of lambda waves on one side should raise a suspicion of an abnormality on the side of lower amplitude. Lambda waves disappear when the patient stares at a point and when the room is not as bright. They are physiological and often associated with saccadic eye movements.

• Rhythmic midtemporal discharge or rhythmic temporal theta burst of drowsiness (see chapter 3)

This unusual activity, present mainly in adolescents and young adults was described in 1952 by Gibbs and Gibbs with the term "psychomotor variant pattern", it was later called "rhythmic midtemporal discharge" and the preferred term is now "rhythmic theta burst of drowsiness". Nevertheless, this activity can persist during non-REM and REM sleep, which is why we still prefer rhythmic midtemporal discharge. Due to this relationship between sleep they are described in chapter 3 "EEG and Sleep".

• Subclinical rhythmic electrographic discharges in adults (SREDA)

SREDA were first described by Naquet *et al.* in 1961 using the term "paroxystic discharges of the parietal and posterior temporal regions". Onset is abrupt, and the sharp waveforms reach maximal amplitude from onset. Pattern frequency of 4 to 7 Hz is sustained, lasting from a few seconds to a few minutes. Contrary to epileptic discharges, topographic distribution of SREDA shows no build-up. Less commonly, the onset involves a build-up of slow waves gradually occurring at shorter intervals. As their name indicates, SREDA concern the parietal and posterior temporal head regions. Although usually bilateral, the discharges can be asymmetrical with spread to the central region. Discharges occur during wakefulness and can be activated by hyperventilation or intermittent photic stimulation. SREDA have also been observed during drowsiness and Fleming *et al.* (2003) have observed their occurrence in REM sleep. SREDA mainly occur in individuals over 50 years. Some authors have described these discharges in patients with a vascular history. This pattern occurs several times in a single routine recording, and will be present in subsequent EEGs with an identical topographic distribution. SREDA are not associated with any clinical diagnosis or with any subjective symptoms. They are of no diagnostic significance.

• Midline theta rhythm (Ciganek)

Midline theta rhythm was described by Ciganek (Ciganek, 1959) and may be observed during wakefulness or drowsiness. This unusual sinusoidal or arciform 4-7 Hz activity occurs predominantly over the vertex (Cz). Sometimes, it resembles mu rhythms but it is not similarly reactive. This pattern has no pathological significance.

• Breach rhythm (rhythms over skull defects)

A breach rhythm is an increase in high-voltage activity of alpha, beta, and mu rhythms or other physiological elements such as wicket spikes, spindles nearby the breach which can occur in persons with a skull defect (e.g. after craniotomy). It is helpful to note that the breach rhythm is unilateral.

The breach rhythm may be associated with faster unilateral alpha background activity with only partial eye reactivity. It often has larger arch-like shaped (mu) waveforms. Increased brain activity can be associated with enhanced unilateral theta activity, but the activity remains monomorphic. Increased fast beta activity admixed with alpha, mu, or theta waveforms may present as an irregular rhythm with some sharp waveforms. Most frequently, beta rhythms and sharp wave activity, generally low amplitude, are admixed in the breach rhythm. These sharply contoured waveforms should not be mistaken for epileptic abnormalities. Indeed, the amplitude of the latter is higher, they can be clearly distinguished from background activity, they occur on more than one electrode, and sometimes they present aftercoming slow wave components. In presence of polymorphic slow delta activity associated with fast breach rhythms, suspicion of brain damage must be raised. Breach rhythm occurs in wakefulness, and is persistent throughout all sleep stages. In rare cases other than with craniotomy, breach rhythm has also been described, for example with bone metastasis on the skull (Tannier *et al.*, 1982).

I • 1 Background activity in a child with posterior slow waves (1)

Context

EEG of a 9-year-old child referred for learning disability.

What to note

On the left, the child's eyes are closed. High-voltage alpha activity (10 Hz), symmetrical over the occipital regions. Alpha rhythm is intermixed with posterior slow waves, presenting sharply-contoured waves that interrupt the sinusoidal pattern of the alpha rhythm. On the right, child hyperventilating. Posterior slow waves are significantly enhanced by hyperventilation.

Comment

Posterior slow waves are a physiological activity in children. They differ from the delta waves sometimes seen in childhood absence epilepsy. In the latter, the delta waves have higher amplitude, are more regular and monomorphic, and without superimposition of the alpha rhythm (see plate I-3).

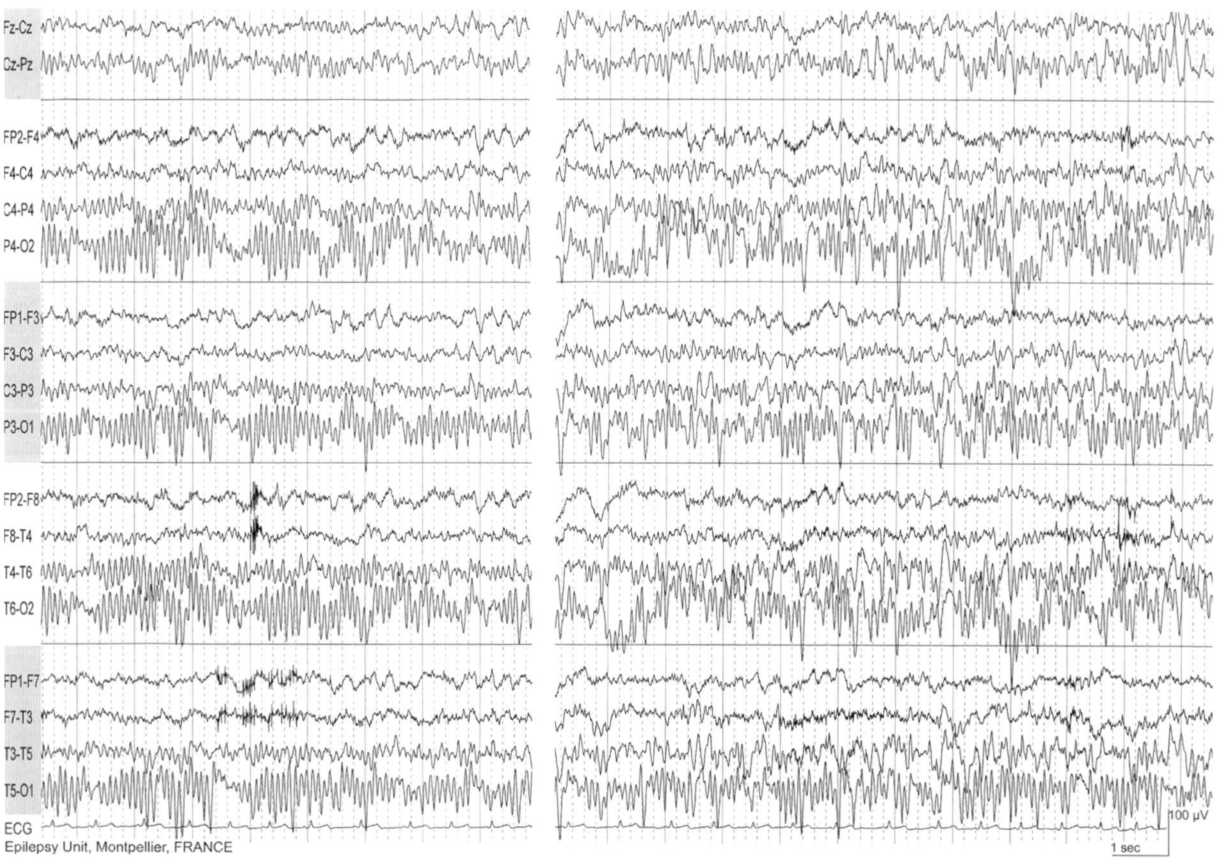

Figure a / Recording at 15 mm/s.

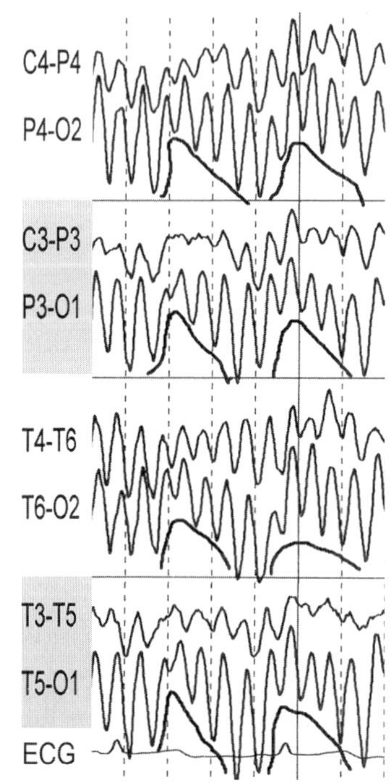

Figure b / Alpha rhythm with superimposed posterior slow waves (underlined).

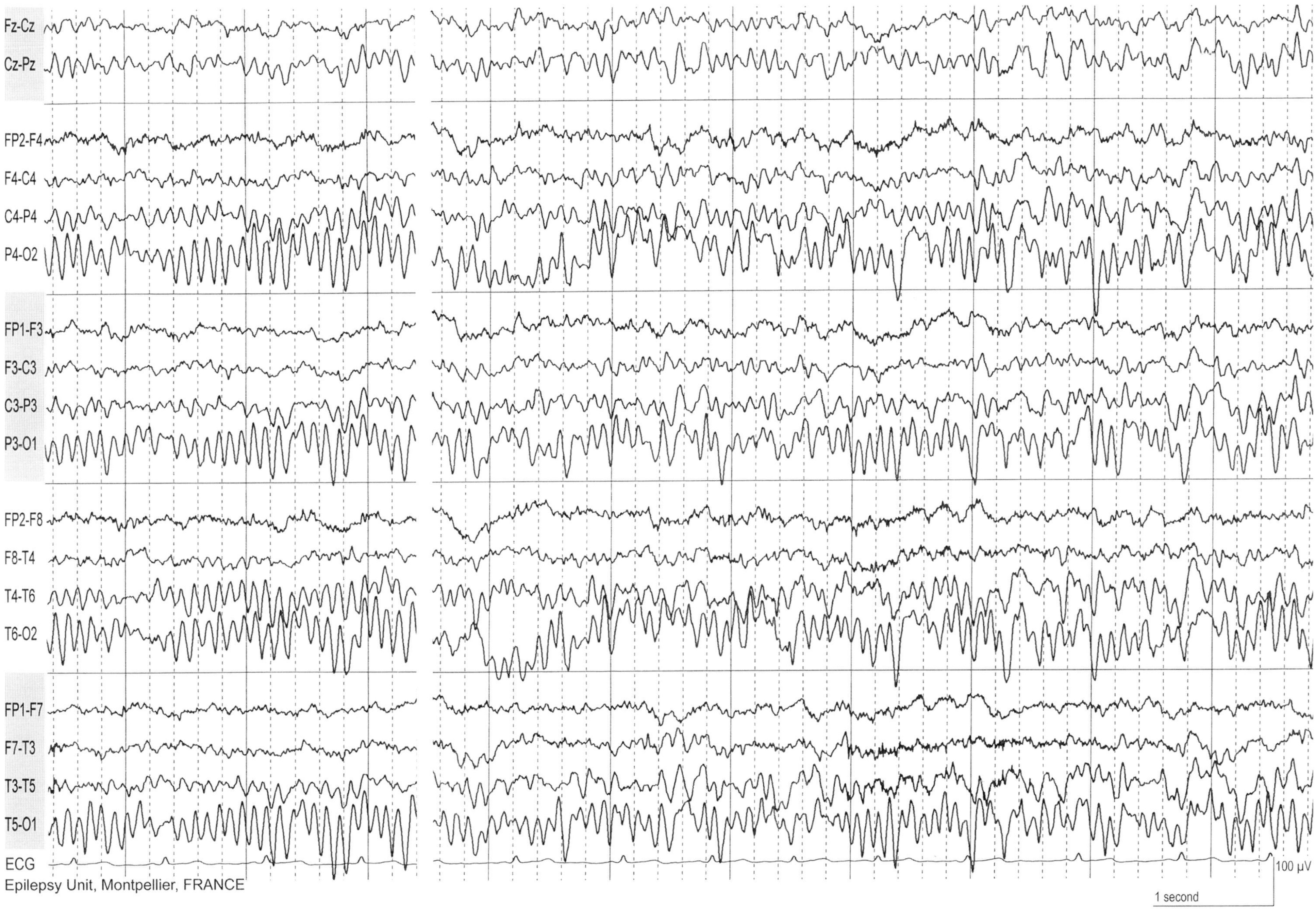
Fz-Cz
Cz-Pz
FP2-F4
F4-C4
C4-P4
P4-O2
FP1-F3
F3-C3
C3-P3
P3-O1
FP2-F8
F8-T4
T4-T6
T6-O2
FP1-F7
F7-T3
T3-T5
T5-O1
ECG
Epilepsy Unit, Montpellier, FRANCE
100 µV
1 second

I • 2 Background activity in a child with posterior slow waves (2)

Context

EEG of a 9-year-old child referred for headache.

What to note

The child starts hyperventilation. High-voltage background alpha activity (9 Hz) predominant in the right occipital region. Alpha rhythm appears irregular. It is intermixed with posterior slow waves. Superimposition of alpha rhythm and posterior slow waves conveys an impression of spike-waves when the alpha wave deflects downward at the beginning or end of the posterior slow wave. This is a common pitfall that must be differentiated from epileptic abnormalities. Moreover, the amplitude of both alpha rhythm and posterior slow waves is higher on the right side so that the background activity conveys an impression of less organization on the left side. Note cardiac arrhythmia, which can be observed with hyperventilation, on the ECG.

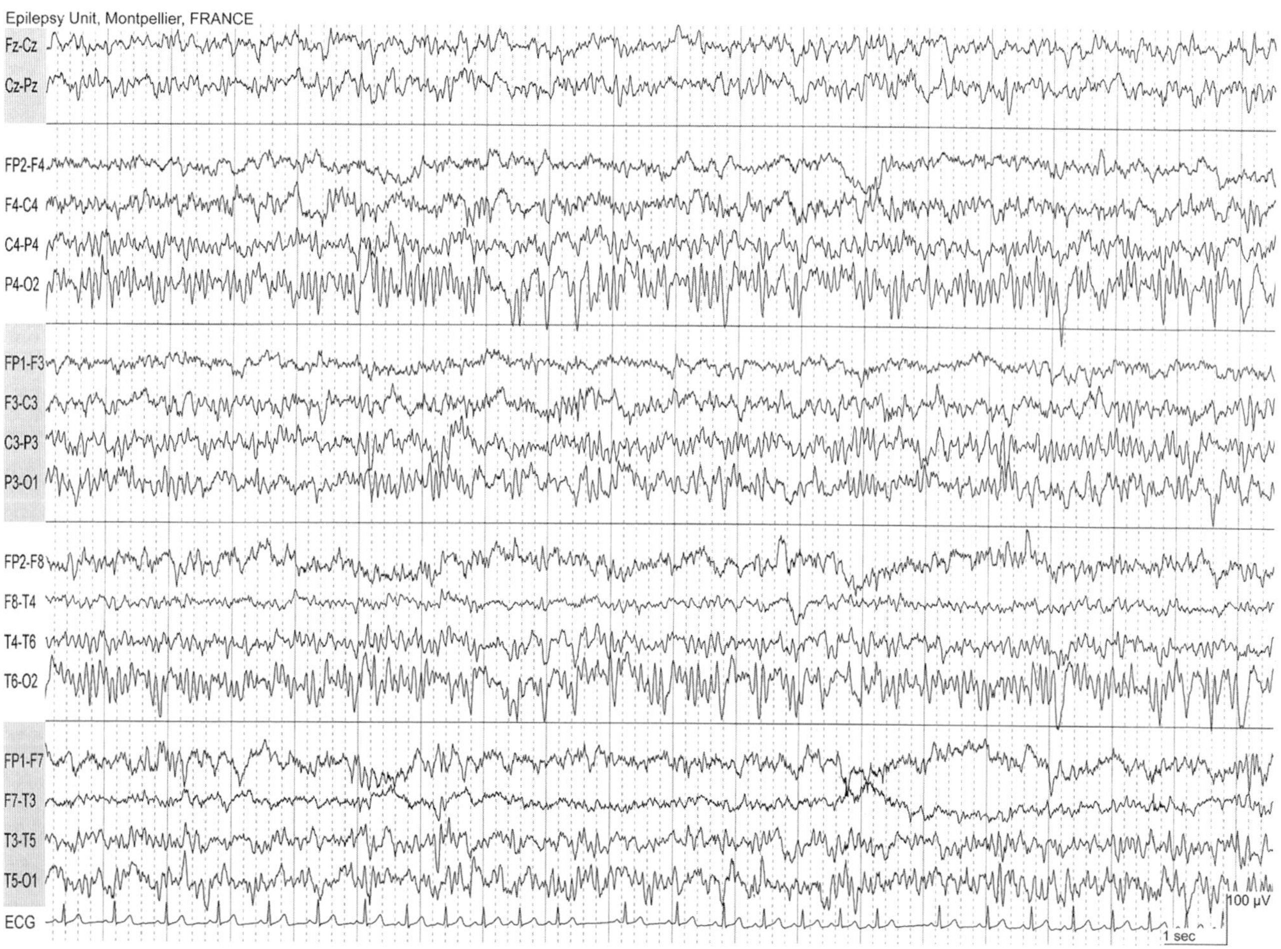

Figure a / Recording at 15 mm/s.

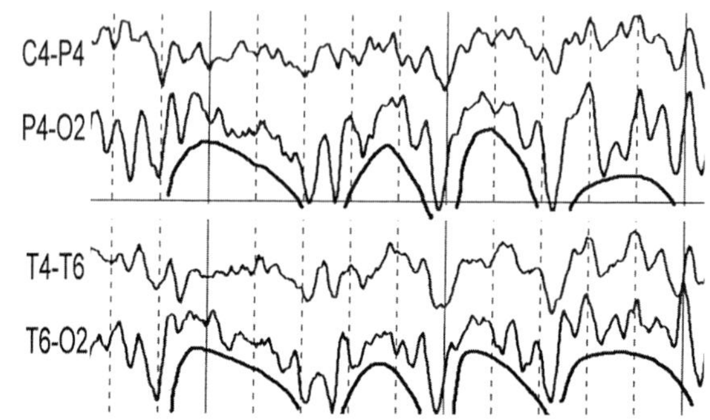

Figure b / Superimposition of alpha rhythm and posterior slow waves (underlined) in the right posterior region.

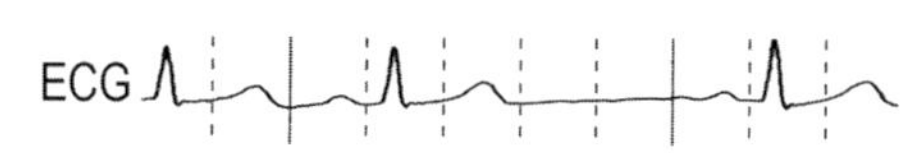

Figure c / Cardiac arrhythmia. ECG derivation must not be forgotten when analyzing an EEG.

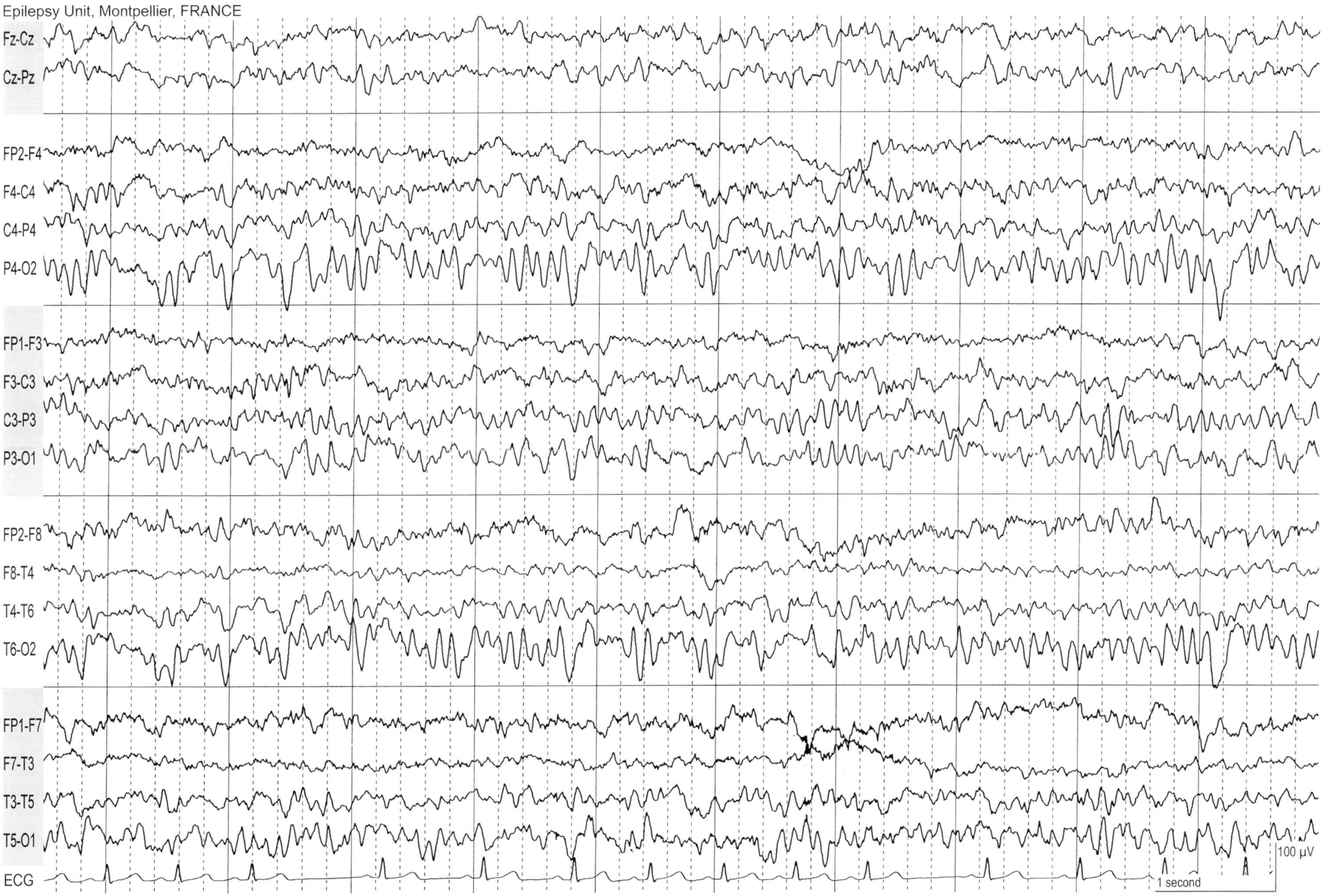
Epilepsy Unit, Montpellier, FRANCE
Fz-Cz
Cz-Pz
FP2-F4
F4-C4
C4-P4
P4-O2
FP1-F3
F3-C3
C3-P3
P3-O1
FP2-F8
F8-T4
T4-T6
T6-O2
FP1-F7
F7-T3
T3-T5
T5-O1
ECG
100 µV
1 second

• 3 Posterior rhythmic delta activity in a child with childhood absence epilepsy

Context

EEG of a 7-year-old child followed for childhood absence epilepsy.

What to note

Theta background activity at 7Hz associated with high amplitude monomorphic posterior delta waves at 3 Hz upon eye closure. The delta waves tend to spread to the centro-parietal regions and are not superimposed with the background activity. Posterior delta waves differ from posterior slow waves in their topographic distribution, amplitude, and frequency as well as in the absence of superimposition with the alpha rhythm. Posterior delta waves are seen above all in childhood absence epilepsy. Whether asynchronous or not, they are bilateral. They are enhanced by hyperventilation and may precede an absence seizure. Note on the plate at 15 mm/s, the occurrence of a spike-wave discharge.

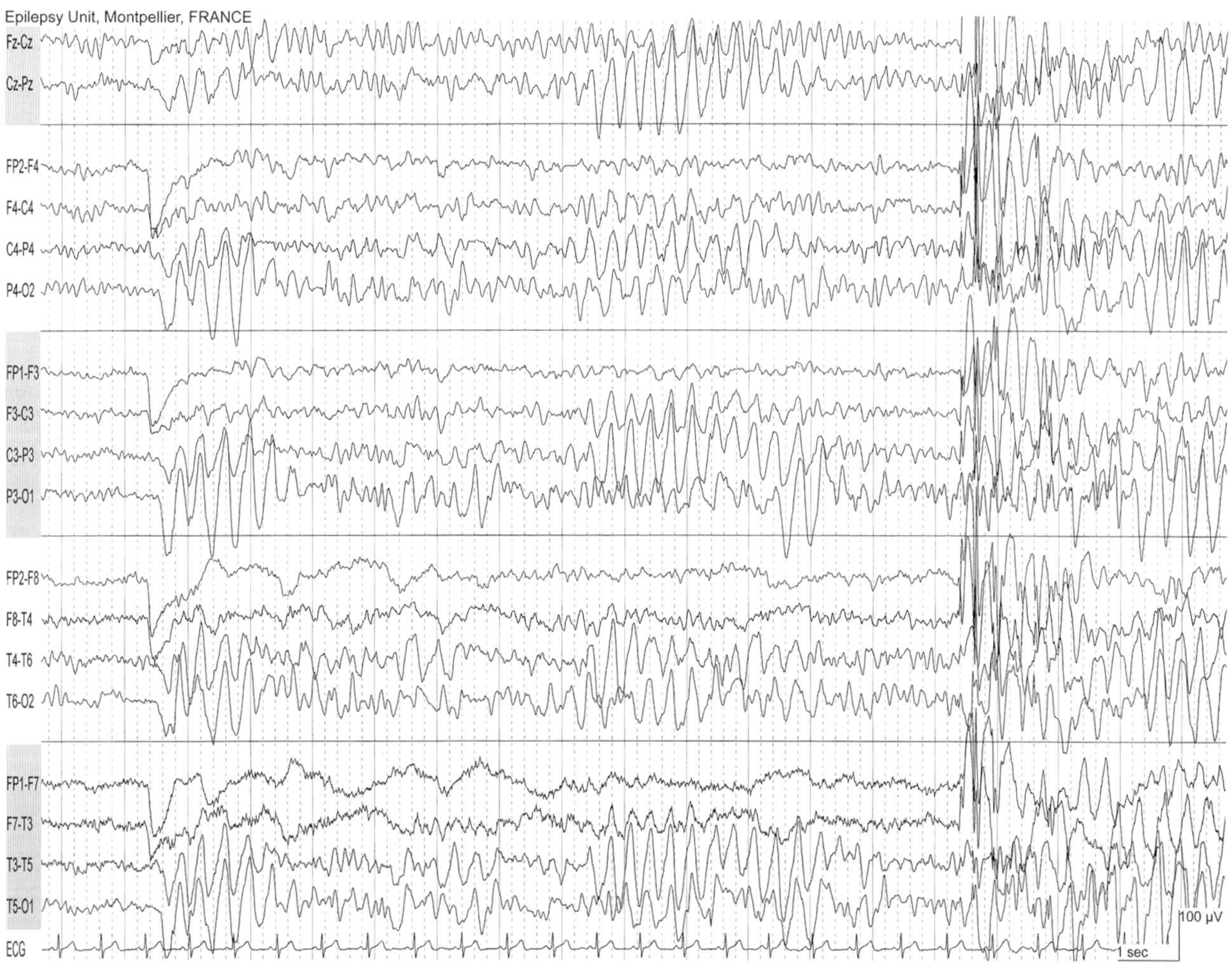

Figure a / Recording at 15 mm/s. Occurrence of a spike-wave discharge four seconds prior to end of plate.

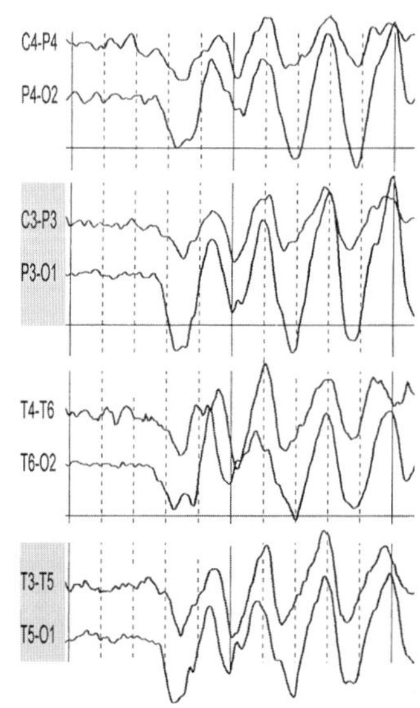

Figure b / Monomorphic posterior delta waves.

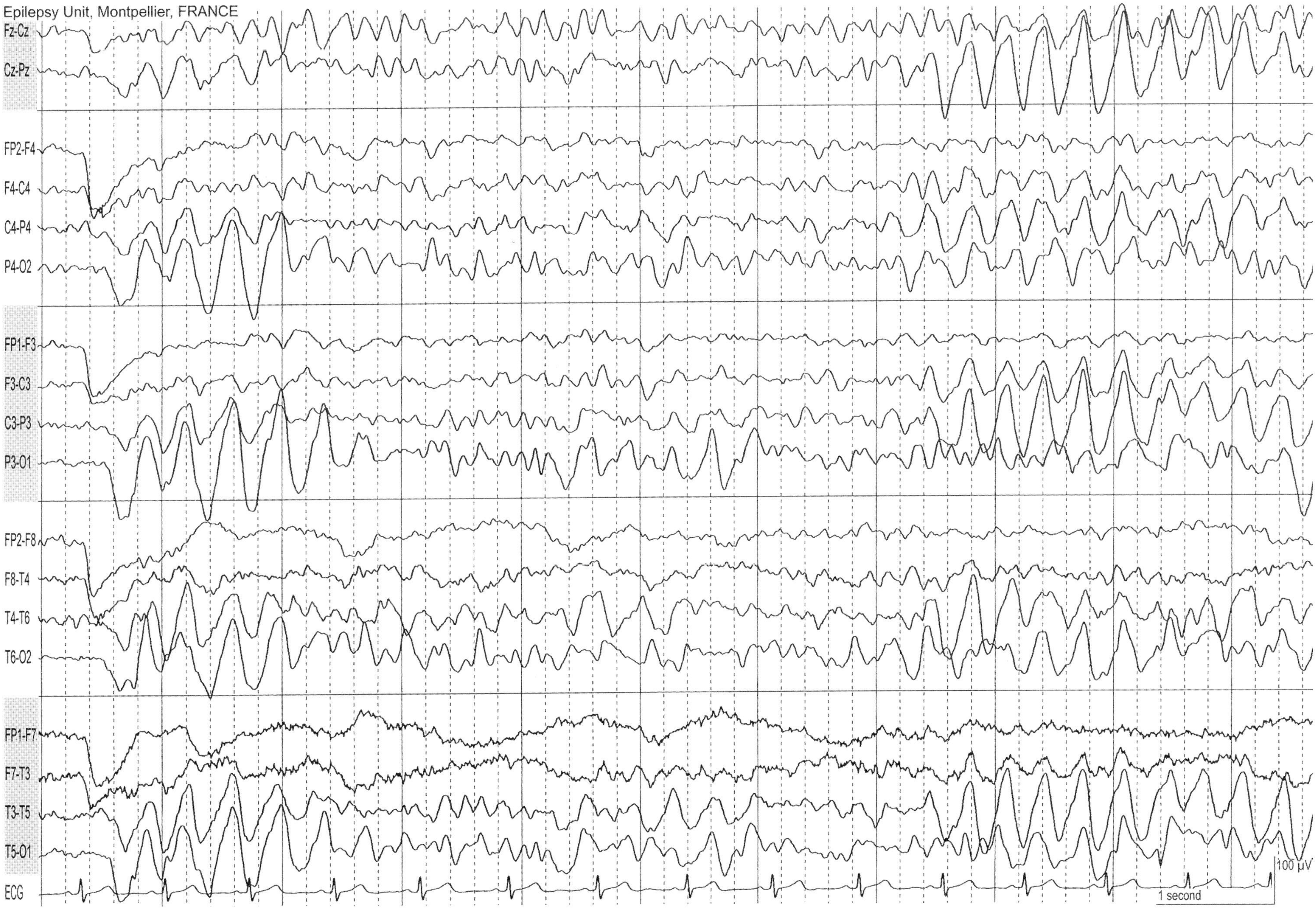
Epilepsy Unit, Montpellier, FRANCE
Fz-Cz
Cz-Pz
FP2-F4
F4-C4
C4-P4
P4-O2
FP1-F3
F3-C3
C3-P3
P3-O1
FP2-F8
F8-T4
T4-T6
T6-O2
FP1-F7
F7-T3
T3-T5
T5-O1
ECG
100 µV
1 second

I • 4 Temporal Intermittent Rythmic Delta Activity (TIRDA) in an adolescent with juvenile absence epilepsy

Context

EEG of a 17-year-old man referred after two generalised tonic-clonic seizures. Typical absences started at age 14.

What to note

The patient's eyes are closed. Background activity with 10 Hz alpha rhythm in the occipital regions. There are delta waves over the right and left temporal region. Note the asynchrony.

Comment

In our series, TIRDA is an EEG pattern observed in 13% of patients with juvenile absence epilepsy (Gelisse *et al.*, 2011). This pattern is activated by hyperventilation and drowsiness. The frequency is around 3 Hz. It decreases in NREM sleep and reappeared in REM sleep. TIRDA in patients with juvenile absence epilepsy could represent a continuum with the posterior delta waves seen in childhood absence epilepsy but with a more anterior location.

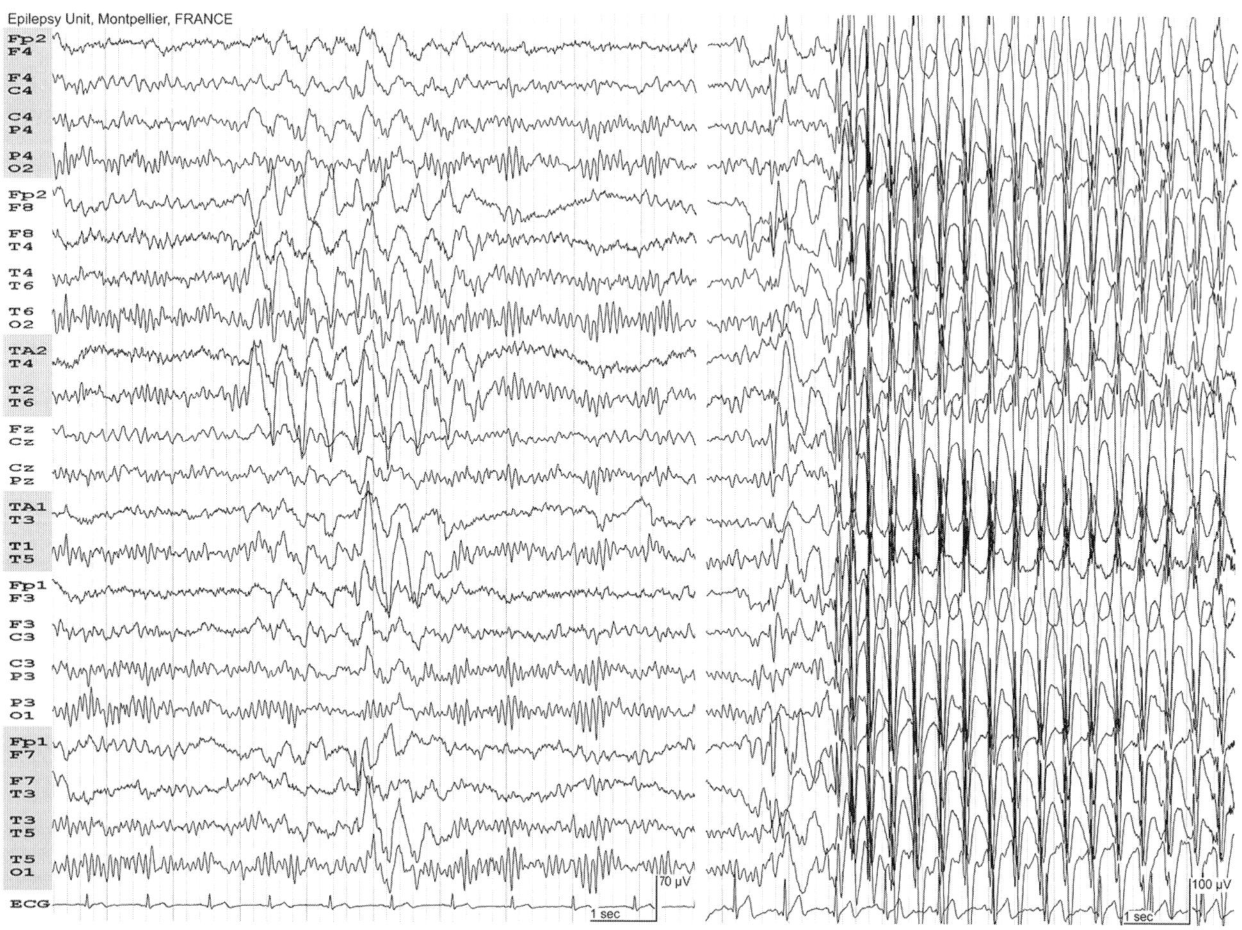

Figure a / Recording at 15 mm/s. On the right segment, a typical absence seizure.

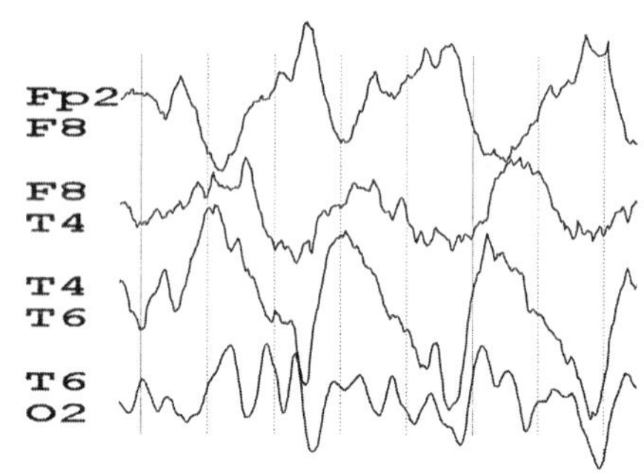

Figure b / TIRDA on the right temporal region.

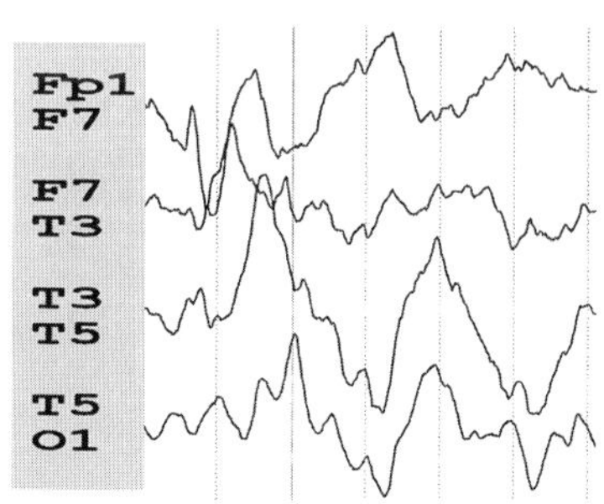

Figure c / TIRDA on the left temporal region.

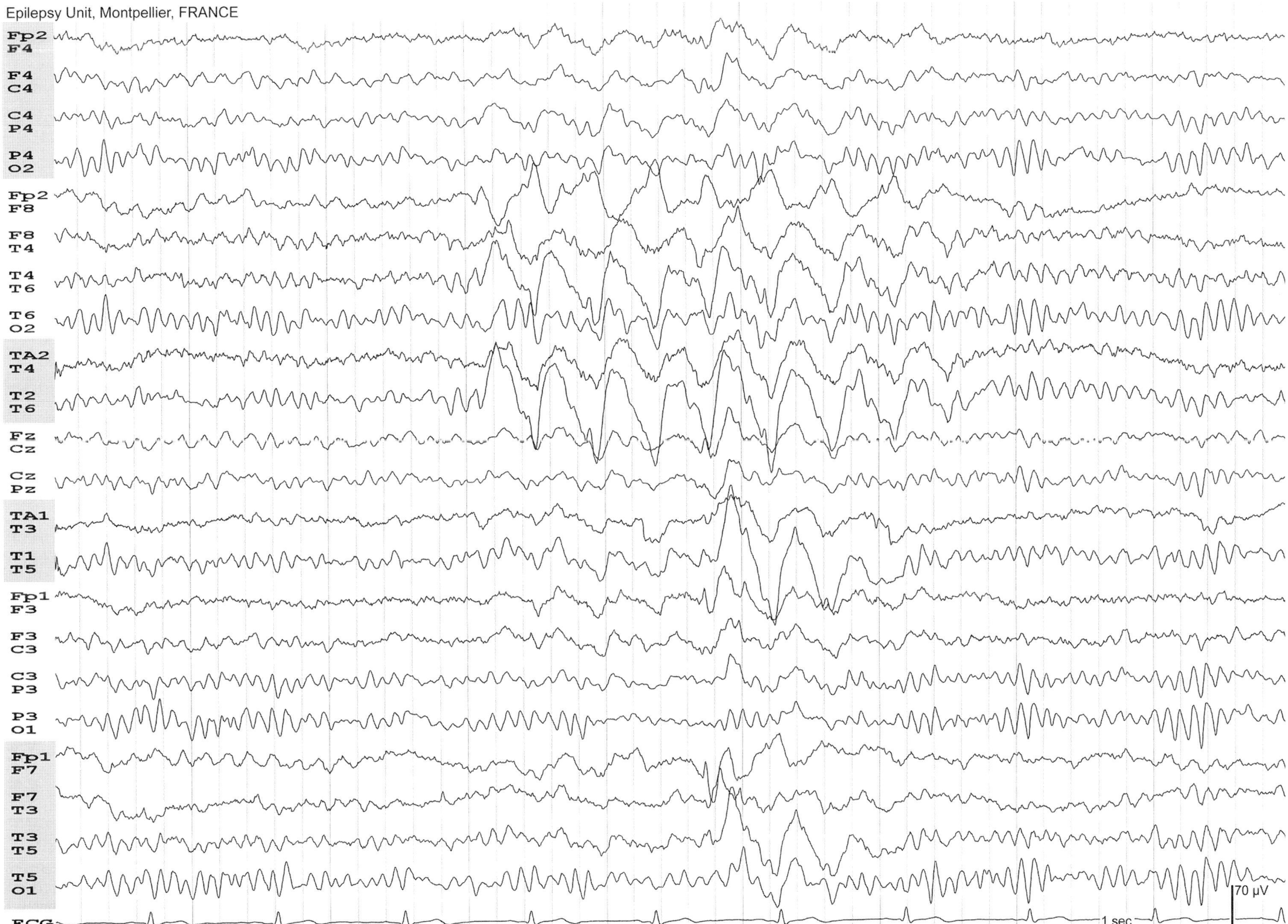
Epilepsy Unit, Montpellier, FRANCE
Fp2 F4
F4 C4
C4 P4
P4 O2
Fp2 F8
F8 T4
T4 T6
T6 O2
TA2 T4
T2 T6
Fz Cz
Cz Pz
TA1 T3
T1 T5
Fp1 F3
F3 C3
C3 P3
P3 O1
Fp1 F7
F7 T3
T3 T5
T5 O1
ECG
70 µV
1 sec

I • 5 Background activity in an adult, reactivity of the alpha rhythm and beta rhythms

Context

EEG in a 43-year-old woman followed for juvenile myoclonic epilepsy.

What to note

The patient's eyes are closed. Background activity with 10 Hz alpha rhythm in the occipital regions. The alpha rhythm blocks when her eyes open. Eyelid blinking artifacts appear. Note on this plate the presence of low voltage fast activities at 22 Hz on the anterior derivations. They correspond to physiological beta rhythms.

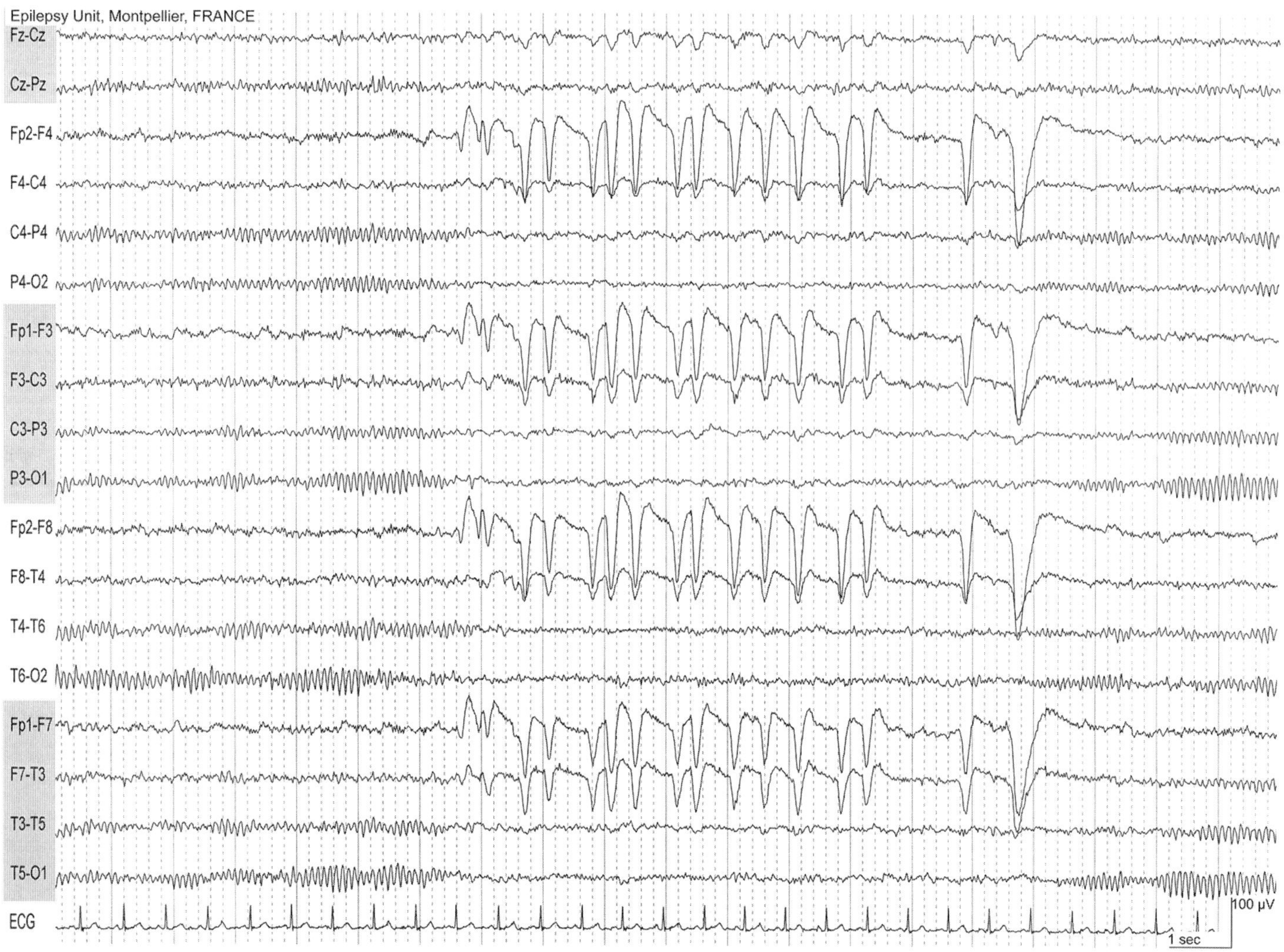

Figure a / Recording at 15 mm/s. Note the reactivity of the alpha rhythm upon eye opening and eye closure. As soon as she closes her eyes, alpha background activity with sinusoidal waves reappears.

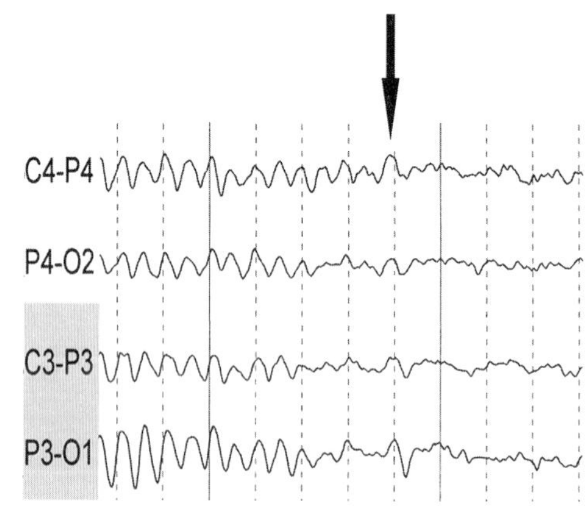

Figure b / Opening of eyes (arrow): disappearance of alpha rhythm.

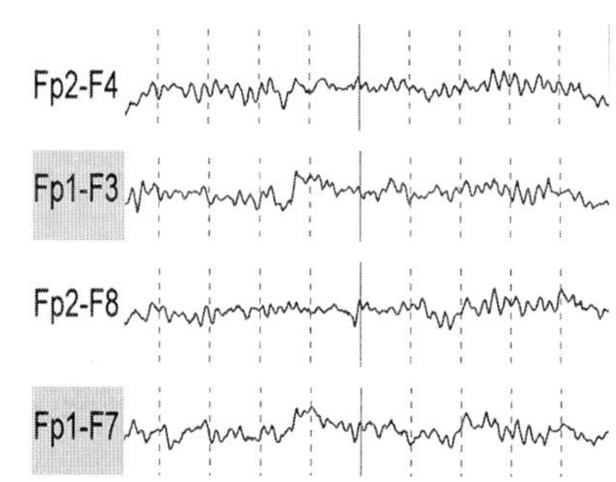

Figure c / Beta rhythms.

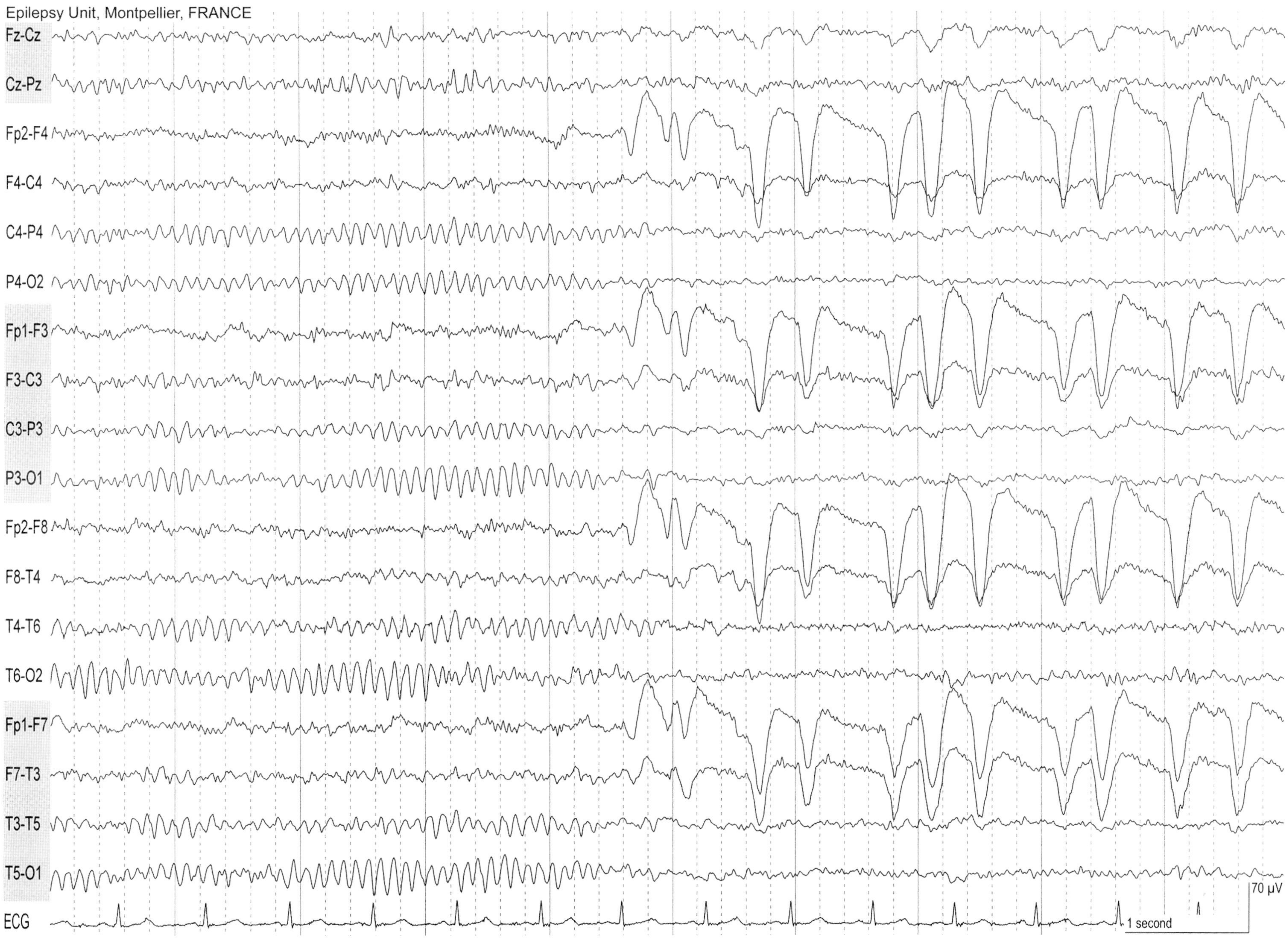
Epilepsy Unit, Montpellier, FRANCE
Fz-Cz
Cz-Pz
Fp2-F4
F4-C4
C4-P4
P4-O2
Fp1-F3
F3-C3
C3-P3
P3-O1
Fp2-F8
F8-T4
T4-T6
T6-O2
Fp1-F7
F7-T3
T3-T5
T5-O1
ECG
70 µV
1 second

I • 6 Beta rhythms in a child with posterior slow waves

Context

EEG of a 12-year-old child followed for epilepsy.

What to note

The child's eyes are closed. Background activity with an alpha rhythm (8-9 Hz) associated with posterior slow waves. Note a superimposition of the two rhythms (alpha rhythm and posterior slow waves) conveying an impression of sharp waves. Fast activities at 21 Hz can be seen on the anterior derivations with predominance on the right. These are beta rhythms. The amplitude is unusually high here. The patient was not treated with benzodiazepines or barbiturates.

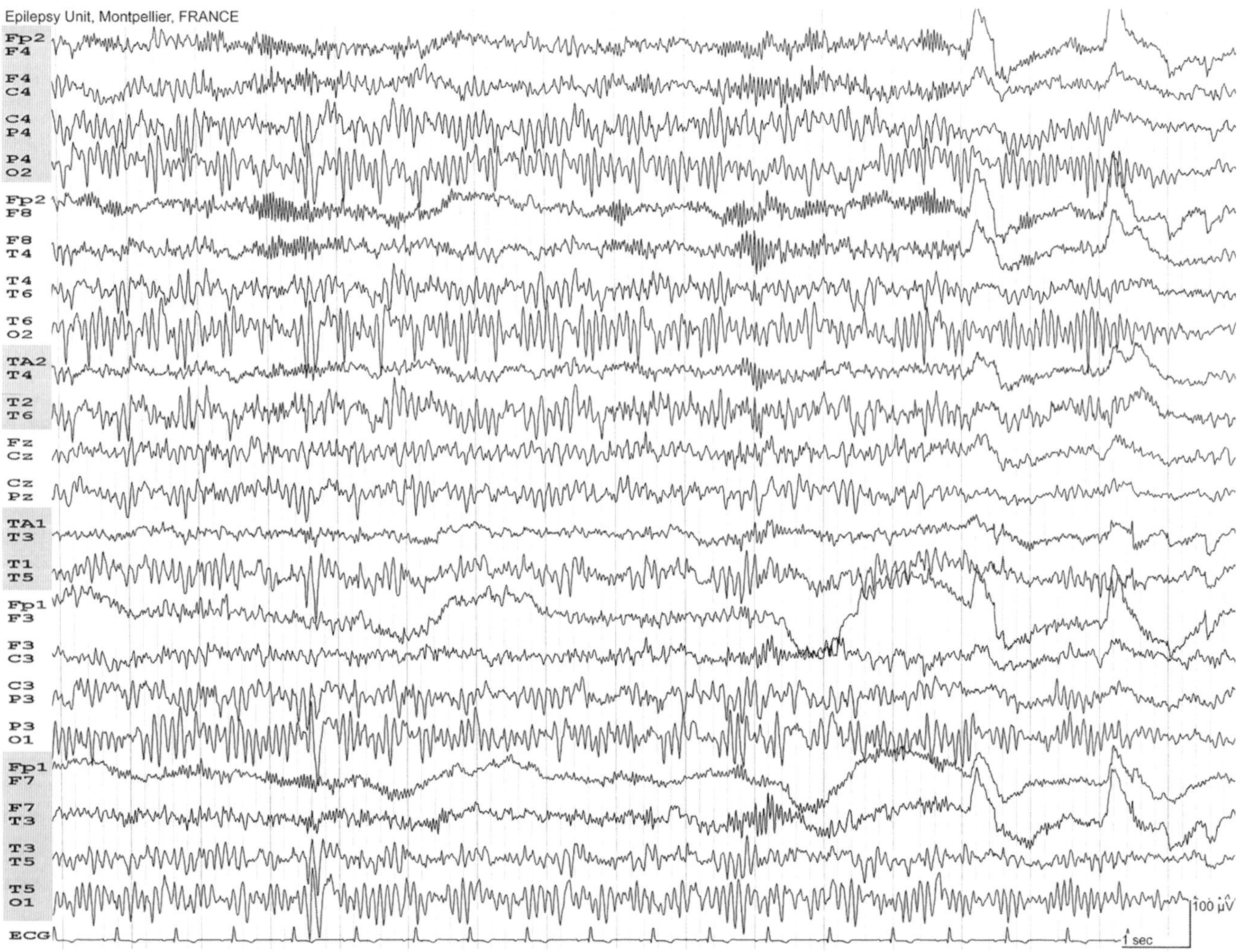

Figure a / Recording at 15 mm/s.

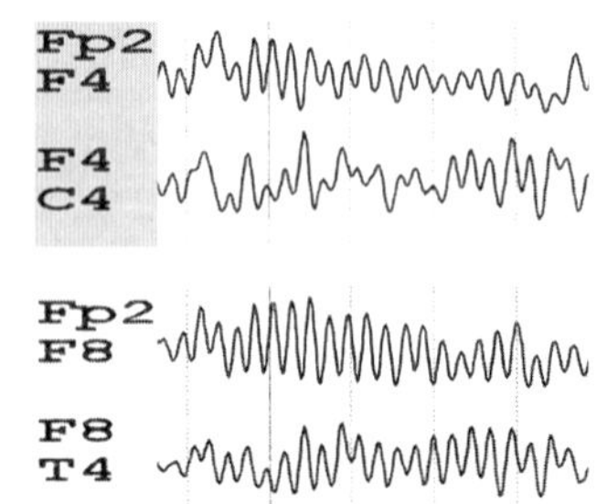

Figure b / Beta activity on anterior regions.

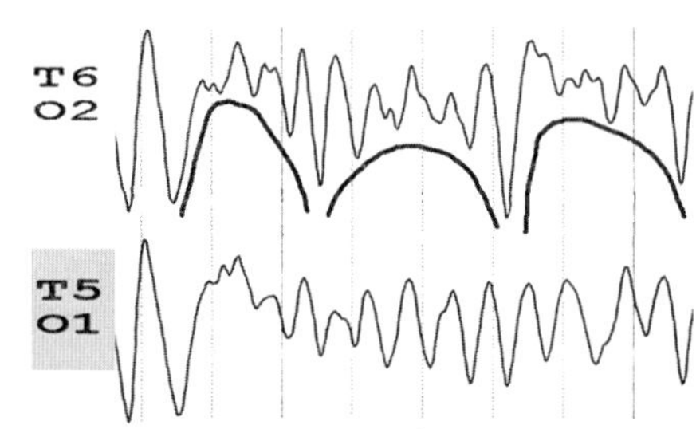

Figure c / Superimposed alpha rhythm and posterior slow waves, underlined here, in the right posterior region.

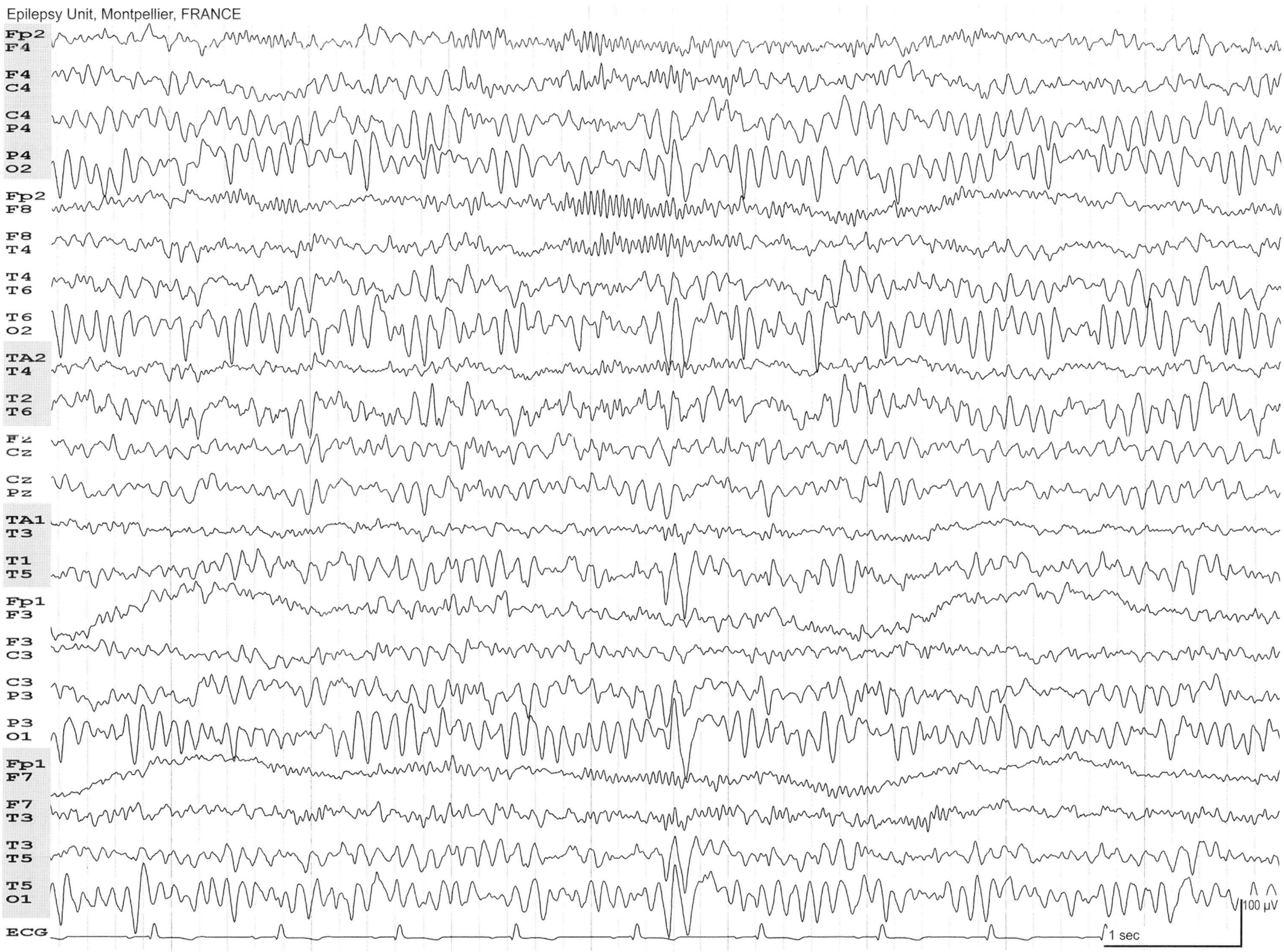
Epilepsy Unit, Montpellier, FRANCE
Fp2
F4
F4
C4
C4
P4
P4
O2
Fp2
F8
F8
T4
T4
T6
T6
O2
TA2
T4
T2
T6
Fz
Cz
Cz
Pz
TA1
T3
T1
T5
Fp1
F3
F3
C3
C3
P3
P3
O1
Fp1
F7
F7
T3
T3
T5
T5
O1
ECG
100 µV
1 sec

• 7 Background activity in an adult, notched alpha waves and beta rhythms

Context

42-year-old man referred after a first generalized tonic-clonic seizure. He was treated with a benzodiazepine.

What to note

The patient's eyes are closed. Background activity with posterior alpha rhythm (8 Hz). Benzodiazepines increase anterior beta activity creating a pharmacological rhythm. These beta rhythms spread to the posterior regions. Some alpha waves are clearly forked due to the superimposed beta waves. See with the following plates, the differences with the slow and fast alpha variant.

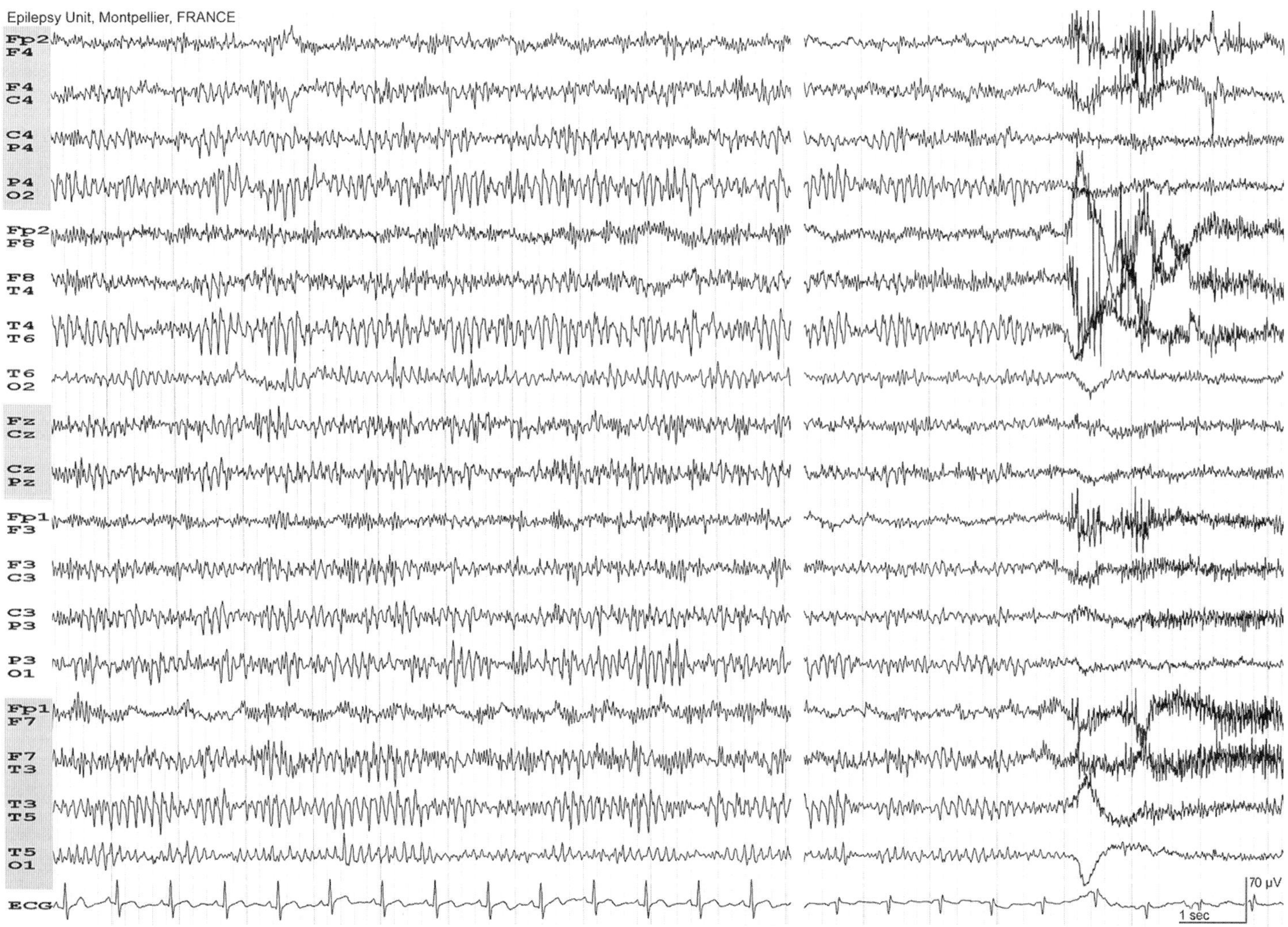

Figure a / Recording at 15 mm/s. Right segment, reactivity of the alpha rhythm upon eye opening.

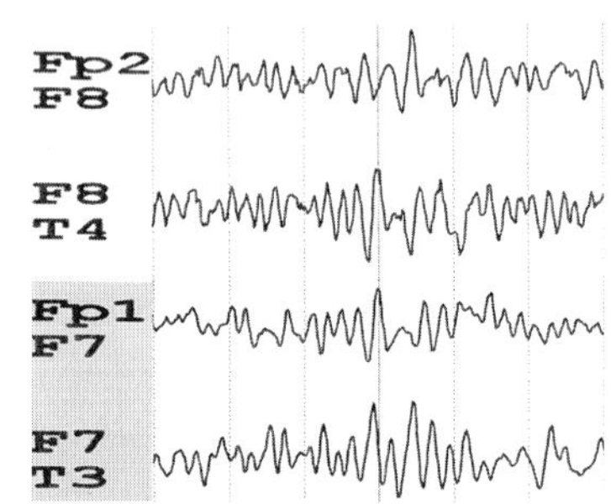

Figure b / Beta rhythm at 20 Hz.

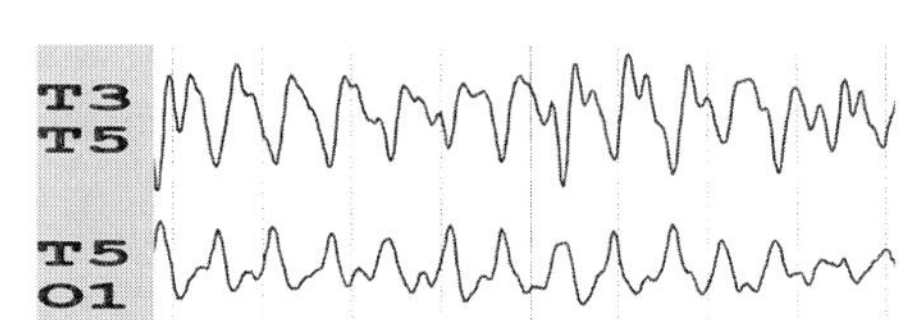

Figure c / Notched alpha waves.

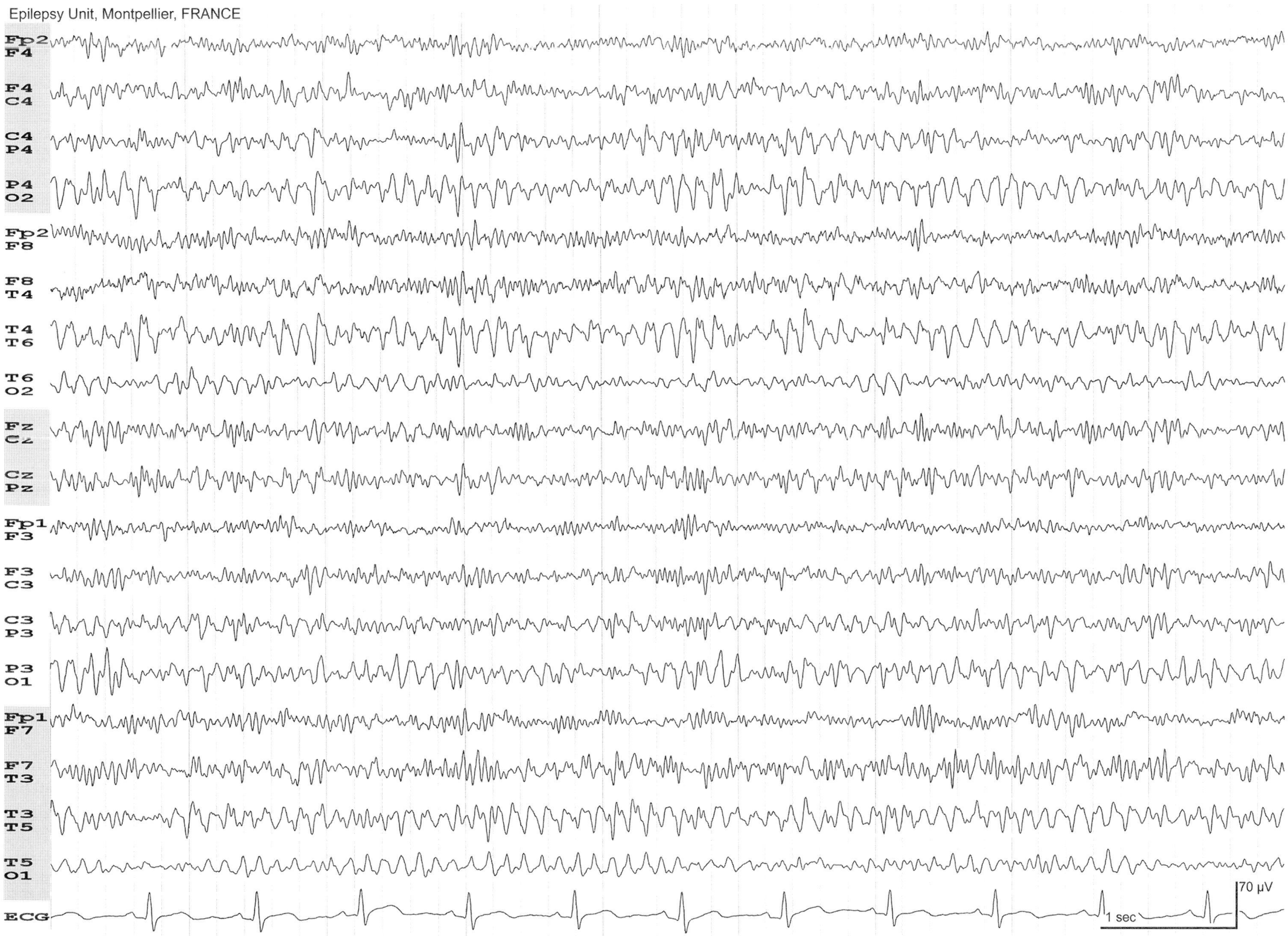
Epilepsy Unit, Montpellier, FRANCE
Fp2 F4
F4 C4
C4 P4
P4 O2
Fp2 F8
F8 T4
T4 T6
T6 O2
Fz Cz
Cz Pz
Fp1 F3
F3 C3
C3 P3
P3 O1
Fp1 F7
F7 T3
T3 T5
T5 O1
ECG
70 µV
1 sec

I • 8 Slow alpha variant: subharmonic (1)

Context

49-year-old woman referred for epilepsy follow-up.

What to note

Background activity with posterior alpha rhythm at 10 to 11 Hz during 1 second. The rhythm drops to a 5.5 Hz frequency corresponding to a slow alpha variant, also referred to as a subharmonic alpha rhythm. In this patient, slow alpha variant was also observed in REM sleep (see plate III-35).

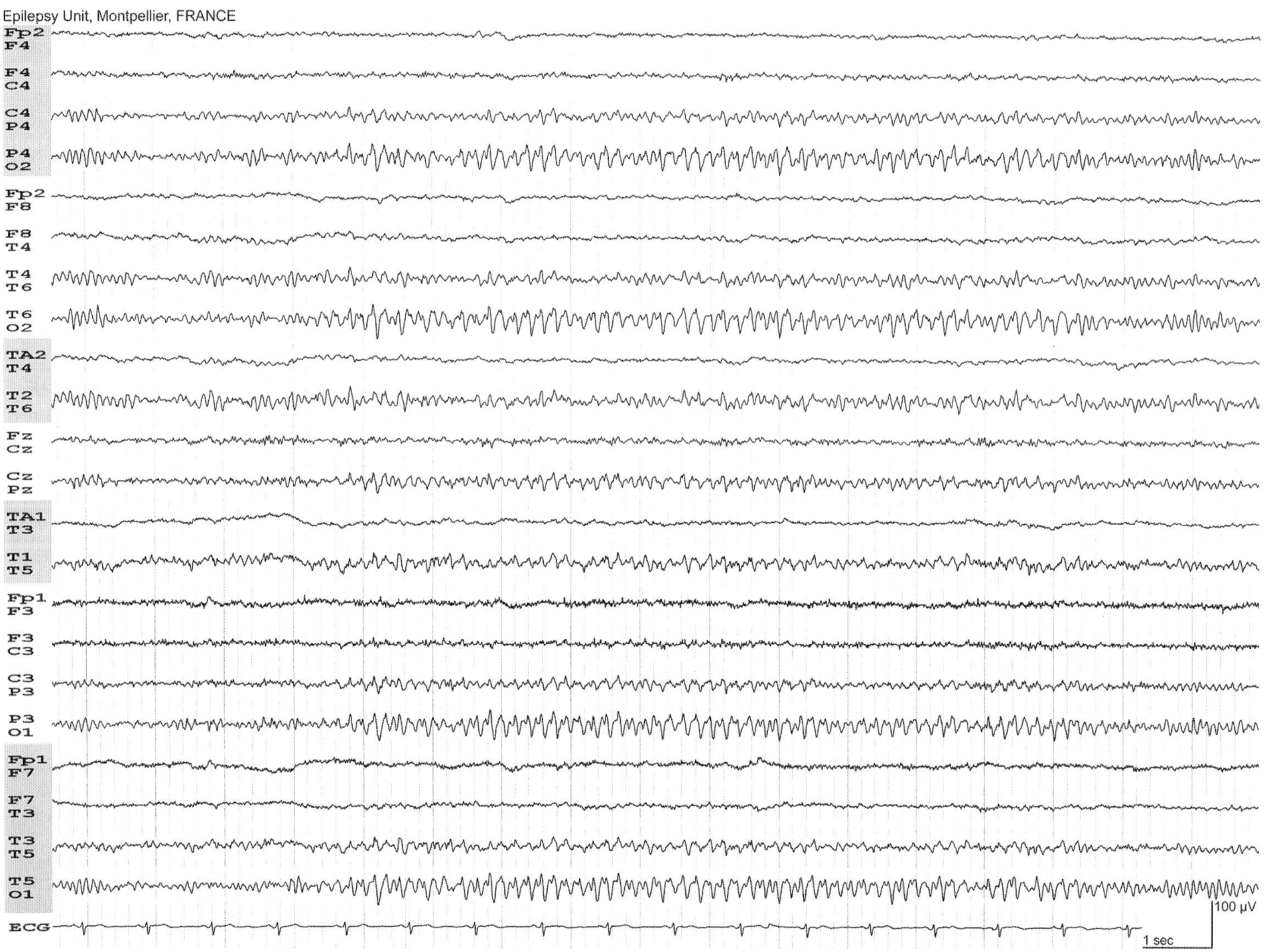

Figure a / Recording at 15 mm/s. Normal alpha and subharmonic alpha rhythm are intermixed in this patient.

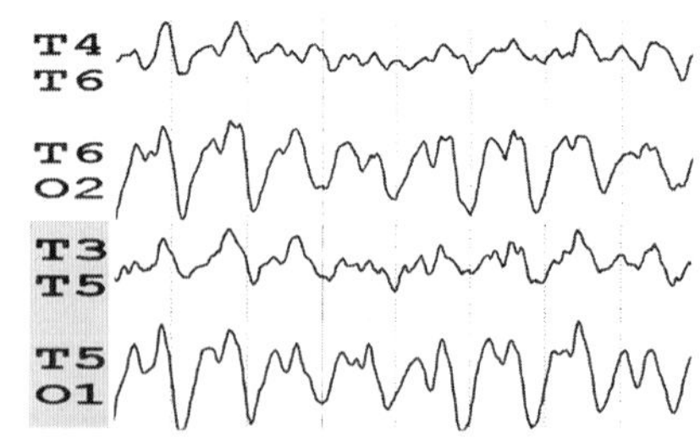

Figure b / Notched theta waves corresponding to a slow alpha variant.

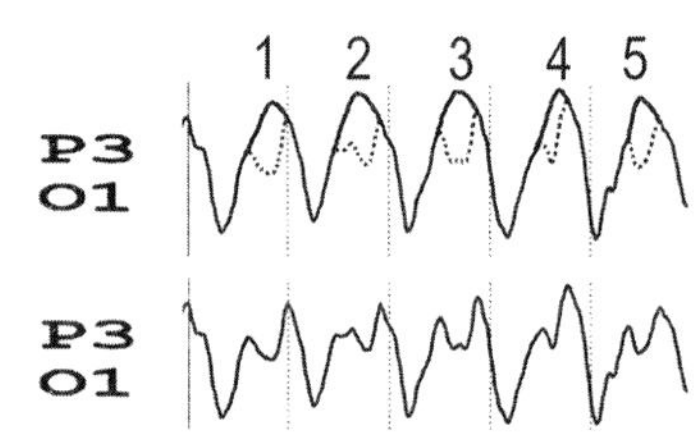

Figure c / A 5.5 Hz rhythm (top), and it has been traced over. At the bottom, the wave is clearly forked but it does not mark the end of the cycle. By counting the "peaks", you obtain 10-11, which corresponds to the patient's alpha rhythm.

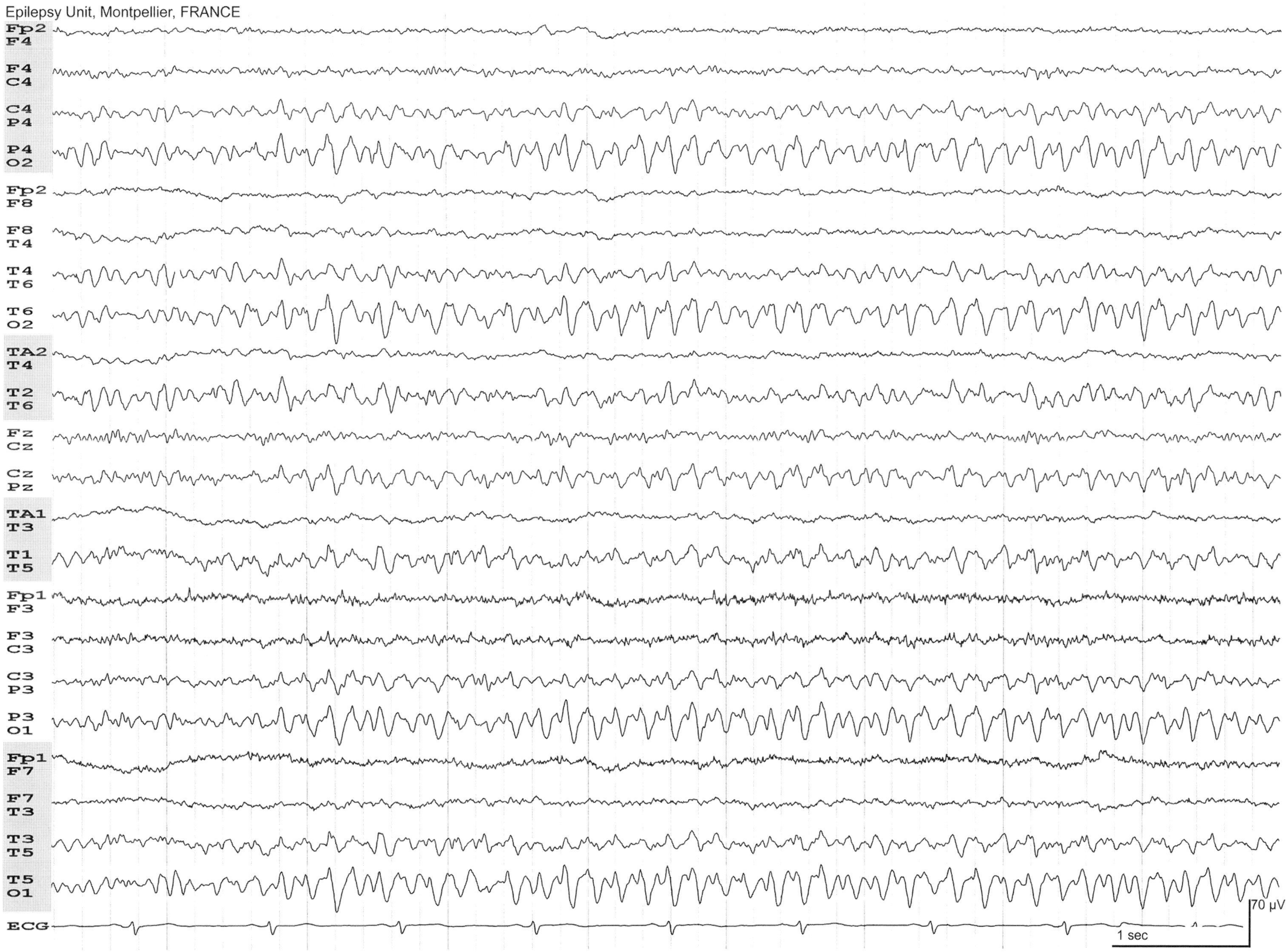
Epilepsy Unit, Montpellier, FRANCE
Fp2 F4
F4 C4
C4 P4
P4 O2
Fp2 F8
F8 T4
T4 T6
T6 O2
TA2 T4
T2 T6
Fz Cz
Cz Pz
TA1 T3
T1 T5
Fp1 F3
F3 C3
C3 P3
P3 O1
Fp1 F7
F7 T3
T3 T5
T5 O1
ECG
70 µV
1 sec

• 9 Slow alpha variant: subharmonic (2)

Context

EEG of a 52-year-old woman referred for assessment after an episode of loss of consciousness.

What to note

Background activity with a high-amplitude theta rhythm (5 Hz). The rhythm is clearly posterior when the patient's eyes are closed and amplitude is greater on the right hemisphere. On the right side of the plate, the rhythm disappears upon eye opening. Although some of the waveforms are notched as in the preceding example, the alpha variant pattern is much more monomorphic in this patient.

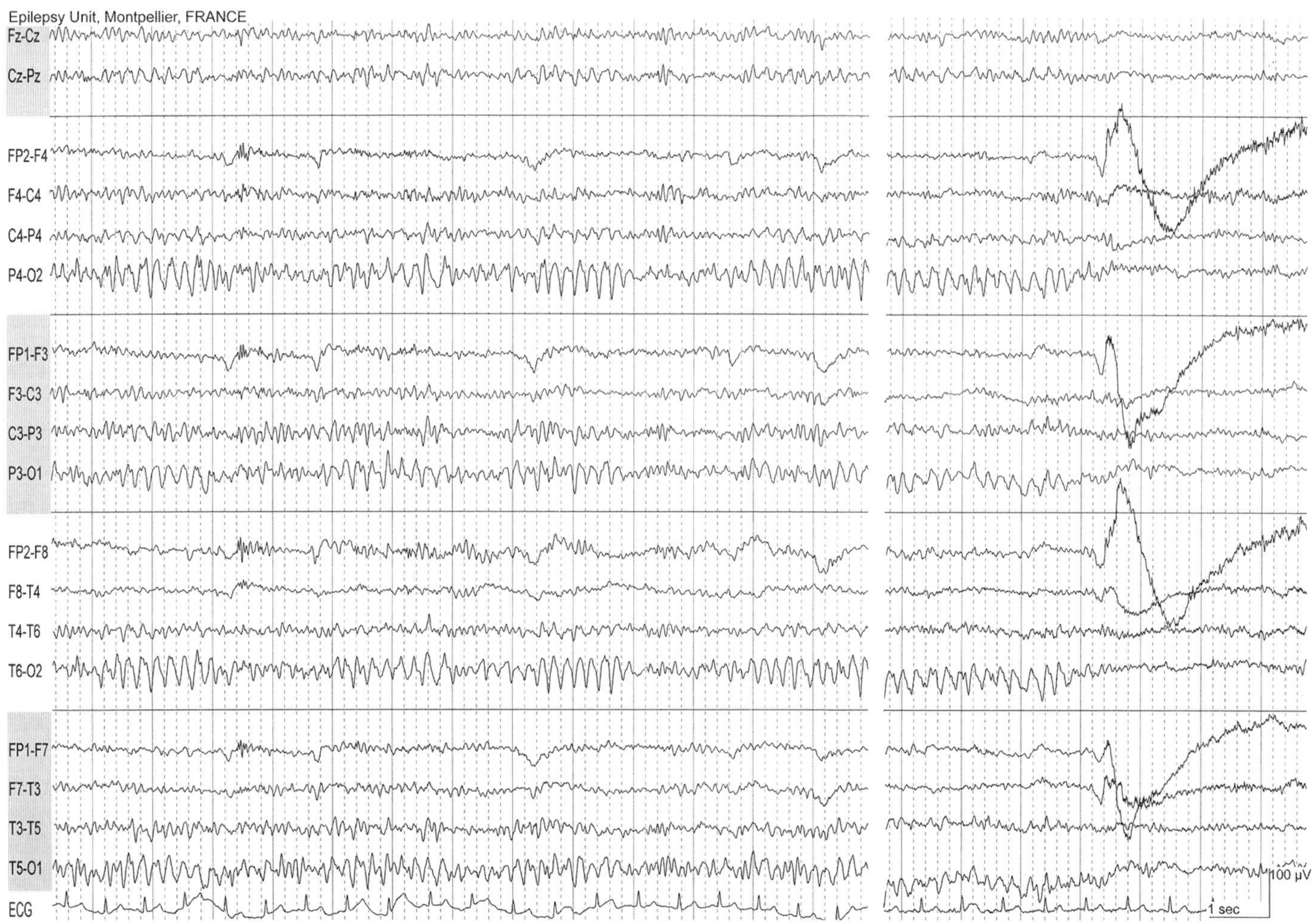

Figure a / Recording at 15 mm/s. Note the reactivity upon eye opening.

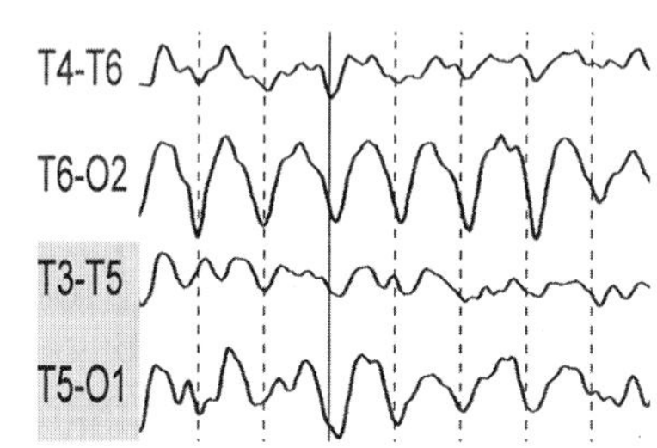

Figure b / Posterior theta activity (5 Hz).

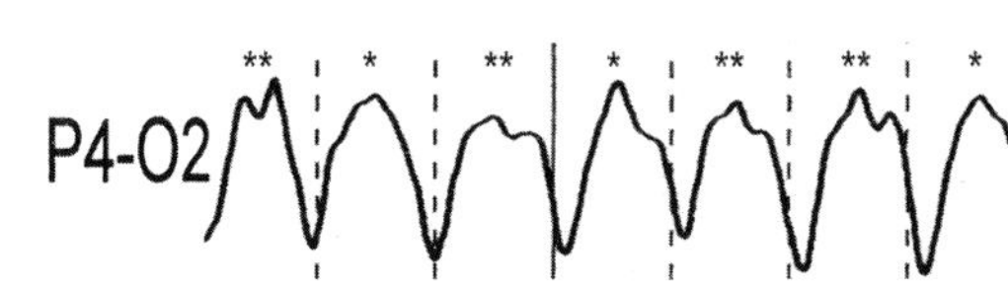

Figure c / * Monomorphic theta wave.
** Notched theta wave (bifid aspect).

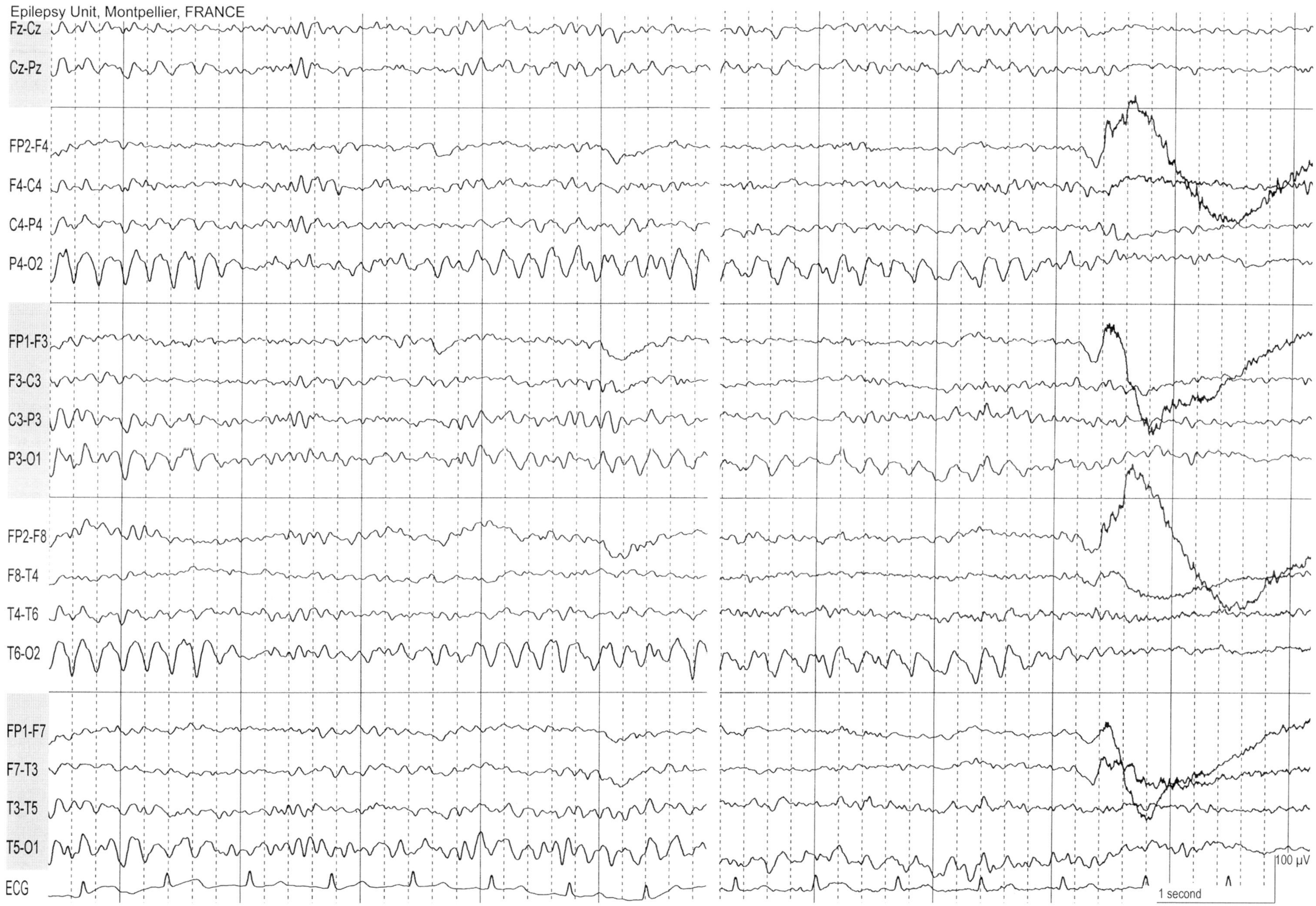
Epilepsy Unit, Montpellier, FRANCE
Fz-Cz
Cz-Pz
FP2-F4
F4-C4
C4-P4
P4-O2
FP1-F3
F3-C3
C3-P3
P3-O1
FP2-F8
F8-T4
T4-T6
T6-O2
FP1-F7
F7-T3
T3-T5
T5-O1
ECG
100 µV
1 second

I • 10 Slow alpha variant: subharmonic (3)

Context

59-year-old man with focal epilepsy (right insular cavernoma).

What to note

The patient is awake, closed eyes. Background activity with theta rhythm can be observed. The rhythm is irregular with sharp-contoured waves, and disappears completely as soon as the eyes are opened.

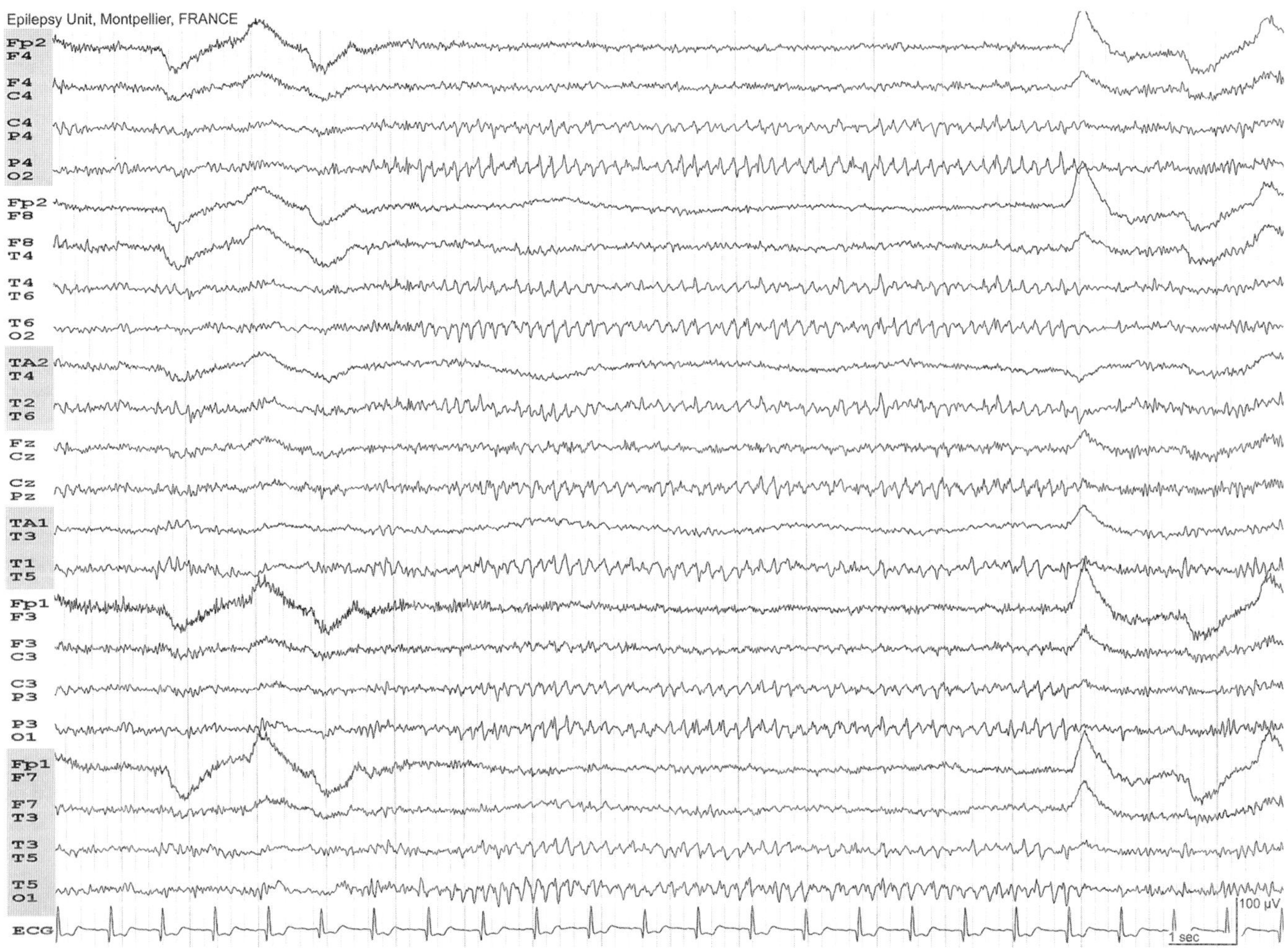

Figure a / Recording at 15 mm/s. Note the reactivity upon eye closure and eye opening.

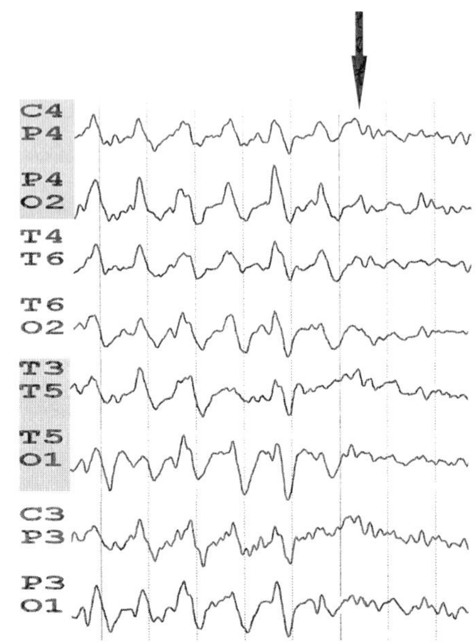

Figure b / Irregular and sharp-contoured waveforms over the posterior regions corresponding to a subharmonic alpha rhythm. Disappearance of the slow alpha variant upon opening of eyes (arrow).

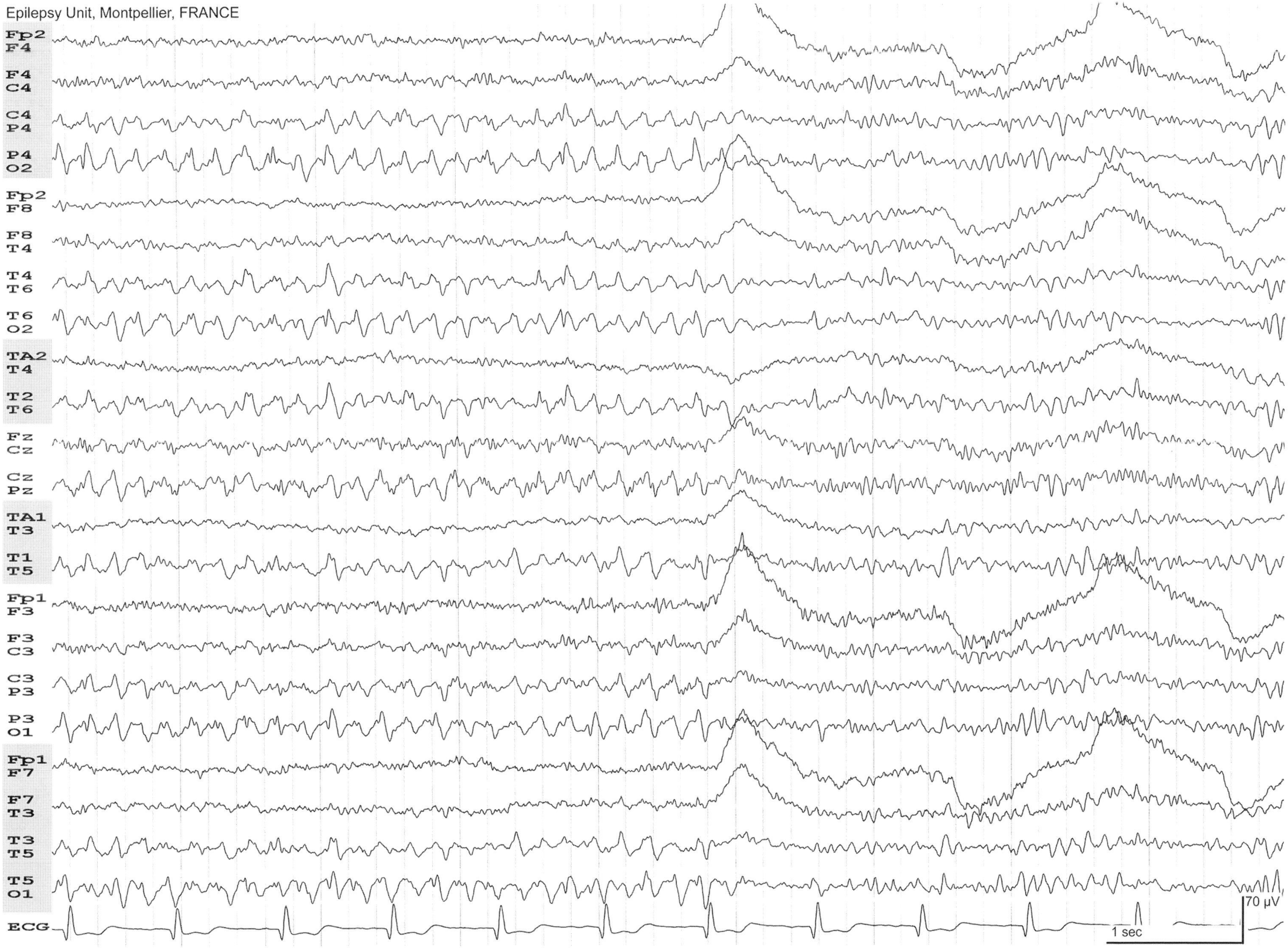
Epilepsy Unit, Montpellier, FRANCE
Fp2 F4
F4 C4
C4 P4
P4 O2
Fp2 F8
F8 T4
T4 T6
T6 O2
TA2 T4
T2 T6
Fz Cz
Cz Pz
TA1 T3
T1 T5
Fp1 F3
F3 C3
C3 P3
P3 O1
Fp1 F7
F7 T3
T3 T5
T5 O1
ECG
70 µV
1 sec

I • 11 Fast alpha variant (1)

Context

36-year-old man followed for epilepsy.

What to note

On the left, the patient's eyes are open. An eyelid movement artifact occurs on the fronto-polar derivations when he is asked to close his eyes. As soon as he closes his eyes, a posterior background activity at 16-18 Hz appears for two seconds, corresponding to a fast alpha variant. Note that some waveforms are notched. On the right, the patient's eyes are closed. Background activity with a 18 Hz sinusoidal rhythm in the occipital regions.

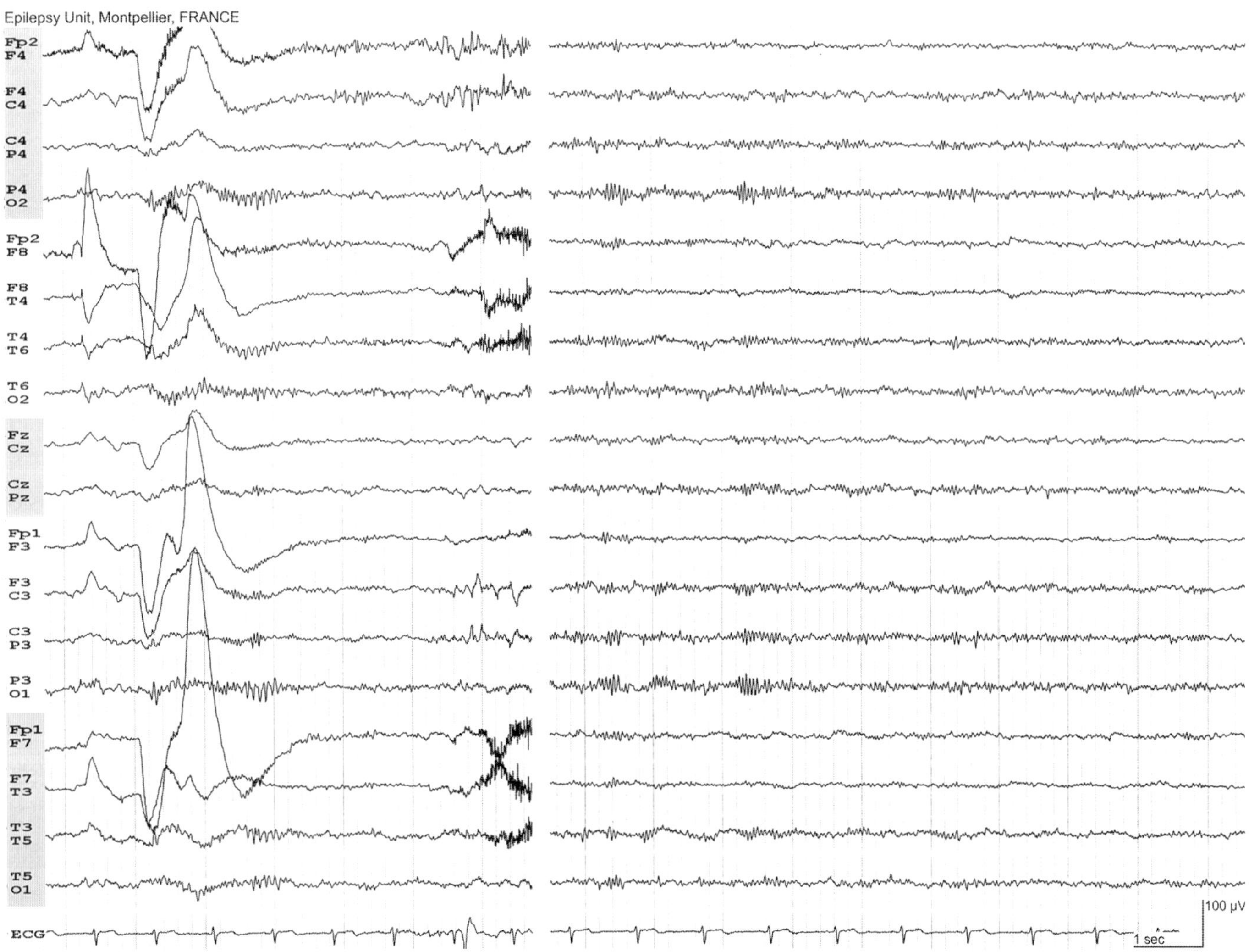

Figure a / Recording at 15 mm/s.

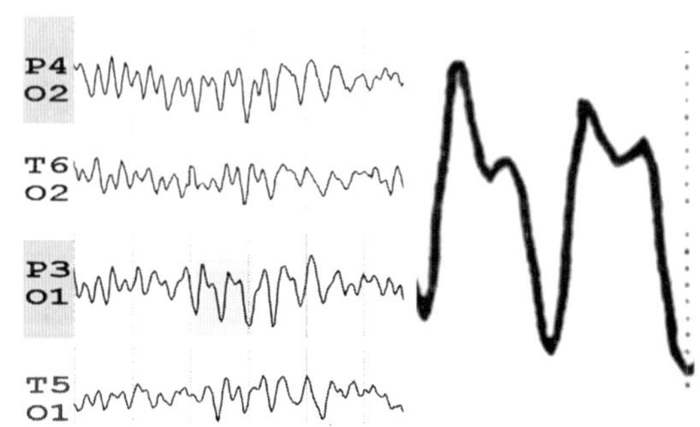

Figure b / Fast alpha variant.
Some waveforms are notched (zoom).

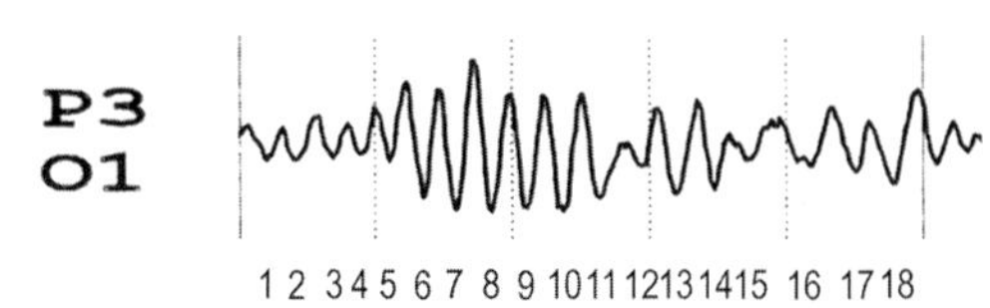

Figure c / Fast alpha variant at 18 Hz. Note the sinusoïdal aspect.

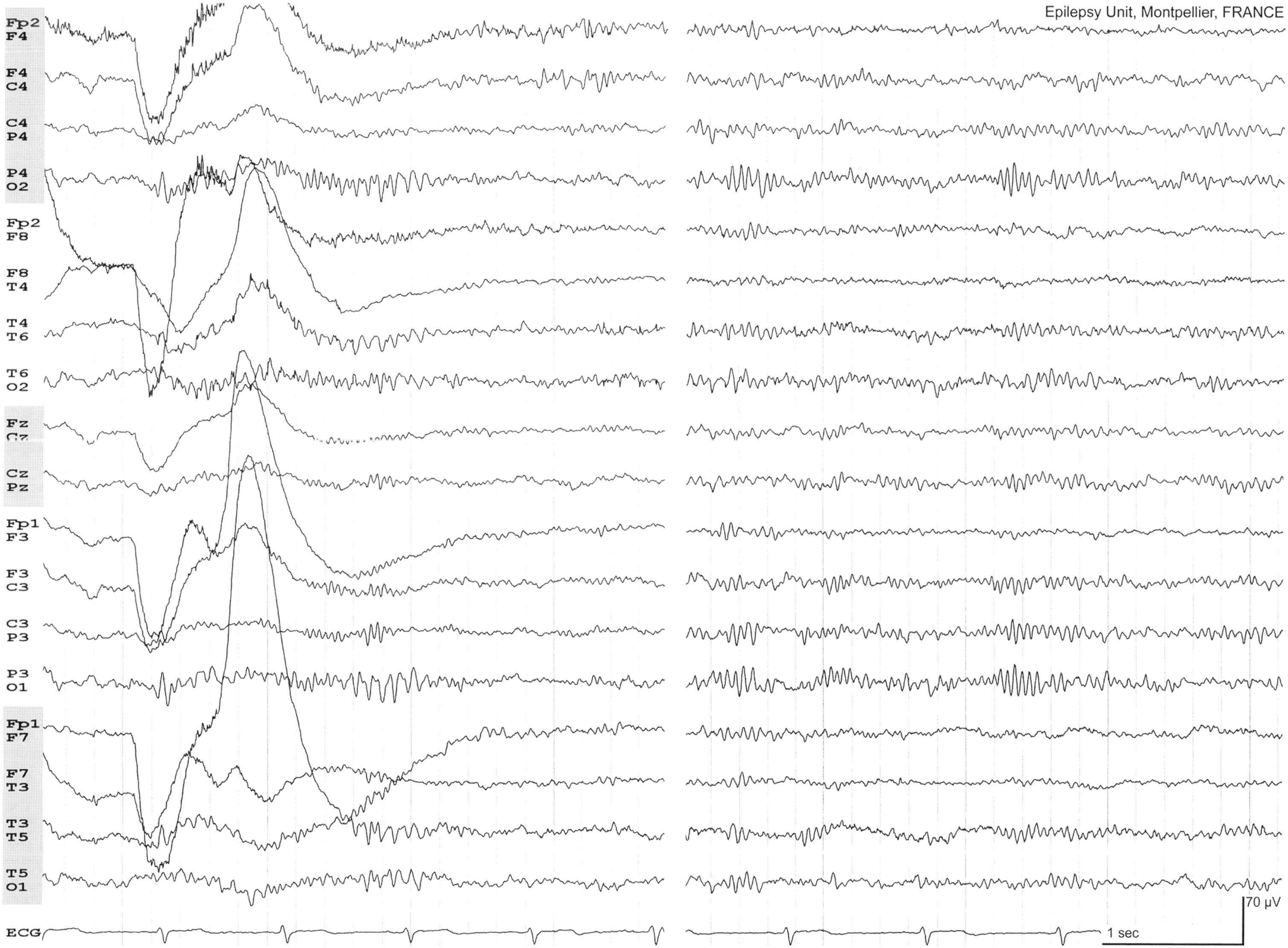
Epilepsy Unit, Montpellier, FRANCE
Fp2 F4
F4 C4
C4 P4
P4 O2
Fp2 F8
F8 T4
T4 T6
T6 O2
Fz Cz
Cz Pz
Fp1 F3
F3 C3
C3 P3
P3 O1
Fp1 F7
F7 T3
T3 T5
T5 O1
ECG
70 µV
1 sec

I • 12 Fast alpha variant (2)

Context

49-year-old woman followed for epilepsy.

What to note

The patient's eyes are closed. Low-voltage 17 Hz rhythm can be observed over the occipital regions. It disappears upon eye opening. Presence of eyelid movement artifacts.

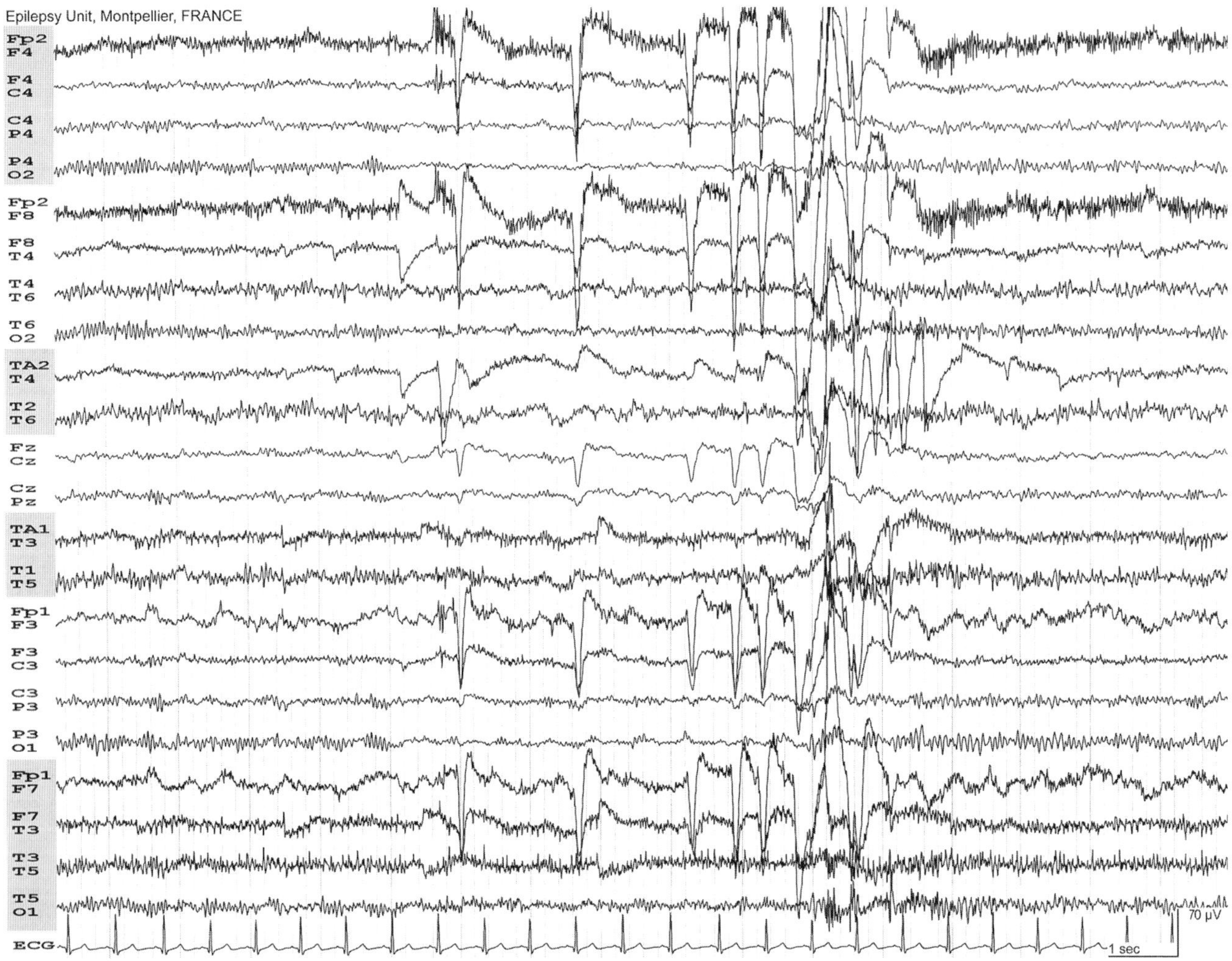

Figure a / Recording at 15 mm/s. Note the reactivity upon eye opening and eye closure.

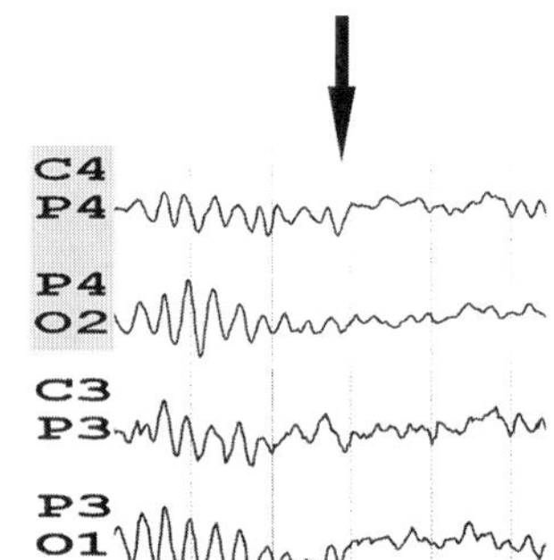

Figure b / Disappearance of the fast alpha variant upon eye opening (arrow).

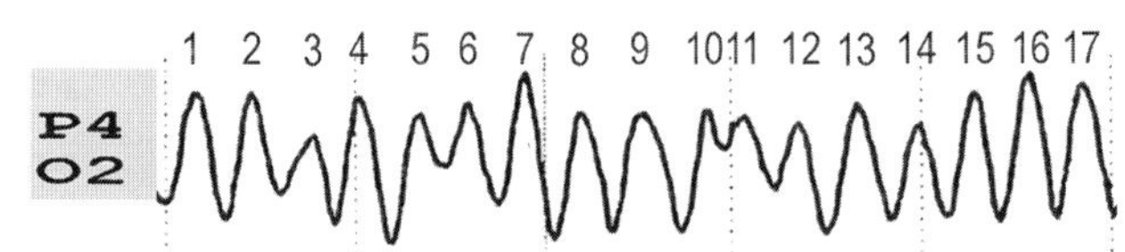

Figure c / Fast alpha variant at 17 Hz.

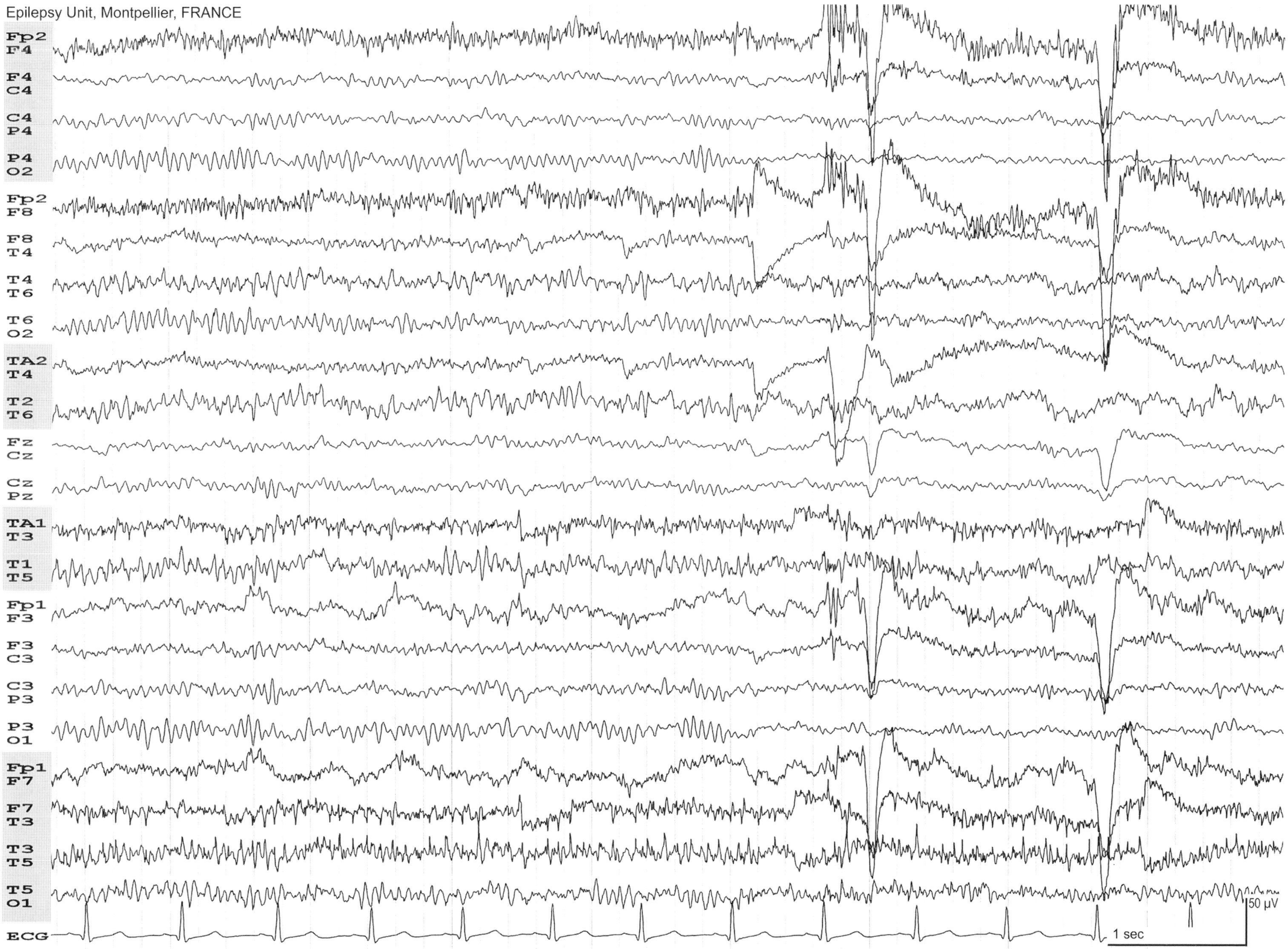
Epilepsy Unit, Montpellier, FRANCE
Fp2 F4
F4 C4
C4 P4
P4 O2
Fp2 F8
F8 T4
T4 T6
T6 O2
TA2 T4
T2 T6
Fz Cz
Cz Pz
TA1 T3
T1 T5
Fp1 F3
F3 C3
C3 P3
P3 O1
Fp1 F7
F7 T3
T3 T5
T5 O1
ECG
50 µV
1 sec

• 13 Mu rhythm in an infant

Context

18-month-old girl referred after several episodes of loss of consciousness with revulsion of eyes.

What to note

Awake recording, with infant's eyes open. On the left side of the recording, an arch-like rhythm (8 Hz) can be seen on the left central region. This is a mu rhythm in an 18-month-old infant. On the right side, the mu rhythm can be seen on the right central region. Detection of a mu rhythm in an infant is very unusual. On the right side, the recording is superimposed with anterior muscular activities. Electrode artifact at P3-O1 and T5-O1.

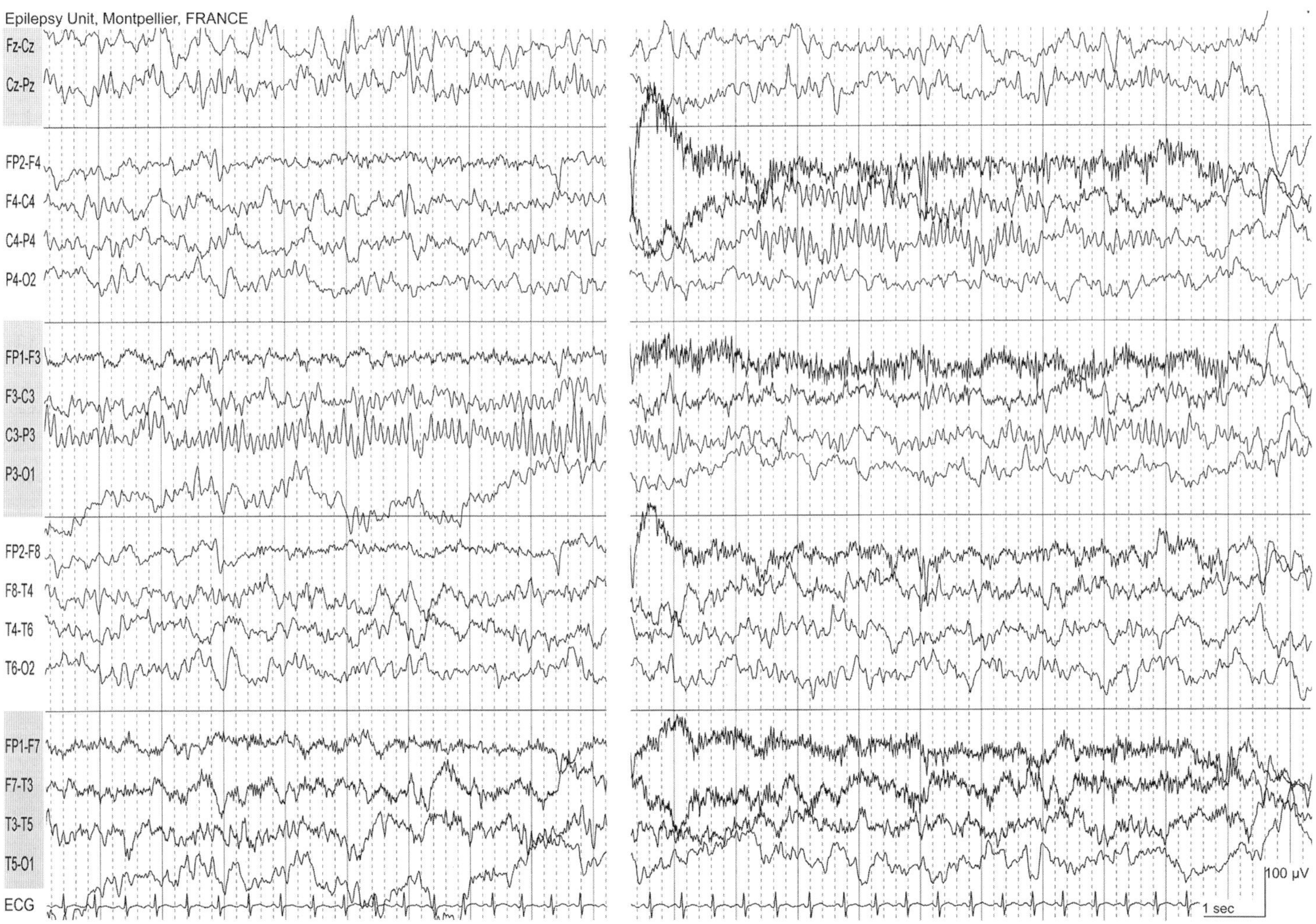

Figure a / Recording at 15 mm/s.

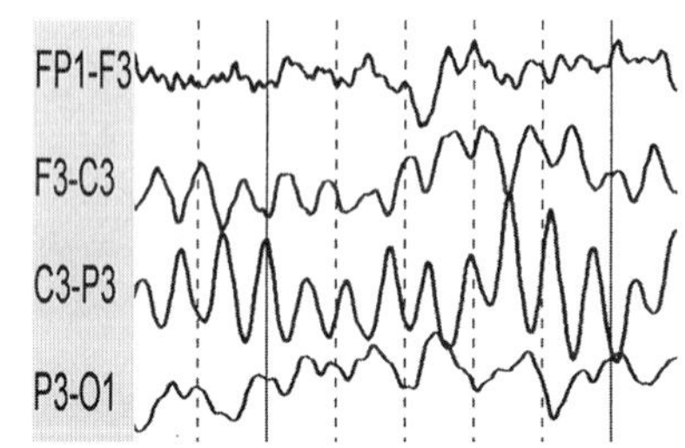

Figure b / Mu rhythm on the left central region.

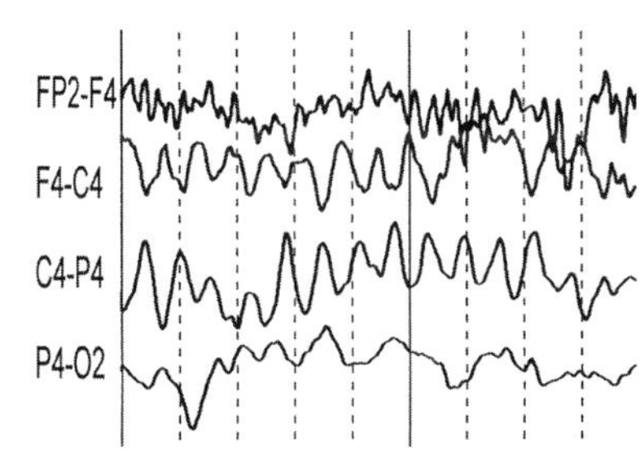

Figure c / Mu rhythm on the right central region. Muscular activities at Fp2-F4.

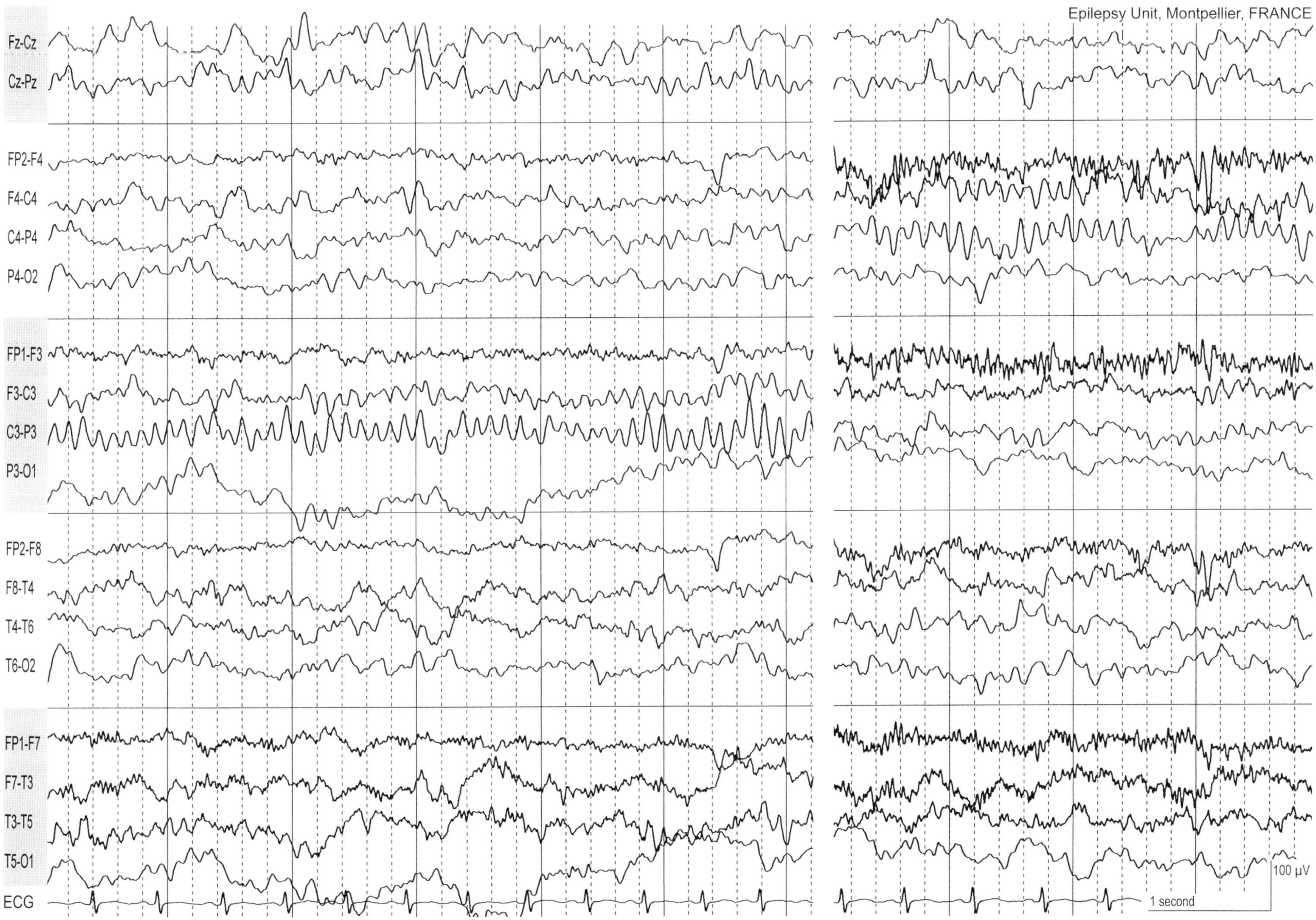
Epilepsy Unit, Montpellier, FRANCE
Fz-Cz
Cz-Pz
FP2-F4
F4-C4
C4-P4
P4-O2
FP1-F3
F3-C3
C3-P3
P3-O1
FP2-F8
F8-T4
T4-T6
T6-O2
FP1-F7
F7-T3
T3-T5
T5-O1
ECG
100 µV
1 second

• 14 Mu rhythm in a child

Context

9-year-old child referred for childhood absence epilepsy.

What to note

The alpha rhythm and posterior slow waves disappear after eye opening. Then, a rhythm with a central arch-like shaped wave (9 Hz) appears. The rhythm is bilateral at first, then there is a shift to left central predominance. The mu rhythm is unusual due to its sharp-contoured waves, but this is not pathological. It can be observed more commonly with background activity of greater amplitude. Generally speaking, the greater the amplitude of the alpha rhythm, the greater the other physiological rhythms tend to be. They must not be misinterpreted as pathological patterns.

What to do

Ask the child to clench his fists in order to test reactivity of the rhythm (disappearance during clenching).

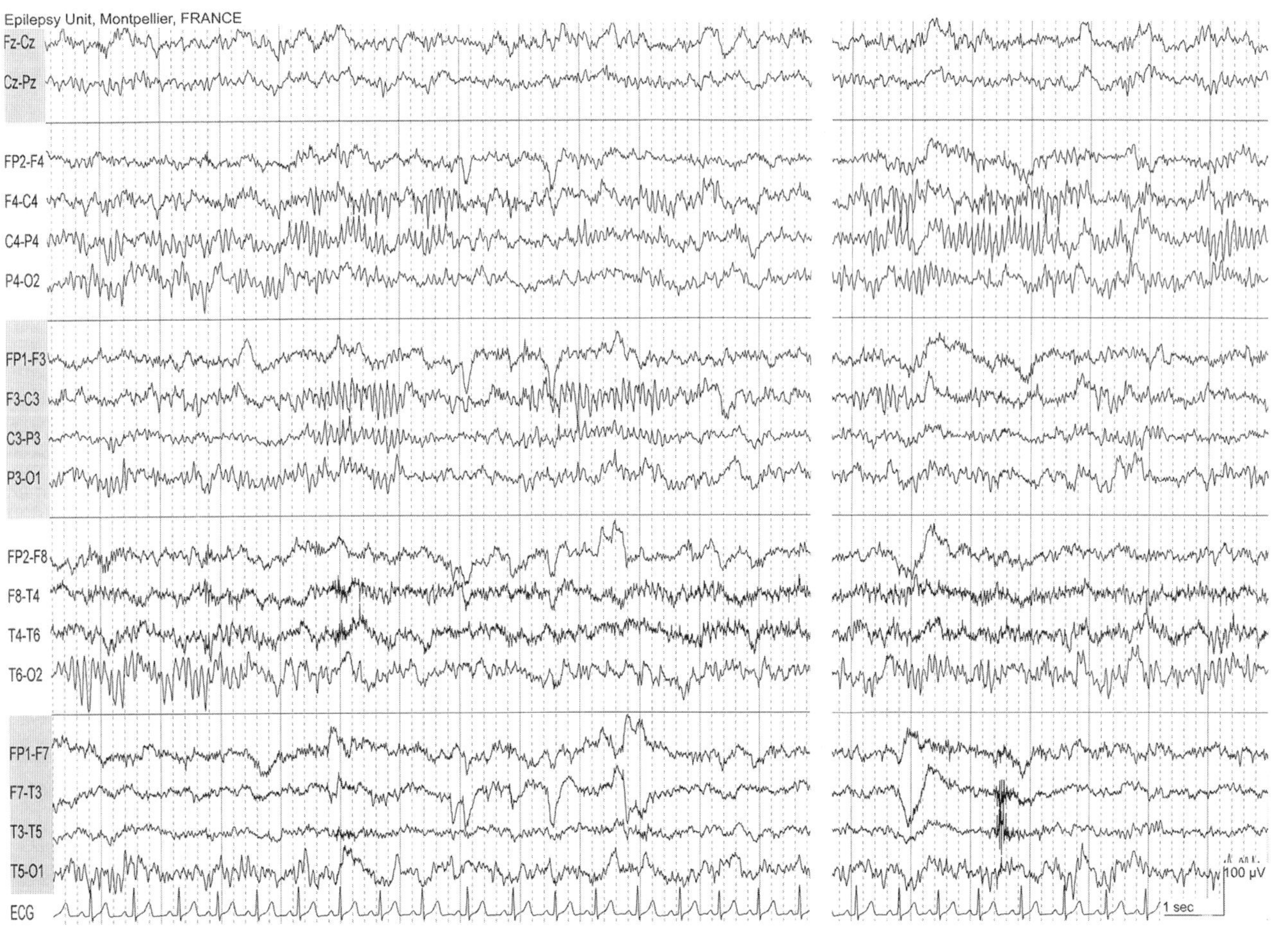

Figure a / Recording at 15 mm/s. On the right plate, the mu rhythm can be observed on the right central region.

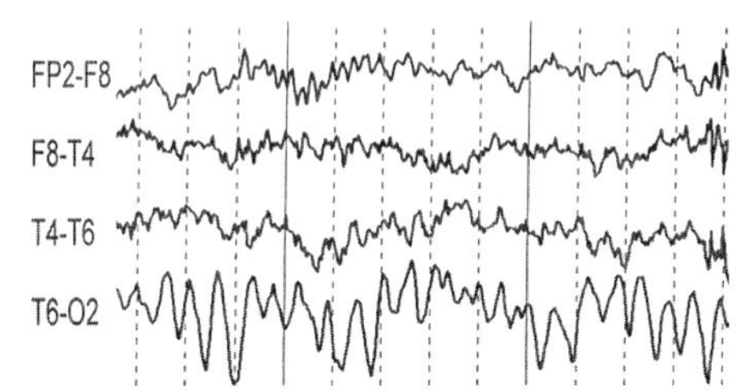

Figure b / Alpha rhythm and posterior slow waves of youth.

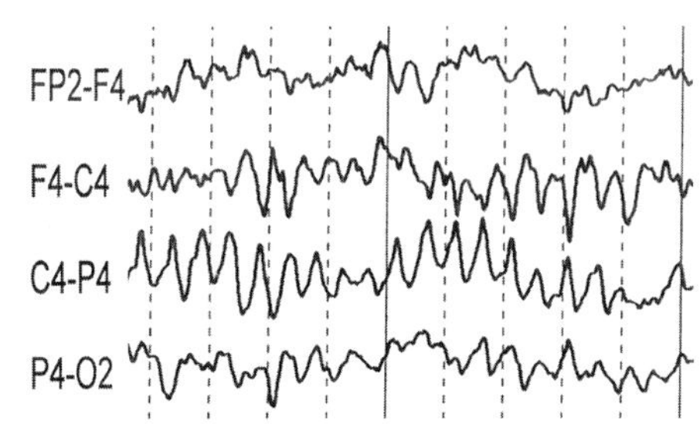

Figure c / Mu rhythm of high amplitude with sharp-contoured waves on the right central region.

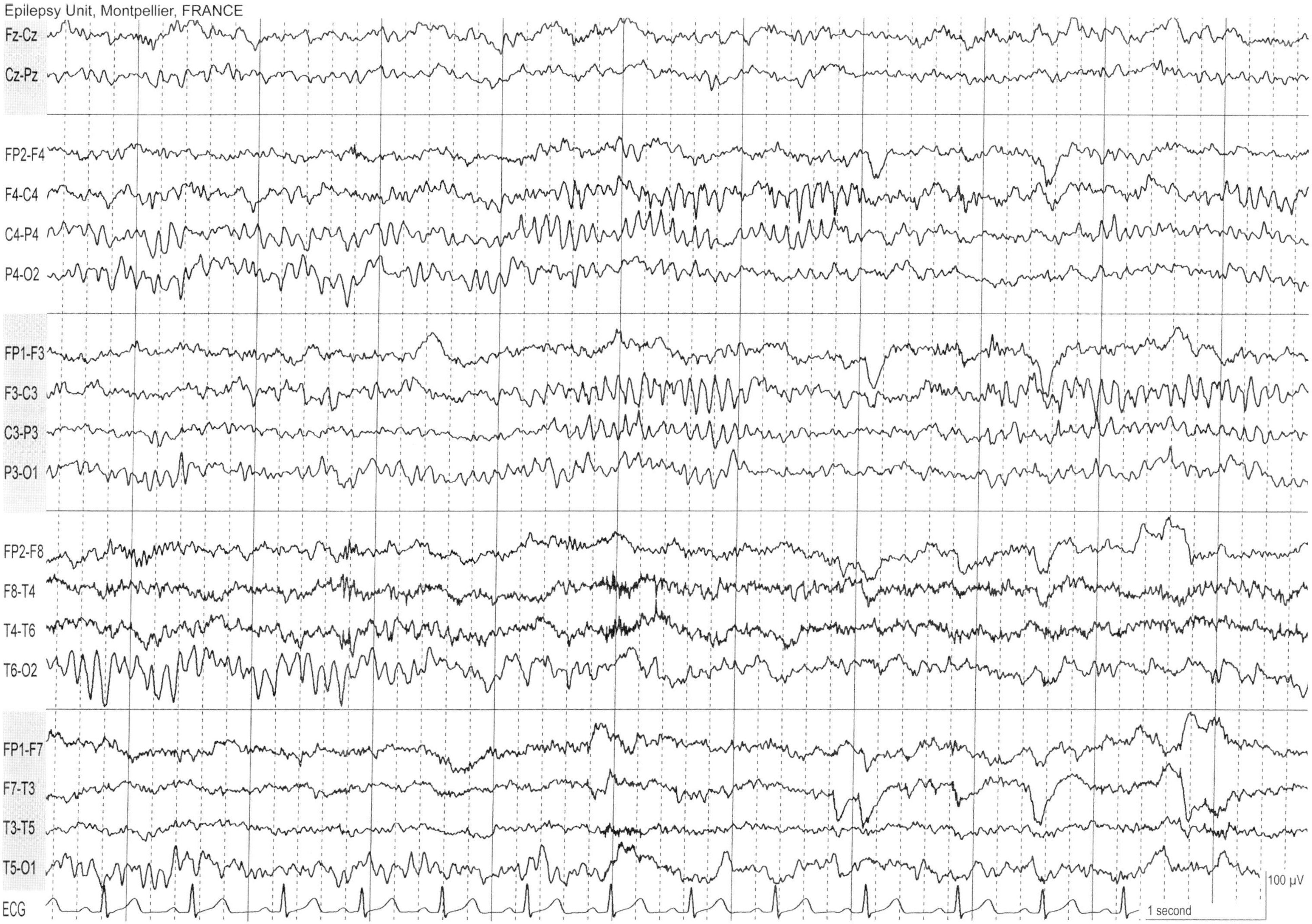
Epilepsy Unit, Montpellier, FRANCE
Fz-Cz
Cz-Pz
FP2-F4
F4-C4
C4-P4
P4-O2
FP1-F3
F3-C3
C3-P3
P3-O1
FP2-F8
F8-T4
T4-T6
T6-O2
FP1-F7
F7-T3
T3-T5
T5-O1
ECG
100 µV
1 second

• 15 Mu rhythm and alpha reactivity in an adult

Context

EEG of 38-year-old woman followed for epilepsy.

What to note

At the beginning of the plate, background activity with alpha rhythm of great amplitude can be observed with predominance on the right posterior region. The mu rhythm continues with an asynchronous pattern first on the right central region for 5 seconds after opening of eyes, then on the left central region (see plate at 15 mm/second). On close examination, it appears that the mu rhythm was already present at the beginning but it conveyed a false impression of an alpha rhythm with anterior spread. In fact, by counting the waves in the central region, it appears that the mu rhythm is slower than the alpha rhythm. Note eyelid movement artifacts upon eye opening.

What to do

Ask the patient to clench his/her fists in order to test reactivity of the mu rhythm (disappearance during clenching).

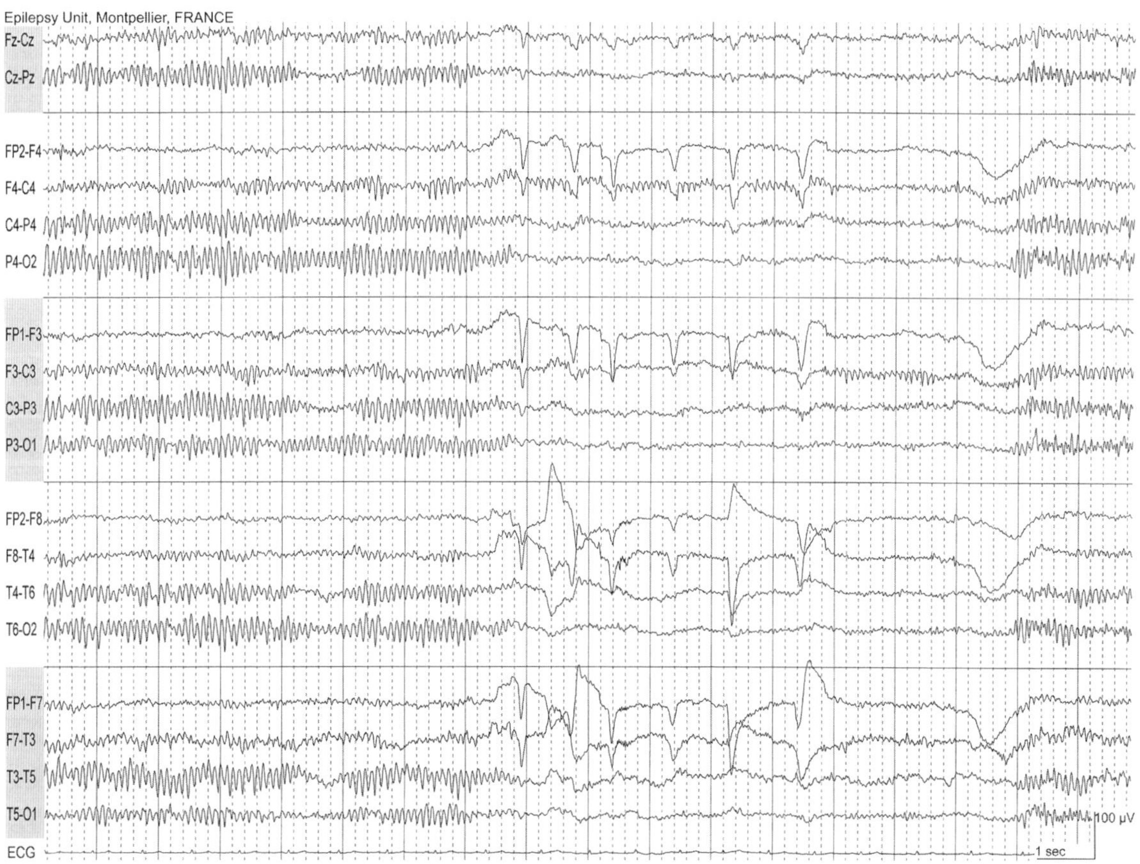

Figure a / Recording at 15 mm/s. Mu rhythm on the right central region then on the left central region.

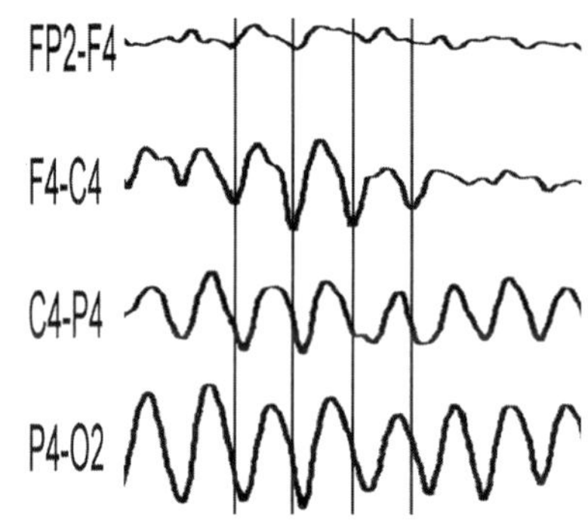

Figure b / Zoom. Posterior alpha rhythm with a false impression of posterior-anterior spread. Mu rhythm at F4-C4. Note that the frequency is different.

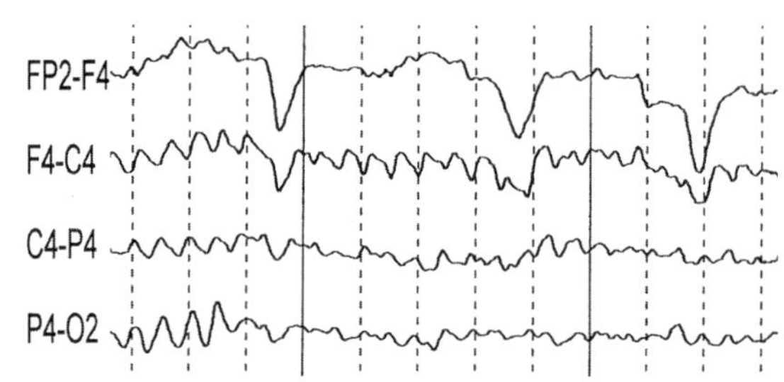

Figure c / The alpha rhythm disappears with eye opening. Mu rhythm clearly detectable on the right central region. Presence of eyelid movement artifacts at Fp2-F4.

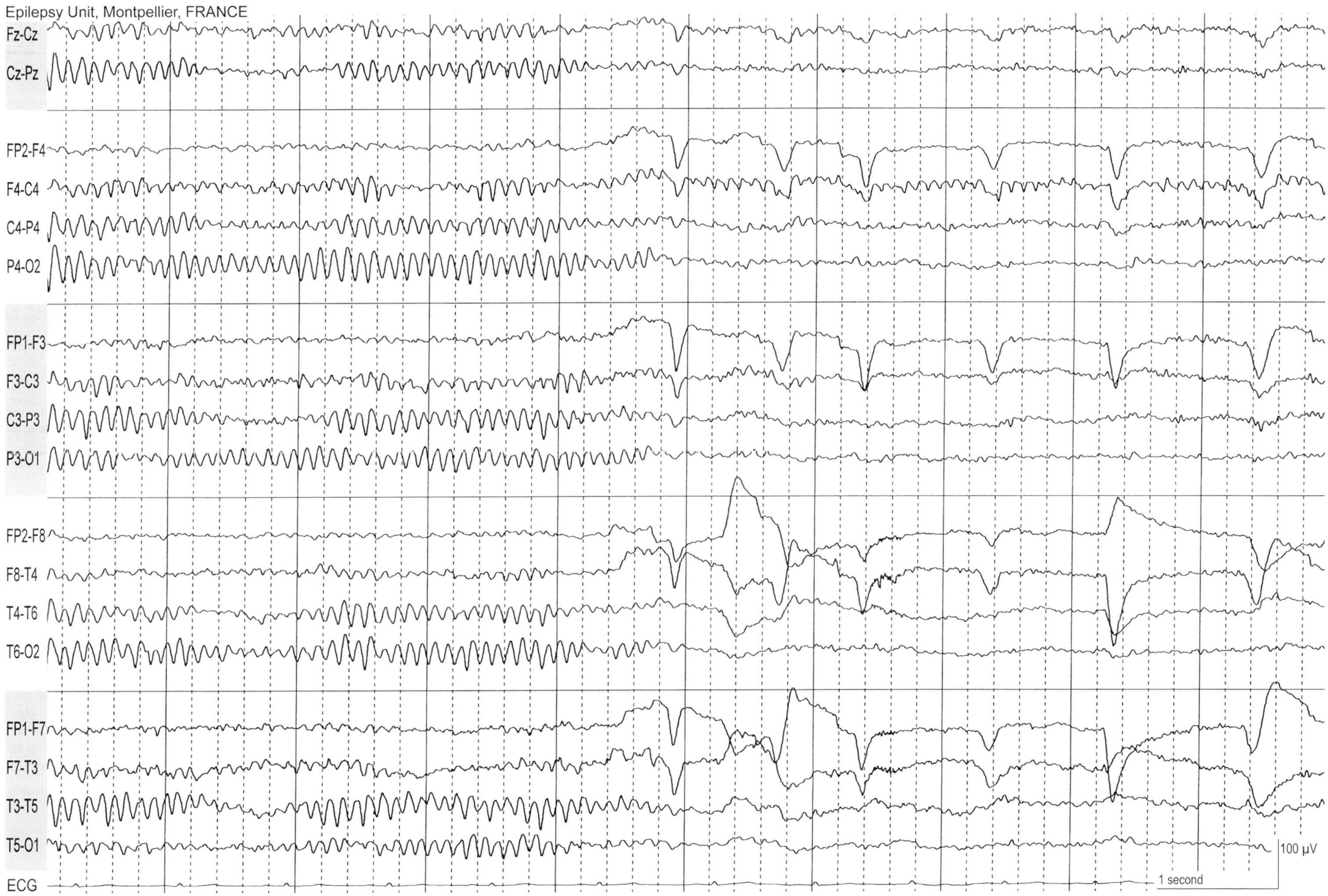
Epilepsy Unit, Montpellier, FRANCE
Fz-Cz
Cz-Pz
FP2-F4
F4-C4
C4-P4
P4-O2
FP1-F3
F3-C3
C3-P3
P3-O1
FP2-F8
F8-T4
T4-T6
T6-O2
FP1-F7
F7-T3
T3-T5
T5-O1
ECG
100 µV
1 second

I • 16 Reactivity of the mu rhythm in an adult

Context

52-year-old woman with right temporal lobe epilepsy.

What to note

The eyes are open with eyelids movement artifacts on the frontopolar derivations. A mu rhythm with predominance on the right fronto-central region can be observed. The patient is asked to clench her left fist. A muscular contraction can be seen on the left hand EMG lead. The mu rhythm disappears.

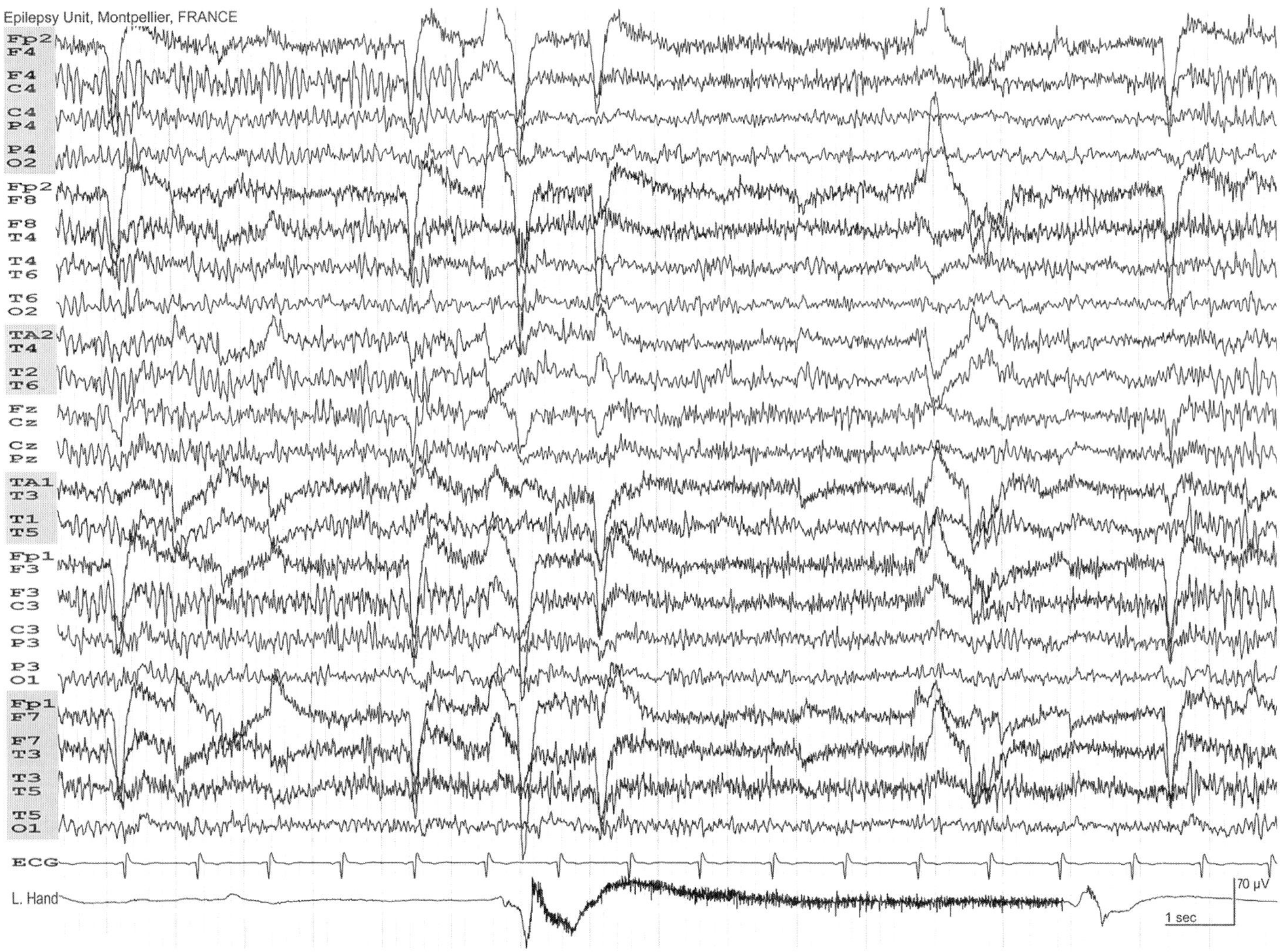

Figure a / Recording at 15 mm/s. Mu rhythm reappears at the end of the plate when the patient is asked to stop clenching.

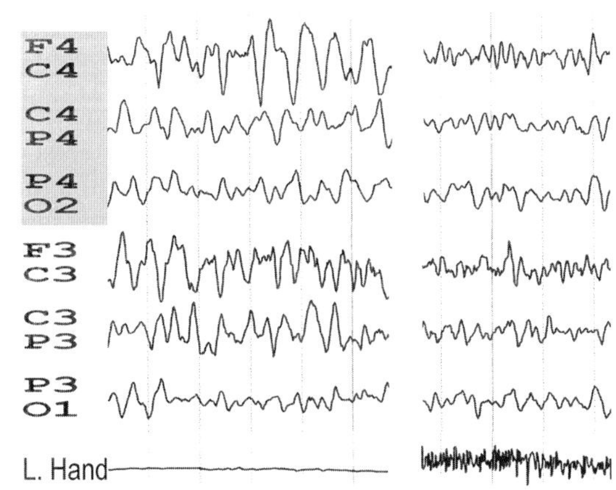

Figure b / Reactivity of mu rhythm upon contraction of the left hand.

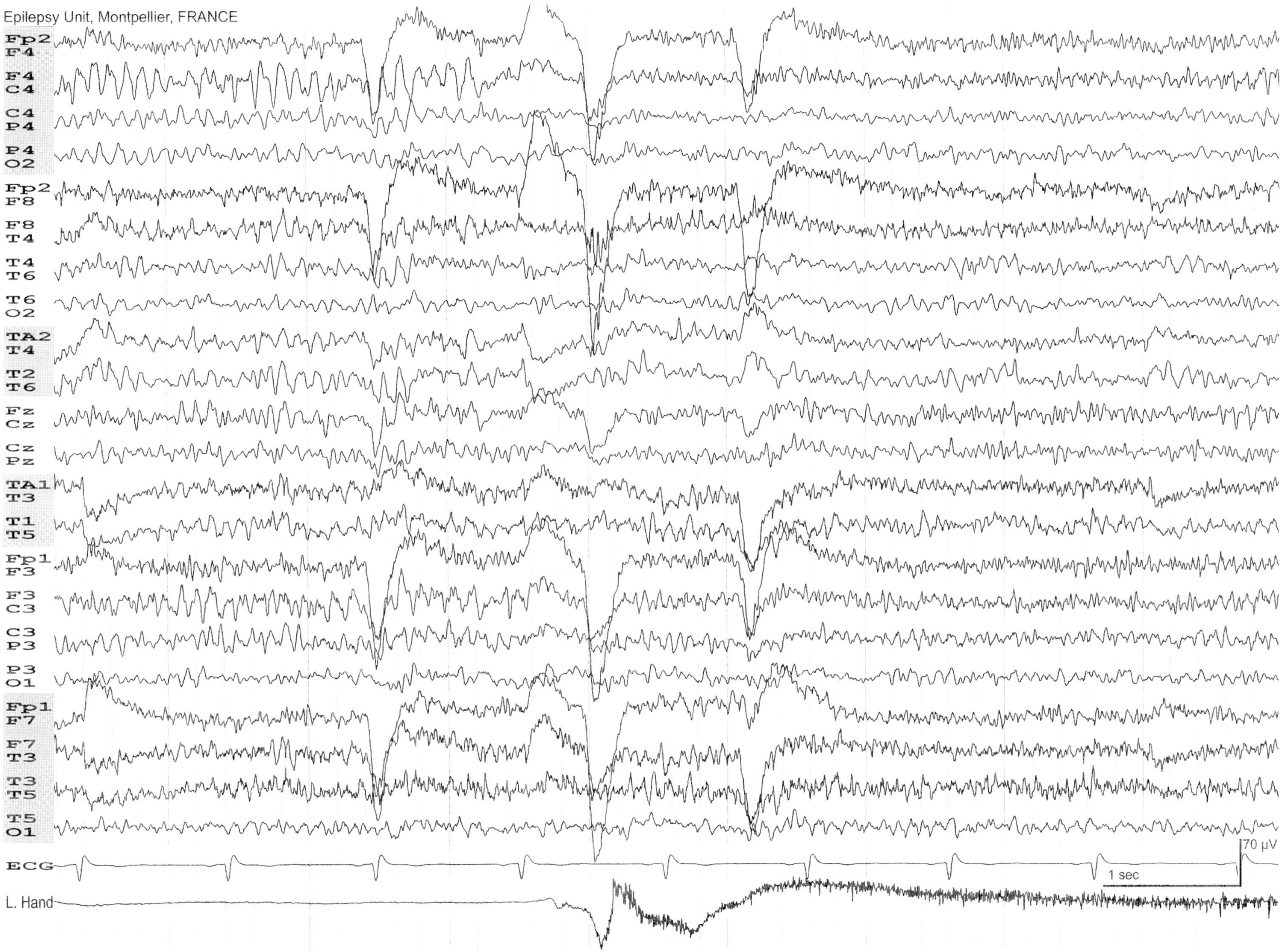
Epilepsy Unit, Montpellier, FRANCE
Fp2 F4
F4 C4
C4 P4
P4 O2
Fp2 F8
F8 T4
T4 T6
T6 O2
TA2 T4
T2 T6
Fz Cz
Cz Pz
TA1 T3
T1 T5
Fp1 F3
F3 C3
C3 P3
P3 O1
Fp1 F7
F7 T3
T3 T5
T5 O1
ECG
L. Hand
70 µV
1 sec

I • 17 Posterior mu rhythm in an adult

Context
EEG of 18-year-old woman with confusional arousals.

What to note
The patient's eyes are open. Bilateral mu rhythm with predominance on the vertex region. Frequency is at 8 Hz. Interestingly, the topographic distribution is not limited to the central region and spreads to the parietal regions. To test reactivity of the mu rhythm, it would have been necessary to have the patient move her feet due to its localization near the vertex.

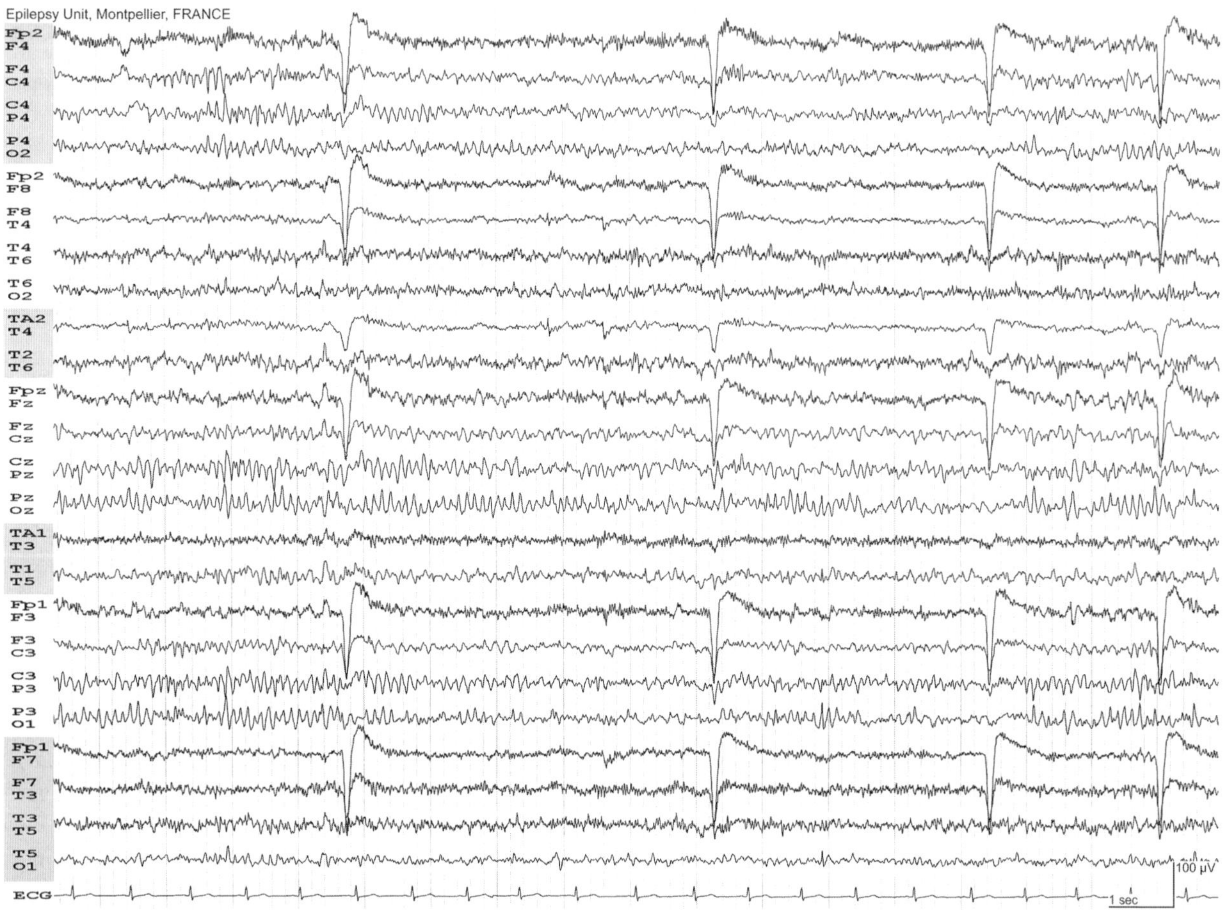

Figure a / Recording at 15 mm/s. Mu rhythm. Eyelid movement artifacts on the fronto-polar derivations.

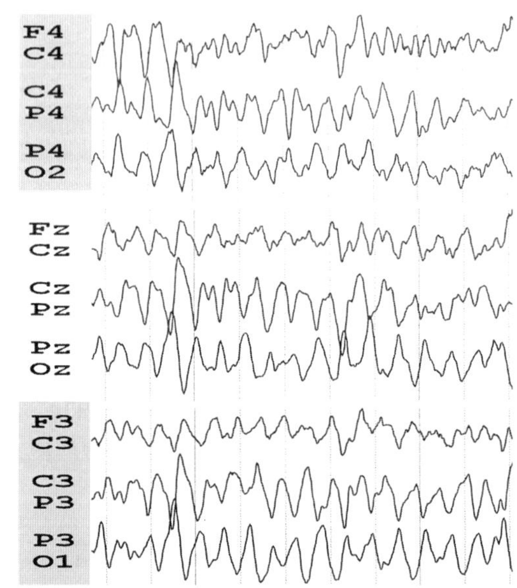

Figure b / Bilateral mu rhythm with parietal predominance.

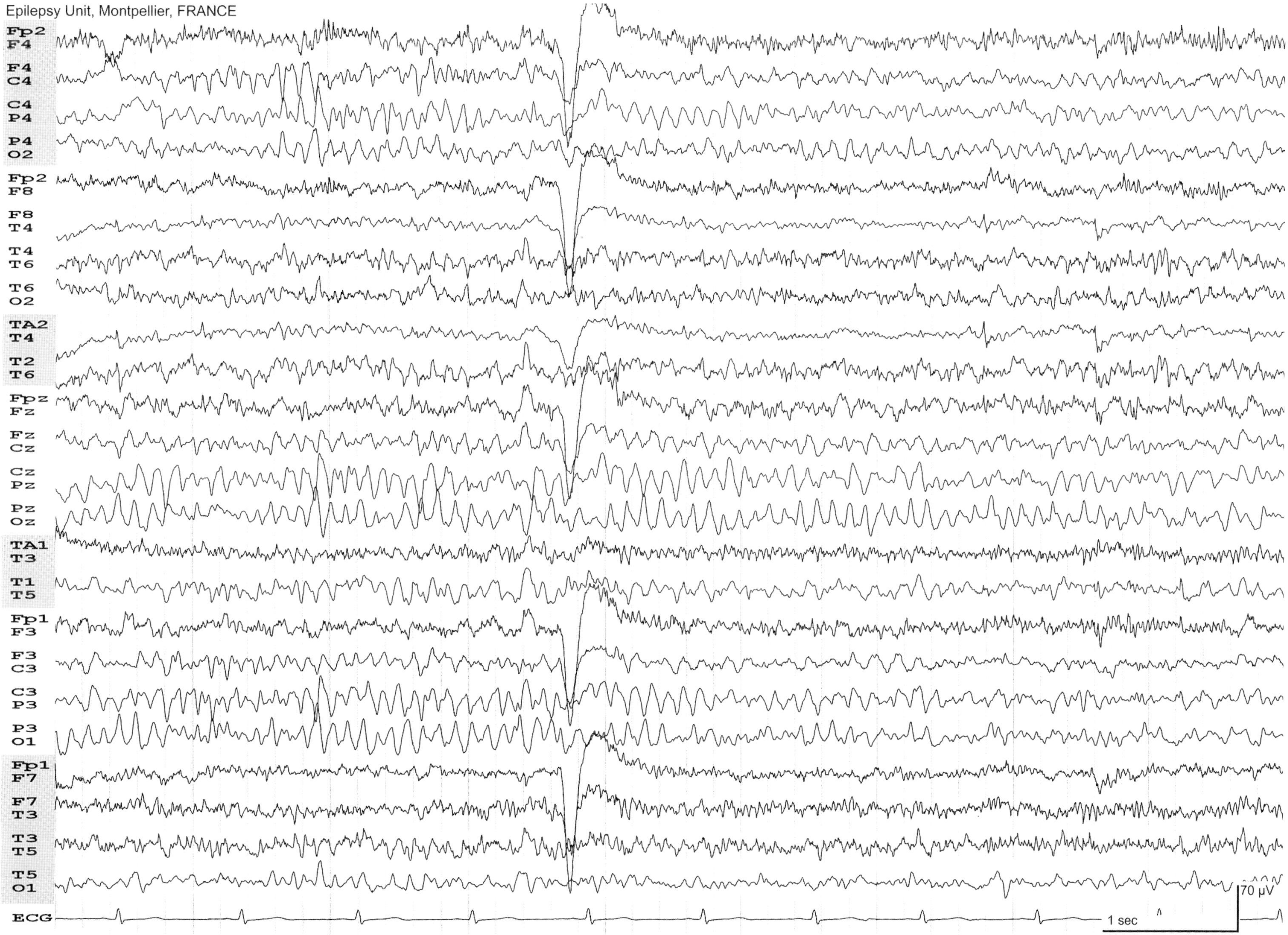
Epilepsy Unit, Montpellier, FRANCE
Fp2 F4
F4 C4
C4 P4
P4 O2
Fp2 F8
F8 T4
T4 T6
T6 O2
TA2 T4
T2 T6
Fpz Fz
Fz Cz
Cz Pz
Pz Oz
TA1 T3
T1 T5
Fp1 F3
F3 C3
C3 P3
P3 O1
Fp1 F7
F7 T3
T3 T5
T5 O1
ECG
70 µV
1 sec

I • 18 Slow mu variant

Context

42-year-old woman, presurgical assessment for cryptogenic medial right temporal lobe epilepsy.

What to note

Background activity with an alpha rhythm (11 Hz) of slightly higher amplitude on the left side and a false impression of spread to the central regions. When she opens her eyes, a mu rhythm can be seen on the central and vertex regions. However, the mu rhythm on the vertex region does not present its usual arch-like shaped morphology. It is rather like a subharmonic mu rhythm.

Comment

To test reactivity of the mu rhythm, it would have been necessary to have the patient move her feet due to its localization near the vertex.

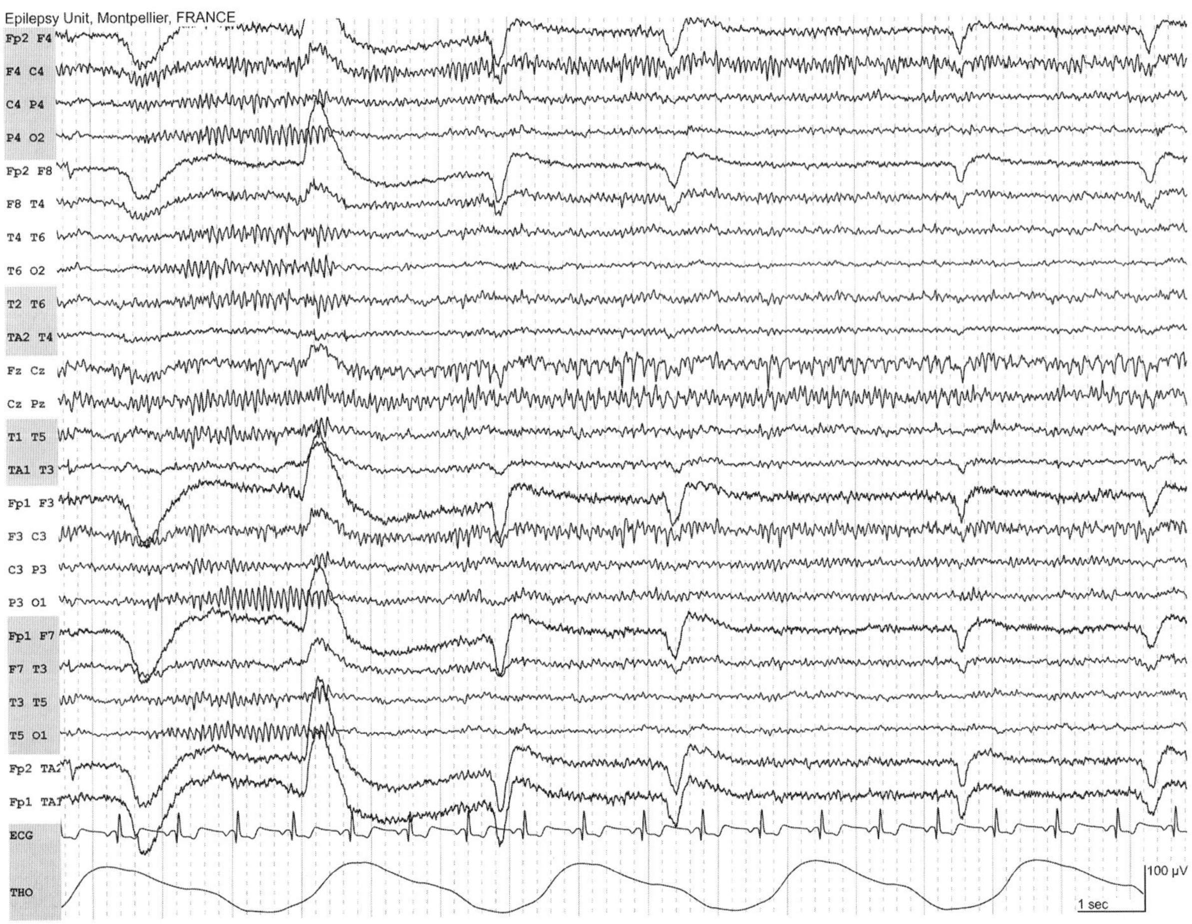

Figure a / Recording at 15 mm/s.

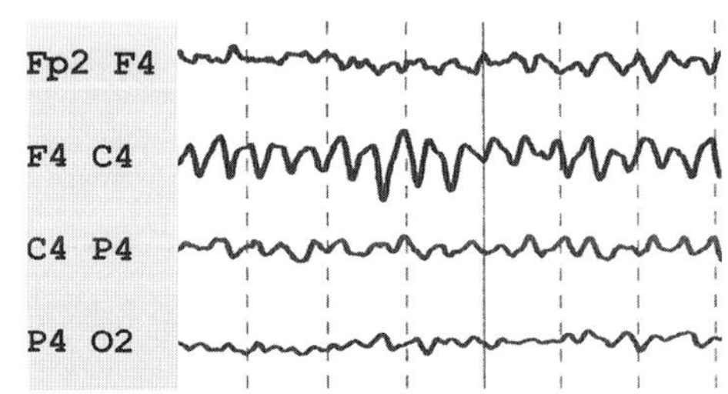

Figure b / Mu rhythm on the right central region.

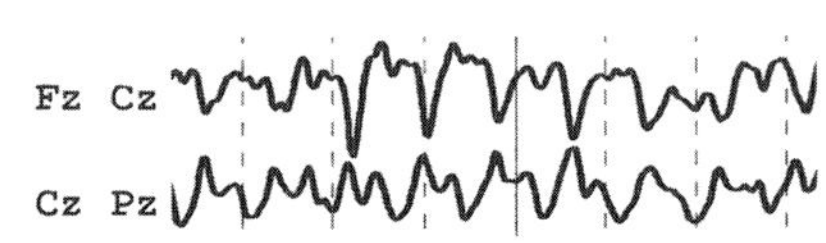

Figure c / Mu rhythm: subharmonic pattern on the vertex.

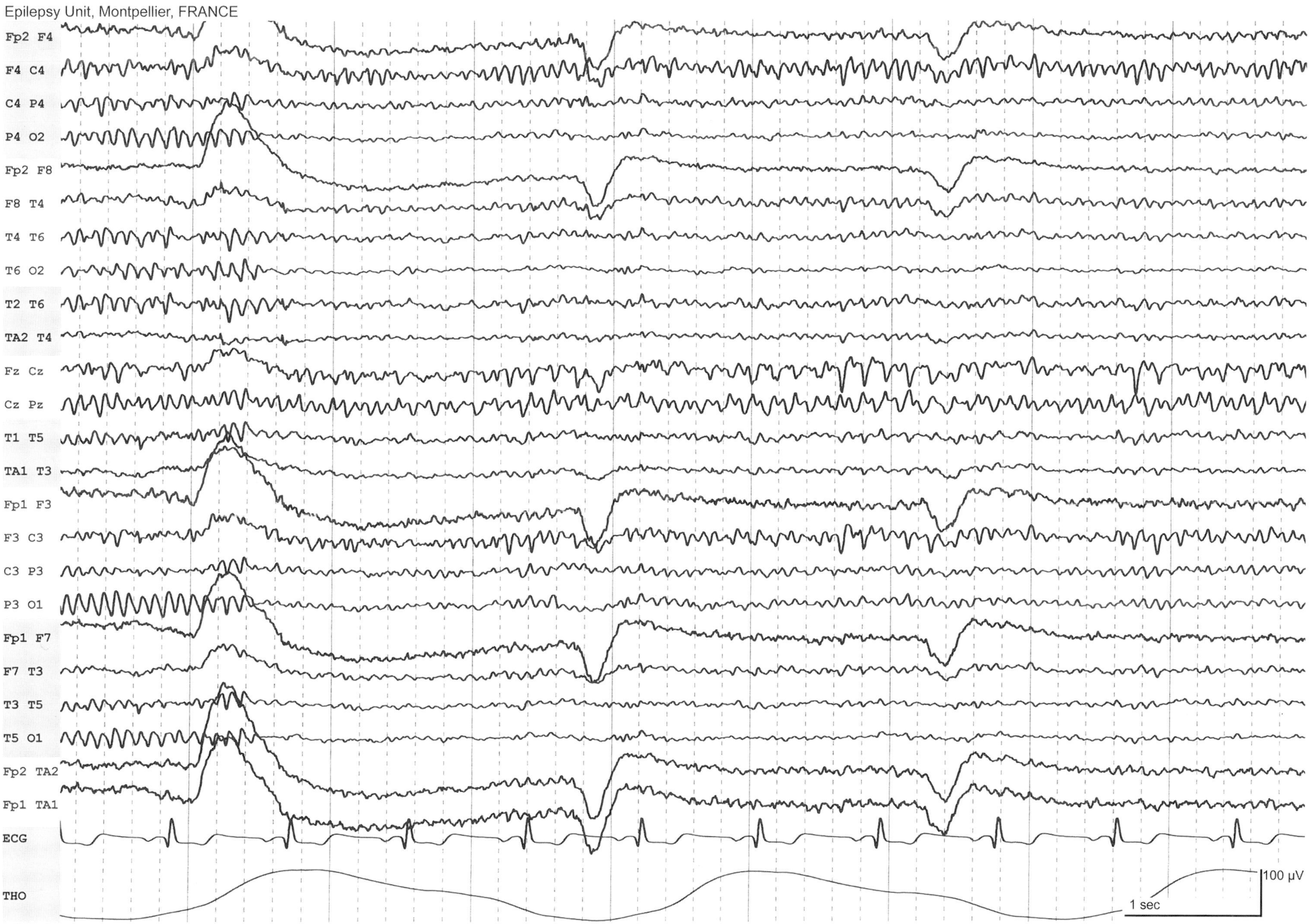
Epilepsy Unit, Montpellier, FRANCE
Fp2 F4
F4 C4
C4 P4
P4 O2
Fp2 F8
F8 T4
T4 T6
T6 O2
T2 T6
TA2 T4
Fz Cz
Cz Pz
T1 T5
TA1 T3
Fp1 F3
F3 C3
C3 P3
P3 O1
Fp1 F7
F7 T3
T3 T5
T5 O1
Fp2 TA2
Fp1 TA1
ECG
THO
100 µV
1 sec

I • 19 Lambda waves in an adult

Context

27-year-old woman with cryptogenic left temporo-parieto-occipital junction epilepsy. Same patient as plates III-47 and III-50.

What to note

The patient's eyes are open. There are eyelid movement artifacts. Some clearly sharp waves can be seen on the occipital regions. These are typical lambda waves, which are physiological. On the frontal-polar derivations and on the left temporal region, the fast low-amplitude activity corresponds to muscle activity.

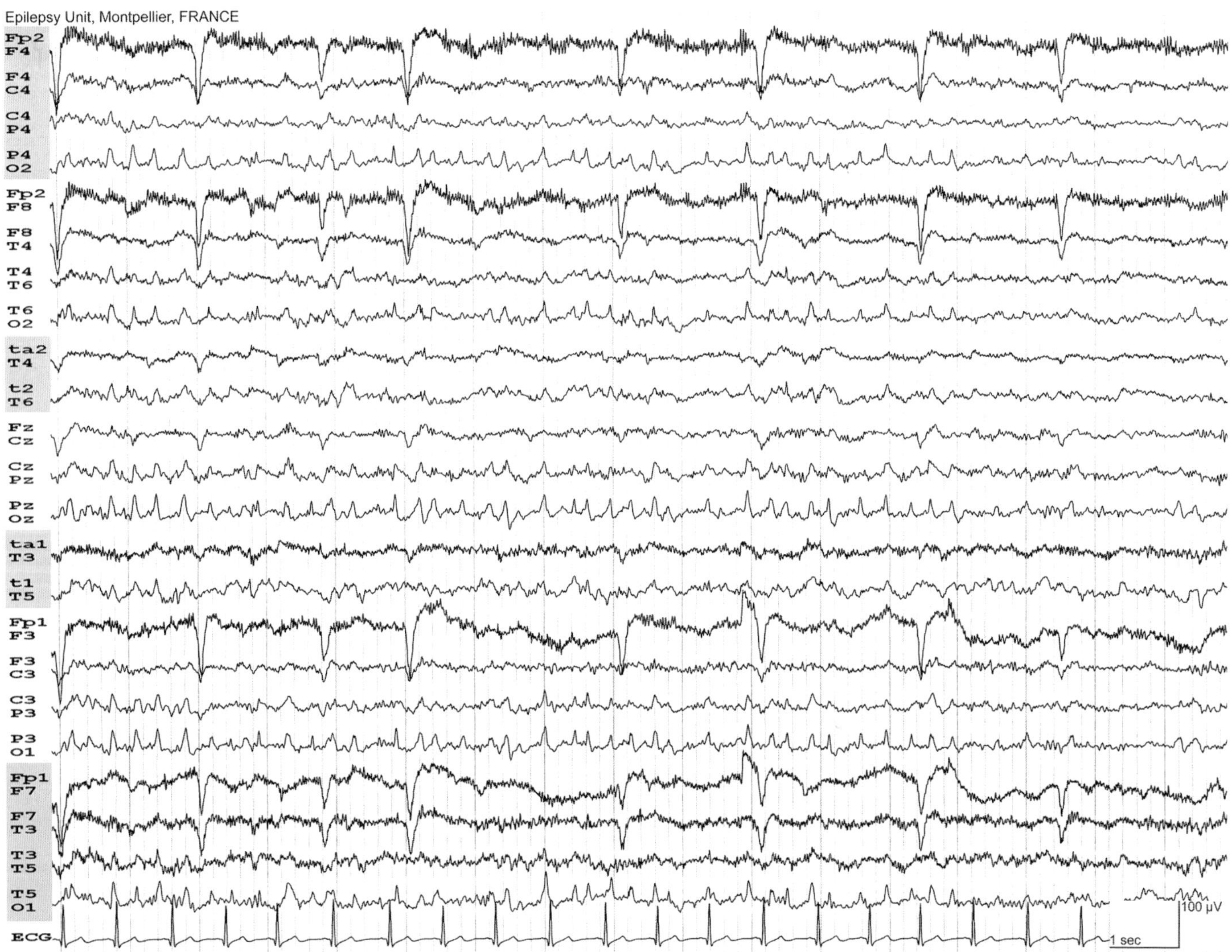

Figure a / Recording at 15 mm/s.

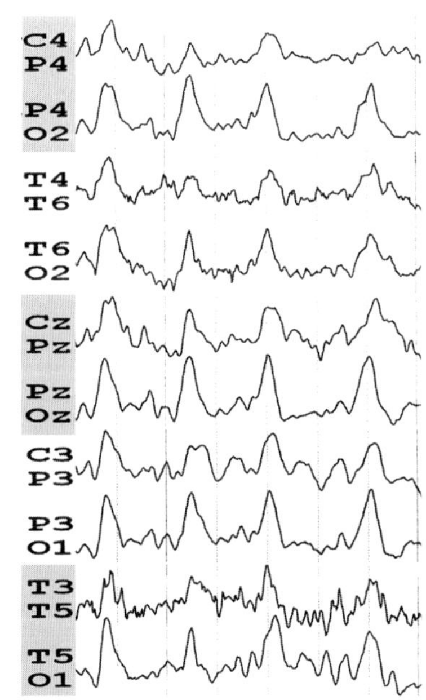

Figure b / Lambda waves on the occipital regions.

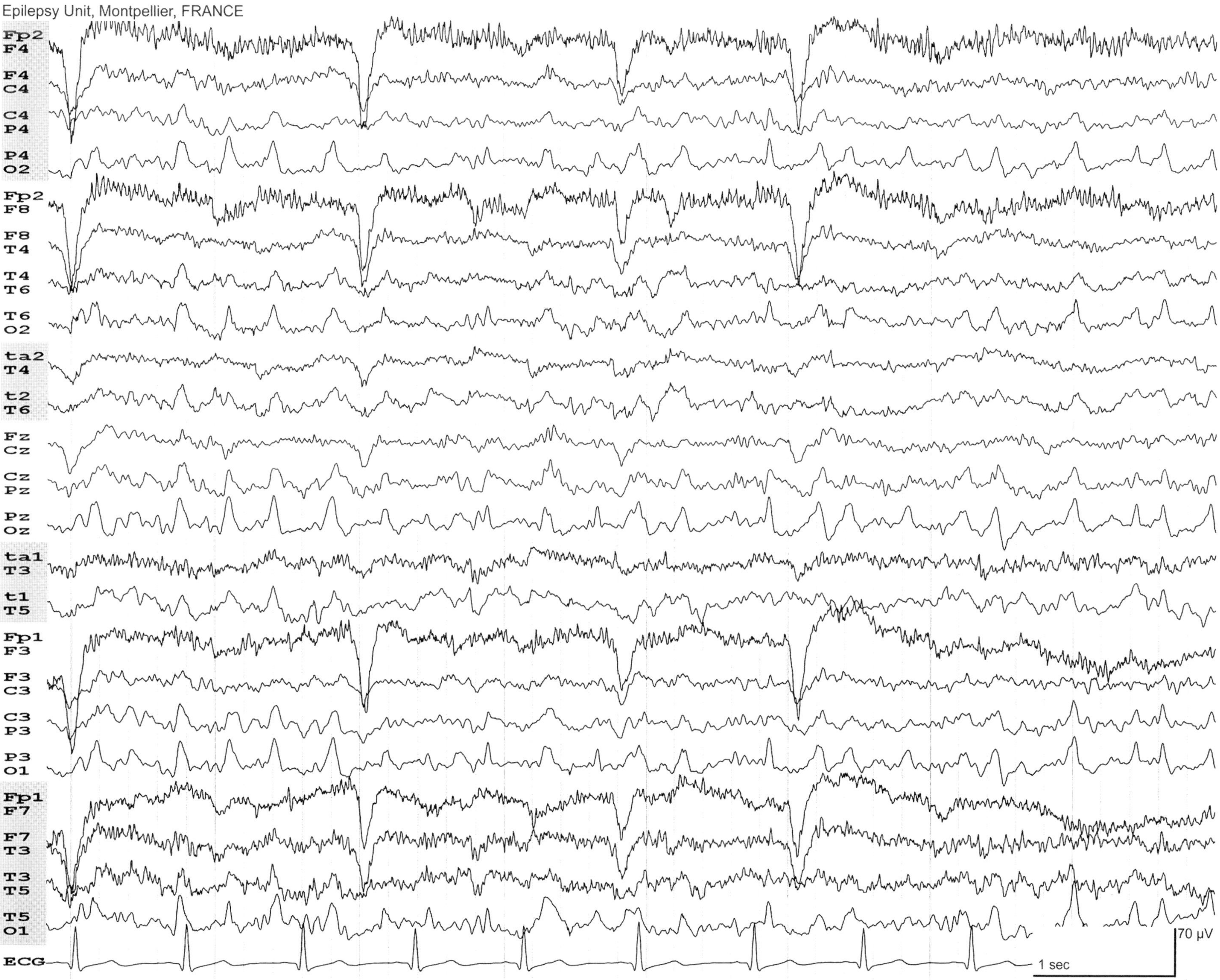
Epilepsy Unit, Montpellier, FRANCE
Fp2 F4
F4 C4
C4 P4
P4 O2
Fp2 F8
F8 T4
T4 T6
T6 O2
ta2 T4
t2 T6
Fz Cz
Cz Pz
Pz Oz
ta1 T3
t1 T5
Fp1 F3
F3 C3
C3 P3
P3 O1
Fp1 F7
F7 T3
T3 T5
T5 O1
ECG
70 µV
1 sec

I • 20 Lambda waves in an adult which disappear with point fixation and paradoxical alpha

Context

24-year-old woman with juvenile myoclonic epilepsy.

What to note

During the first 4 seconds, the patient is reading with presence of saccadic eye movements (upward and downward deflections). There are also over the frontal anterior regions (phase reversal at F8 and F7) fast potentials corresponding to contraction of the lateral rectus muscle. This muscle artifact is termed lateral rectus spike. Some clearly diphasic sharp waves can be seen on the posterior regions. These are lambda waves of unusually high amplitude. The patient is then asked to stare at a letter (eyelid artifact). The lambda waves disappear. A brief burst of alpha rhythm at 12 Hz over the occipital regions can be seen that corresponds to paradoxical alpha rhythm. The fixation that normally blocks the alpha produced in this patient a transient quiet wakefulness. Note the presence of muscle activity on the temporal and fronto-polar derivations.

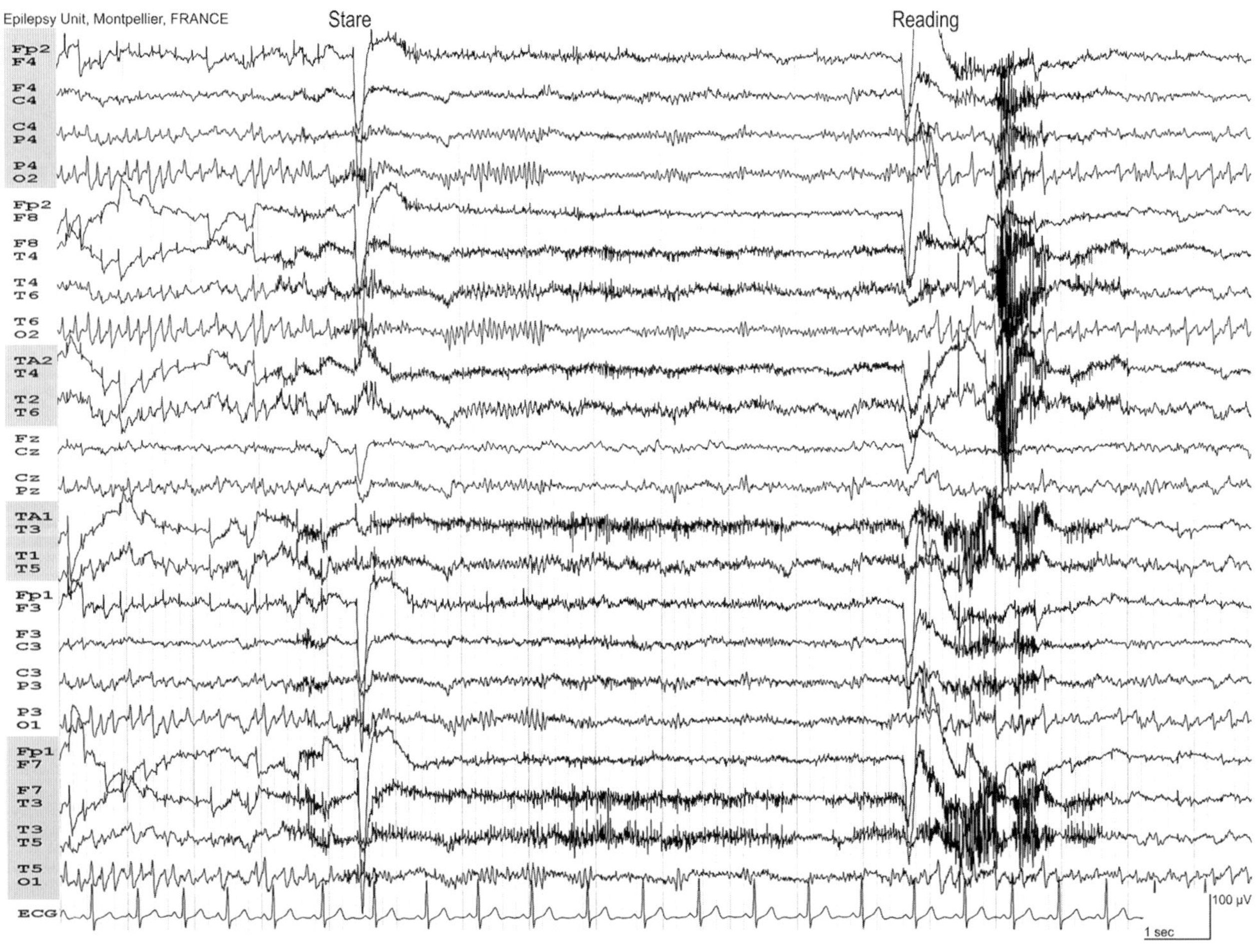

Figure a / Recording at 15 mm/s. Note the recurrence of lambda waves when the patient is asked to read again.

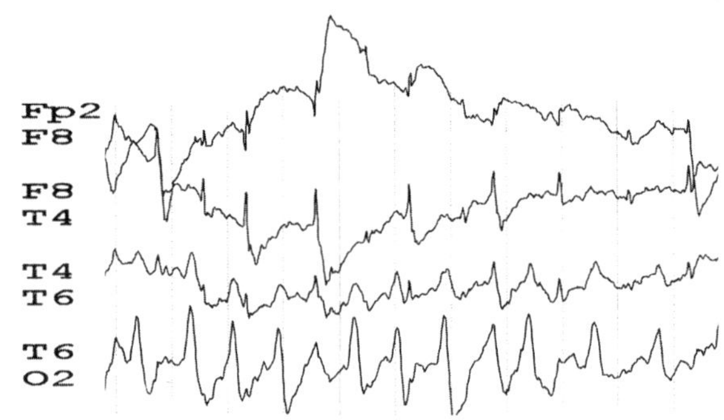

Figure b / Lambda waves at T6-O2. Saccadic eye movements with rectus lateral spikes at F8.

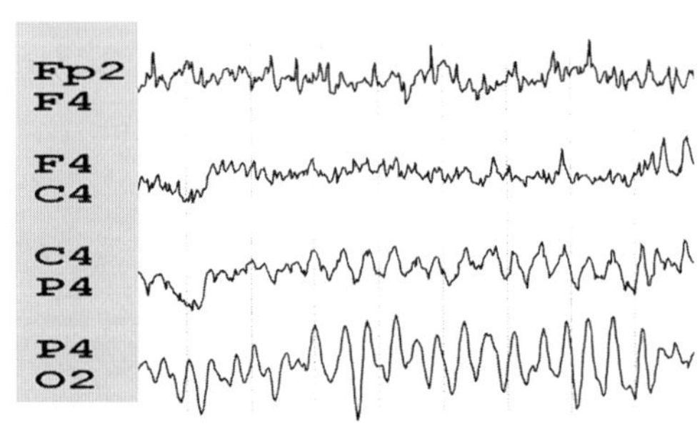

Figure c / Alpha rhythm at 12 Hz at P4-O2. Muscular activities on the frontal derivations.

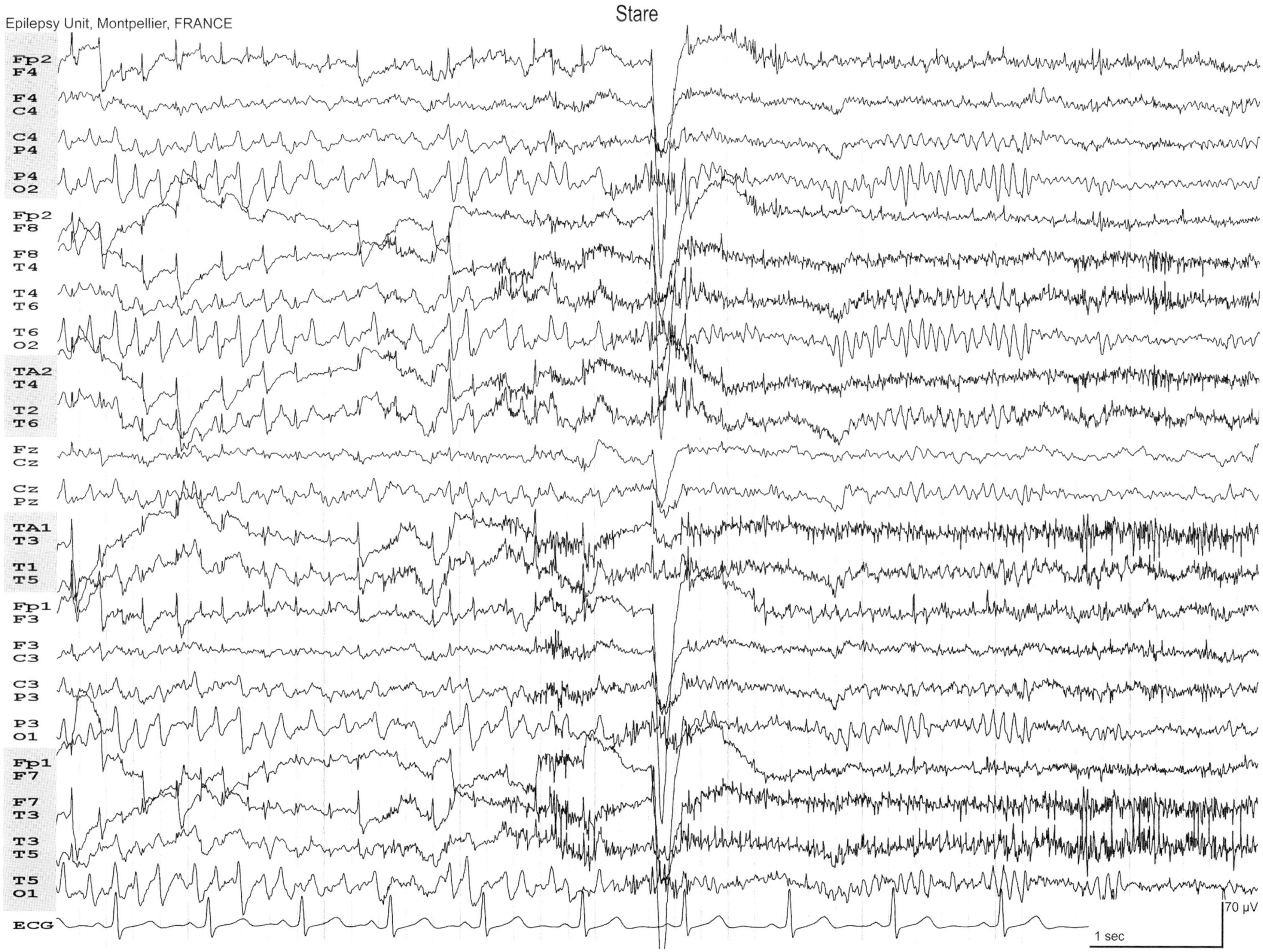
Epilepsy Unit, Montpellier, FRANCE
Stare
Fp2 F4
F4 C4
C4 P4
P4 O2
Fp2 F8
F8 T4
T4 T6
T6 O2
TA2 T4
T2 T6
Fz Cz
Cz Pz
TA1 T3
T1 T5
Fp1 F3
F3 C3
C3 P3
P3 O1
Fp1 F7
F7 T3
T3 T5
T5 O1
ECG
70 µV
1 sec

I • 21 Lambda waves in an adult which disappear with point fixation

Context

37-year-old woman, presurgical assessment for right mesial temporal lobe epilepsy.

What to note

The patient's eyes are open throughout the recording. During the first 4 seconds, the patient is reading. Theta activity with low amplitude, subcontinuous and slightly sharp-contoured waves can be observed on the occipital derivations. The patient is then asked to stare at a letter, and eyelid movement artifacts appear at the fronto-polar derivations. The theta activity disappears as soon as she begins to stare at the letter. Note the unusual theta-like and sub-continuous wave morphology.

Comment

Lambda waves can be observed during reading activities, they disappear when the person stares at a point.

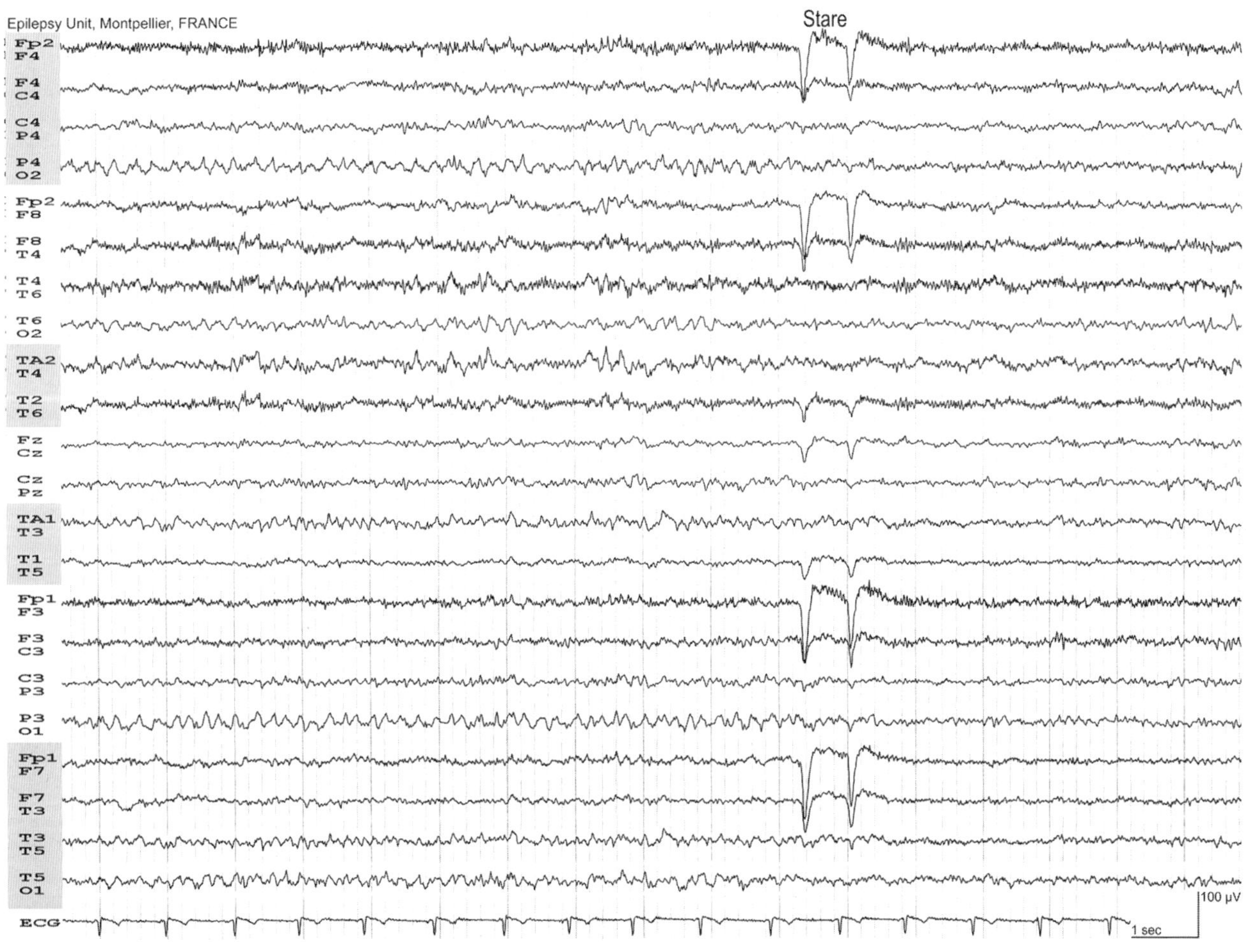

Figure a / Recording at 15 mm/s. Subcontinuous theta activity on the occipital derivations.

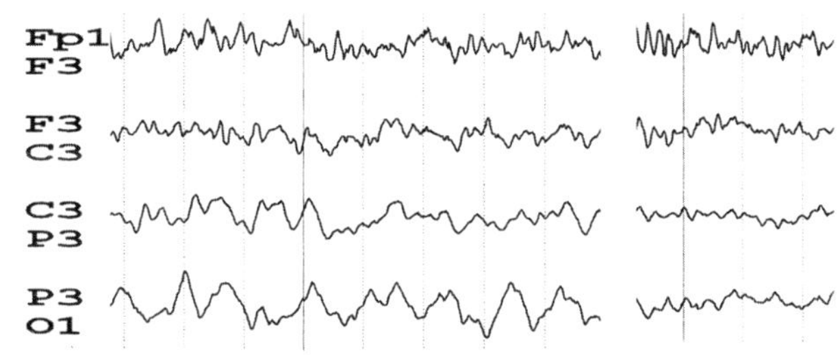

Figure b / Sub-continuous theta-like lambda waves on P3-O1 (first segment). When the patient is asked to stare at a point, the lambda waves disappear (second segment).

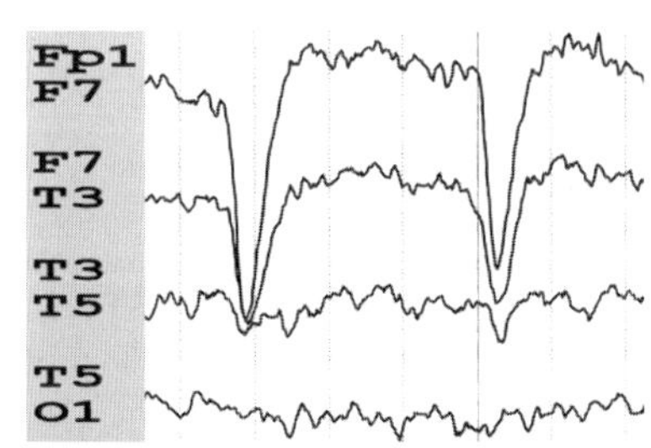

Figure c / Eyelid movement artifacts at Fp1-F7.

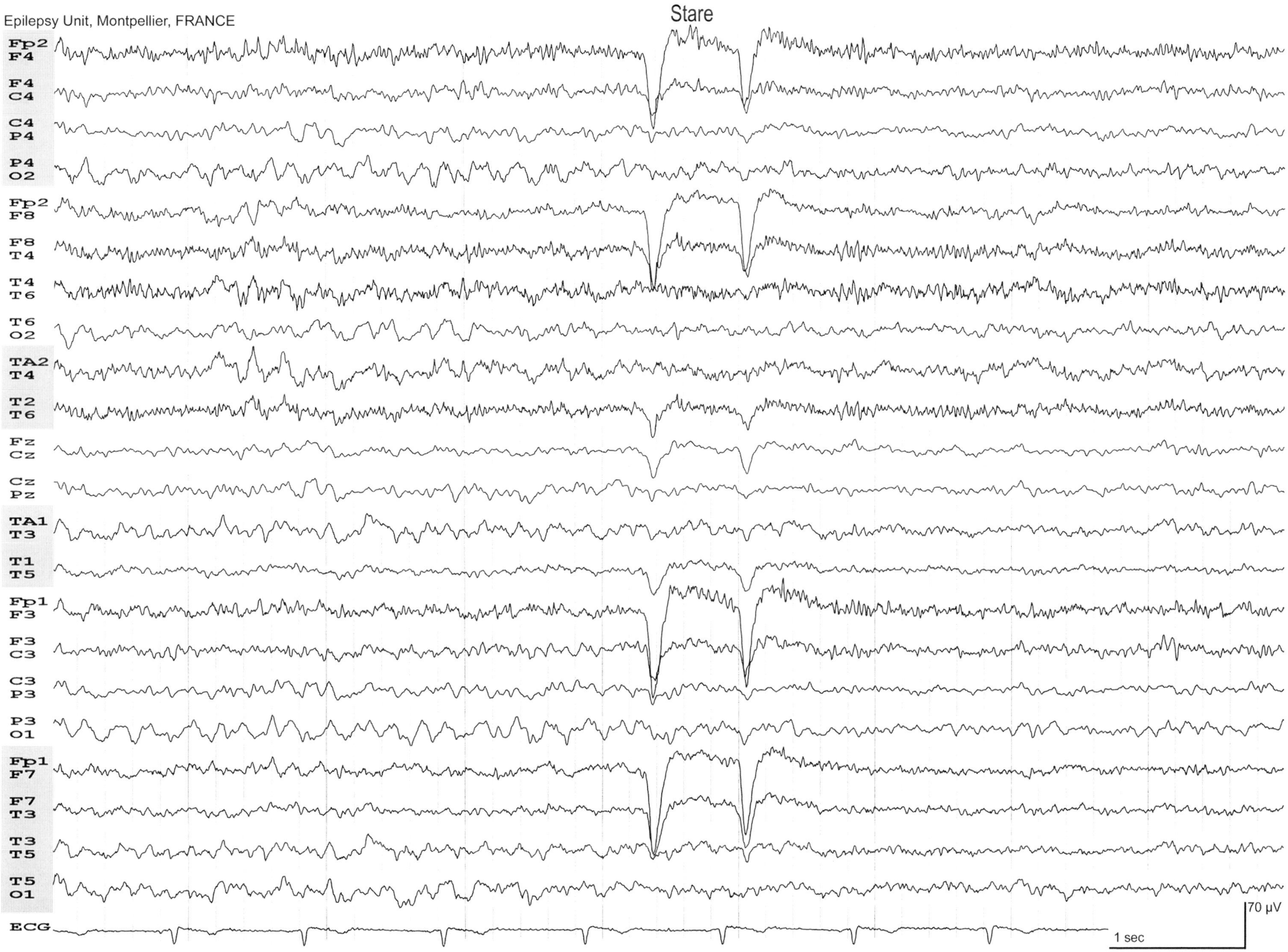
Epilepsy Unit, Montpellier, FRANCE
Stare
Fp2 F4
F4 C4
C4 P4
P4 O2
Fp2 F8
F8 T4
T4 T6
T6 O2
TA2 T4
T2 T6
Fz Cz
Cz Pz
TA1 T3
T1 T5
Fp1 F3
F3 C3
C3 P3
P3 O1
Fp1 F7
F7 T3
T3 T5
T5 O1
ECG
70 µV
1 sec

I • 22 Midline theta rhythm (Cigánek rhythm) (1)

Context

18-year-old woman with confusional arousals. Same patient as plate I-17.

What to note

The patient's eyes are open. Theta waves can be observed in phase reversal under Fz. They spread to the left and right frontal regions. The frequency is around 6 Hz. These waveforms correspond to midline theta rhythm.

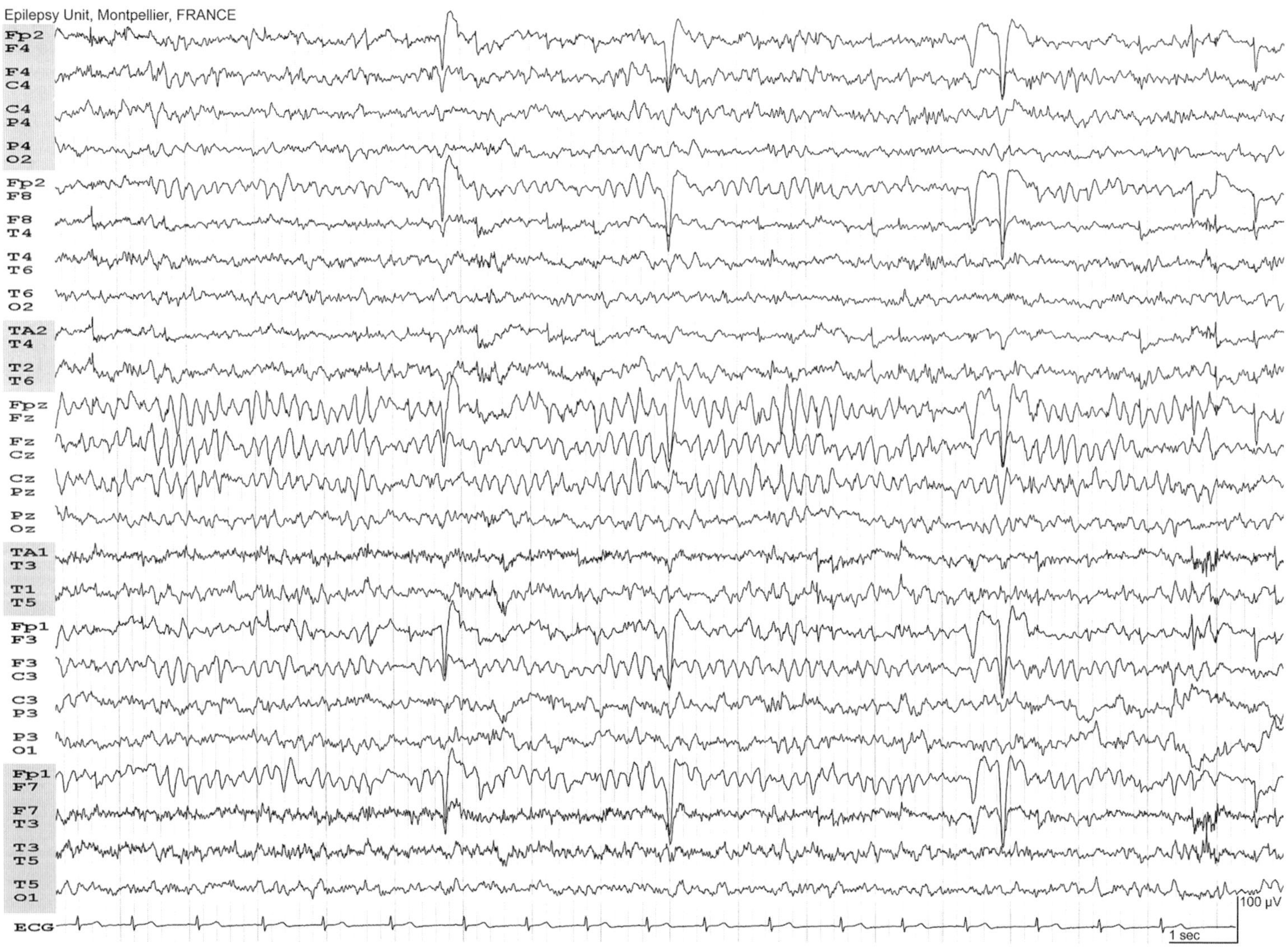

Figure a / Recording at 15 mm/s.

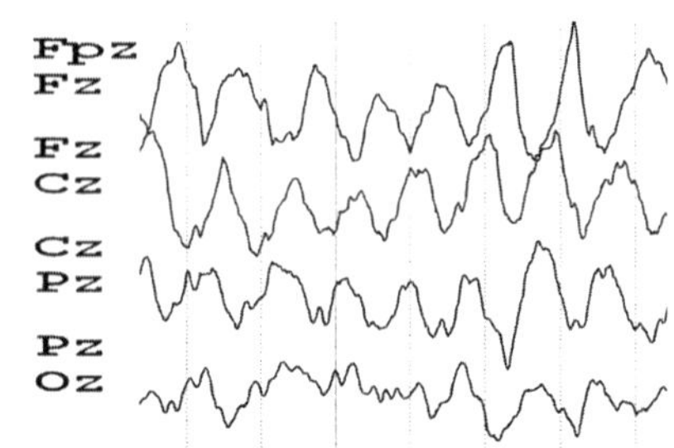

Figure b / Midline theta rhythm.

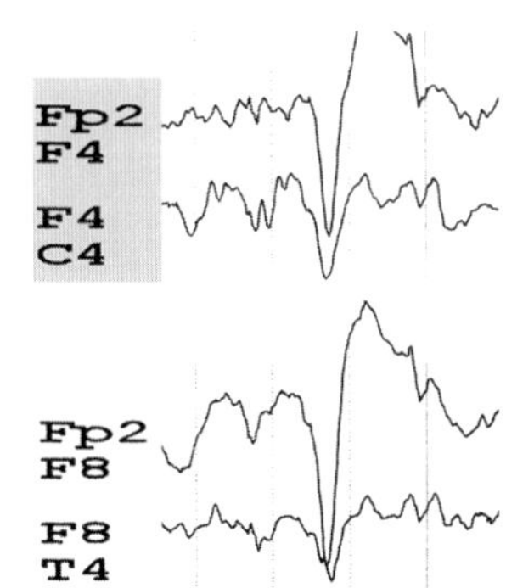

Figure c / Eyelid movement artifact.

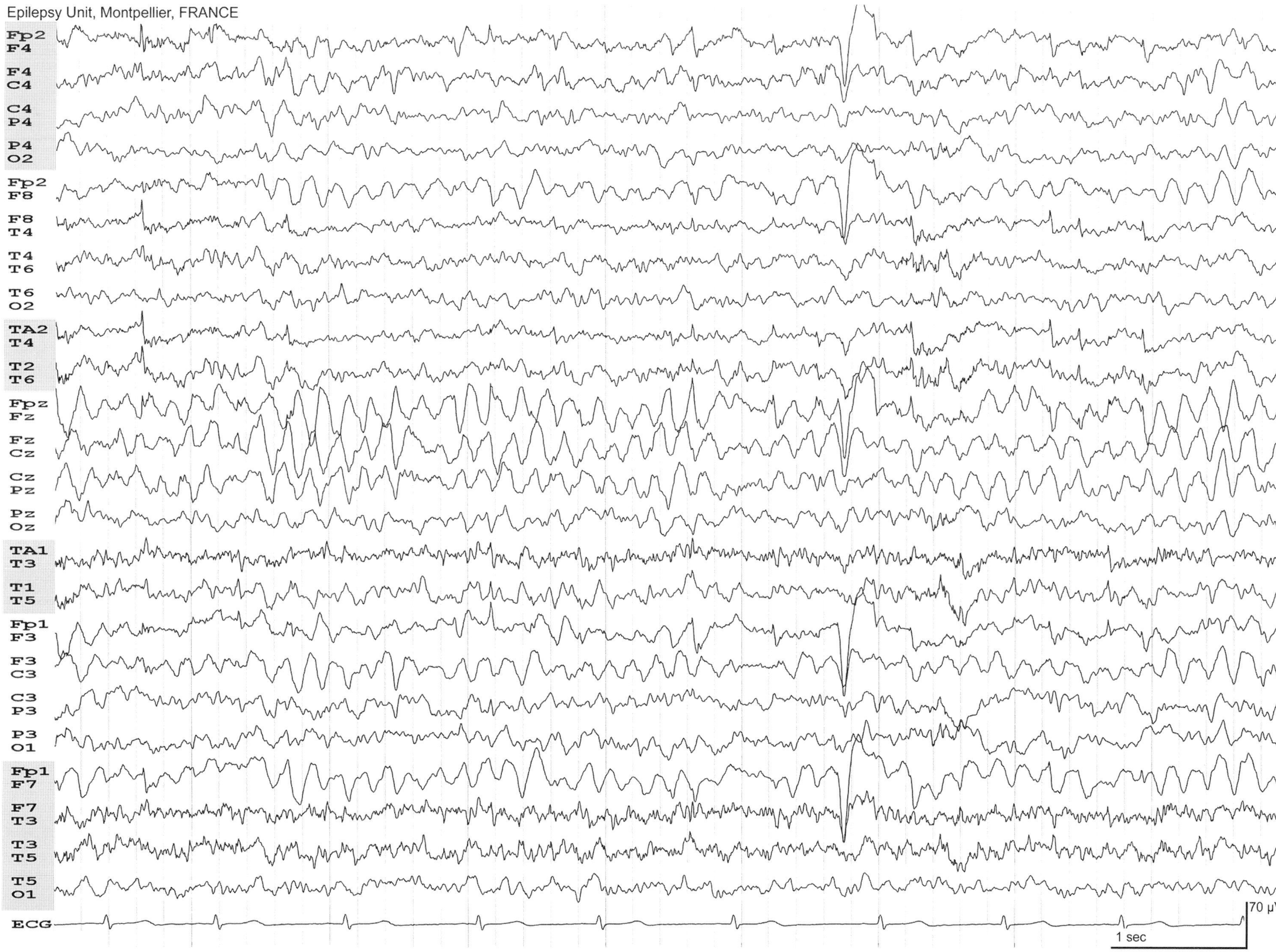
Epilepsy Unit, Montpellier, FRANCE
Fp2 F4
F4 C4
C4 P4
P4 O2
Fp2 F8
F8 T4
T4 T6
T6 O2
TA2 T4
T2 T6
Fpz Fz
Fz Cz
Cz Pz
Pz Oz
TA1 T3
T1 T5
Fp1 F3
F3 C3
C3 P3
P3 O1
Fp1 F7
F7 T3
T3 T5
T5 O1
ECG
70 µV
1 sec

• 23 Midline theta rhythm (Cigánek rhythm) (2)

Context

33-year-old woman with parietal lobe epilepsy.

What to note

The patient's eyes are open. Subcontinuous monomorphic theta activity at 6-7 Hz at Cz.

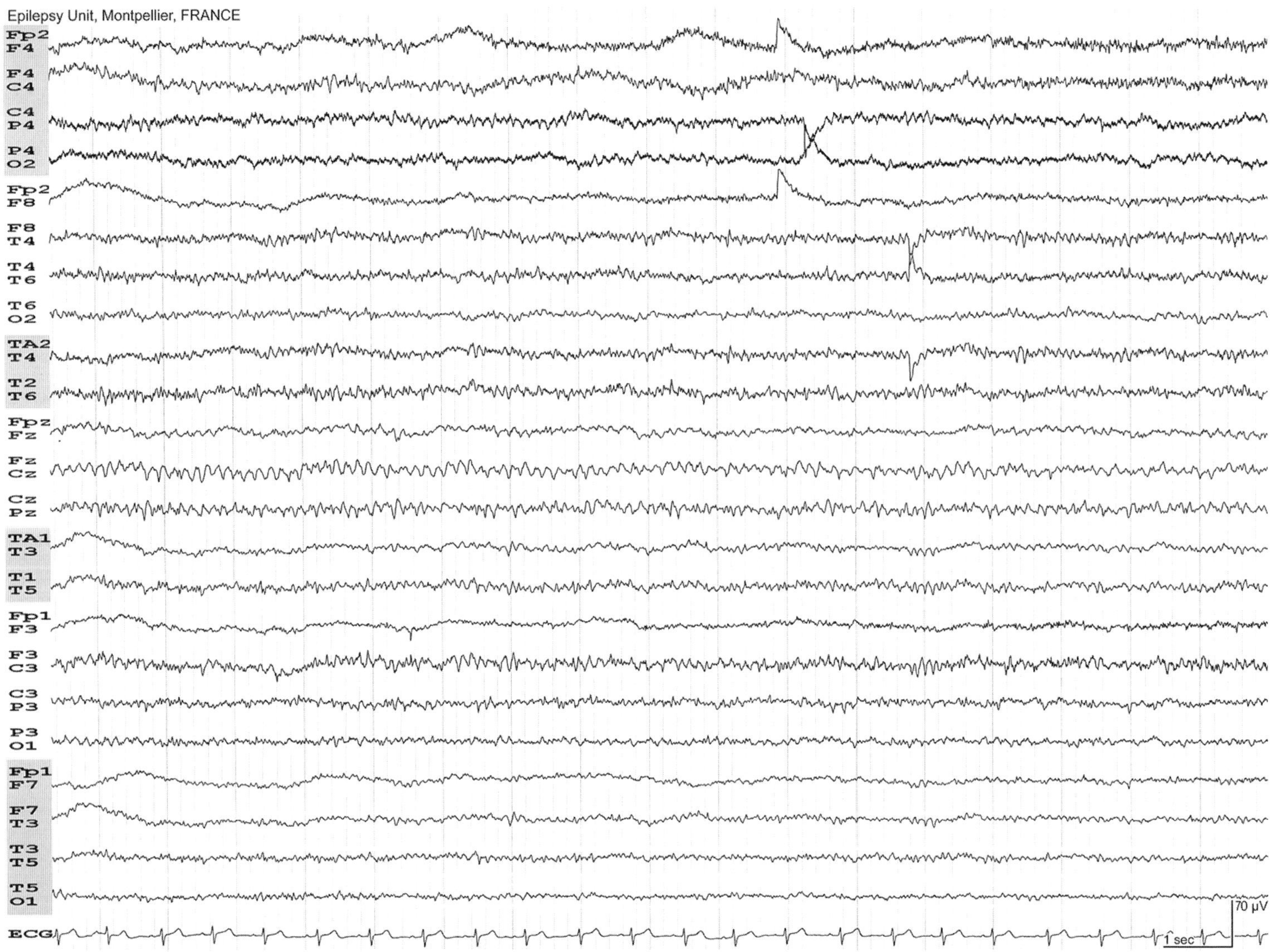

Figure a / Recording at 15 mm/s. Note electrode pop artifacts at Fp2, P4 and T4.

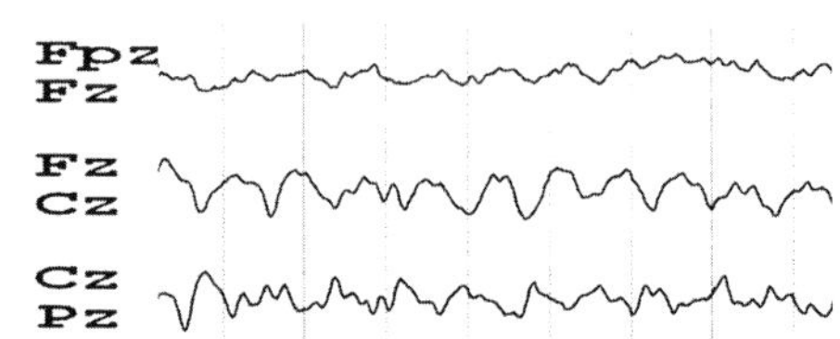

Figure b / Midline theta rhythm at 6 to 7 Hz.

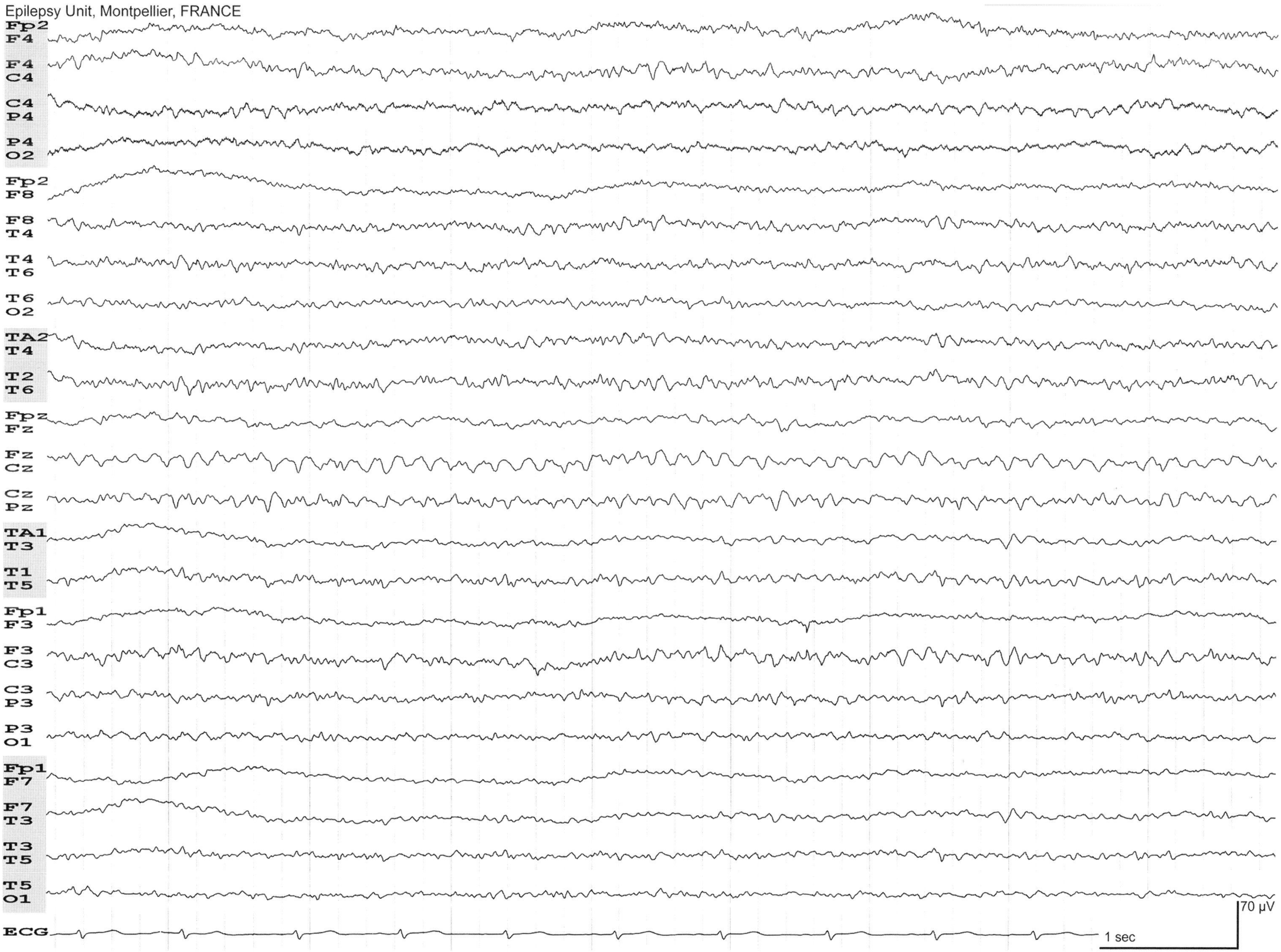
Epilepsy Unit, Montpellier, FRANCE
Fp2 F4
F4 C4
C4 P4
P4 O2
Fp2 F8
F8 T4
T4 T6
T6 O2
TA2 T4
T2 T6
Fpz Fz
Fz Cz
Cz Pz
TA1 T3
T1 T5
Fp1 F3
F3 C3
C3 P3
P3 O1
Fp1 F7
F7 T3
T3 T5
T5 O1
ECG
70 µV
1 sec

I • 24 Subclinical Rhythmic Electrographic Discharges in Adults (SREDA) (1)

Context

55-year-old man with a history of transient ischemic attack and auricular fibrillation.

What to note

The patient's eyes are closed. Low-amplitude posterior background activity can be seen within the alpha frequency range. During hyperventilation, slow waves appear bilaterally on the mid and posterior regions at gradually shorter intervals until there is a continuous discharge. Amplitude is maximal from onset and it remains constant, throughout the following plate. SREDA are a non-pathological activity often observed in people with a past vascular history, and often occurring with hyperventilation or intermittent photic stimulation.

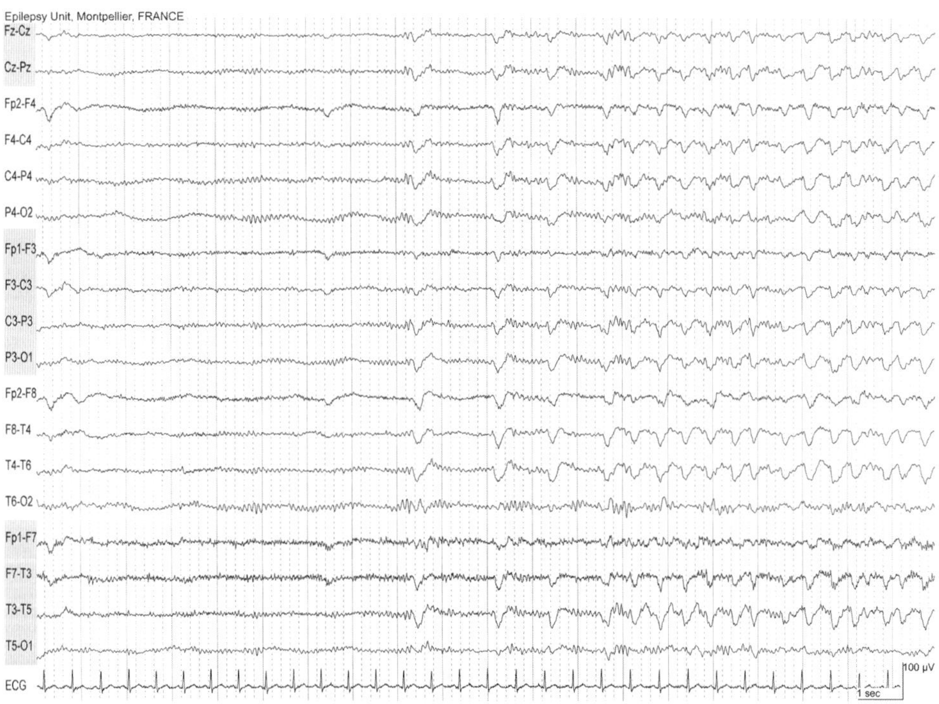

Figure a / Recording at 15 mm/s.

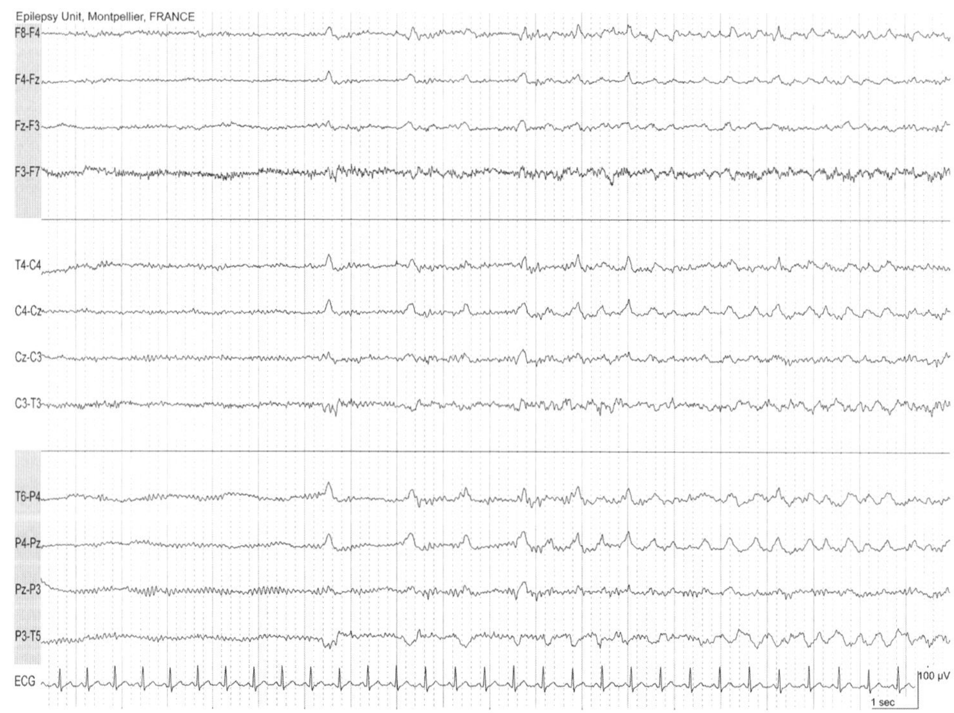

Figure b / Recording at 15 mm/s. Transverse montage of the same plate. Greater amplitude over the posterior regions with predominance on the right hemisphere.

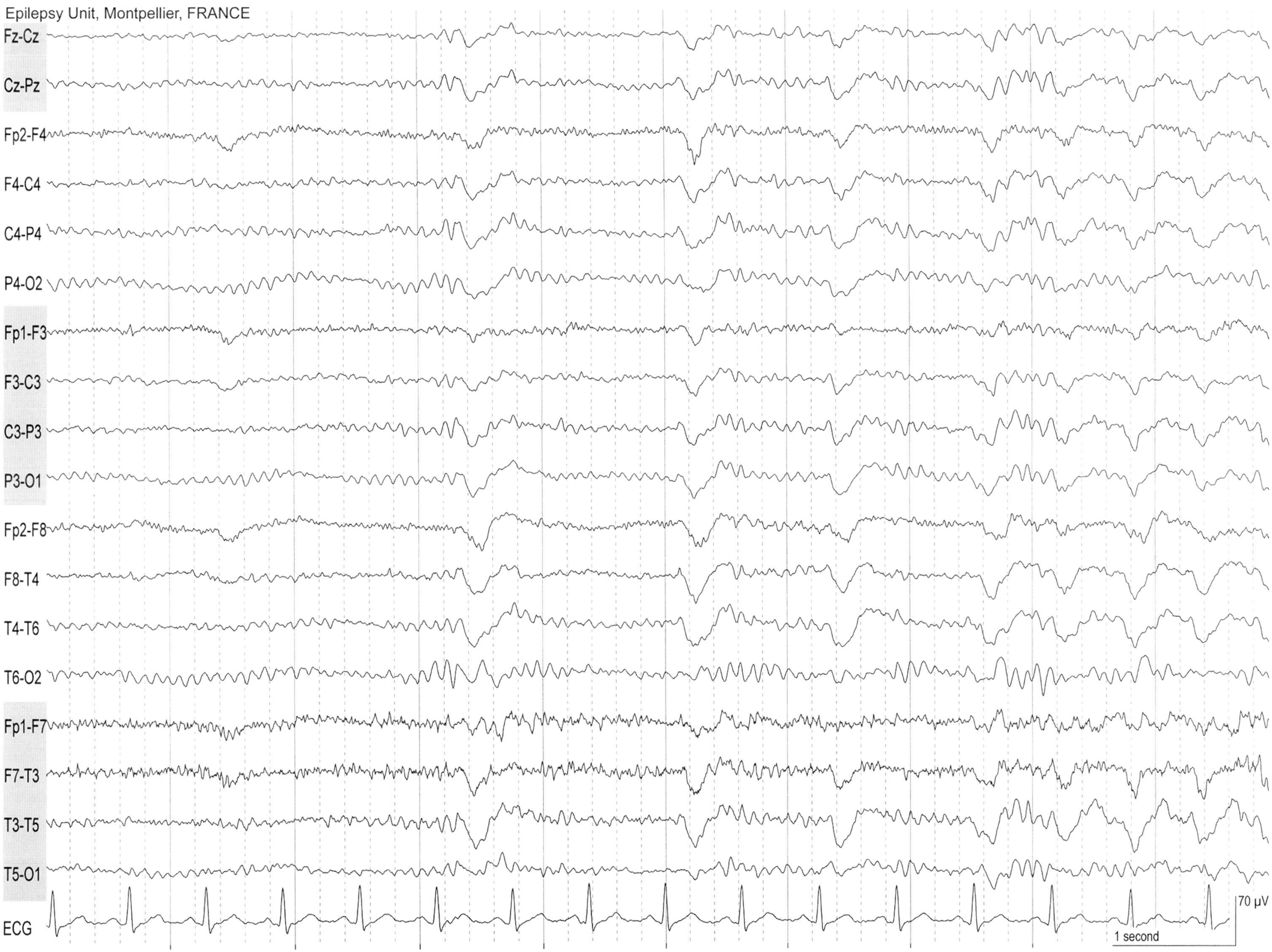
Epilepsy Unit, Montpellier, FRANCE
Fz-Cz
Cz-Pz
Fp2-F4
F4-C4
C4-P4
P4-O2
Fp1-F3
F3-C3
C3-P3
P3-O1
Fp2-F8
F8-T4
T4-T6
T6-O2
Fp1-F7
F7-T3
T3-T5
T5-O1
ECG
70 µV
1 second

• 25 Subclinical Rhythmic Electrographic Discharges in Adults (SREDA) (2)

Context

55-year-old man, same patient as on I-24, continued.

What to note

Continuation of identical monomorphic delta activity with constant amplitude. The activity stops progressively when hyperventilation is stopped (see plate at 15 mm/s).

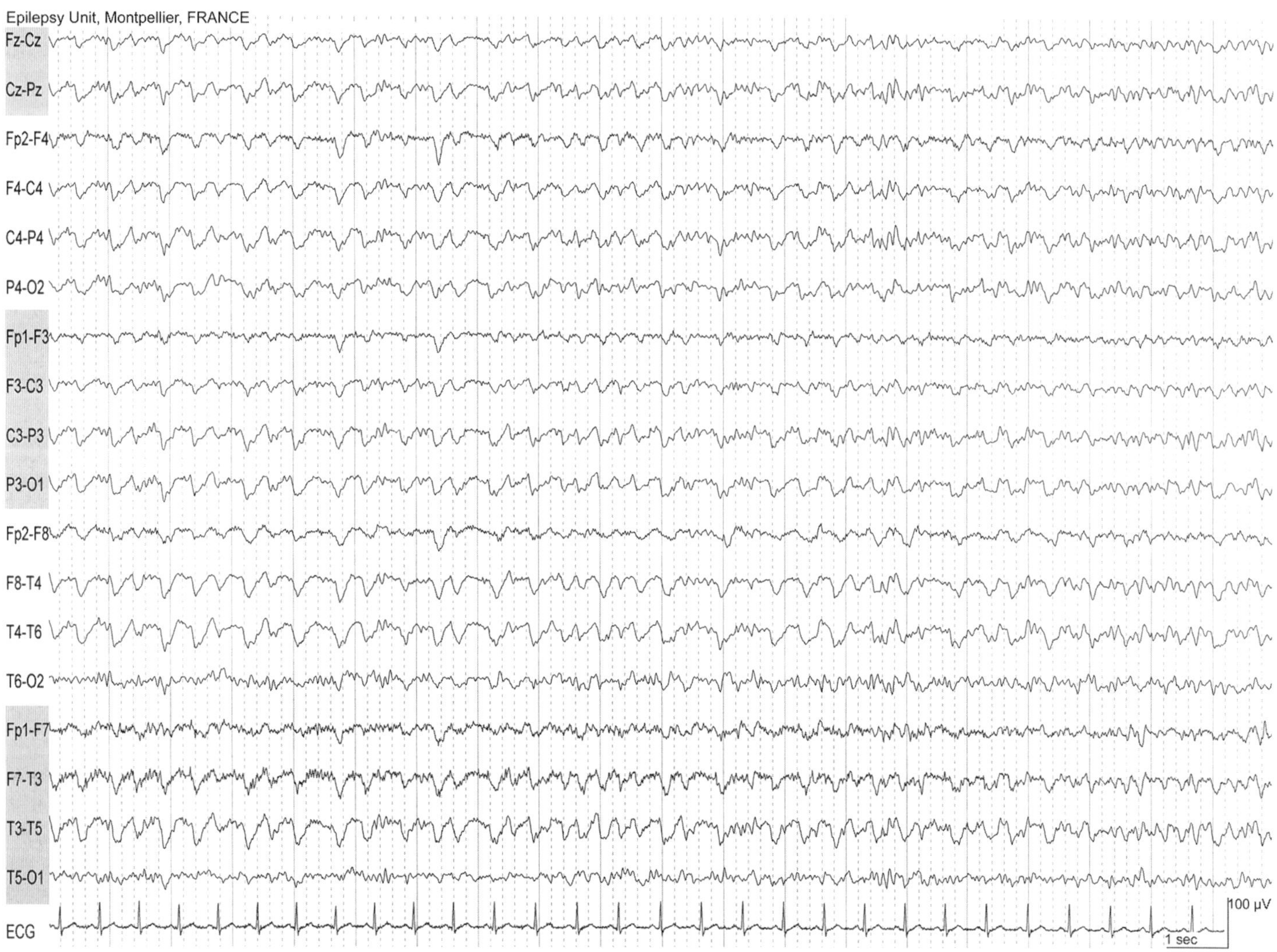

Figure a / Recording at 15 mm/s. The activity stops progressively when it is asked to stop hyperventilation.

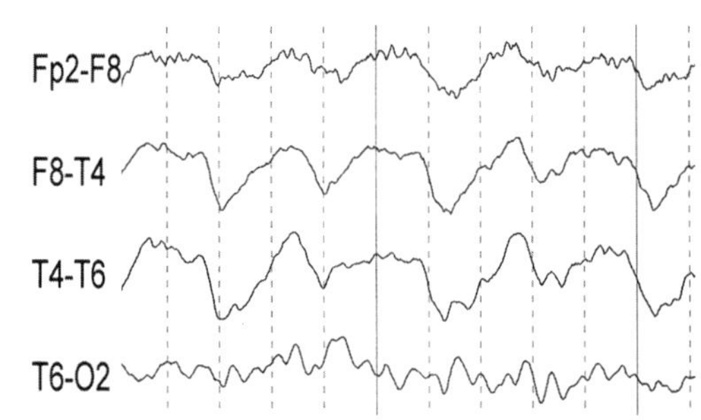

Figure b / Monomorphic slow activity and alpha rhythm at T6-O2.

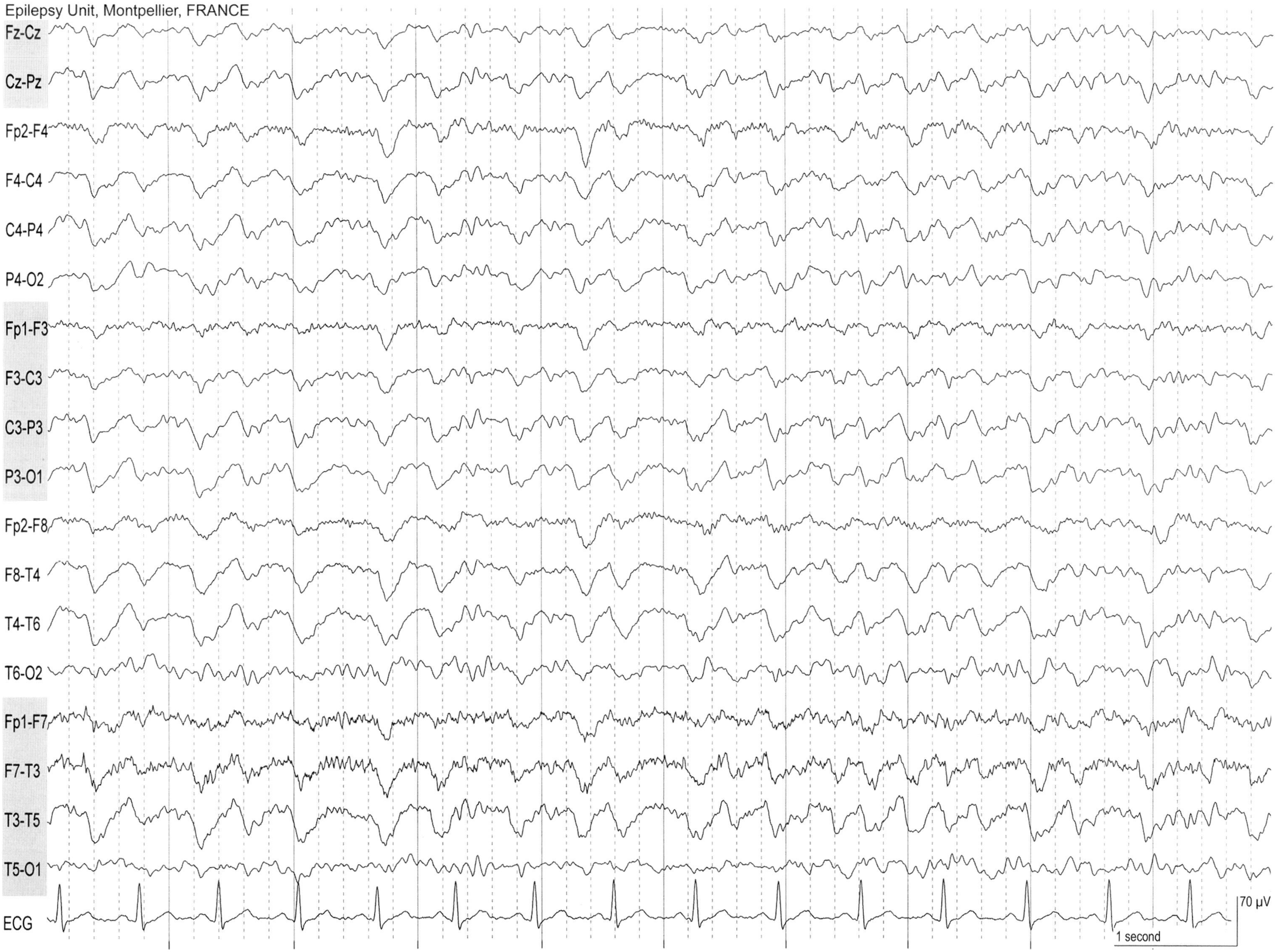
Epilepsy Unit, Montpellier, FRANCE
Fz-Cz
Cz-Pz
Fp2-F4
F4-C4
C4-P4
P4-O2
Fp1-F3
F3-C3
C3-P3
P3-O1
Fp2-F8
F8-T4
T4-T6
T6-O2
Fp1-F7
F7-T3
T3-T5
T5-O1
ECG
70 µV
1 second

I • 26 Subclinical Rhythmic Electrographic Discharges in Adults (SREDA) (3)

Context

39-year-old man referred after two episodes of loss of consciousness.

What to note

The patient's eyes are closed and he is relaxed. Slow waves appear on the right posterior temporal region followed by a delta frequency discharge on the right cento-parieto-temporal region followed by a theta discharge with predominance on the right hemisphere. Amplitude is maximal from onset and it remains constant.

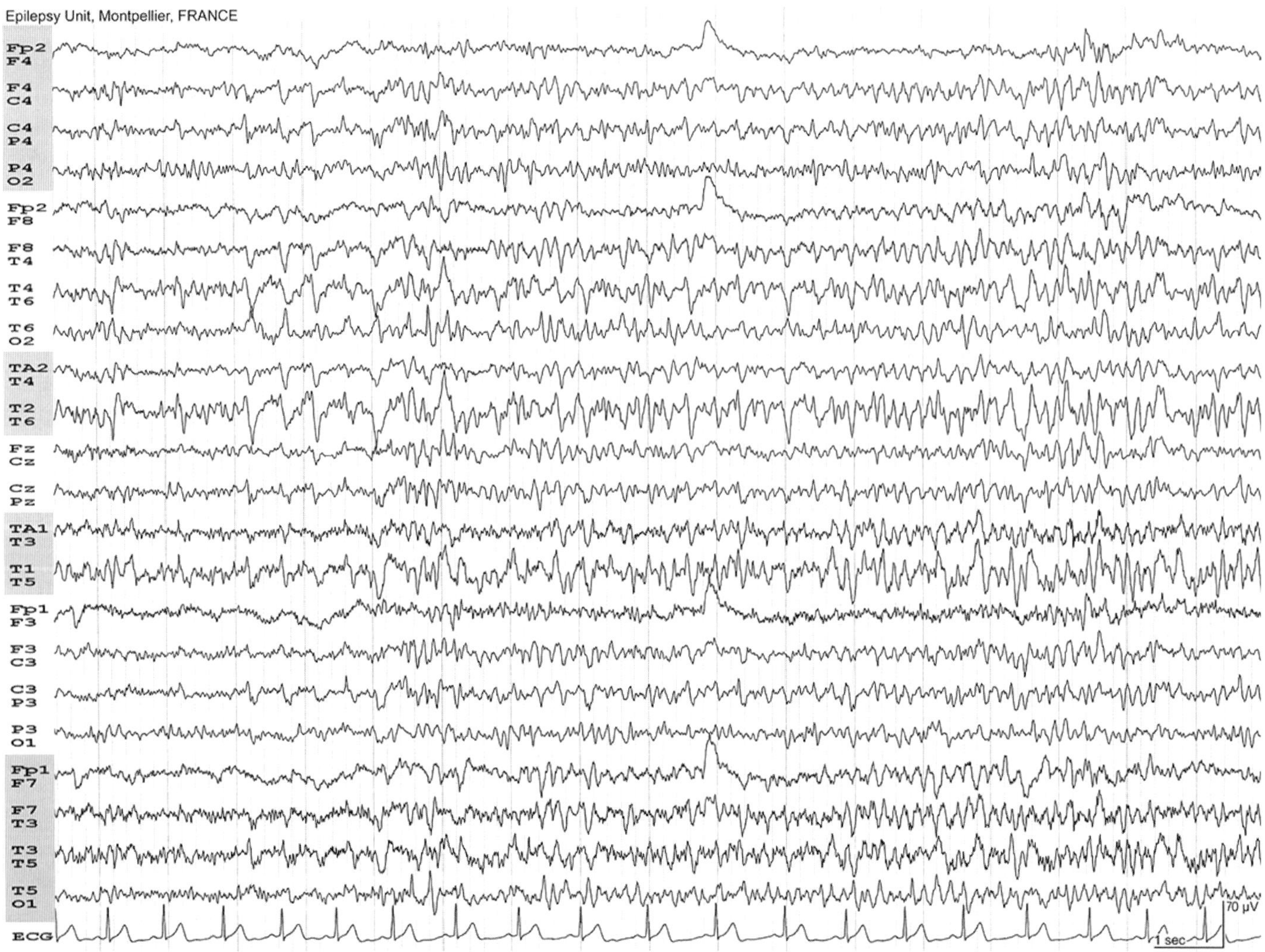

Figure a / Recording at 15 mm/s.

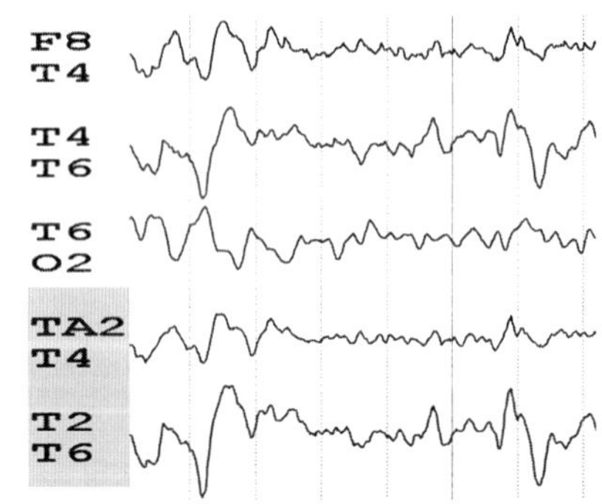

Figure b / Onset of SREDA.

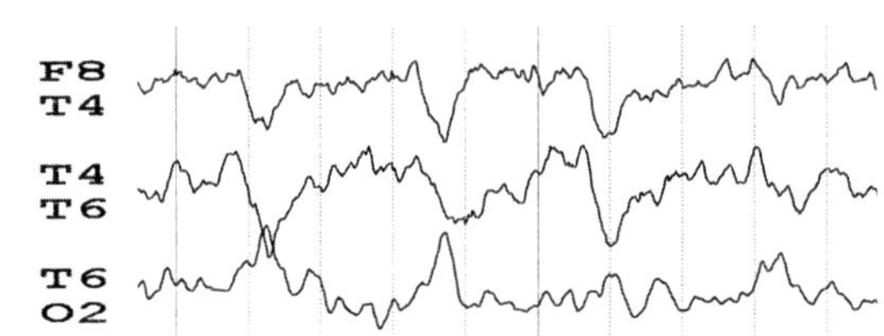

Figure c / Delta waves.

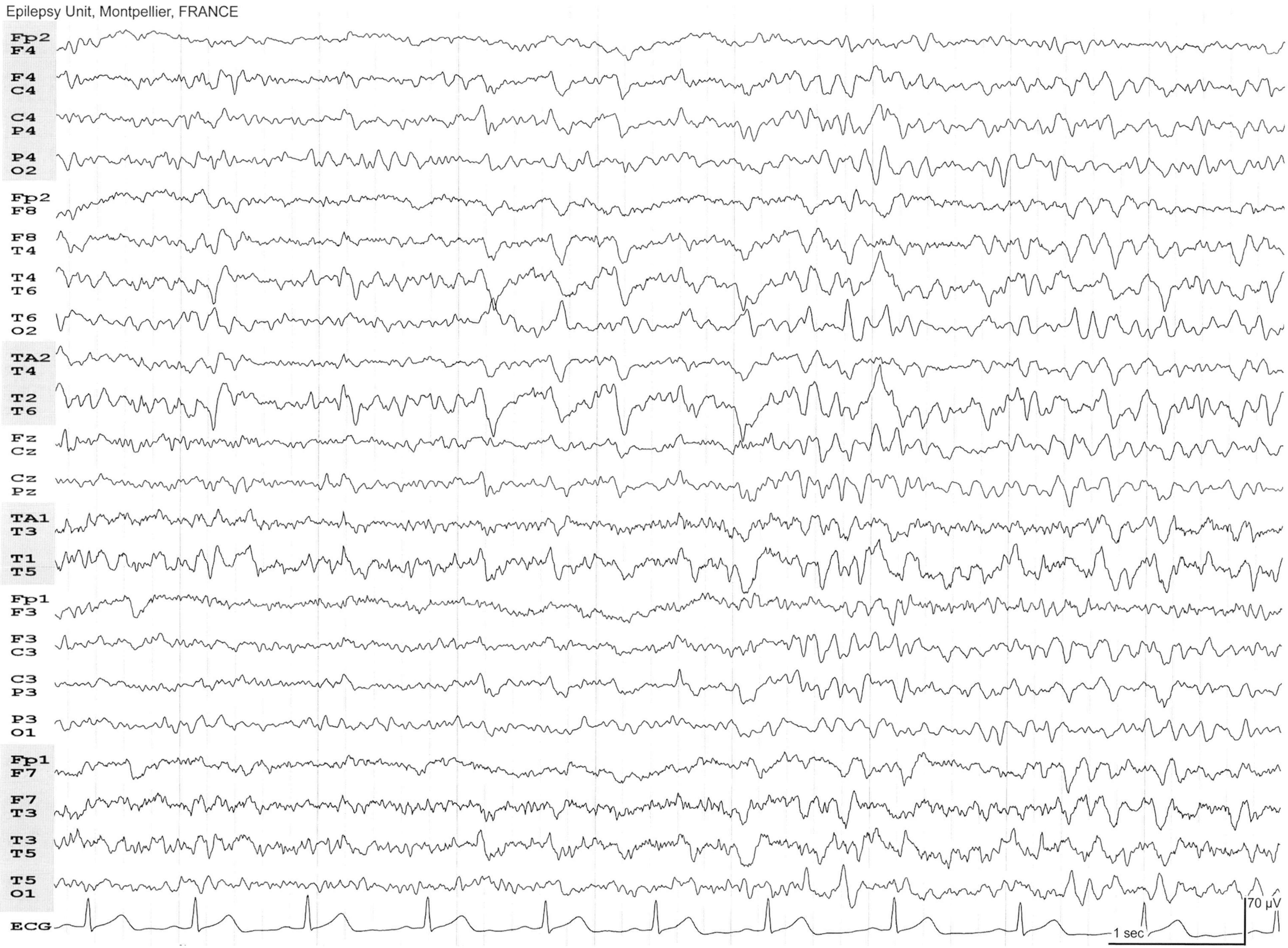
Epilepsy Unit, Montpellier, FRANCE
Fp2 F4
F4 C4
C4 P4
P4 O2
Fp2 F8
F8 T4
T4 T6
T6 O2
TA2 T4
T2 T6
Fz Cz
Cz Pz
TA1 T3
T1 T5
Fp1 F3
F3 C3
C3 P3
P3 O1
Fp1 F7
F7 T3
T3 T5
T5 O1
ECG
70 µV
1 sec

• 27 Subclinical Rhythmic Electrographic Discharges in Adults (SREDA) (4)

Context

39-year-old man, same patient as on I-26, continued.

What to note

Continuation of identical monomorphic theta-delta activity with constant amplitude on the centro-parieto-temporal regions. In this patient, SREDA were observed during relaxation but also in sleep during the transition phases from NREM sleep stage 2 into REM sleep (see plates III-74 and 75).

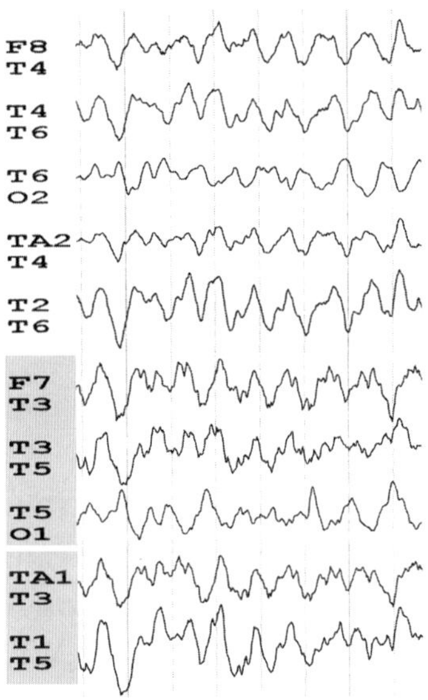

Figure a / Monomorphic theta-delta activity.

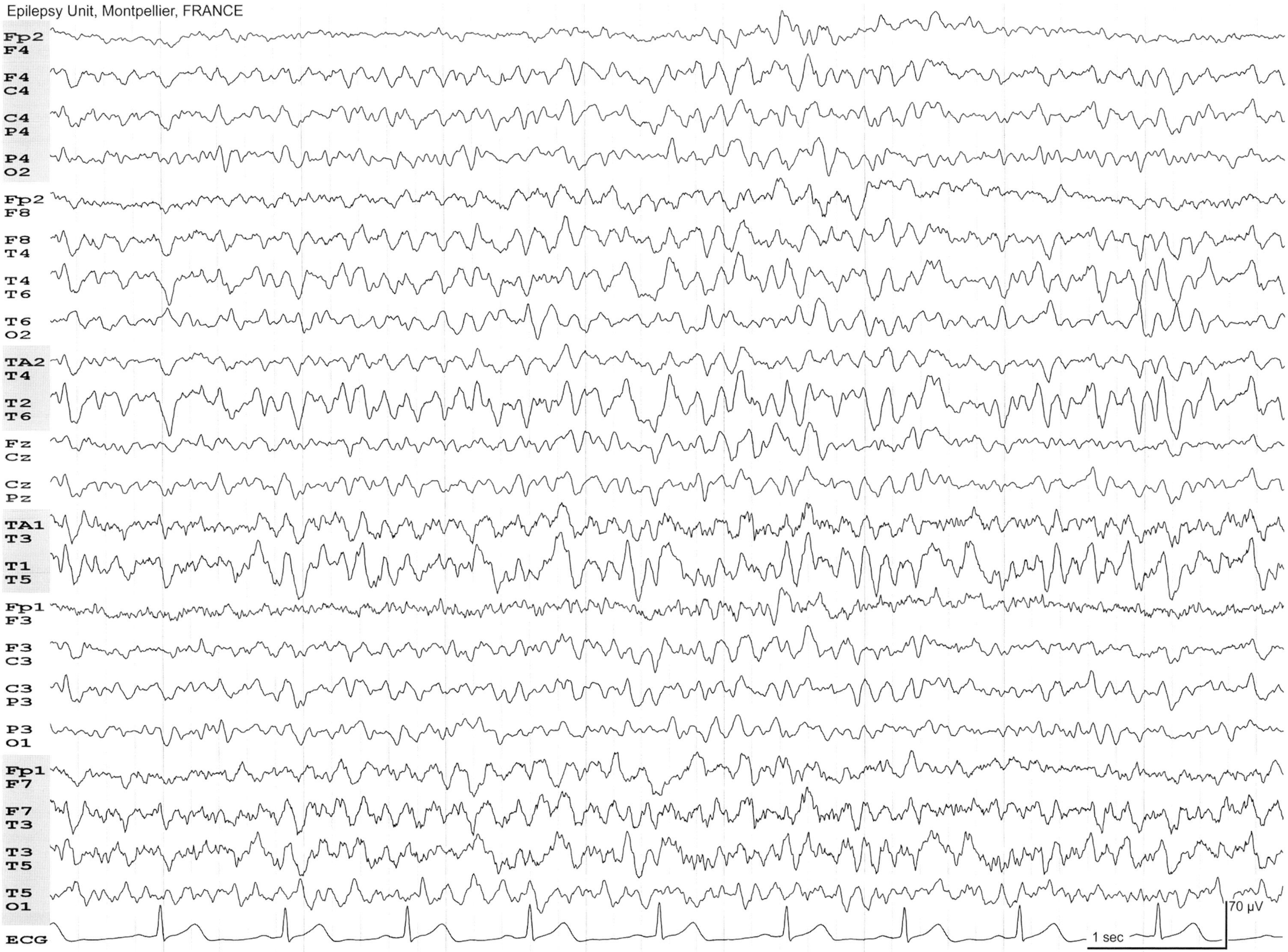
Epilepsy Unit, Montpellier, FRANCE
Fp2 F4
F4 C4
C4 P4
P4 O2
Fp2 F8
F8 T4
T4 T6
T6 O2
TA2 T4
T2 T6
Fz Cz
Cz Pz
TA1 T3
T1 T5
Fp1 F3
F3 C3
C3 P3
P3 O1
Fp1 F7
F7 T3
T3 T5
T5 O1
ECG
70 µV
1 sec

• 28 Subclinical Rhythmic Electrographic Discharges in Adults (SREDA) (5)

Context

76-year-old woman seen after an episode of loss of consciousness.

What to note

During hyperventilation, bilateral theta activity over the parietal regions. In this patient, SREDA were recorded during hyperventilation but also could reappear spontaneously without any activation. Note superimposed temporal muscular activities (T3).

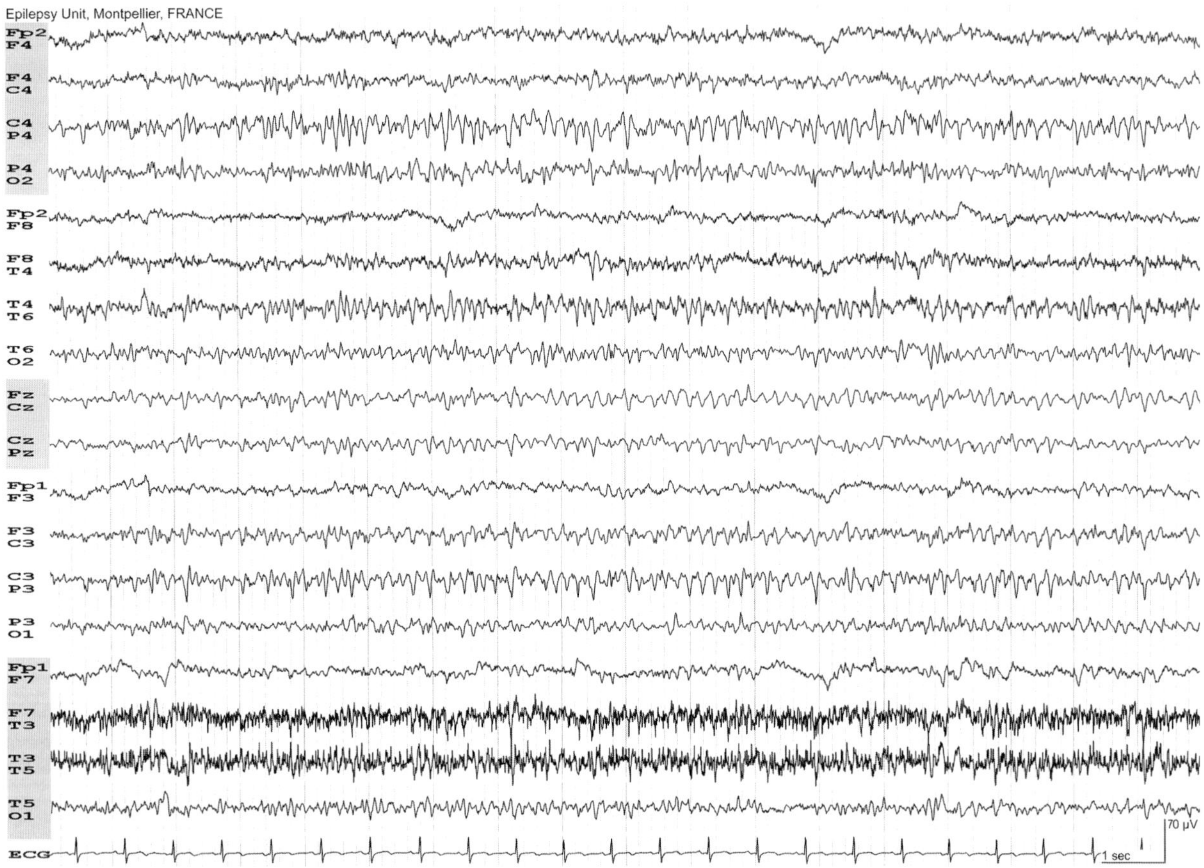

Figure a / Recording at 15 mm/s.

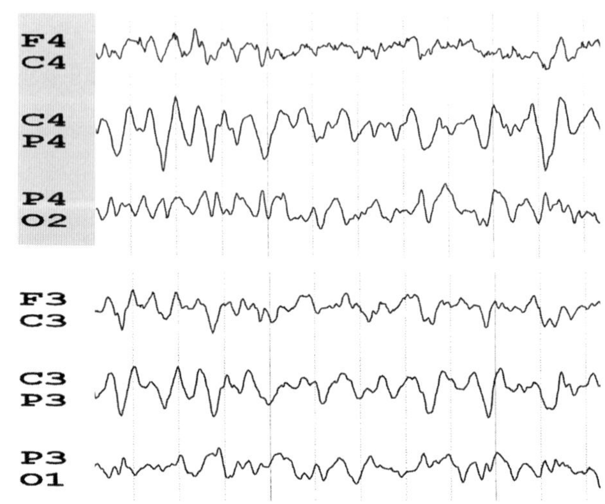

Figure b / SREDA: theta activity over the parietal regions.

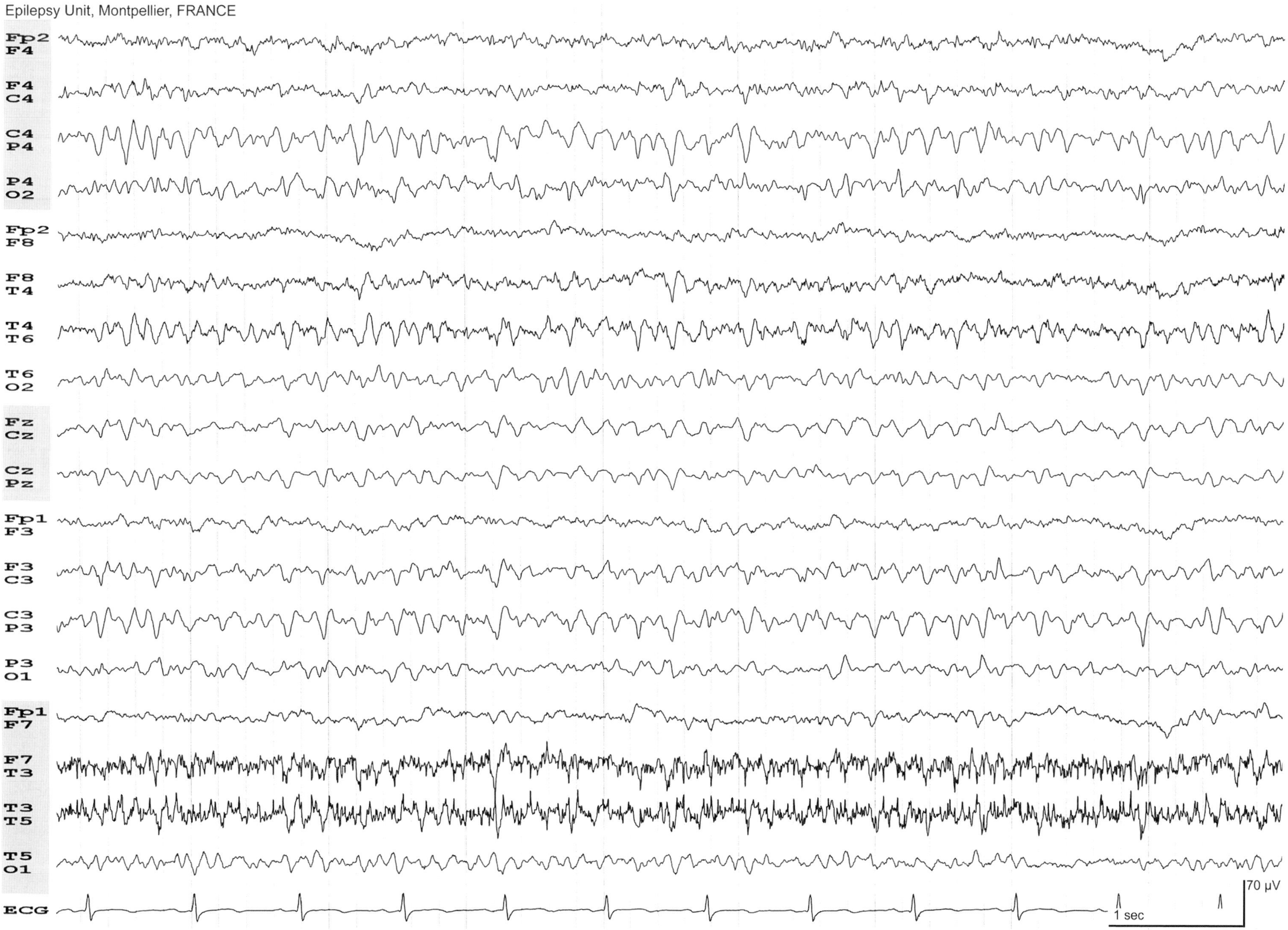
Epilepsy Unit, Montpellier, FRANCE
Fp2 F4
F4 C4
C4 P4
P4 O2
Fp2 F8
F8 T4
T4 T6
T6 O2
Fz Cz
Cz Pz
Fp1 F3
F3 C3
C3 P3
P3 O1
Fp1 F7
F7 T3
T3 T5
T5 O1
ECG
70 µV
1 sec

• 29 Temporal theta acitivity (wicket spikes)

Context

49-year-old woman referred for episodes of loss of consciousness later diagnosed as vagal syncopes.

What to note

Left segment: the patient's eyes are open with eyelid movement artifacts on the fronto-polar derivations and fast rhythms corresponding to muscular activities. A burst of irregular theta waves over the left temporal region can be seen. Right segment: the patient is in NREM sleep stage II with typical wicket spikes on the left temporal region. The slow wave activity over the left temporal region observed during wakefulness corresponds to wicket spikes but the morphology in this state of vigilance is not typical. During wakefulness, the wicket spikes are often irregular with a theta-like morphology. Typical wicket spikes appear during drowsiness and sleep.

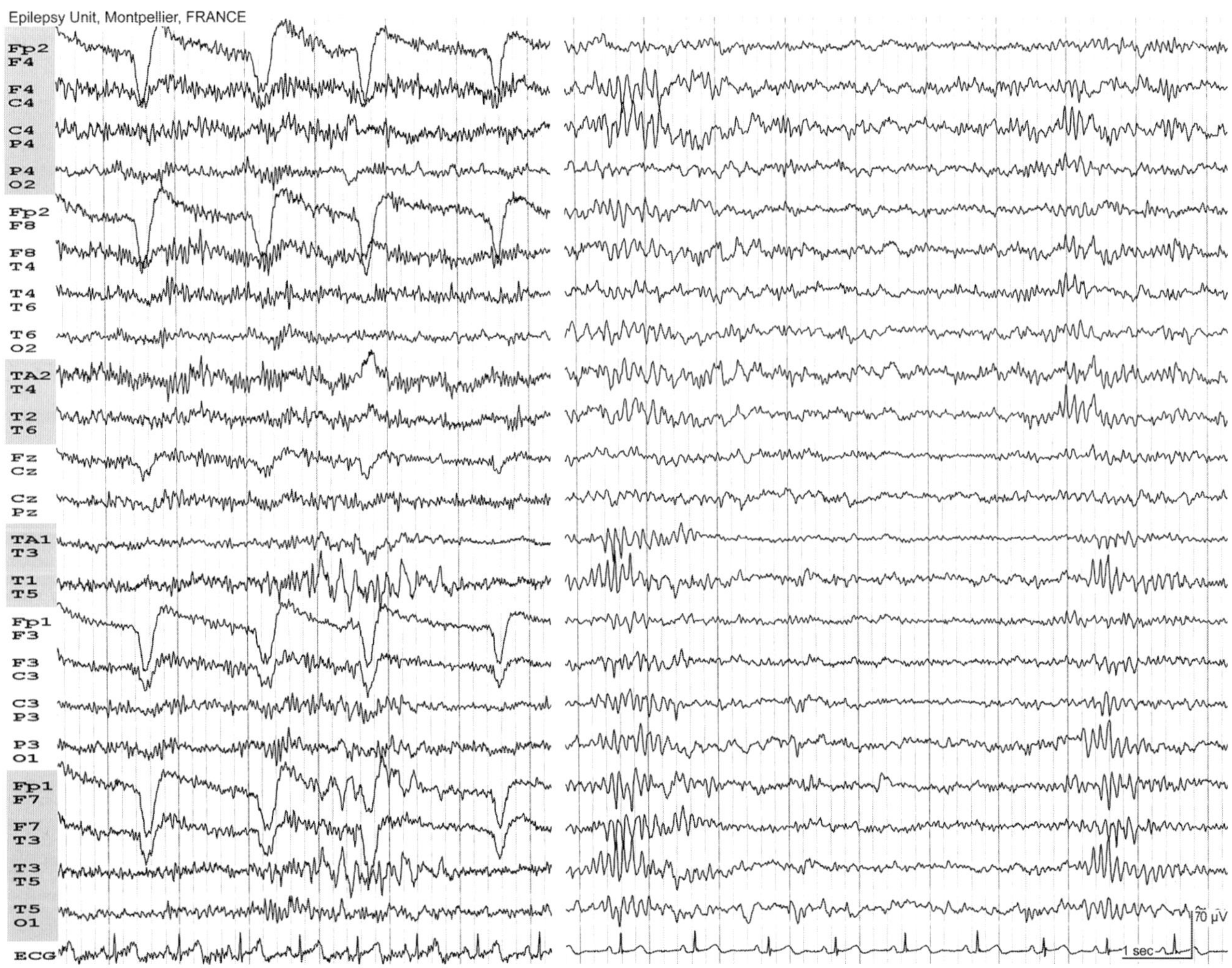

Figure a / Recording at 15 mm/s.

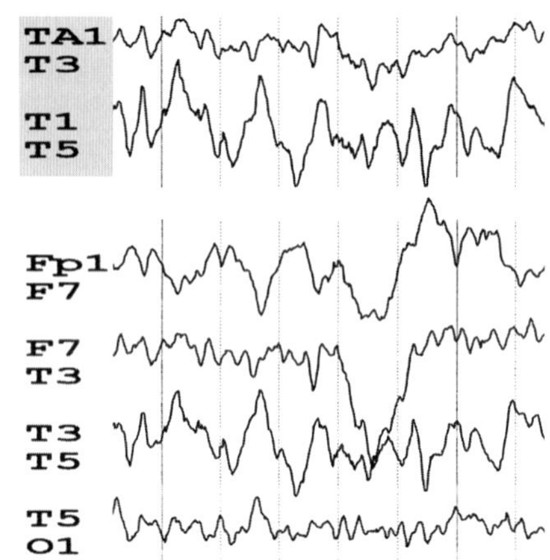

Figure b / Theta waves at 4 Hz.

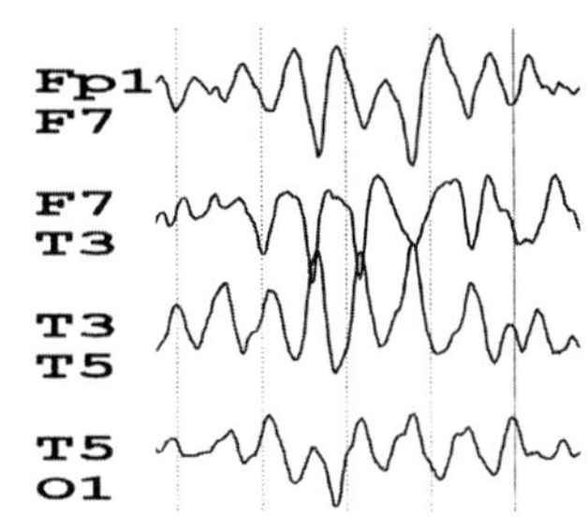

Figure c / Typical wicket spikes during NREM sleep stage II.

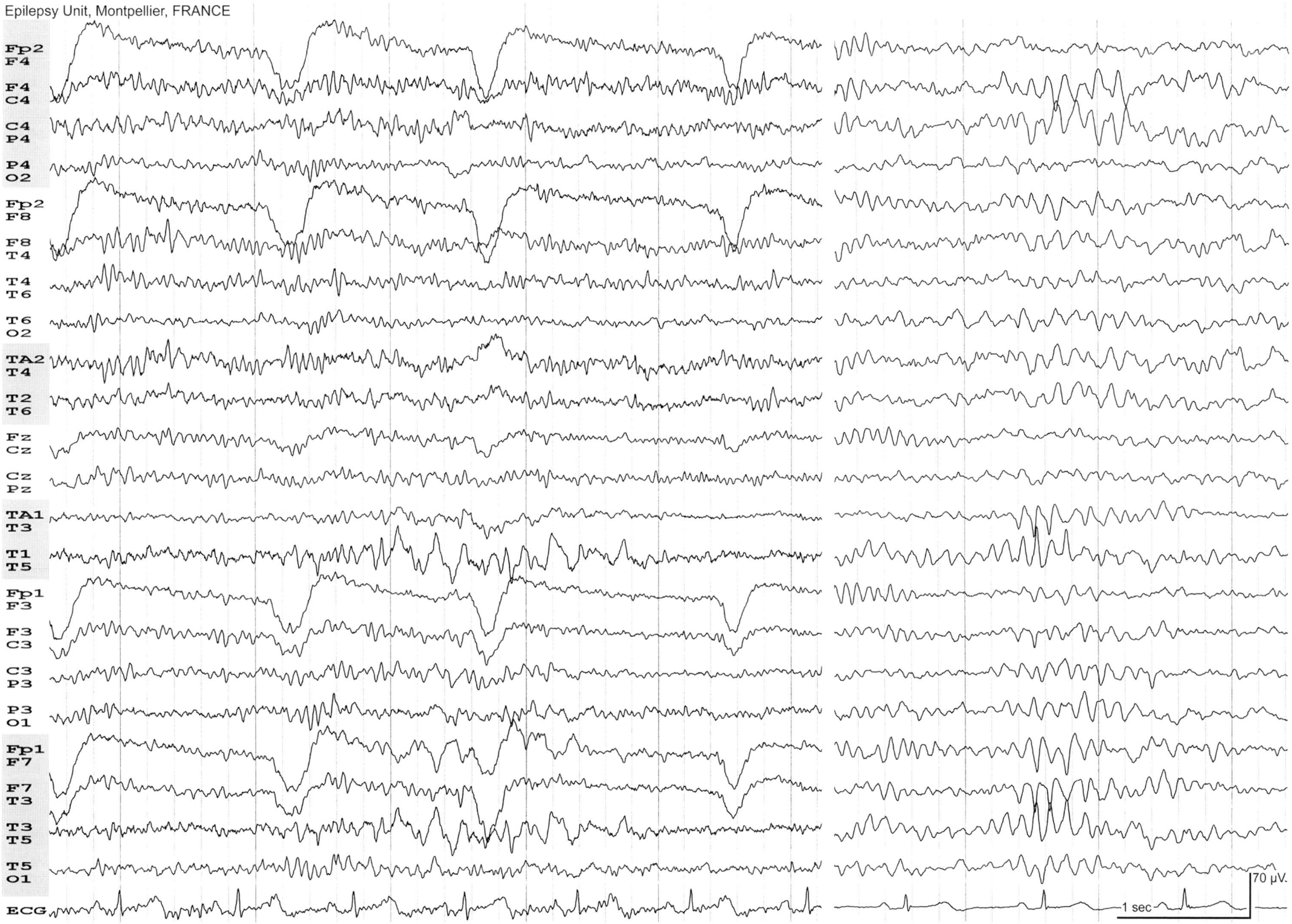
Epilepsy Unit, Montpellier, FRANCE
Fp2 F4
F4 C4
C4 P4
P4 O2
Fp2 F8
F8 T4
T4 T6
T6 O2
TA2 T4
T2 T6
Fz Cz
Cz Pz
TA1 T3
T1 T5
Fp1 F3
F3 C3
C3 P3
P3 O1
Fp1 F7
F7 T3
T3 T5
T5 O1
ECG
70 µV.
1 sec

I • 30 Temporal theta-delta activity (wicket spikes)

Context

60-year-old woman referred for episodes of loss of consciousness.

What to note

Left segment: awake, eyes are closed. Posterior alpha background activity can be seen. A burst of theta-delta waves occurs on the right temporal region. The slow waves are forked because they are intermixed with the alpha waves. In the central and right segment, the patient is in NREM sleep stage II. Wicket spikes over the right and left temporal regions can be observed. Here again, the sleep recording is particularly interesting. The slow temporal waves observed during wakefulness are not pathological and correspond to wicket spikes.

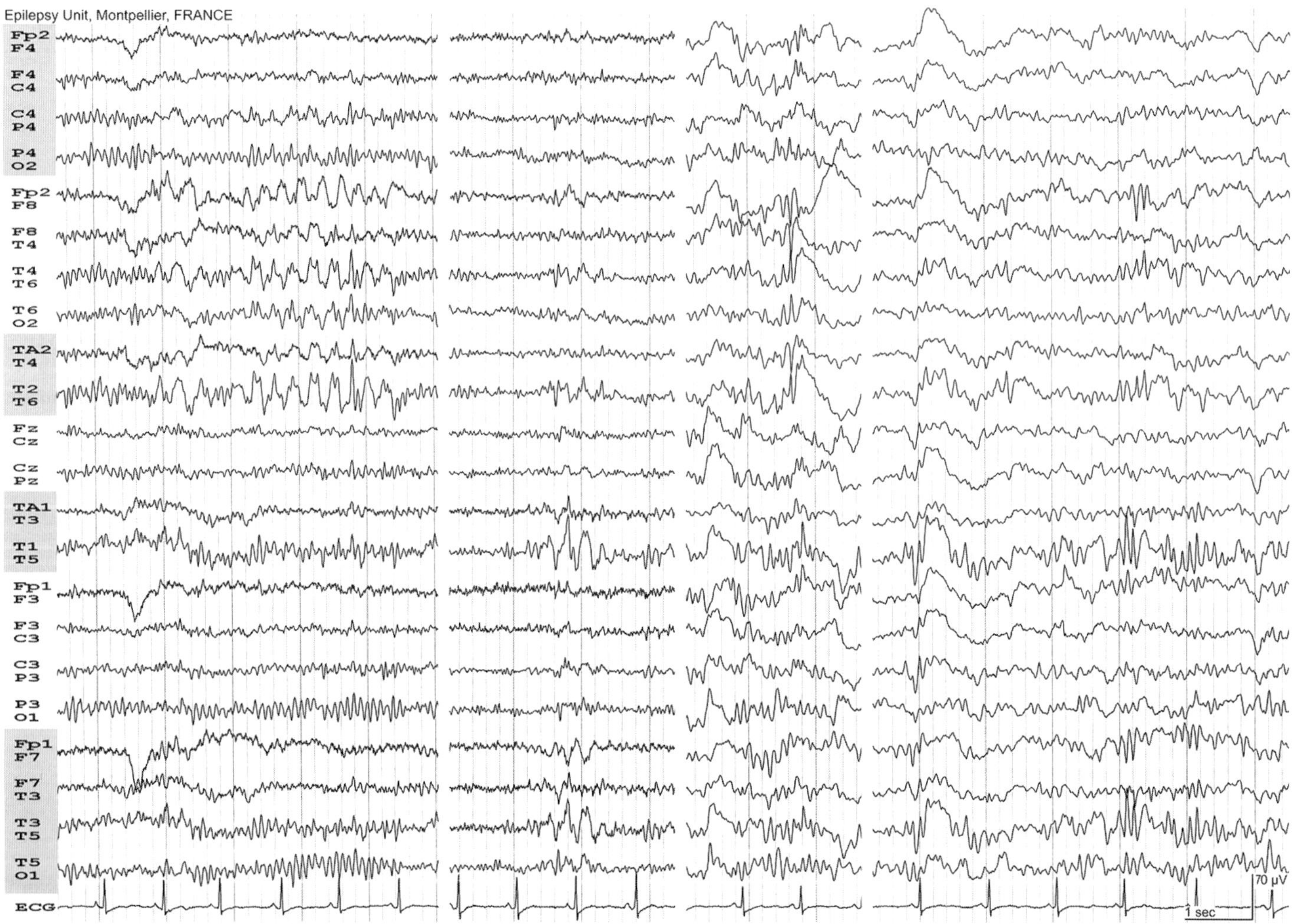

Figure a / Recording at 15 mm/s. Second segment: eyes open. Sharp waves over the left temporal region.

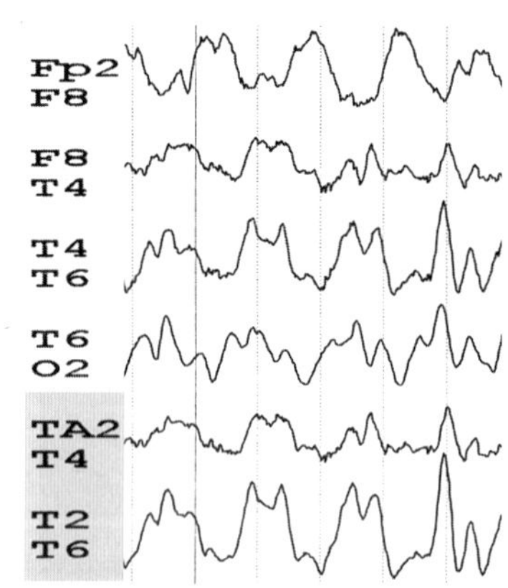

Figure b / Temporal slow waves. The last element, if taken alone can be mistaken for an "epileptic" spike. But the same element, when seen during sleep is clearly a wicket spike.

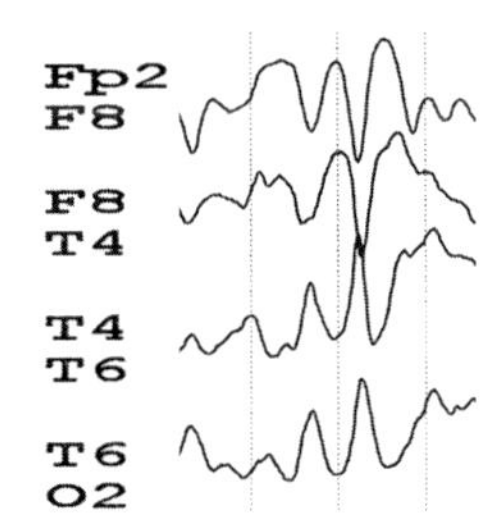

Figure c / Wicket spikes on the right temporal region.

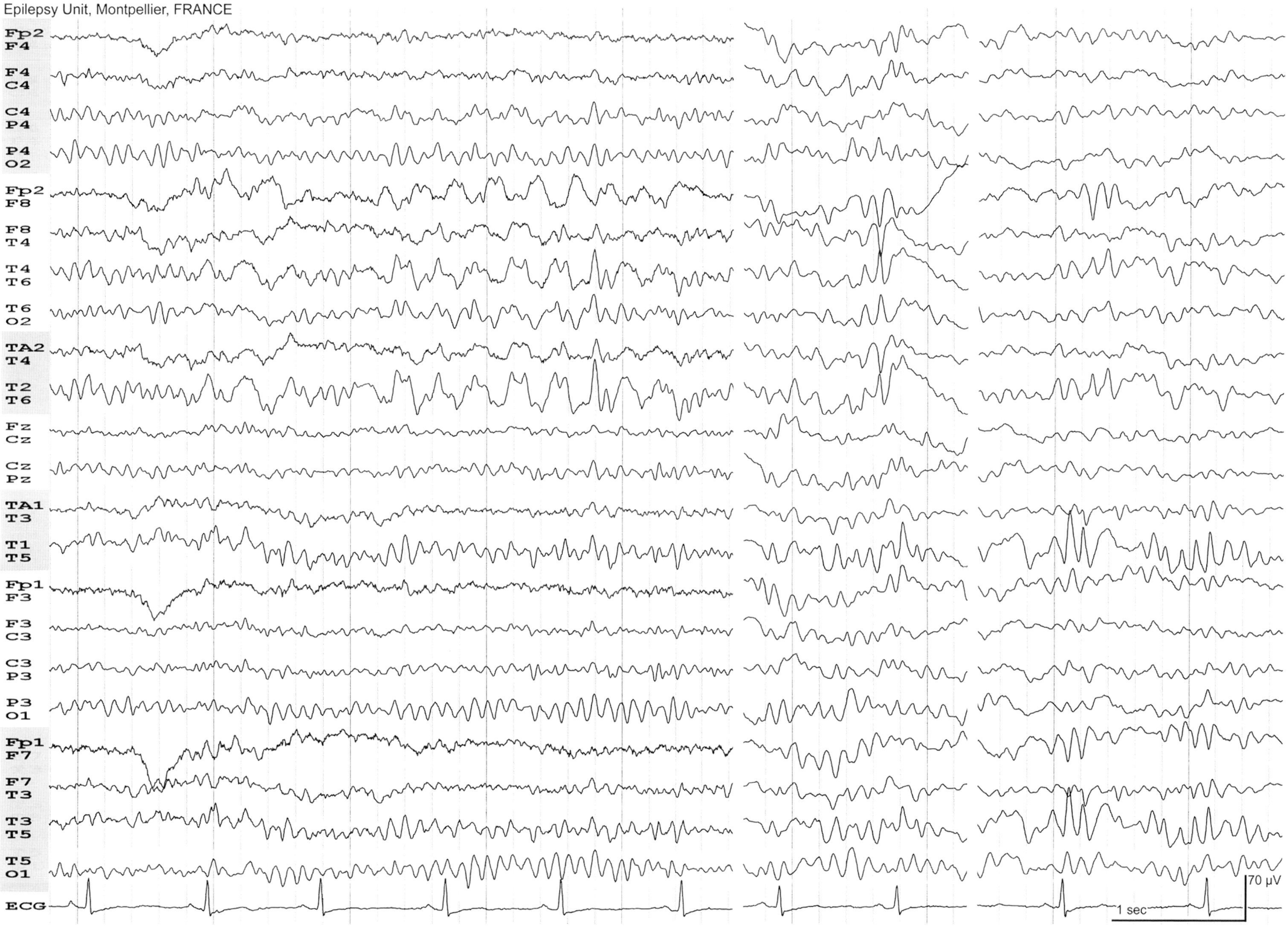
Epilepsy Unit, Montpellier, FRANCE
Fp2 F4
F4 C4
C4 P4
P4 O2
Fp2 F8
F8 T4
T4 T6
T6 O2
TA2 T4
T2 T6
Fz Cz
Cz Pz
TA1 T3
T1 T5
Fp1 F3
F3 C3
C3 P3
P3 O1
Fp1 F7
F7 T3
T3 T5
T5 O1
ECG
70 µV
1 sec

I • 31 Temporal theta-delta activity (rhythmic midtemporal discharges)

Context

43-year-old woman with temporal lobe epilepsy.

What to note

The woman is awake. A theta activity at 4 Hz appears on the right temporal region. It is difficult with this tracing to determine whether this activity is paraphysiological or pathological, i.e. an interictal abnormality in this patient with temporal lobe epilepsy. The monomorphic and bilateral aspects are in favor of a paraphysiological activity. In fact, in these difficult cases, a sleep recording is necessary. This patient had typical rhythmic midtemporal discharges during drowsiness and sleep (see below). Theta activity in this patient corresponds to rhythmic midtemporal discharges observed during wakefulness.

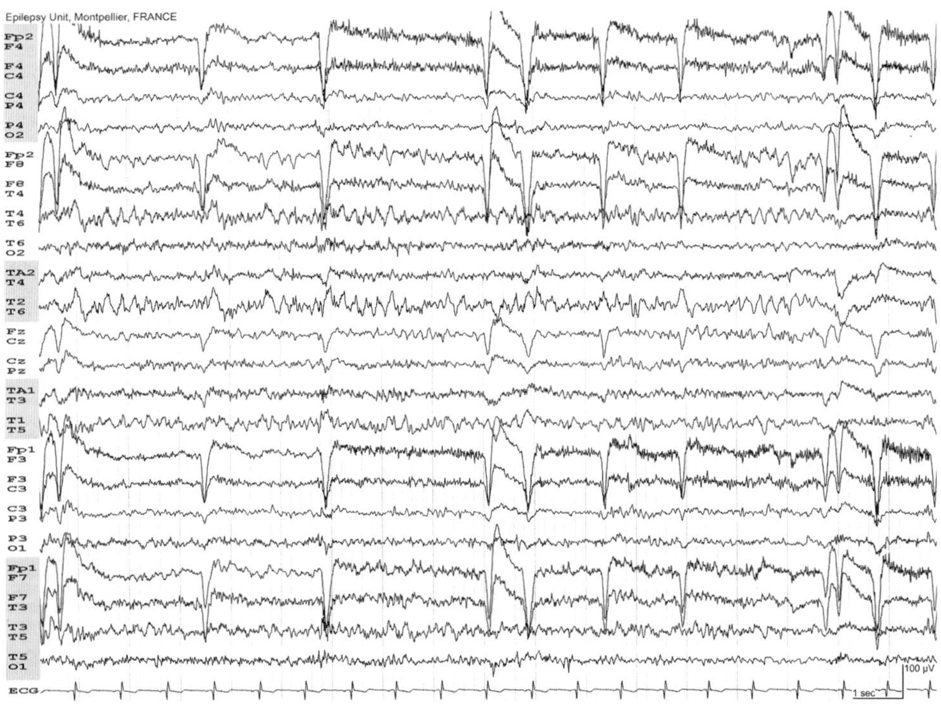

Figure a / Recording at 15 mmm/s.

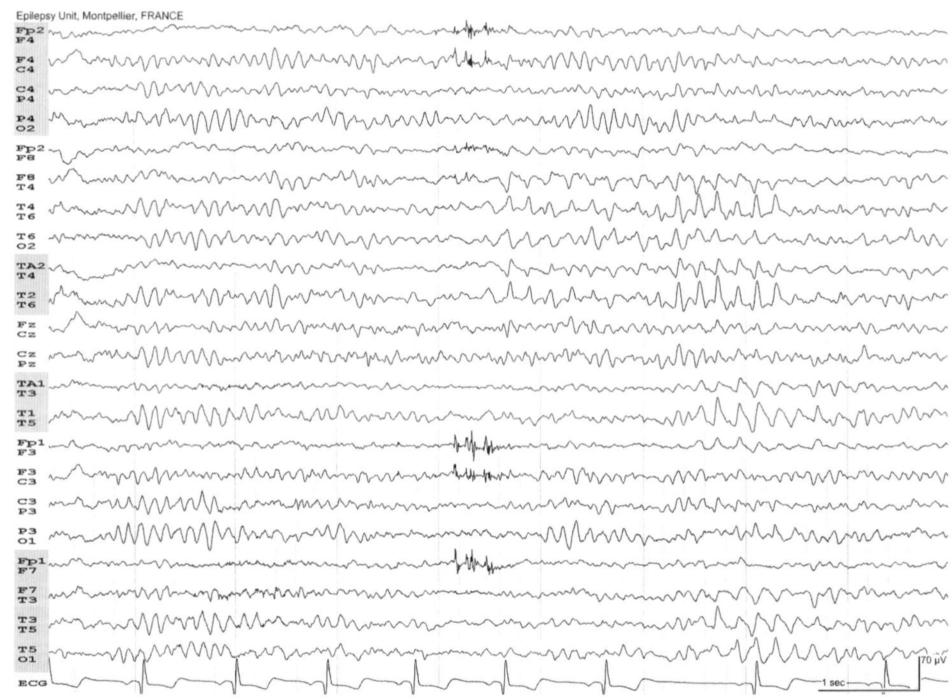

Figure b / Same patient. Typical rhythmic midtemporal discharges over the right and left temporal regions in REM sleep. Note the presence of muscular twitches and mu rhythm.

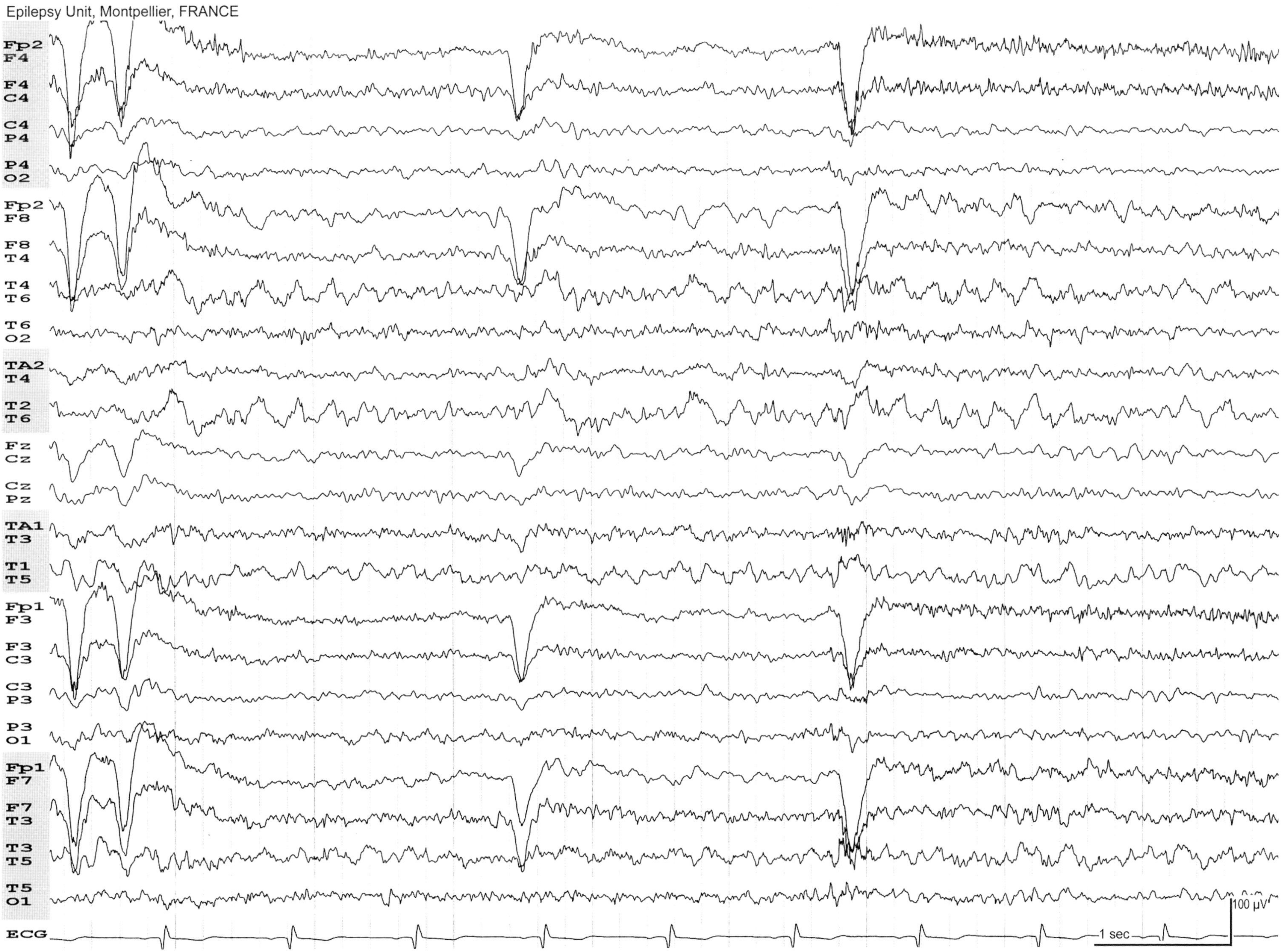
Epilepsy Unit, Montpellier, FRANCE
Fp2 F4
F4 C4
C4 P4
P4 O2
Fp2 F8
F8 T4
T4 T6
T6 O2
TA2 T4
T2 T6
Fz Cz
Cz Pz
TA1 T3
T1 T5
Fp1 F3
F3 C3
C3 P3
P3 O1
Fp1 F7
F7 T3
T3 T5
T5 O1
ECG
1 sec
100 µV

I • 32 Breach rhythm (1)

Context

35-year-old woman, history of surgery for a left parietal meningioma.

What to note

Background activity with a high-amplitude 9.5 Hz rhythm on the left parietal region, which disappears upon eye opening and corresponds to an enhanced alpha rhythm due to the breach. Note the eyelid movement artifacts over the fronto-polar derivations.

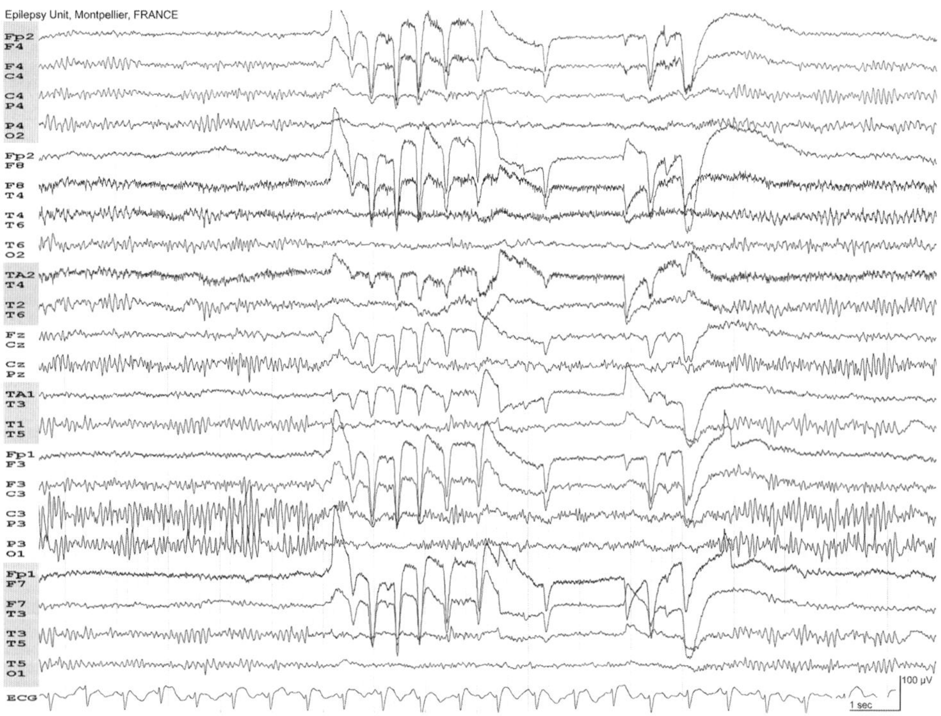

Figure a / Recording at 15 mm/s. Note the reactivity of the breach rhythm upon eye opening and eye closure.

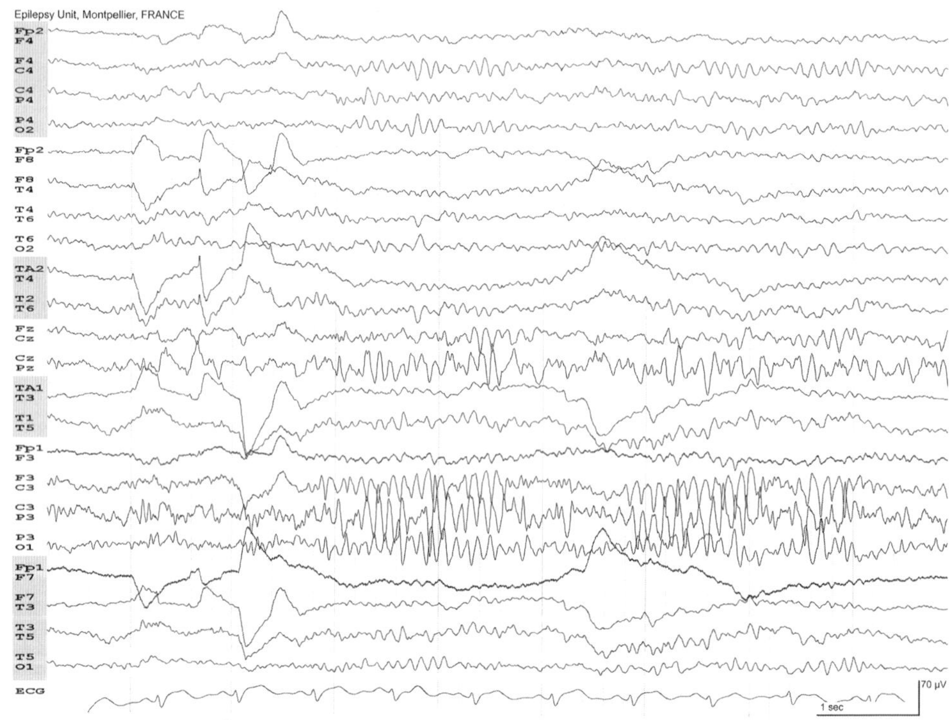

Figure b / REM sleep with rapid eye movements over the fronto-polar derivations. Note the presence of breach rhythm over the left parietal region.

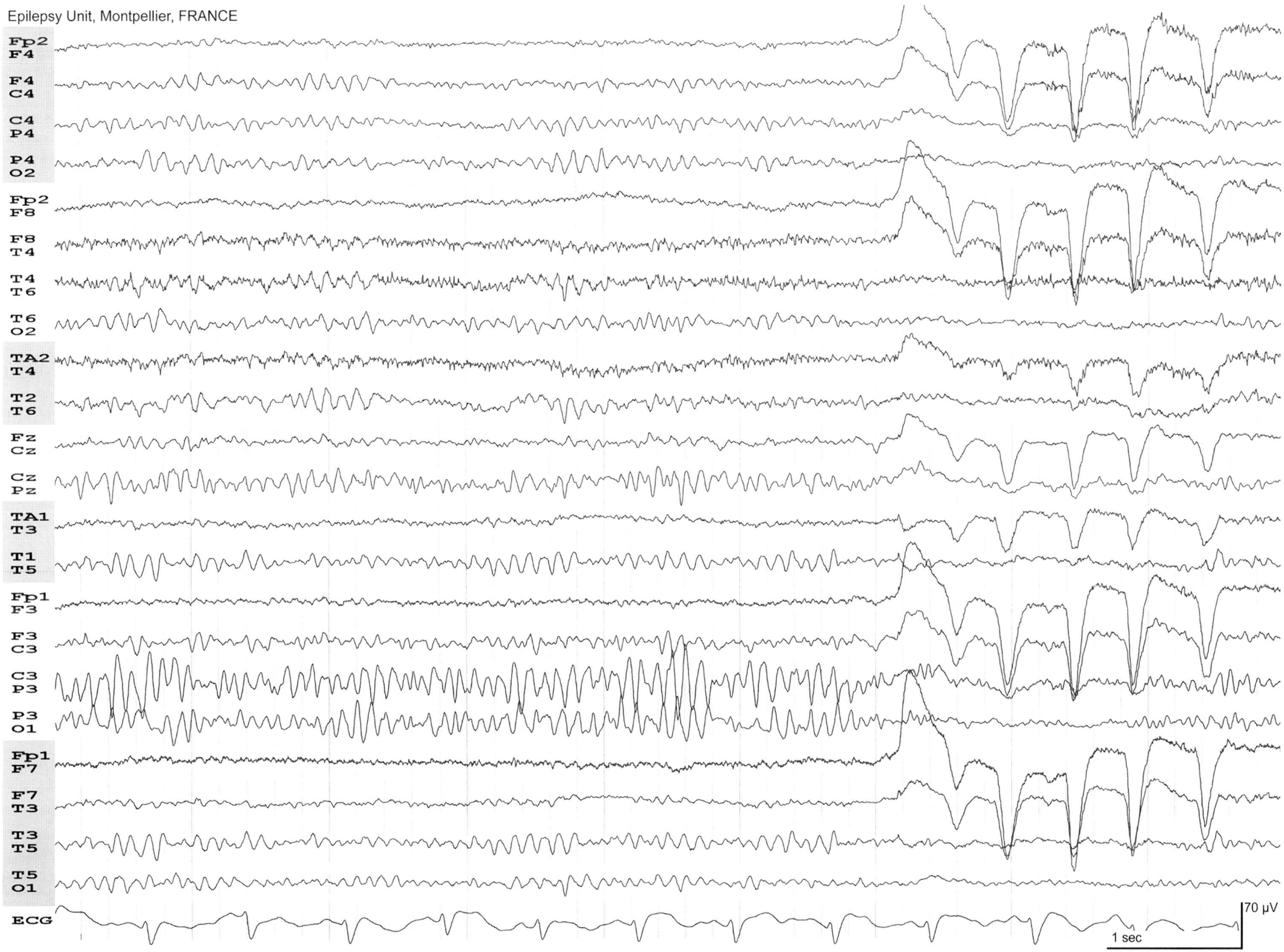
Epilepsy Unit, Montpellier, FRANCE
Fp2 F4
F4 C4
C4 P4
P4 O2
Fp2 F8
F8 T4
T4 T6
T6 O2
TA2 T4
T2 T6
Fz Cz
Cz Pz
TA1 T3
T1 T5
Fp1 F3
F3 C3
C3 P3
P3 O1
Fp1 F7
F7 T3
T3 T5
T5 O1
ECG
70 µV
1 sec

I • 33 Breach rhythm (2)

Context

69-year-old man who had surgery 3 years earlier for a right central meningioma, well-controlled epilepsy.

What to note

Over the central region at C4 (transverse montage) the high-amplitude arch-like shaped 8 Hz activity corresponds to an enhanced mu rhythm due to the presence of a breach. The breach rhythm spreads to the right parietal region.

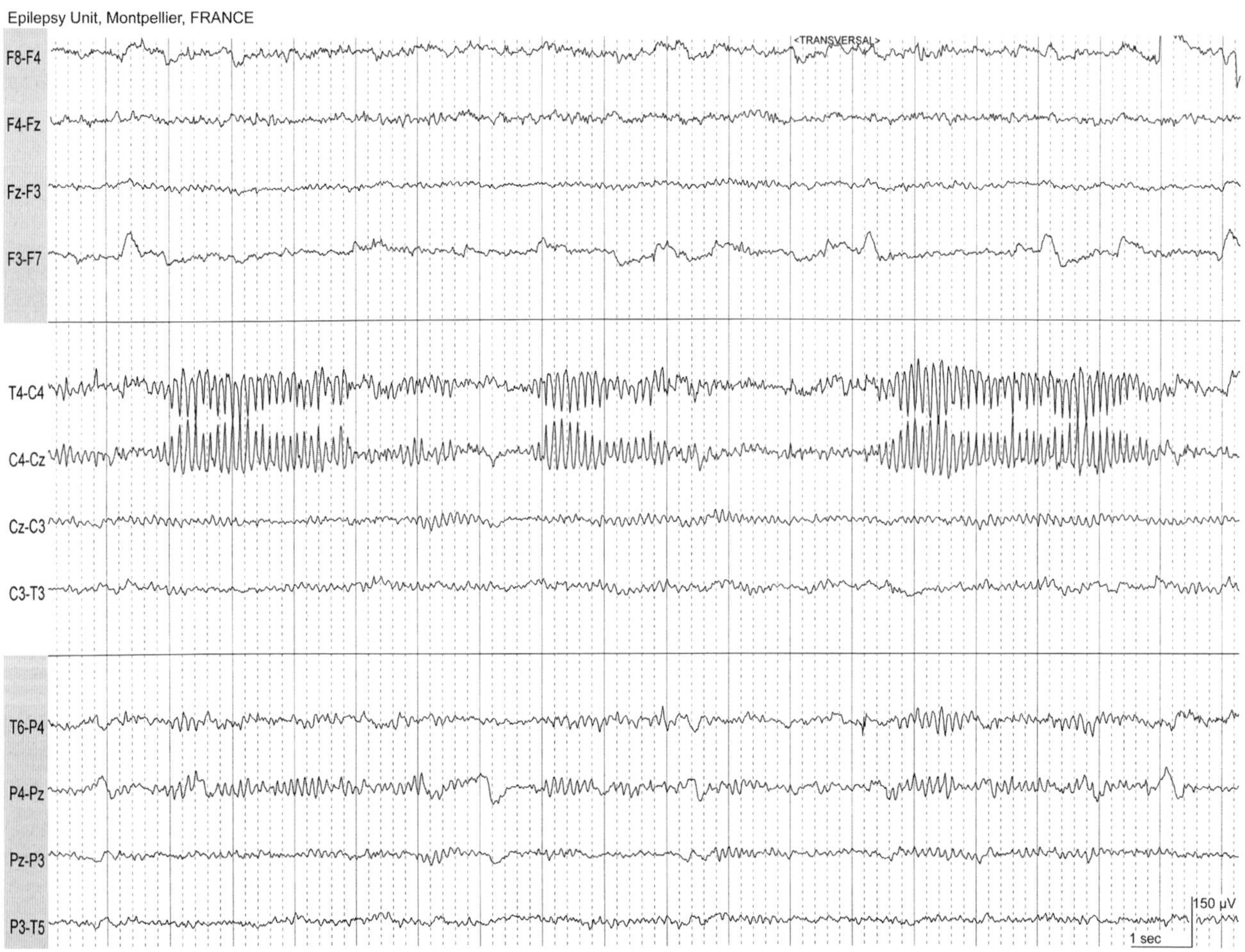

Figure a / Recording at 15 mm/s.

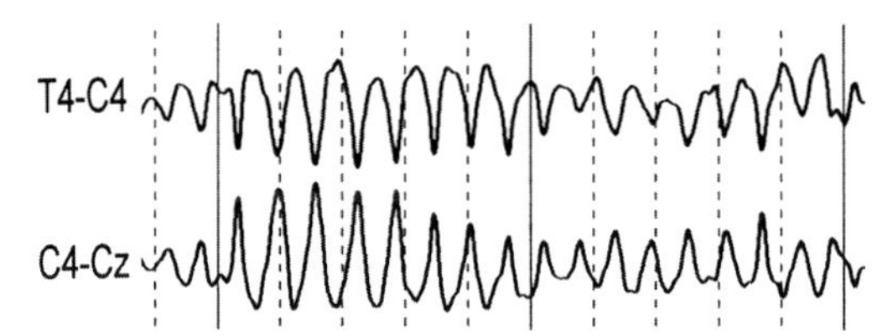

Figure b / At C4, mu rhythm enhanced due to the presence of a breach.

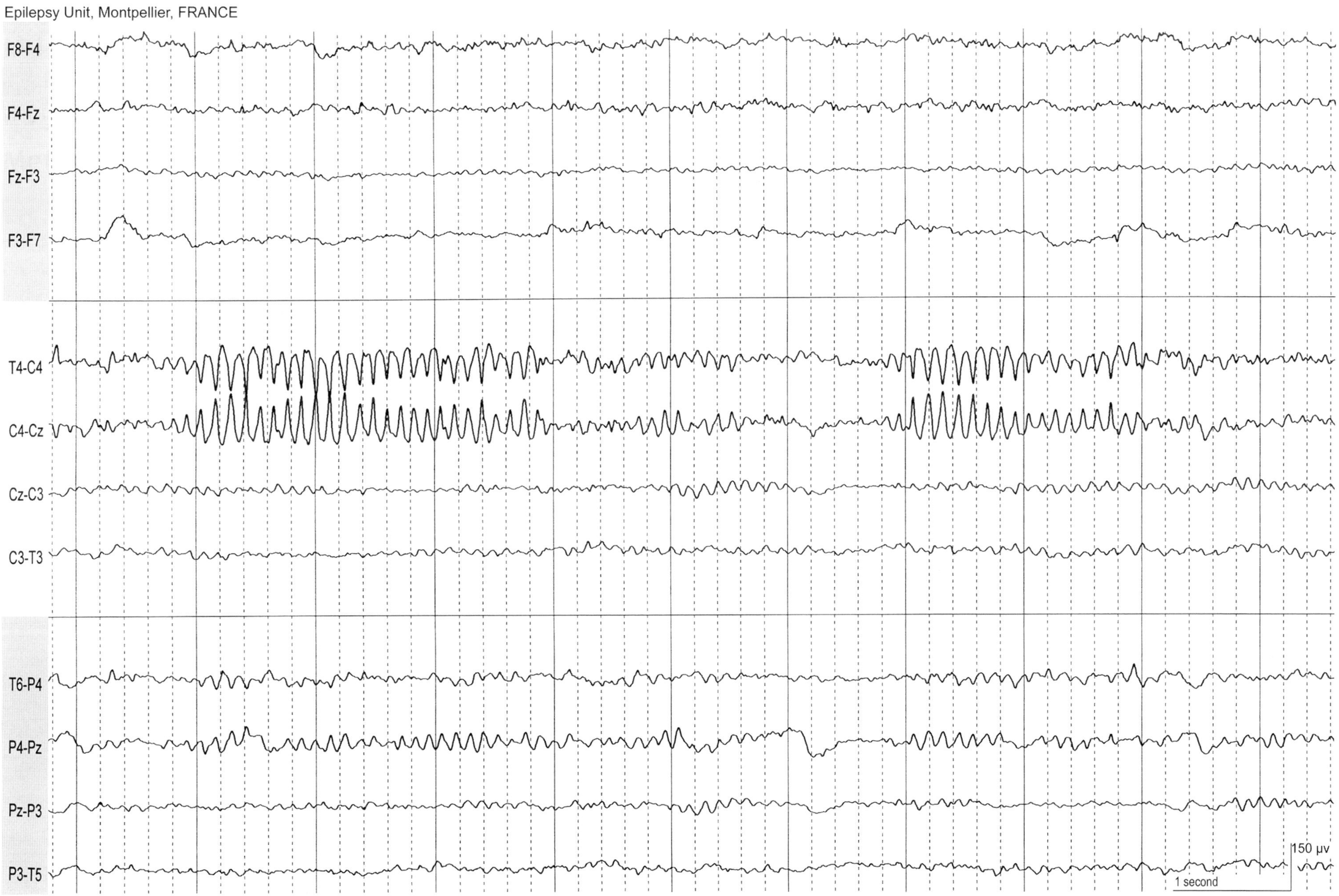
Epilepsy Unit, Montpellier, FRANCE
F8-F4
F4-Fz
Fz-F3
F3-F7
T4-C4
C4-Cz
Cz-C3
C3-T3
T6-P4
P4-Pz
Pz-P3
P3-T5
150 µv
1 second

I • 34 Breach rhythm (3)

Context

49-year-old woman with medial temporal lobe epilepsy, 5 years after surgery for a right cavernous sinus meningioma.

What to note

Eyes open. On the right temporal region, 9 Hz activity with sharply-contoured waveforms, in phase reversal on T4. These are not epileptiform abnormalities, but a typical breach rhythm. These elements mimic of wicket spikes.

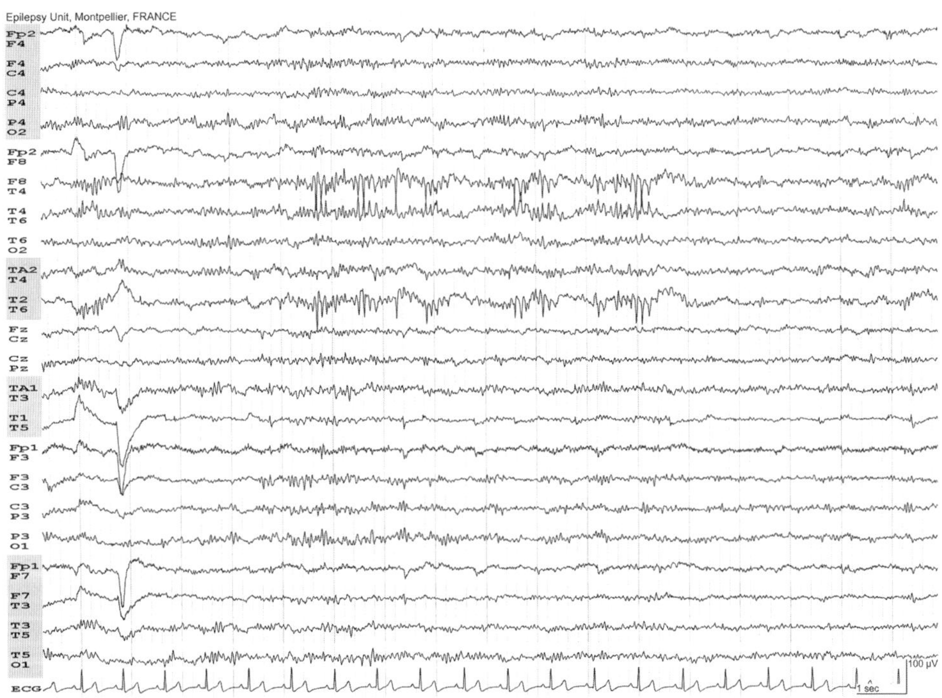

Figure a / Recording at 15 mm/s.

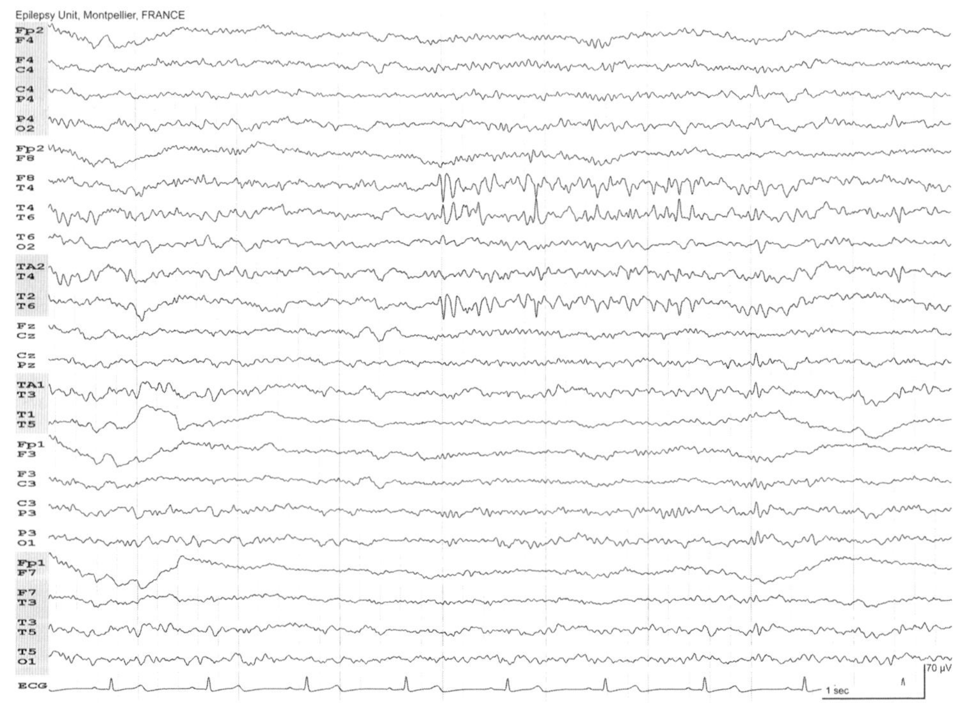

Figure b / REM sleep with rapid eye movements at the beginning of the plate. Breach rhythm over the right temporal region.

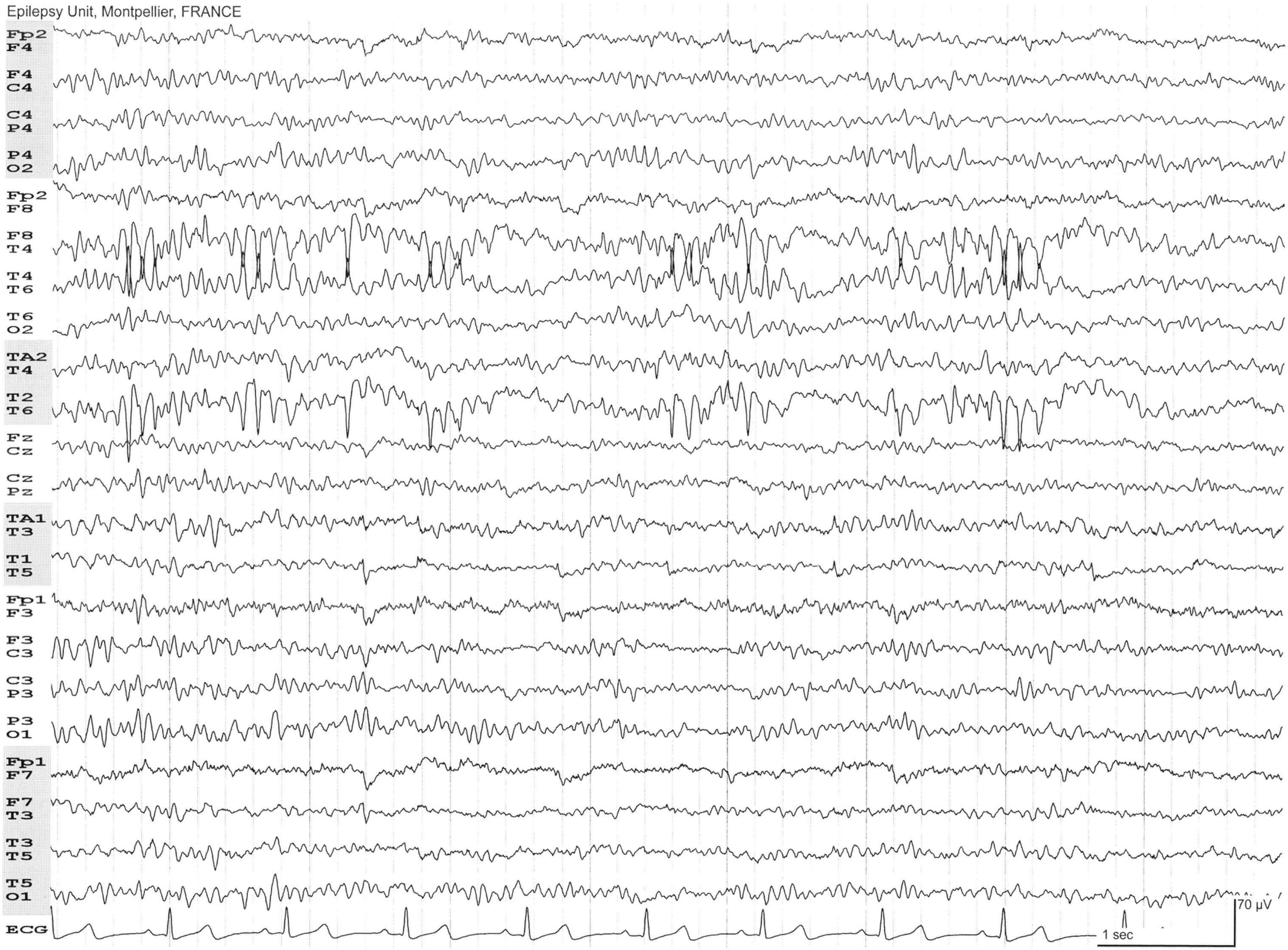
Epilepsy Unit, Montpellier, FRANCE
Fp2 F4
F4 C4
C4 P4
P4 O2
Fp2 F8
F8 T4
T4 T6
T6 O2
TA2 T4
T2 T6
Fz Cz
Cz Pz
TA1 T3
T1 T5
Fp1 F3
F3 C3
C3 P3
P3 O1
Fp1 F7
F7 T3
T3 T5
T5 O1
ECG
70 µV
1 sec

I • 35 Breach rhythm (4)

Context

38-year-old woman, underwent surgery for a left temporal lobe epilepsy, also presenting non-epileptic seizures (psychogenic).

What to note

The patient is awake subsequently with open eyes, then closed eyes (eyelid closing artifacts). Amplitude of the posterior alpha (9-10 Hz) wave is higher on the right side. Beta rhythms can be observed on the anteriorly regions. On the left fronto-temporal region, the breach rhythm corresponds to higher amplitude activity with sub-continuous sharp-contoured waveforms. Amplitude of the spread to the right frontal region is very low (Fp2-F8). The morphology of this breach rhythm was not typical during wakefulness but became typical in NREM sleep (see below).

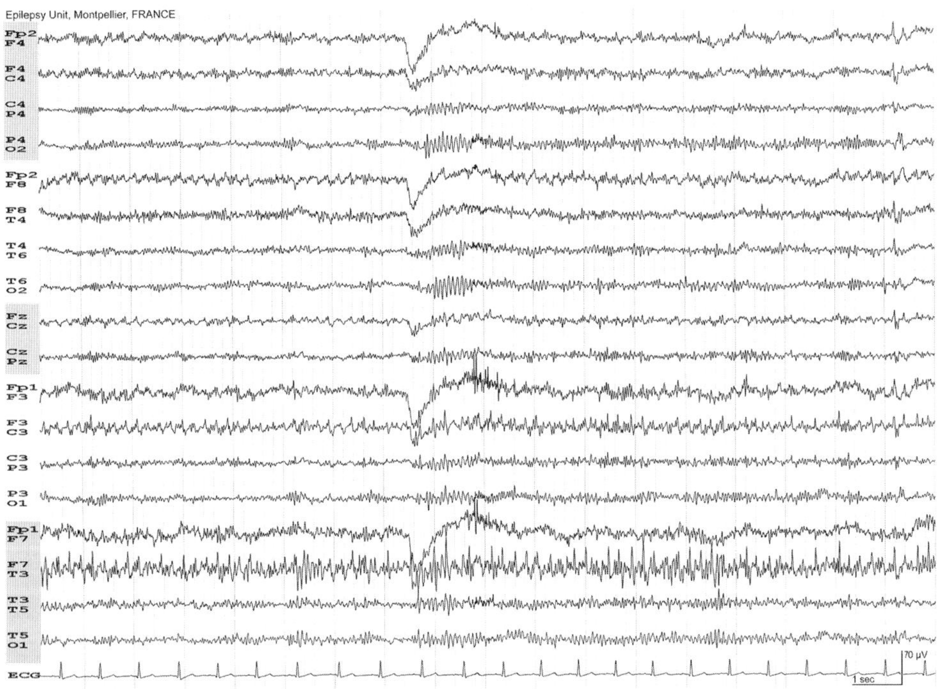

Figure a / Recording at 15 mm/s. Morphology of the breach rhythm remains unchanged after eye closure.

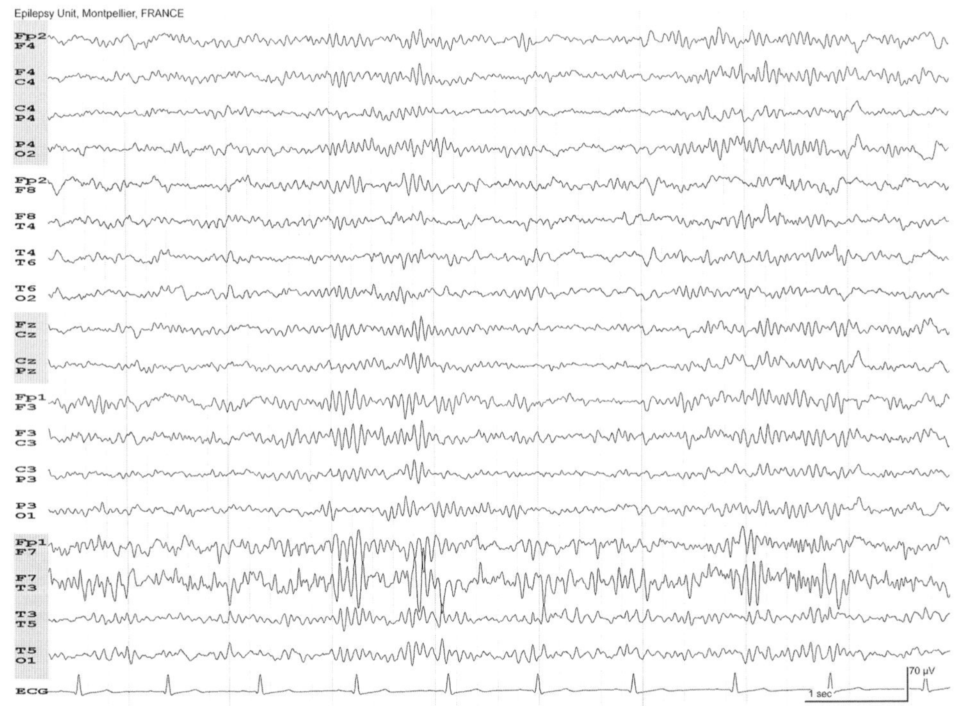

Figure b / Recording at 30 mm/s. The woman is in NREM sleep stage II (sleep spindles over the fronto-central regions, with higher amplitude on the left). A subcontinuous activity admixing sharp and ample activities can be seen at Fp1-F7 and F7-T3, corresponding to a typical breach rhythm.

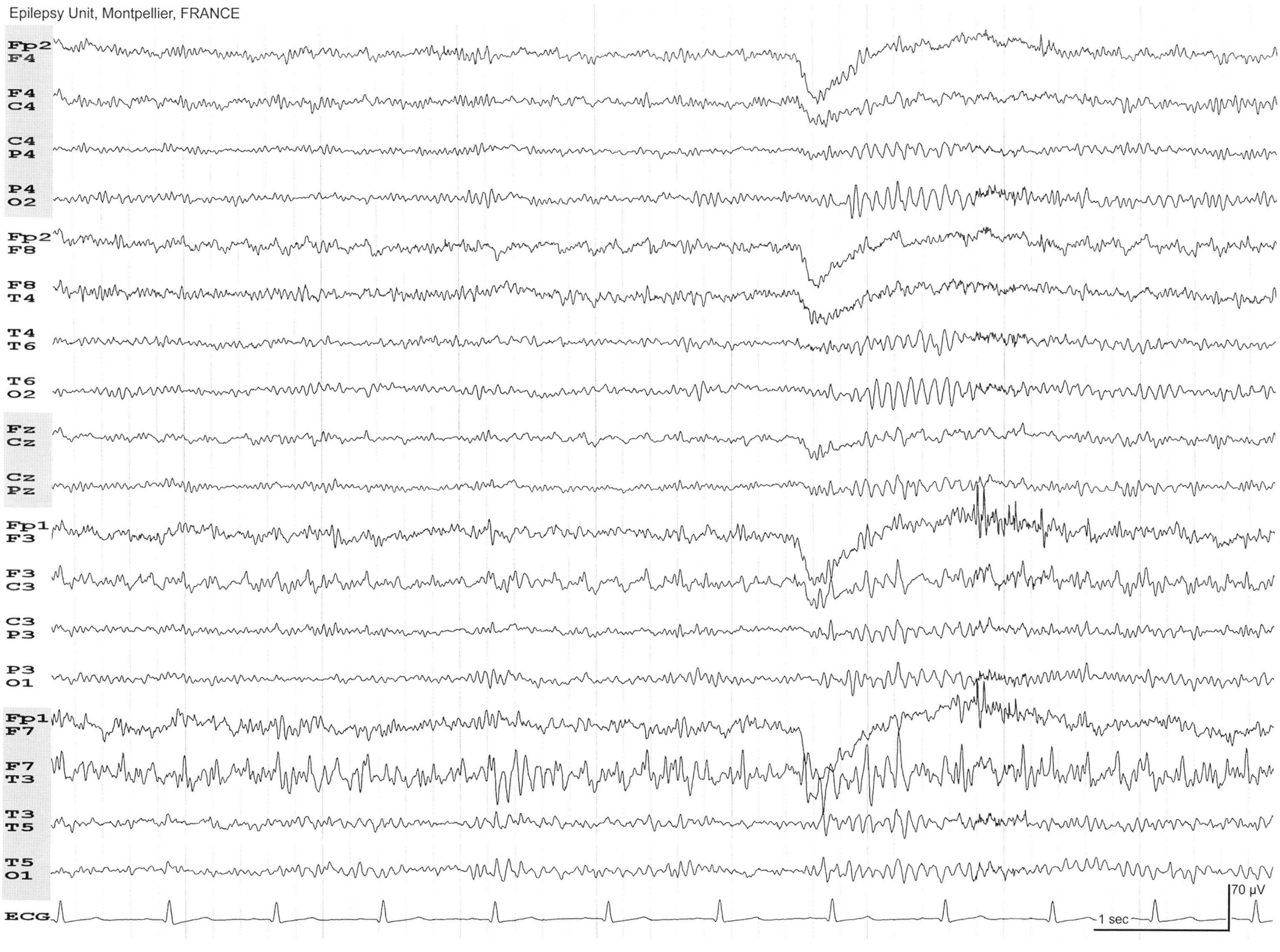
Epilepsy Unit, Montpellier, FRANCE
Fp2 F4
F4 C4
C4 P4
P4 O2
Fp2 F8
F8 T4
T4 T6
T6 O2
Fz Cz
Cz Pz
Fp1 F3
F3 C3
C3 P3
P3 O1
Fp1 F7
F7 T3
T3 T5
T5 O1
ECG
70 µV
1 sec

• 36 Breach rhythm in a patient after cortectomy with sequelae of brain trauma

Context

22-year-old woman, after right temporal parietal cortectomy 4 years earlier for drug-resistant focal epilepsy following severe trauma at age 4 years. The patient has been seizure free on antiepileptic drugs.

What to note

The patient's eyes are closed until the 5th second. Eyelid movement artifacts can be seen on the frontal-polar derivations when she opens her eyes (EO). The background activity is not well-developed. It is slower on the right, but reactivity to eye opening is visually detectable. Superimposed slow waves can be observed on the right temporal region (sequellae of brain insult). In the right suprasylvian region, the rhythm is composed of waveforms that are rather slow and sharp-contoured as well as some beta activity. This corresponds to a breach rhythm as well as sequellae of her brain insults. There are little changes with eye opening. The breach rhythm is a little more typical with sharp waves over F4-C4 and C4-P4.

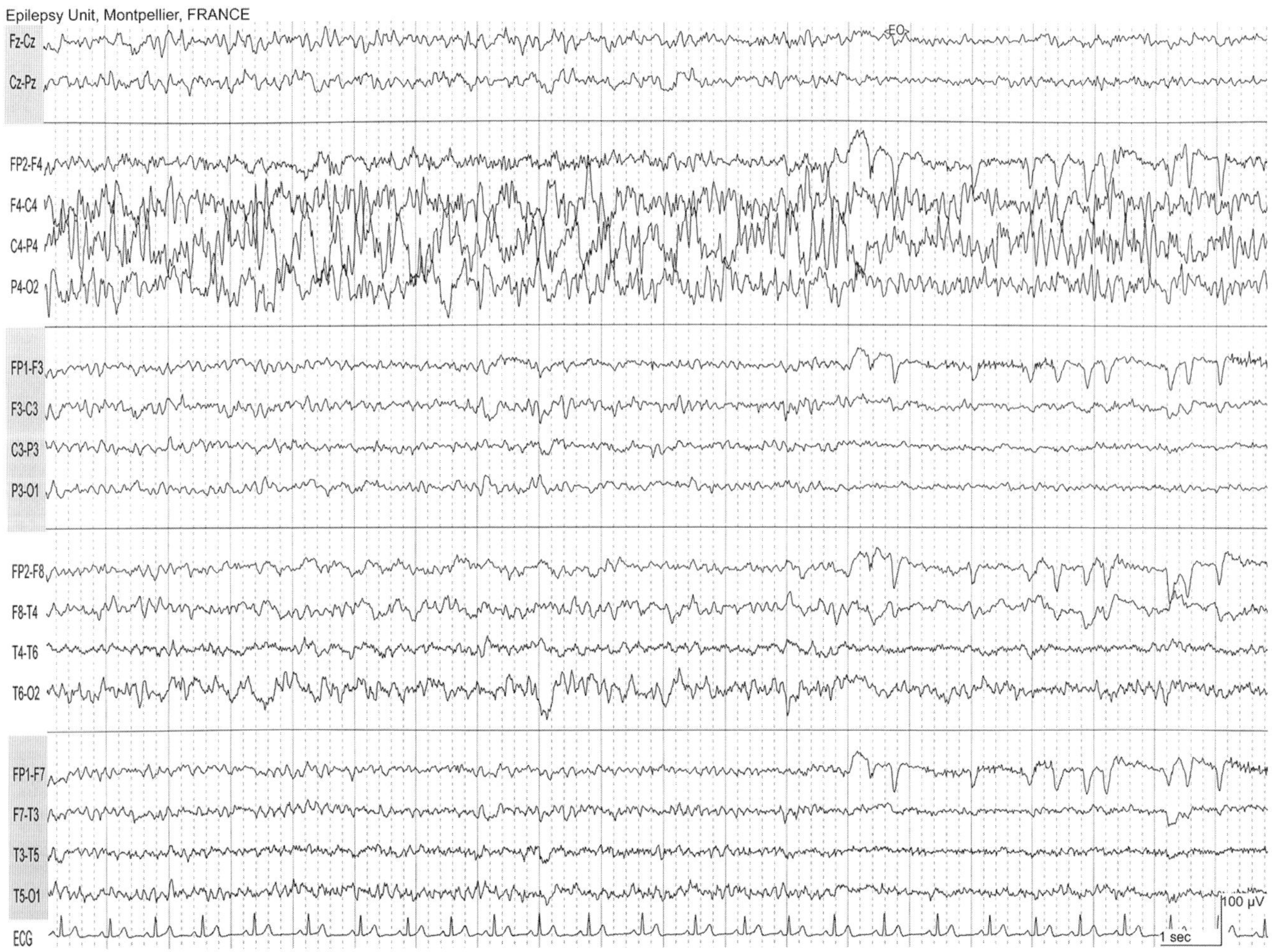

Figure a / Recording at 15 mm/s.

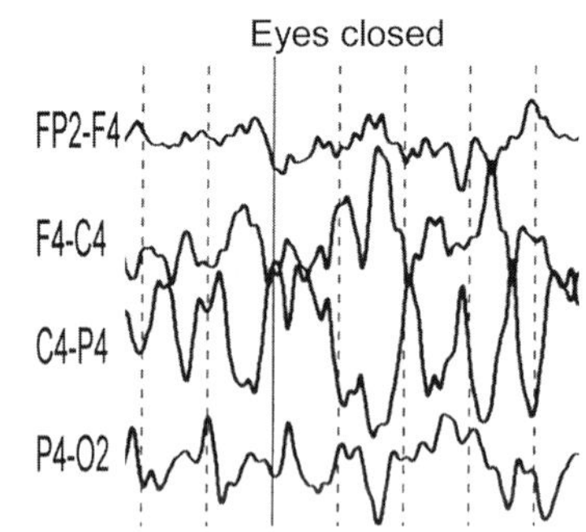

Figure b / Slow and sharp-contoured components at F4-C4, C4-P4 (breach rhythm).

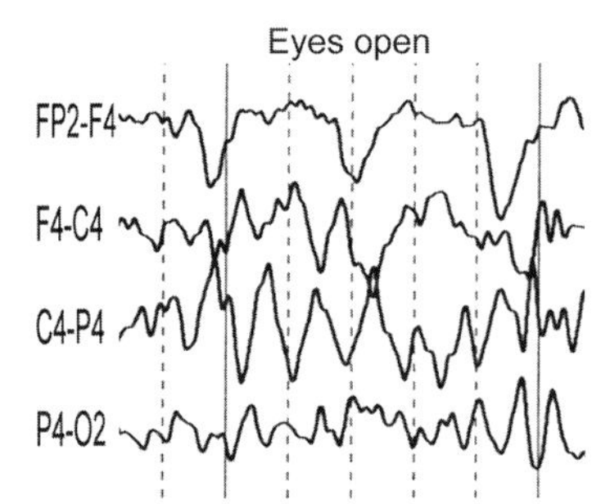

Figure c / Breach rhythm is more typical upon eye opening (eyelid movement artifacts at Fp2-F4).

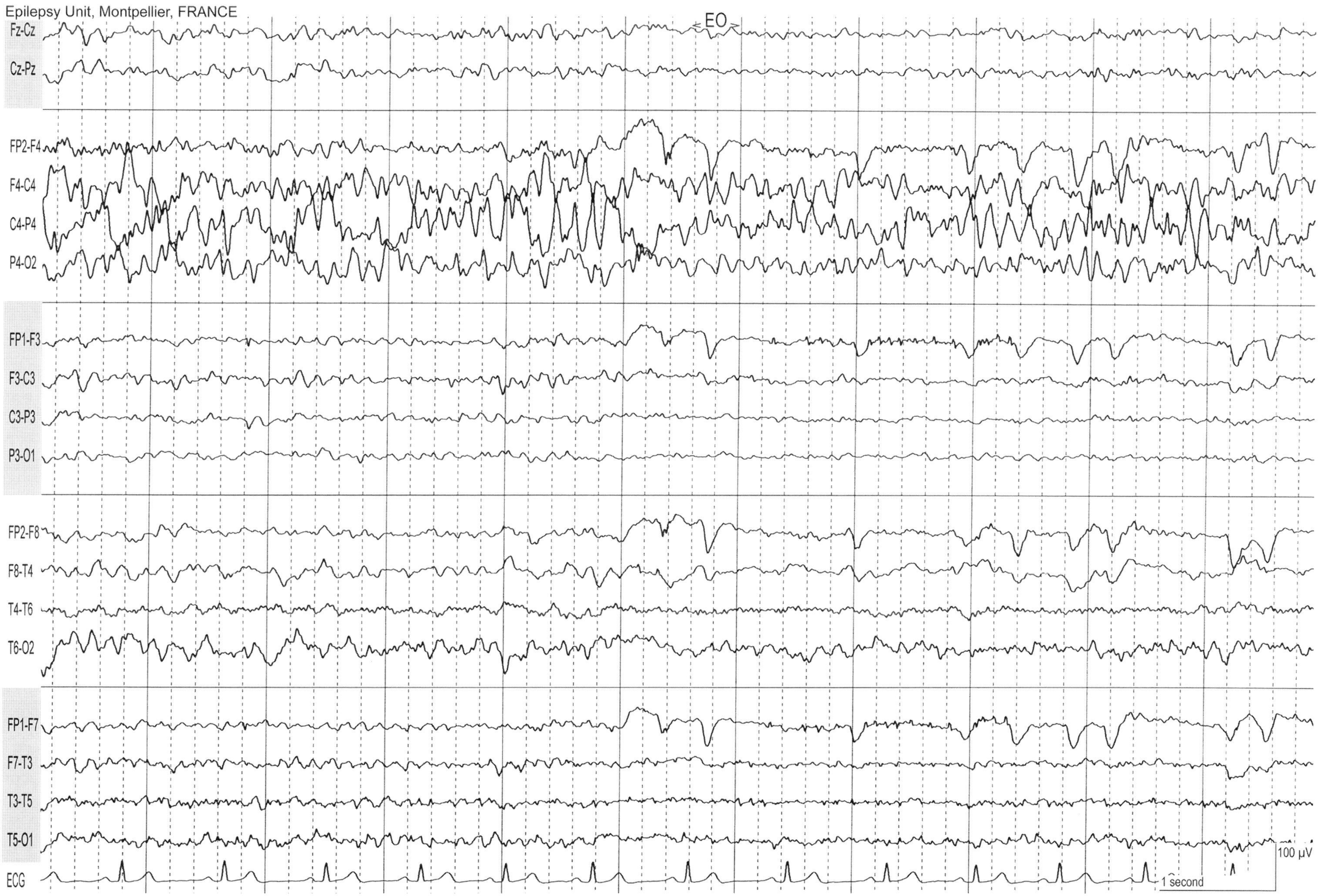
Epilepsy Unit, Montpellier, FRANCE
EO
Fz-Cz
Cz-Pz
FP2-F4
F4-C4
C4-P4
P4-O2
FP1-F3
F3-C3
C3-P3
P3-O1
FP2-F8
F8-T4
T4-T6
T6-O2
FP1-F7
F7-T3
T3-T5
T5-O1
ECG
100 µV
1 second

• 37 When the EEG complicates the situation. Benign spike-waves without epilepsy (1)

Context

3-year-old boy with a typical vasovagal syncope.

What to note

The child is awake, eyes closed. Alpha background activity at 8 Hz intermixed with posterior slow waves of youth. At the frontal polar derivations, irregular waves can be seen corresponding to eye movements. On the right central region, occurrence of diphasic spike-waves, isolated or in a burst. The spikes spread to the right midtemporal region. This presentation in burst is characteristic for idiopathic focal epilepsy with centro-temporal spikes. However, this child had no seizure. His psychomotor development was normal. The changes observed on the EEG evoke age-dependent functional spikes. They can be observed in children who do not display type of epilepsy. The spikes disappear at puberty.

Comment

Beaussart (1972) reported that, in a cohort of 315 children with rolandic spikes, 16% were not epileptic. Cavazzuti *et al.* (1980) observed rolandic spikes in 2.3% of 3,726 healthy children.

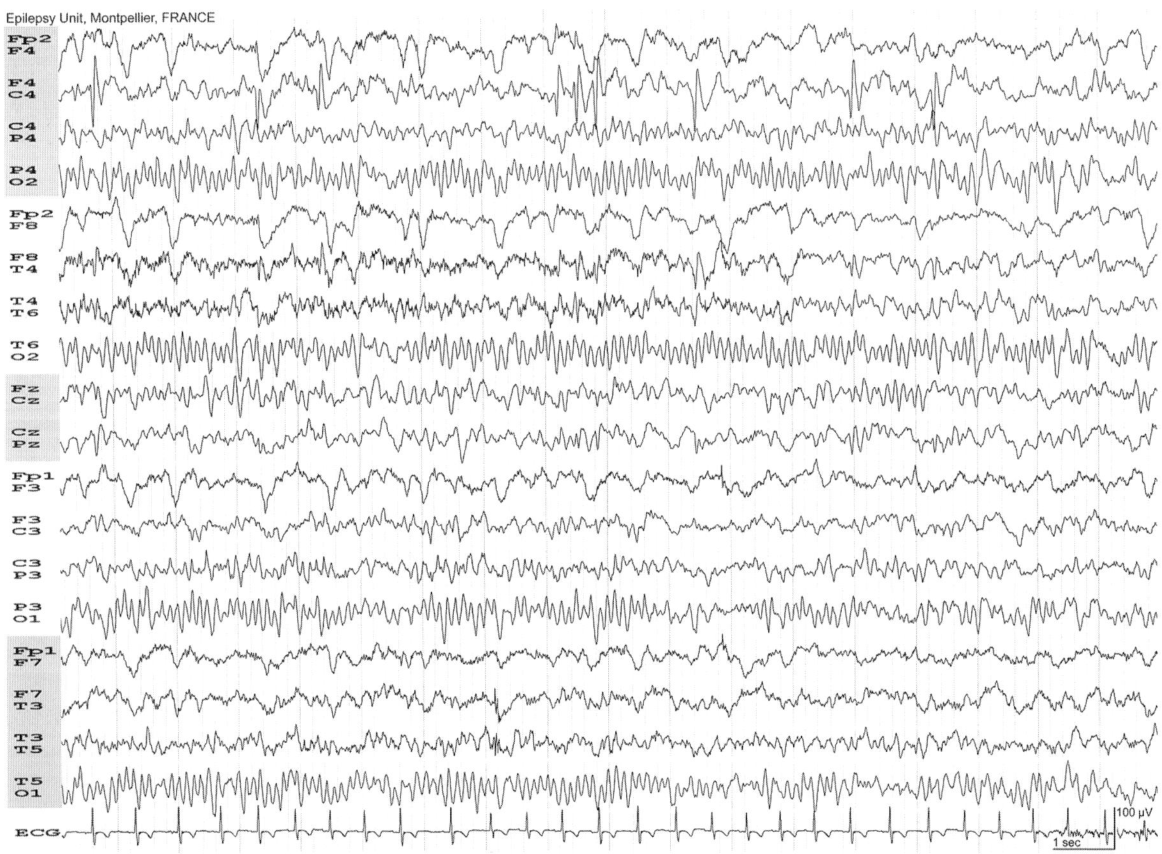

Figure a / Recording at 15 mm/s.

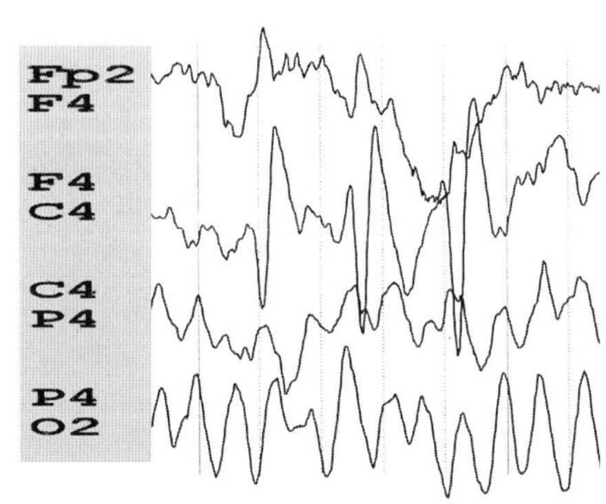

Figure b / Diphasic spike-waves in a burst (F4-C4). Alpha rhythm at 8 Hz.

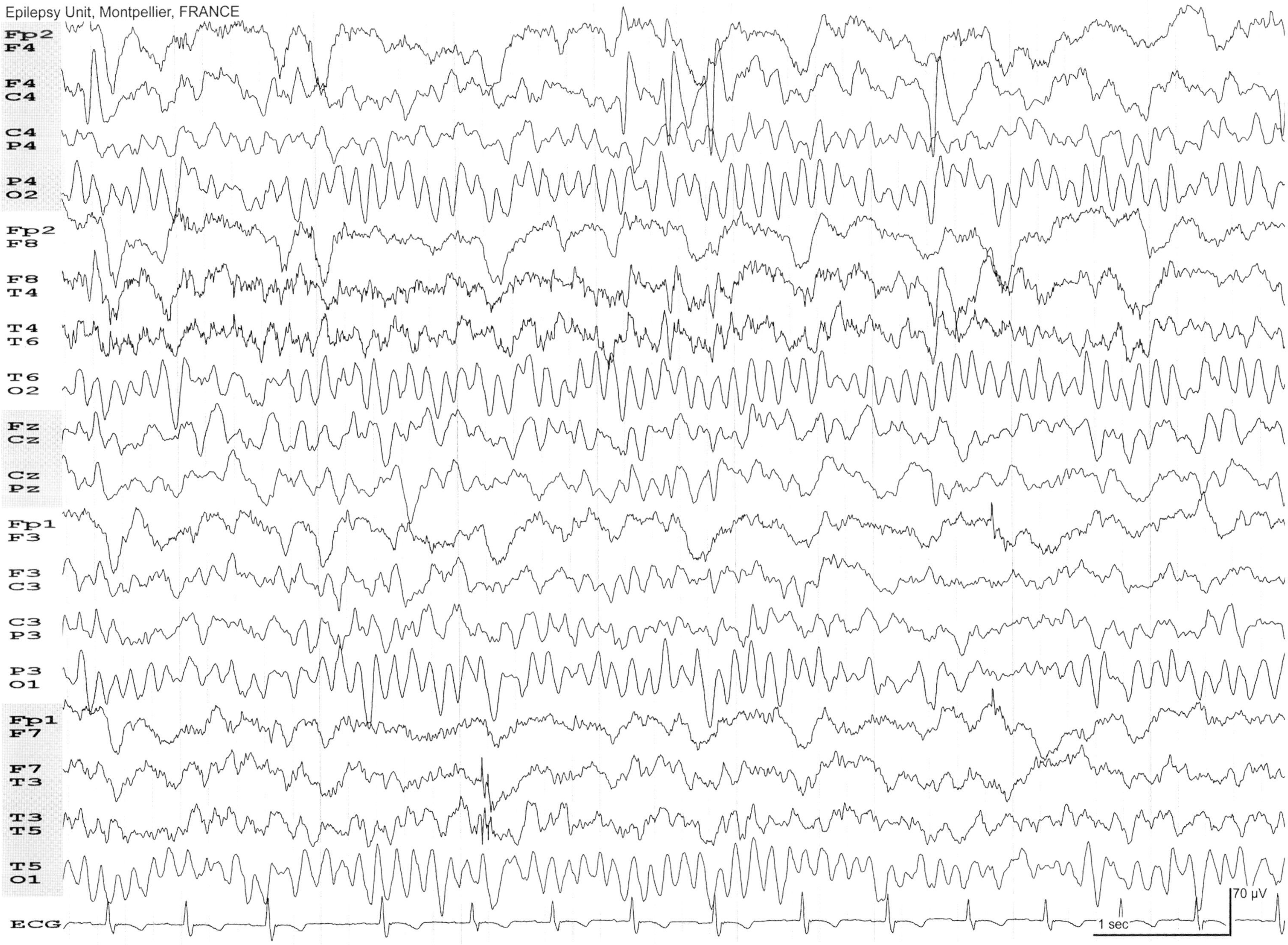
Epilepsy Unit, Montpellier, FRANCE
Fp2 F4
F4 C4
C4 P4
P4 O2
Fp2 F8
F8 T4
T4 T6
T6 O2
Fz Cz
Cz Pz
Fp1 F3
F3 C3
C3 P3
P3 O1
Fp1 F7
F7 T3
T3 T5
T5 O1
ECG
70 µV
1 sec

• 38 When the EEG complicates the situation. Benign spike-waves without epilepsy (2)

Context

3-year-old boy with typical vasovagal syncopes.

What to note

Amplitude is reduced to 15 µV/mm. Eyes closed for 6.5 seconds. Background activity with a 6 to 7 Hz theta rhythm. The theta rhythm blocks on eye opening (eyelid movement artifact on the frontal-polar derivations). When the eyes are closed, high voltage spike-waves over the right occipital region that spread to the left occipital region, and are blocked the eyes open. The morphology of the spike-waves and the reactivity upon eye opening evoked an idiopathic focal epilepsy of childhood (Panayiotopoulos syndrome). This child was asymptomatic with a follow-up of 3 years. The syncopes were typical. They were always triggered to an acute pain. They did not correspond to an ictal syncope sometimes seen in Panayiotopoulos syndrome. Cardiologic assessment was normal.

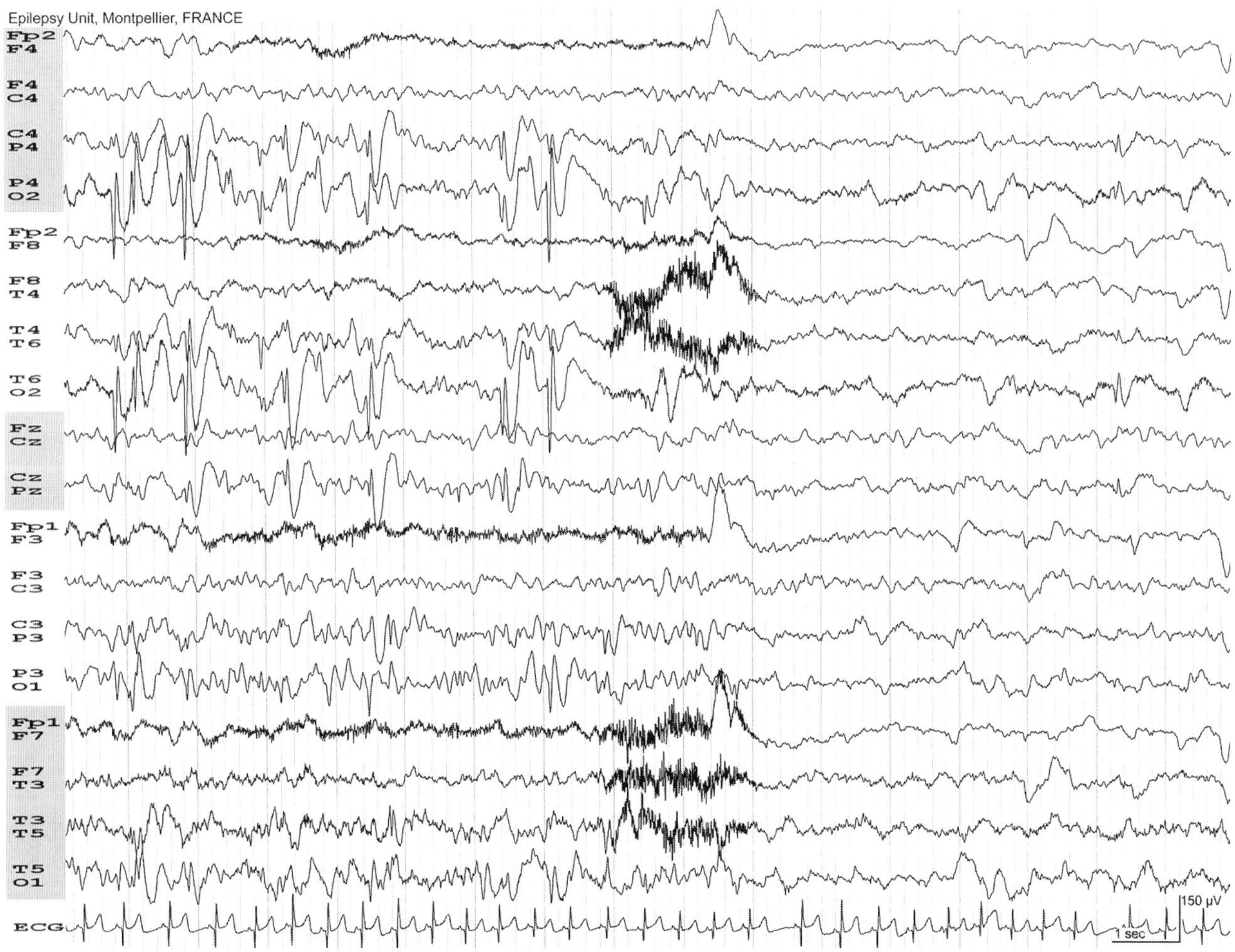

Figure a / Recording at 15 mm/s. Note the reactivity of the spike-waves upon eye opening.

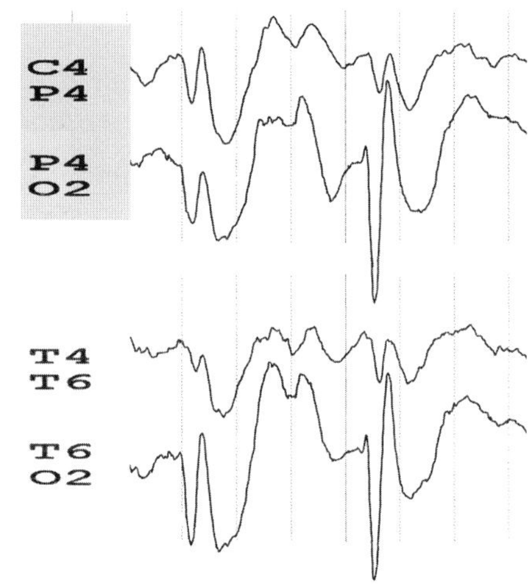

Figure b / Diphasic spike-waves.

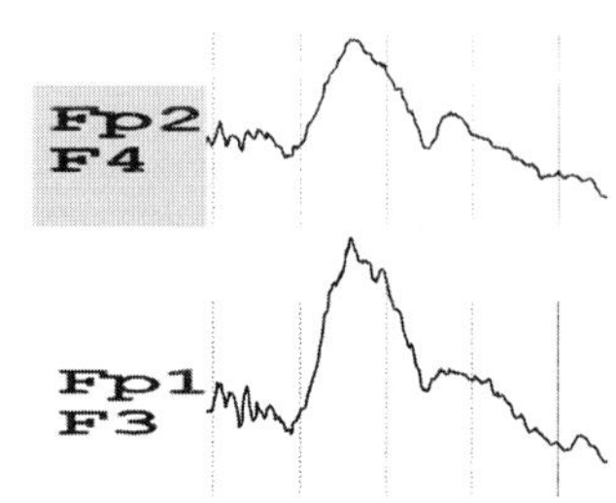

Figure c / Eyelid movement artifact.

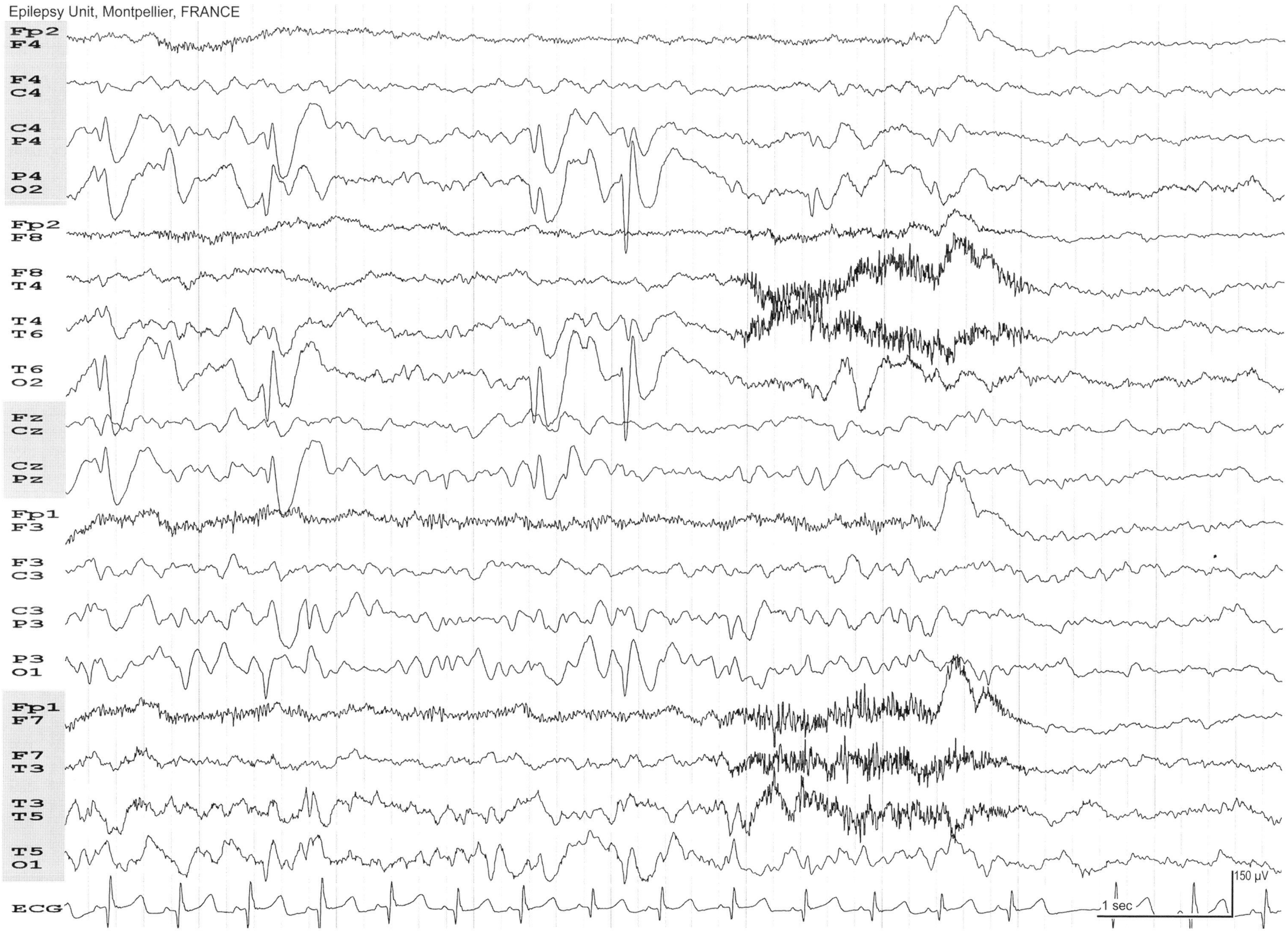
Epilepsy Unit, Montpellier, FRANCE
Fp2 F4
F4 C4
C4 P4
P4 O2
Fp2 F8
F8 T4
T4 T6
T6 O2
Fz Cz
Cz Pz
Fp1 F3
F3 C3
C3 P3
P3 O1
Fp1 F7
F7 T3
T3 T5
T5 O1
ECG
150 µV
1 sec

• 39 When the EEG complicates the situation. Generalized spike-waves without epilepsy

Context

19-year-old woman with a typical vasovagal syncope.

What to note

The patient's eyes are open. Burst of generalized spike-waves. The morphology evokes an idiopathic generalized epilepsy but the patient had no seizure (myoclonic jerks, absence or generalized tonic-clonic seizure). She had a typical vasovagal syncope, misdiagnosed as a seizure and after a first EEG with generalized spike-waves, she received antiepileptic drugs. After this EEG, the treatment was stopped. This patient had a genetic predisposition to idiopathic generalized epilepsy but no epilepsy. She was advised to avoid sleep deprivation and alcohol abuse.

Comment

These three examples indicate how important the clinical context is when interpreting an EEG. The presence of spikes or spike-waves does not necessarily indicate that a patient has epilepsy.

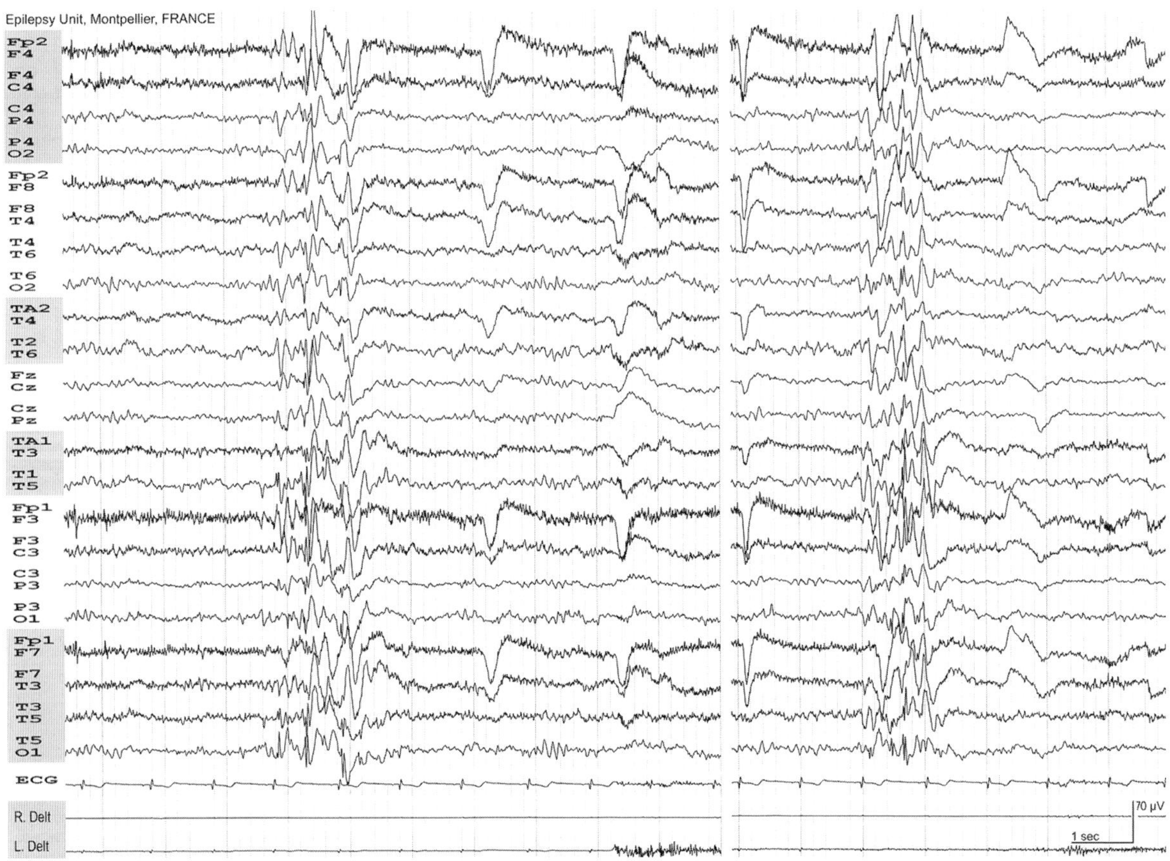

Figure a / Recording at 15 mm/s. Right segment, another example of generalized spike-waves for this patient during the same recording.

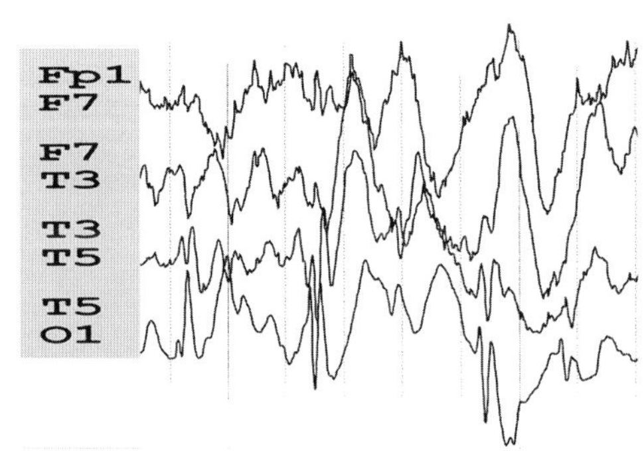

Figure b / Burst of spike-waves. Predominance of the spikes over the posterior region.

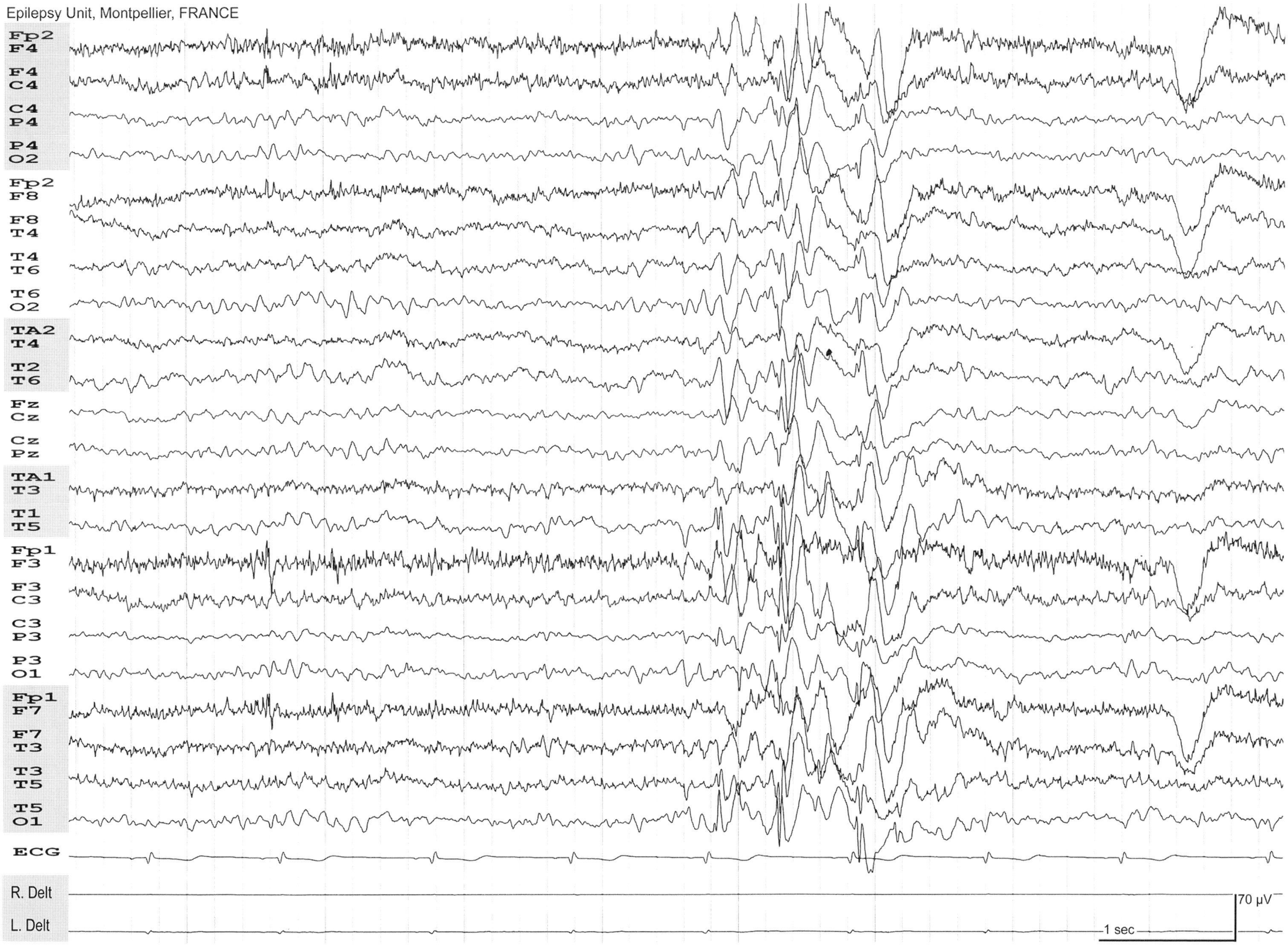
Epilepsy Unit, Montpellier, FRANCE
Fp2 F4
F4 C4
C4 P4
P4 O2
Fp2 F8
F8 T4
T4 T6
T6 O2
TA2 T4
T2 T6
Fz Cz
Cz Pz
TA1 T3
T1 T5
Fp1 F3
F3 C3
C3 P3
P3 O1
Fp1 F7
F7 T3
T3 T5
T5 O1
ECG
R. Delt
L. Delt
70 µV
1 sec

Activation procedures

CHAPITRE II

HYPERVENTILATION

Hyperventilation is routinely performed by asking the patient to accelerate and amplify his breathing until he reaches a frequency of 20 per minute. It is considered an activation procedure since it increases the likelihood of abnormalities. Cerebral hypocapnia is obtained with deep breathing both in and out, but breathing out must be deeper.

Mechanism

The precise mechanism by which hyperventilation provokes EEG changes remains unknown. It is supposed that cerebral hypocapnia-induced vasoconstriction leads to hypoxia of some degree.

Method

• Contra-indications

Prior to an EEG recording, all contra-indications for carrying out hyperventilation must be ruled out in the patient. Recent subarachnoidal hemorrhage (risk of arterial spasms), intracranial hypertension, sickle-cell disease or trait, and moyamoya disease are strict contra-indications. Cardiac insufficiency, respiratory insufficiency, and old age in some cases can be contra-indications as well.

• Hyperventilation procedure

Inspiration must be deep and exhalation deeper than the inspiration, until accelerated respiratory frequency reaches 20 per minute. It is often necessary to do a short test before starting to make sure the patient has understood the procedure. Miming the way to breathe in and out can be useful. It is important to give the patient active support because hyperventilation, when carried out correctly, is tiresome.

Hyperventilation should be performed for at least 3 minutes, but it can be shorter when the patient finds it too unpleasant. The test can be prolonged up to 5 minutes in some cases. After 5 minutes, there is a risk of tiredness or even a fainting spell so that hyperventilation cannot be performed correctly. Hyperventilation can also trigger finger and/or peribuccal paresthesias as well as anxiety attacks.

Hyperventilation should be performed a second time at the end of the recording session. A third or even fourth hyperventilation may be required in some cases (e.g. due to poor conditions in previous hyperventilations or a suspicion of childhood absence epilepsy). It is important to continue the recording several minutes after the end of the last hyperventilation.

Having children blow on pinwheels or imagine they are blowing out candles can be helpful with children as young as age 4 or even 3 years provided they are calm. Crying, which often occurs during EEG recording sessions, can provide useful hyperventilation conditions in very young children.

• When the procedure should be interrupted

The procedure should be interrupted if a significantly abnormal heart beat is observed, if the patient does not feel well, and of course if an acute event occurs.

Observed patterns: slow waves and paroxysmal discharges

Cerebral hypoxia can activate localized or more generalized slowing, which can be physiological or pathological, epileptic paroxysms, or eventually focal or generalized seizures.

• EEG slowing

An increase in amplitude of theta and delta waves indicates the slowing. In children, the slow waves are postero-anterior dominant. In adults, they are typically antero-posterior dominant.

Although more commonly observed in patients with epilepsy, slowing alone is not a diagnostic criterion. EEG slowing is observed in 97% of epileptic children ages 3 to 5 years versus 70% of normal children ages 3 to 5 years. EEG slowing also occurs in 40% in epileptic adults over age 20 years versus 10% in normal adults (Gibbs *et al.*, 1943).

Deep breathing, hypoglycemia (patients on an empty stomach for the EEG), and prolonged standing up can increase the slowing. EEG slowing continues more or less following termination of hyperventilation. It can persist between 30 and 60 seconds in a normal adult, but the immediate cessation is highly suggestive of a physiological slowing. The term used to describe a high-voltage physiological slowing, which occur typically in children, is hypersynchrony hyperventilation.

• Epileptiform activities

Hyperventilation can induce epileptiform patterns in cases of generalized or focal epilepsies. A wide range of interictal abnormalities can be seen (spikes, spike-waves, polyspikes, polyspike-waves), and sometimes seizures can occur during hyperventilation. Hyperventilation is particularly useful for activating typical absences in childhood or in adolescence. Diagnosis of childhood absence epilepsy should therefore be questioned if no absences are observed despite three hyperventilations performed in satisfactory conditions during one EEG recording session.

INTERMITTENT PHOTIC STIMULATION

Intermittent photic stimulation (IPS) is performed with light flashed at the patient's eyes at different frequencies. Photic stimulation is most effective for inducing and recording physiological or pathological photosensitive activities.

Method

• Contra-indications

Photic stimulation is strictly contra-indicated in recent detachment of the retina, recent eye surgery, keratitis and dilated pupils.

• Equipment and protocols

To perform photic stimulation, a stroboscopic light flash is used to deliver white, yellow, or orange flashes, each flash lasting 200 ms with intensity from 0.5 to 60 Hz. Occipital derivations must be included in the EEG recording. It is interesting to perform an EMG polygraphy concomitant to photic stimulation to assess occurrence of myoclonic seizures.

Several photic stimulation protocols have been used. In Brickford's 1979 protocol, a stroboscope is placed directly in front of the patient's eyes at a distance of 20 to 30 cm. Light flashes occur every 5 seconds, first with open eyes and then with closed eyes. The frequencies used are 1, 3, 6, 9, 10, 15, 20 and 30 Hz. Photic stimulation is carried out in a dimly-lit room. Kasteleijn-Nolst Trenite *et al.* (2012) recommend using a stroboscope placed 30 cm from the nasion. The flash trains last 5 seconds with 5-second intervals at IPS frequencies of 1, 2, 8, 10, 15, 18, 20, 25, 40, 50, 60 Hz in three conditions: eye closure, eyes closed and eyes open. If there is not enough time, choose eye closure only and stimulate for 7 s per flash frequency. When in doubt if a frequency has provoked a generalized response, they recommend to repeat the frequency after a rest of 10 seconds or give a frequency of 1 Hz difference. IPS is carried out in a dimly-lit room.

The protocol we use calls for 5-second flash trains with 7-second rest periods. IPS frequency increases gradually from 1 to 30 Hz by 2 Hz intervals, then decreases gradually in the same way from 30 to 1 Hz. The patient's eyes are closed as the frequencies increase. As the frequencies decrease, the patient closes his/her eyes at the beginning of each train and opens them at the end of each train. If spikes, spike-waves, or polyspike-waves are detected, the flash train must be interrupted immediately and a photosensitivity protocol must be performed.

In the photosensitivity protocol, gradually increasing and decreasing frequencies are tested with the patient's eyes open, closed, and closed at the beginning of each train. The purpose is to obtain the highest and lowest frequencies (when the discharge occurs) in the three latter conditions. It is interesting to use frequencies as high as 60 Hz.

• Photic stimulation procedure

To avoid unpleasantly taking the patient by surprise, he must be warned that lights will be flashed during the recording, and that he will be asked to open and close his eyes. The patient will be asked to avoid additional eyelid movements. Photic stimulation is generally carried out between the two hyperventilations. In some cases, photic stimulation can be performed immediately following hyperventilation to combine two activation procedures.

• When the procedure should be interrupted

If a photoparoxysmal response is obtained, the EEG technologist should not complete photic stimulation. Photic stimulation must be terminated immediately as soon as the photosensitivity range is determined, and of course in case a seizure is triggered.

Observed patterns

In response to photic stimulation, several types of responses can be observed: non pathological or unusual responses, i.e. photic driving or photomyogenic responses, as well as abnormal responses, i.e. paroxysmal photosentive responses (photoparoxysmal responses) and epileptic seizures.

• Photic driving response

Photic driving response consists of rhythmical waveforms over the parieto-occipital regions that run time-locked to a train of repetitive flashes. Photic driving response is obtained at several frequencies. Prevalence of photic driving response varies with age. It increases between 6 years and puberty, decreases in adults and increases again in the elderly.

Photic driving response is generally symmetrical. However, as with background activity, it can be slightly asymmetrical in normal individuals. Asymmetrical photic driving can also be observed in patients presenting a lesion or epilepsy. Driving amplitude is not as high on the side of a lesion but it is higher or occurs only on the side of an epileptic focus. In patients with migraines, driving amplitude is higher than in the general population. In young children, non-pathological driving is often observed at low frequencies.

Nevertheless, photic driving is not always physiological. At low frequencies, it can indicate cerebral vascular disease in the elderly. It can also be observed in individuals with renal failure, metabolic pathologies, as well as in individuals taking lithium. Its amplitude is high in progressive myoclonic epilepsies (Unverricht-Lundborg disease, Lafora disease, ceroido-lipofuschinosis), and in Creutzfeldt-Jakob disease.

• Photomyogenic response

Photomyogenic response corresponds to observable rhythmical contractions of the face and eyelid muscles, which run time-locked with the flashes. Photomyogenic response can also extend to other muscles of the head and neck. The contractions build in intensity as the stimulation continues and cease immediately with the termination of stimulation. Photomyogenic response is observed when the patient's eyes are closed. The formerly used terms were photomyoclonic response or fronto-polar response. It occurs in less than 0.3% of normal individuals and 3% of individuals with epilepsy. Photomyogenic response is more frequently observed in individuals presenting brain stem damage, in individuals with psychiatric disorders, in the elderly, in alcoholics and during withdrawal (alcohol, barbiturates, psychotropics). It often occurs in the range of 12 to 18 Hz.

• Parosysmal photosensitive responses (photoparoxysmal responses)

Paroxysmal photosensitive responses or photoparoxysmal responses (PPRs), also referred to as photoconvulsive responses, are cortical responses. Photoparoxysmal responses to stimulation consist of bilaterally distributed spikes, polyspike-waves or spike-waves. They are most often elicited at flash frequencies ranging from 10 to 30 Hz.

Generalized bilaterally distributed polyspike-waves are observed in 20 to 40% of individuals with idiopathic generalized epilepsies. Myoclonic jerks, absences or a generalized tonic-clonic seizure can also be triggered. A photoparoxysmal response is observed in 3% of focal epilepsies and in 1% of normal individuals. Consequently, observation of a photoparoxysmal response alone should not be used to diagnose epilepsy. However, when an abnormal response continues after termination of stimulation (after-discharge), it does argue strongly for epilepsy. In a normal individual, withdrawal from psychotropic drugs can also induce a photoparoxysmal response.

Other procedures for photosensitivity exploration

Pattern stimulation can also be used to evoke photosensitivity. Geometric patterns with 2 mm black and white stripes are drawn on disks of increasing diameters (6, 12, 24, and 48 cm). The stripes are presented both horizontally and vertically. Photoparoxysmal response can also be triggered by watching television, by passing one's hands in front of the person's eyes, or by repetitive eye blinking. The two latter are sometimes used by patients to trigger seizures intentionally.

EYE COMPRESSION

Eye compression is performed to activate vagal hyperactivity. It may be used to diagnose syncope.

Method

• Contra-indications

This procedure is contra-indicated if the individual has undergone cataract surgery or has a history of severe eye disorders. If the individual has a history of severe cardiac disorders, eye compression should be performed by a cardiologist in a specialized unit. Contact lenses must be removed prior to eye compression.

• Eye compression procedure

Atropine must be kept near at hand, and the procedure explained to the patient. He is asked to close his eyes. The clinician then presses firmly on the closed eyes for 10 seconds. The pressure must be strong enough to obtain whitening of a 2 mm spot on the clinician's fingernail. Intensity of eye compression must be maximal from the onset. If a sinus arrest is obtained, eye compression must be stopped to avoid syncope.

Observed patterns

In individuals presenting vagal hyperactivity, eye compression induces bradycardia with clinical symptoms of varying intensity, the maximum being a syncope. Bradycardia can be delayed, appearing several seconds after termination of eye compression, so it is important to continue the recording even in absence of response concomitant to eye compression.

On the basis of a receiver operating curve, it has been suggested that an abnormal response is six seconds (Stephenson, 1990). However, the development of symptoms recognized by the subject as similar to the spontaneous event, in association with bradycardia or asystole of three to five seconds may be considered positive.

EEG in patients with cardiac arrest was documented long ago (Gastaut and Fischer-Williams 1956, 1957). The sequence is a gradual slowing activity with slow theta waves followed by diffuse delta waves. If the cardiac arrest continues, the EEG becomes isoelectric with no cerebral activity and can show muscle artifacts due to the tonic muscular contraction. Gastaut and Fischer-Williams (1956, 1957) investigated 20 syncopes due to ocular compression (15 seconds), and gave a particularly clear description. Until six seconds, the cardiac arrest had no EEG effect. After six seconds, generalized slow waves appear, the amplitude and duration of which increase to their maximum in a few seconds. If the cardiac arrest does not exceed eight to ten seconds, the EEG manifestations are limited to this "hypersynchrony" with a more or less severe obnubilation (confusion). If the cardiac arrest lasts more than 13 seconds, one or two bilateral jerks appear, preceded by a contraction in opisthotonos, often associated with a deviation of the head, and sometimes followed by one or two jerks but without a regular clonic convulsive phase as in an epileptic seizure. These phenomena are associated with such remarkable electrocerebral inactivity that it abruptly replaces the phase of hypersynchrony. Resumption of heart beat occurs during this 10 to 20 second phase. Immediately after, a new burst of slow waves appears, the amplitude and duration of which decrease progressively. Ten to 30 seconds later, the slow hypersynchrony waves are replaced by an alpha rhythm and the subject becomes regains lucidity.

Another method

It is also possible to perform massages of the carotid sinus. Prior to the massages, the clinician must make sure there is no carotid plaque which could be released due to the procedure. Gentle carotid massages can trigger severe bradycardia and eventually a syncope in predisposed individuals. In this case, the EEG characteristics of the syncope are the same as those obtained with eye compression.

II • 1 Hyperventilation hypersynchrony (1)

Context

7-year-old girl with learning difficulties.

What to note

During hyperventilation. Amplitude is reduced to 15 μV/mm. Burst of high amplitude slow waves that cause blocking at this gain with sharp-contoured waveforms. In this case, hyperventilation hypersynchrony with its sharply-contoured pattern has no pathological signification. This burst of slow angular waveforms can be misinterpreted as a spike-wave discharge.

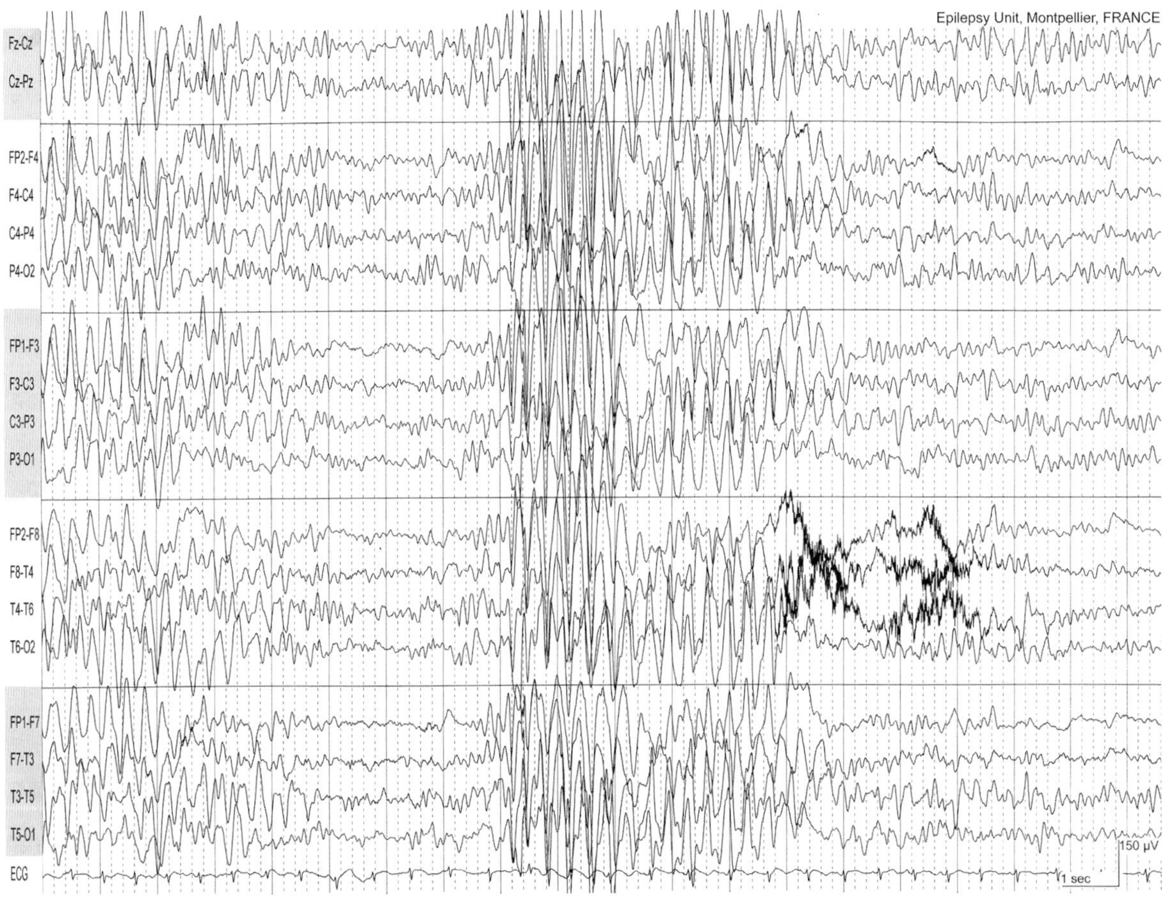

Figure a / Recording at 15 mm/s. At the beginning of the plate, a burst of slow delta waves, then a second burst 3 seconds later.

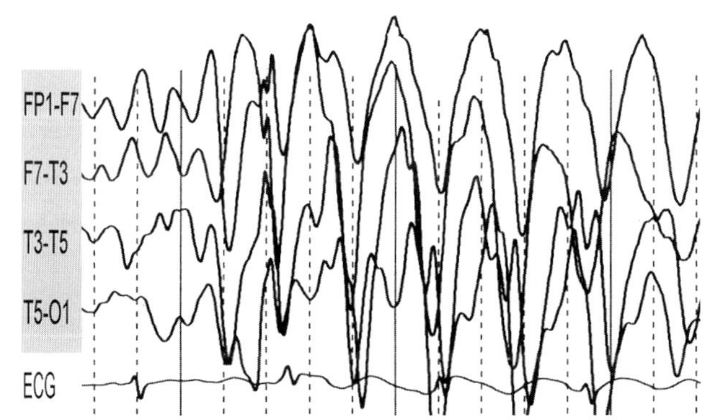

Figure b / Burst with greater amplitude and slow sharp-contoured waveforms; physiological hyperventilation hypersynchrony.

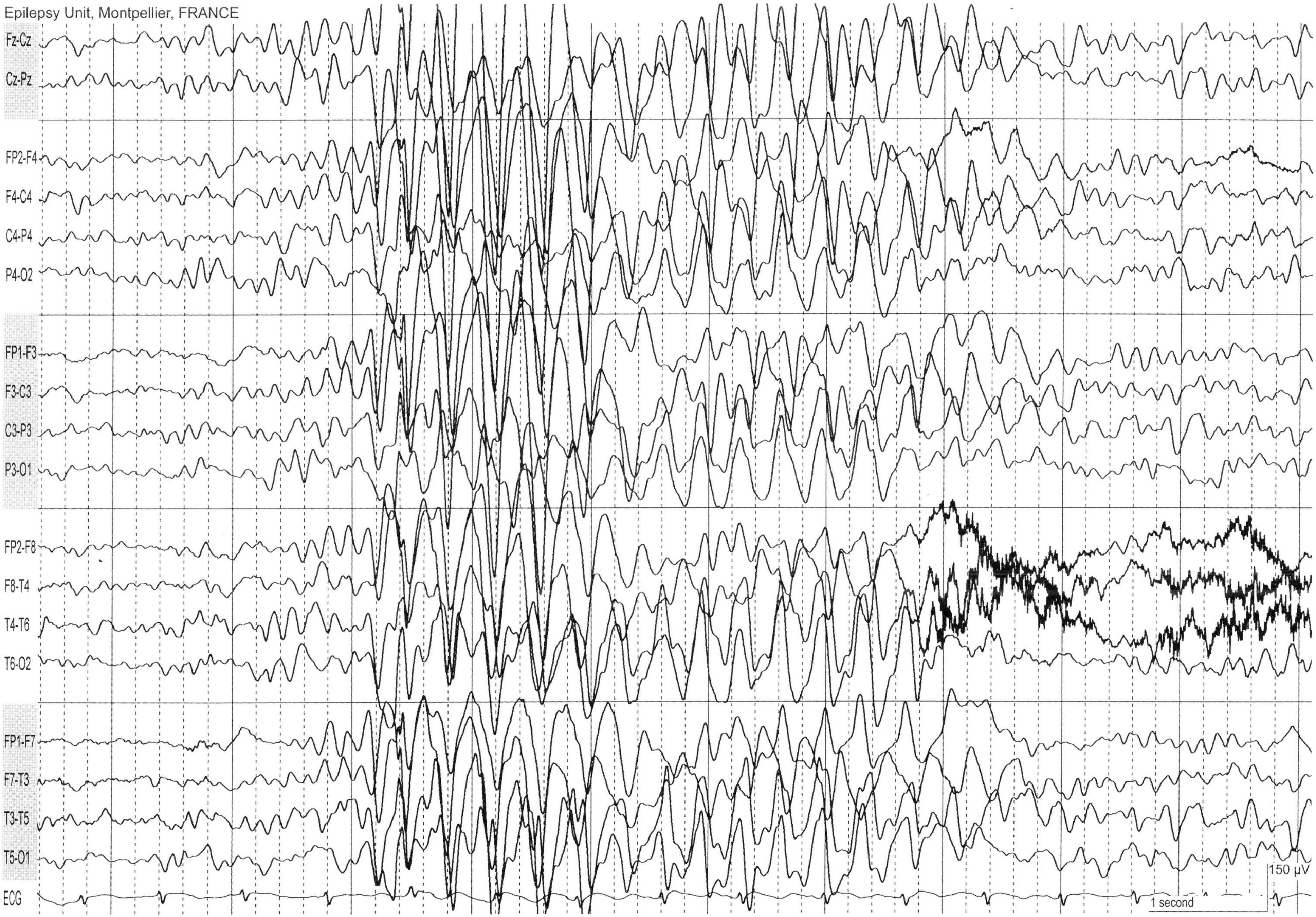
Epilepsy Unit, Montpellier, FRANCE
Fz-Cz
Cz-Pz
FP2-F4
F4-C4
C4-P4
P4-O2
FP1-F3
F3-C3
C3-P3
P3-O1
FP2-F8
F8-T4
T4-T6
T6-O2
FP1-F7
F7-T3
T3-T5
T5-O1
ECG
150 µV
1 second

• 2 Hyperventilation hypersynchrony (2)

Context

10-year-old boy with epilepsy with centro-temporal spikes.

What to note

During hyperventilation. Diffuse slowing including high-amplitude delta waves at 3.5 Hz with a sinusoidal and monomorphic pattern. In this case, hyperventilation hypersynchrony is physiological.

Comment

Hyperventilation hypersynchrony is observed mostly in children and adolescents. It becomes less frequent with age.

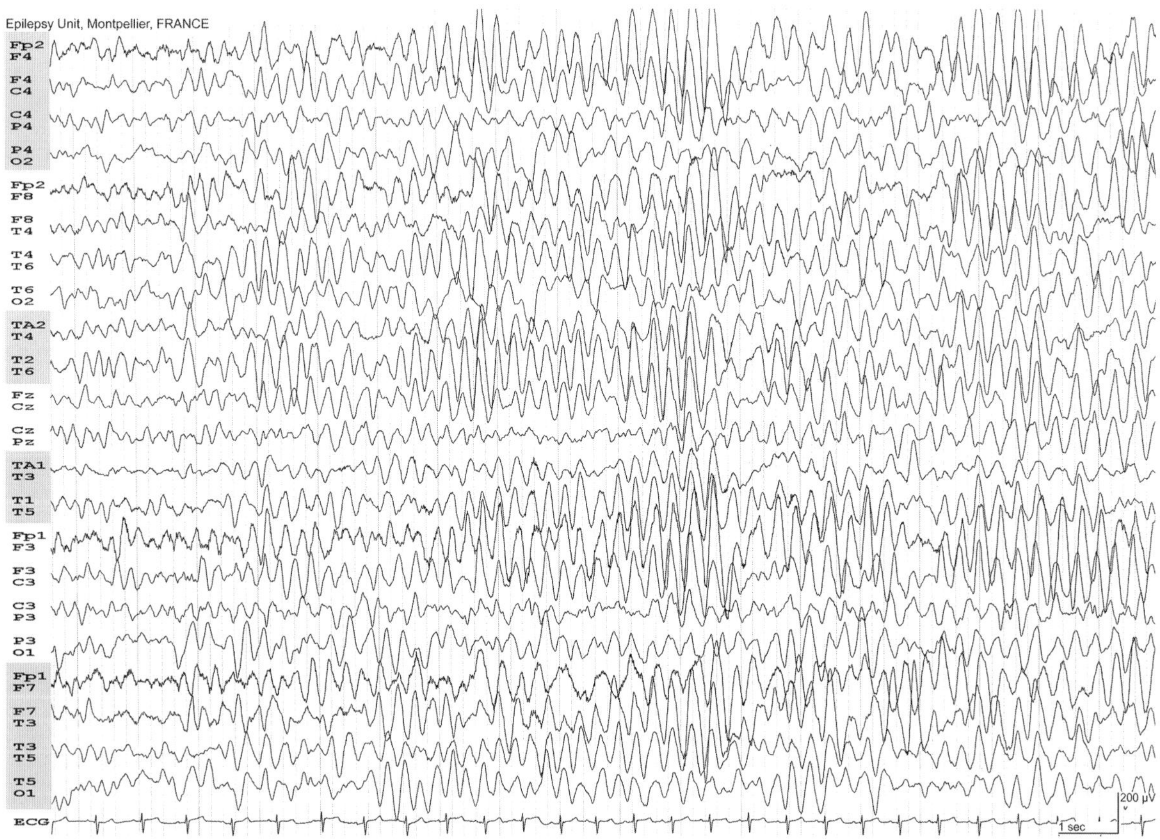

Figure a / Recording at 15 mm/s. Amplitude is reduced to 20 µV/mm. Note the sinusoidal and monomorphic pattern.

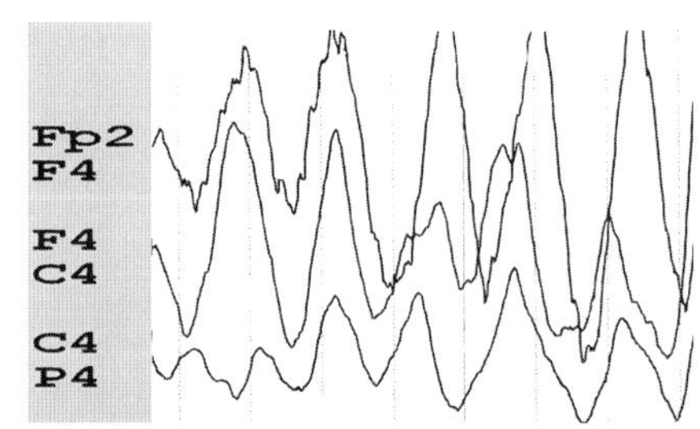

Figure b / Hyperventilation hypersynchrony with slow delta waves at 3.5 Hz.

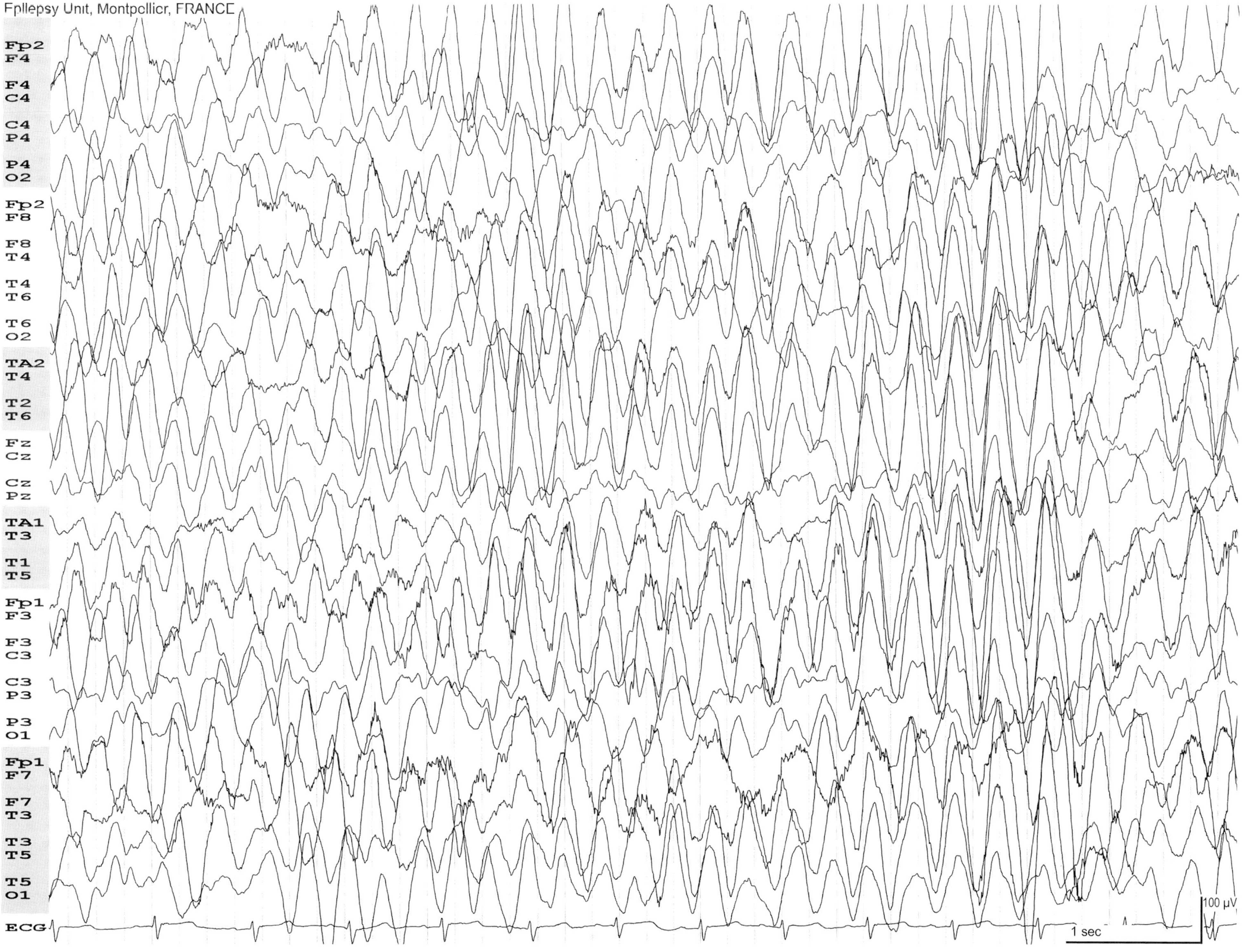
Epilepsy Unit, Montpellier, FRANCE
Fp2 F4
F4 C4
C4 P4
P4 O2
Fp2 F8
F8 T4
T4 T6
T6 O2
TA2 T4
T2 T6
Fz Cz
Cz Pz
TA1 T3
T1 T5
Fp1 F3
F3 C3
C3 P3
P3 O1
Fp1 F7
F7 T3
T3 T5
T5 O1
ECG
100 µV
1 sec

II • 3 Hyperventilation hypersynchrony (3)

Context

38-year-old woman referred for drug resistant epilepsy later diagnosed as vagal syncopes.

What to note

During hyperventilation. A burst of diffuse slow waves at 2.5 Hz. They are no spike-wave. Thus, in this case, hyperventilation hypersynchrony is physiological.

Comment

Hyperventilation hypersynchrony is observed mostly in children and adolescents but can be observed in adults. The burst of slow angular waveforms can be misinterpreted as spike-wave discharge as it was the case in this patient.

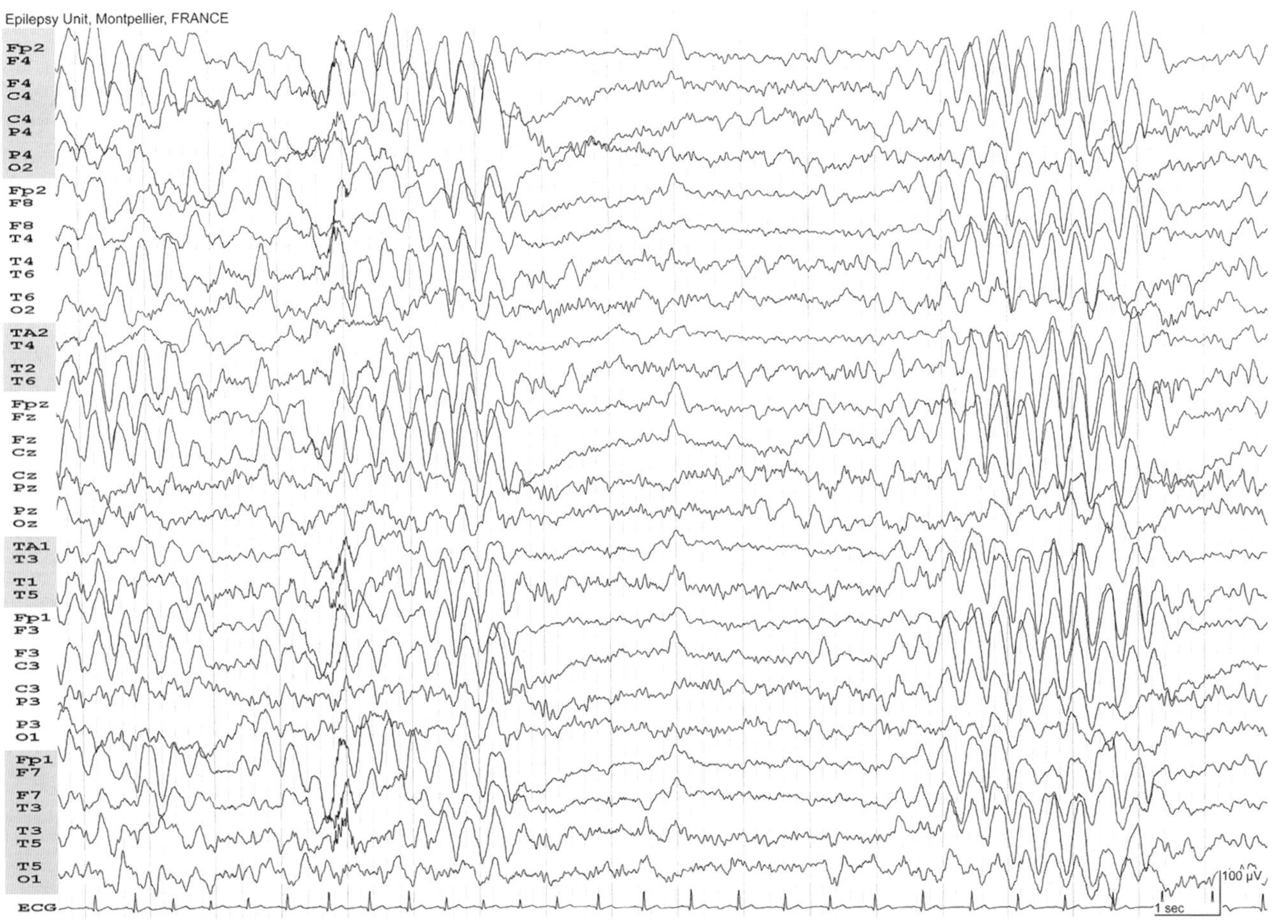

Figure a / Recording at 15 mm/s. At the beginning of the plate, a burst of slow waves, then a second burst and a third burst 6 seconds later. This is typical of physiological hyperventilaton hypersynchrony.

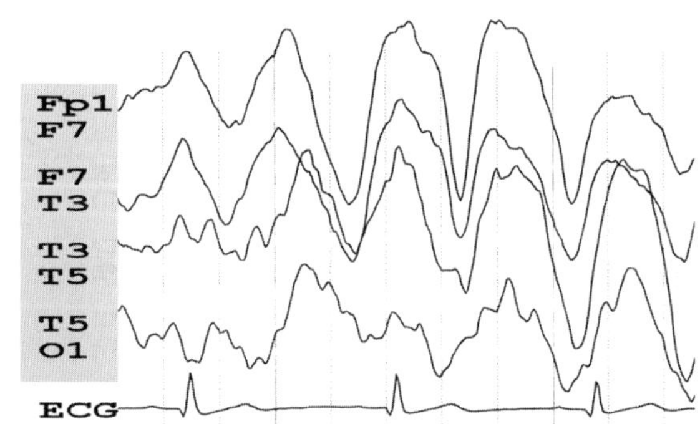

Figure b / Hyperventilation hypersynchrony with slow monomorphic activiy.

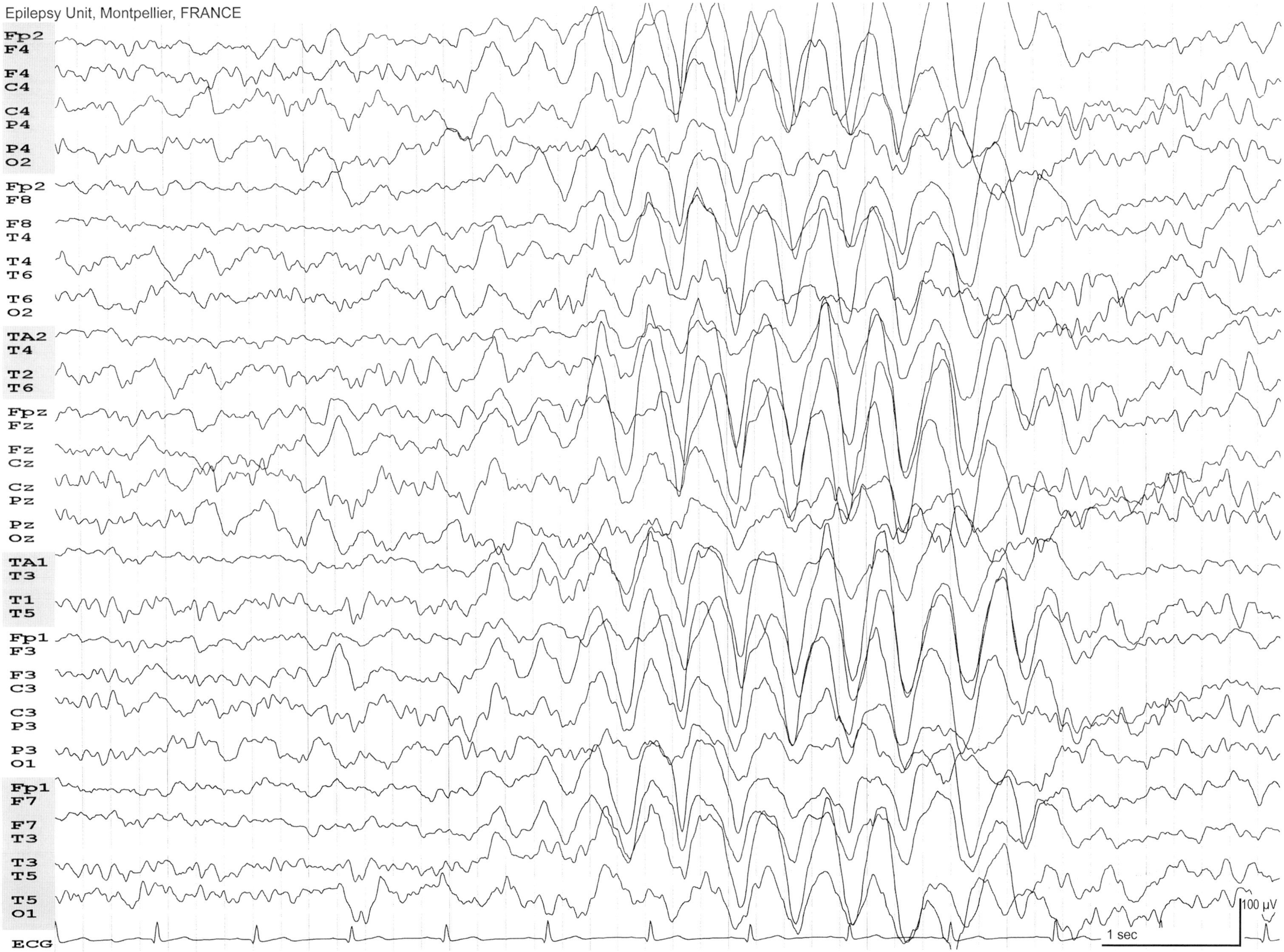
Epilepsy Unit, Montpellier, FRANCE
Fp2 F4
F4 C4
C4 P4
P4 O2
Fp2 F8
F8 T4
T4 T6
T6 O2
TA2 T4
T2 T6
Fpz Fz
Fz Cz
Cz Pz
Pz Oz
TA1 T3
T1 T5
Fp1 F3
F3 C3
C3 P3
P3 O1
Fp1 F7
F7 T3
T3 T5
T5 O1
ECG
100 µV
1 sec

II • 4 Physiological slow waves during hyperventilation

Context

18-year-old boy referred for epilepsy follow-up.

What to note

After 3 minutes of hyperventilation, slowing of background activity and high-voltage diffuse slow waves or anterior activity at 5 Hz. Physiological slowing can be observed during hyperventilation. When slowing occurs on the alpha rhythm it conveys a false impression of spike-waves. An electrode artifact can be seen on T3.

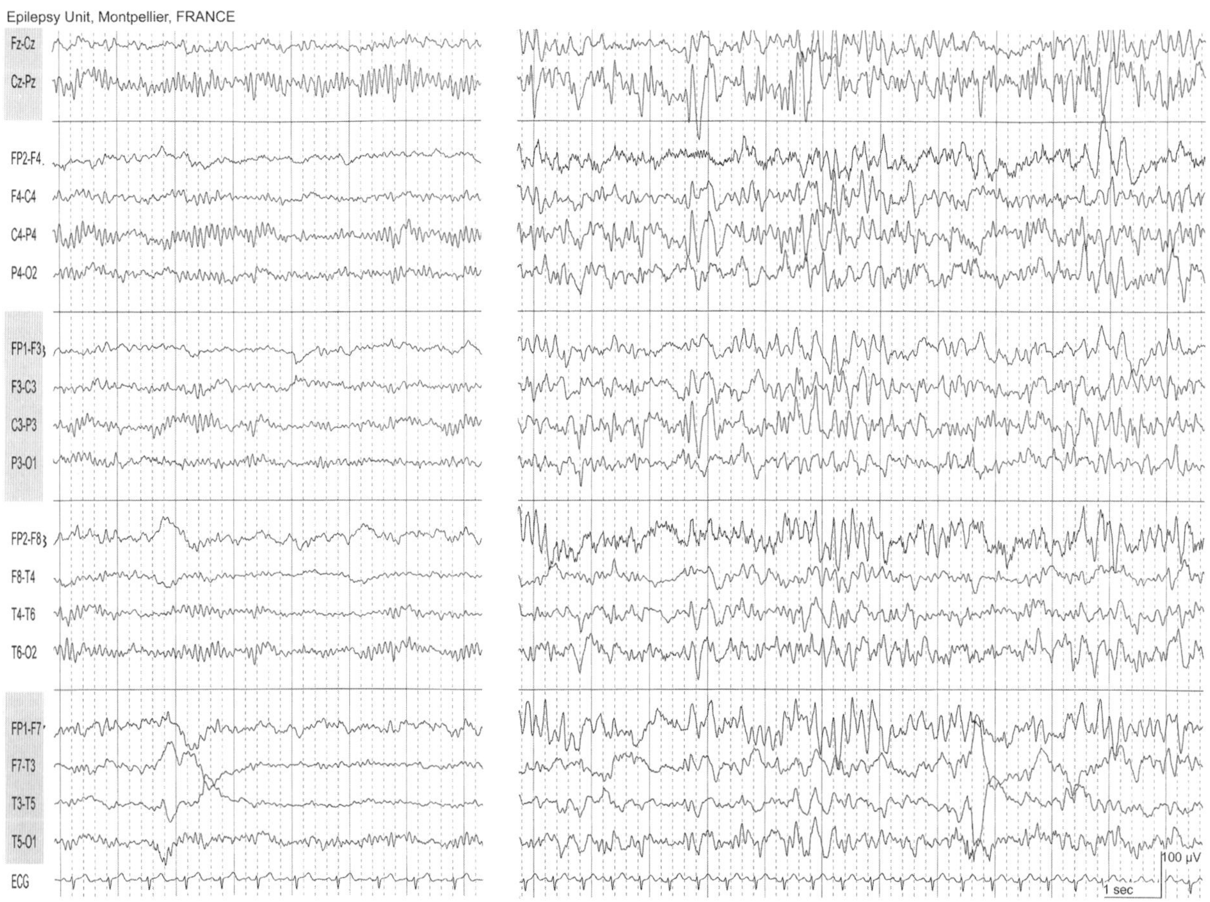

Figure a / Recording at 15 mm/s. On the left plate with eye closed, posterior activity with an alpha rhythm. On the right plate, after 3 minutes of hyperventilation.

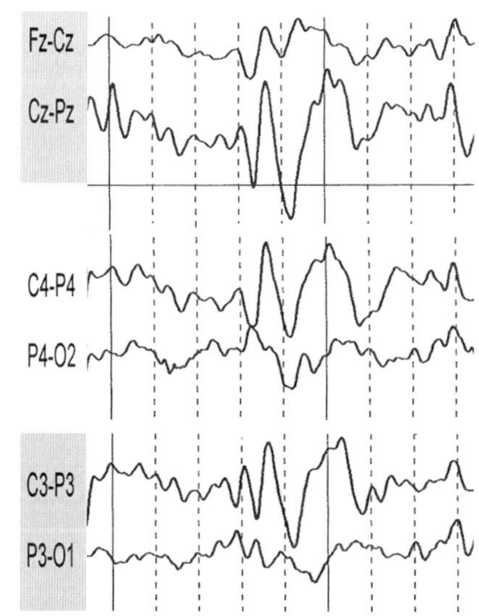

Figure b / Slowing superimposed on the alpha rhythm conveying an impression of spike-waves.

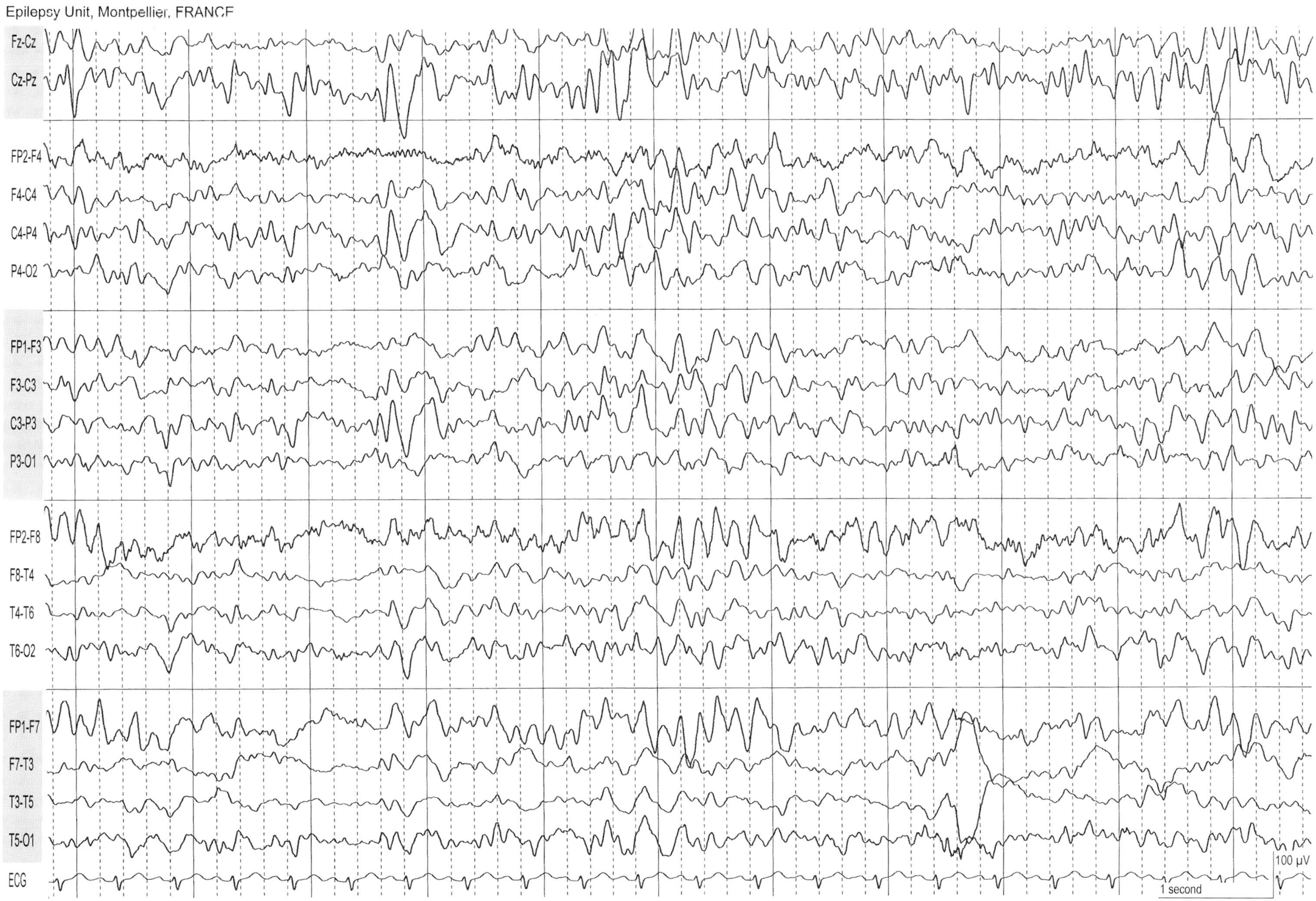
Epilepsy Unit, Montpellier, FRANCE
Fz-Cz
Cz-Pz
FP2-F4
F4-C4
C4-P4
P4-O2
FP1-F3
F3-C3
C3-P3
P3-O1
FP2-F8
F8-T4
T4-T6
T6-O2
FP1-F7
F7-T3
T3-T5
T5-O1
ECG
100 µV
1 second

II • 5 Generalized spike-waves during hyperventilation

Context

19-year-old woman with idiopathic generalized epilepsy.

What to note

After 2 minutes of hyperventilation, slowing of background activity and high-voltage diffuse slow waves corresponding to hypersynchrony. Inside the burst of slow activity, a spike-wave with posterior predominance can be observed. This is an interictal abnormality.

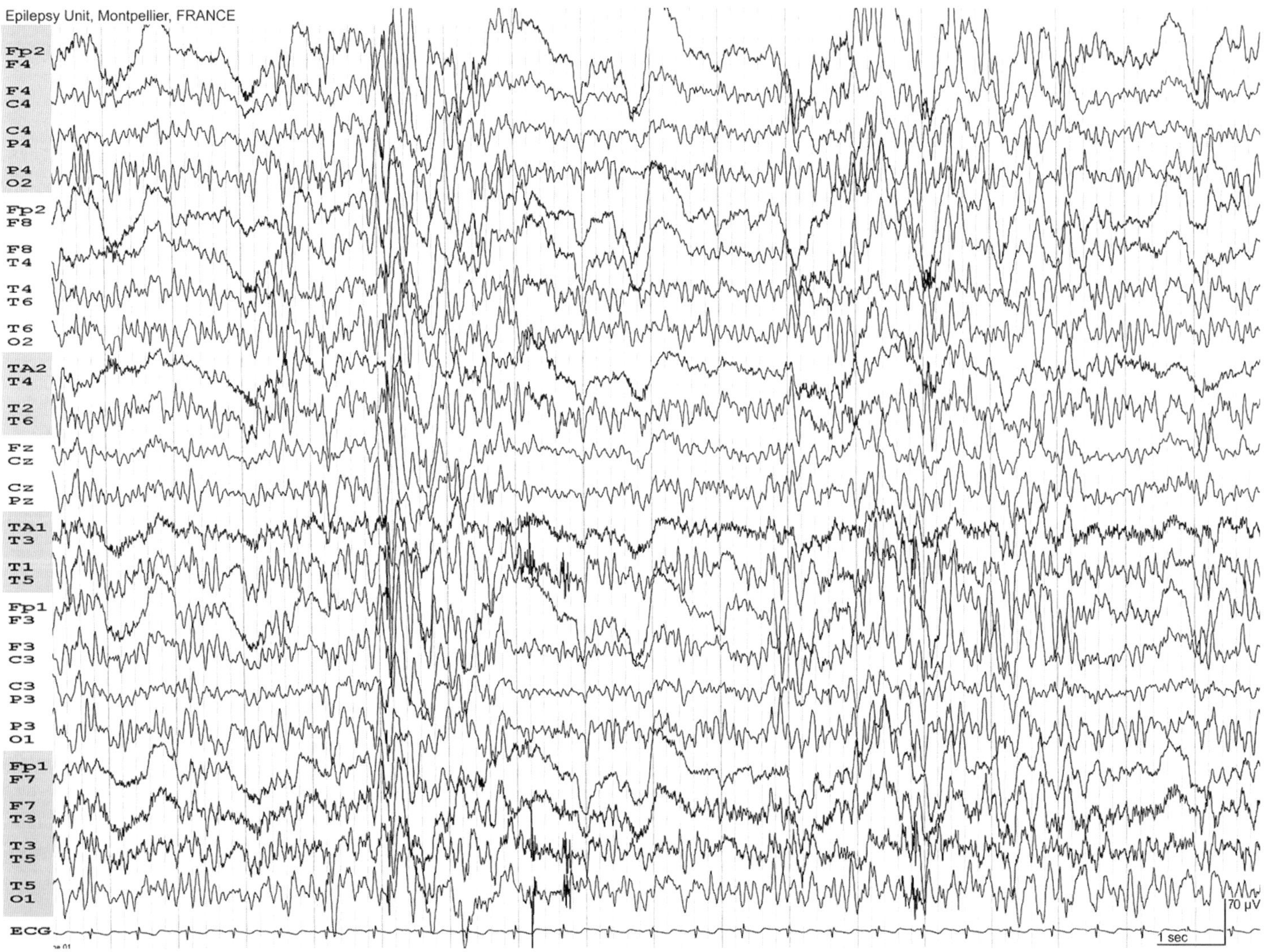

Figure a / Recording at 15 mm/s. Typical physiological hypersynchrony with a spike-wave inside the first burst of high-voltage diffuse slow waves.

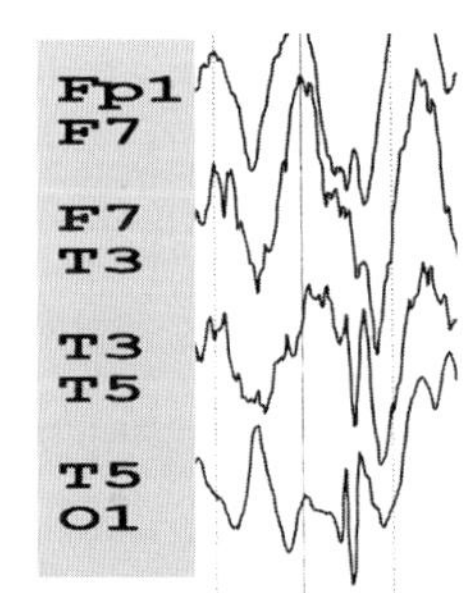

Figure b / Spike-wave.

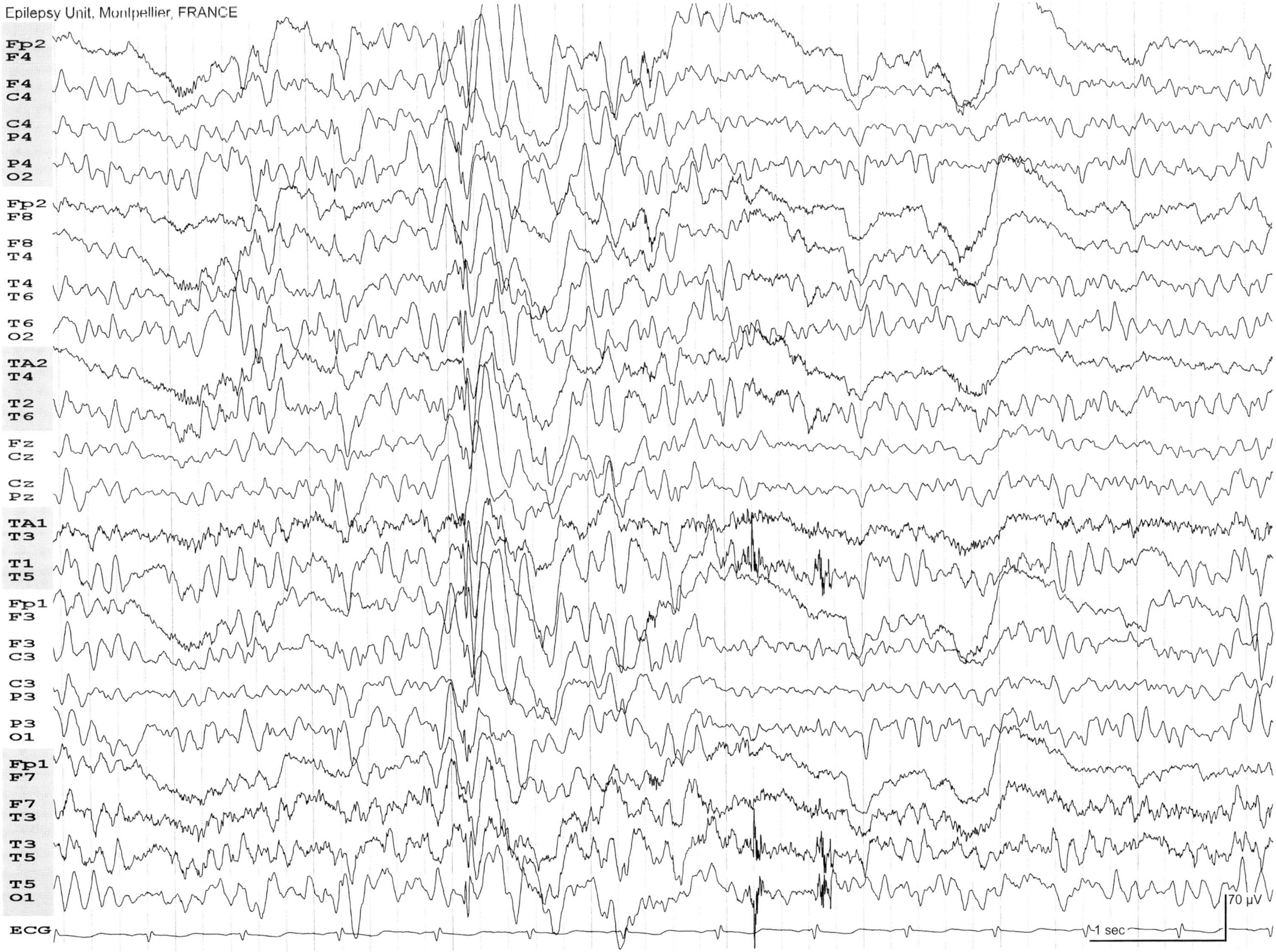
Epilepsy Unit, Montpellier, FRANCE
Fp2
F4
F4
C4
C4
P4
P4
O2
Fp2
F8
F8
T4
T4
T6
T6
O2
TA2
T4
T2
T6
Fz
Cz
Cz
Pz
TA1
T3
T1
T5
Fp1
F3
F3
C3
C3
P3
P3
O1
Fp1
F7
F7
T3
T3
T5
T5
O1
ECG
70 µV
1 sec

II • 6 A typical absence seizure occurring during hyperventilation

Context

9-year-old child referred for drug-resistant childhood absence epilepsy.

What to note

During hyperventilation. Overall background activity is slow and ample. In the middle of this plate, a 4-second burst of very-high-voltage activity with sharp waves. The child's eyes are half closed, he stops breathing, then immediately resumes at the end of the burst. Despite saturation, spike-waves can be detected during the burst. Compare appearance here with hyperventilation hypersynchrony on the preceding plates. Input had to be recalibrated to decrease the amplitude so that the spikes can be more clearly detected. This was performed on the right side of the plate recorded at 15 mm/s. Amplitude was reduced to 30 µV/mm. During the next hyperventilation, the child can be asked to repeatedly tap with his hand throughout the test. If a discharge occurs, the clinician can also pronounce words. If a typical absence occurs, he will stop breathing, will stop tapping and will be unable to repeat the words.

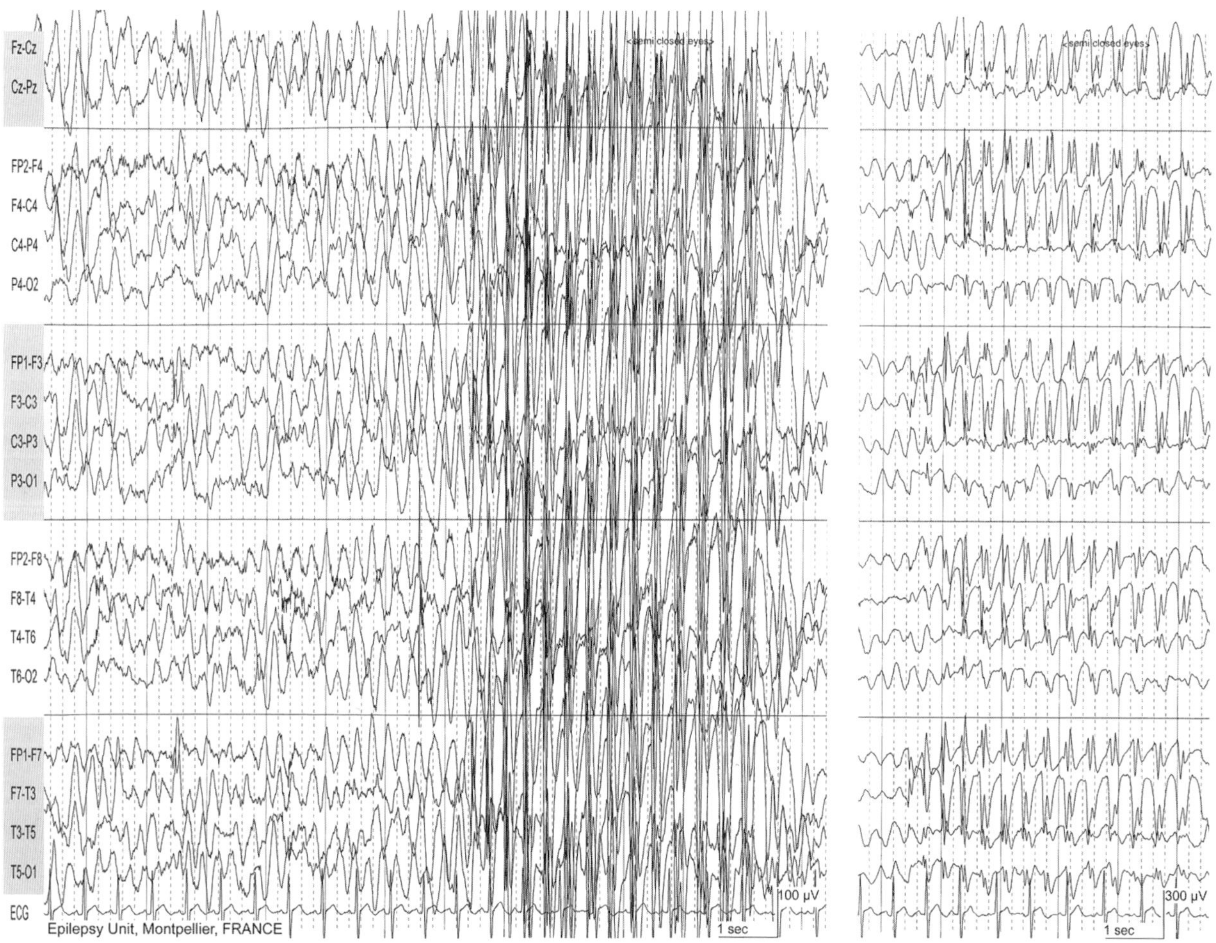

Figure a / Recording at 15 mm/s. Spike-waves are more clearly detectable with lower amplitude at 30 µV/mm.

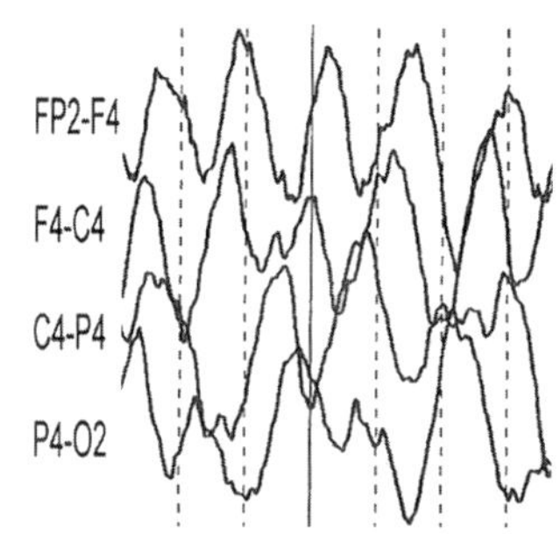

Figure b / Slow background activity during hyperventilation.

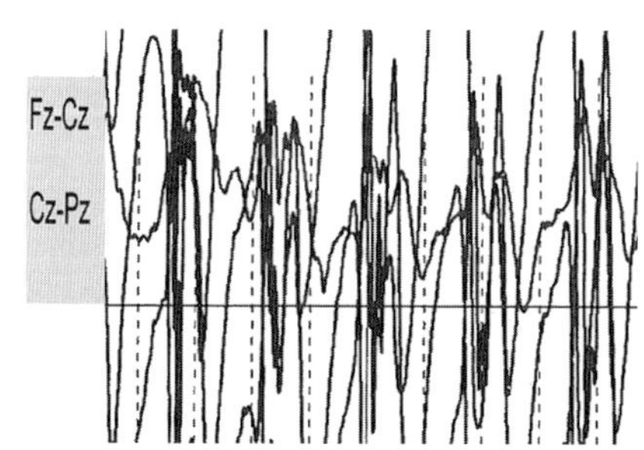

Figure c / Spike-waves occurring during hyperventilation.

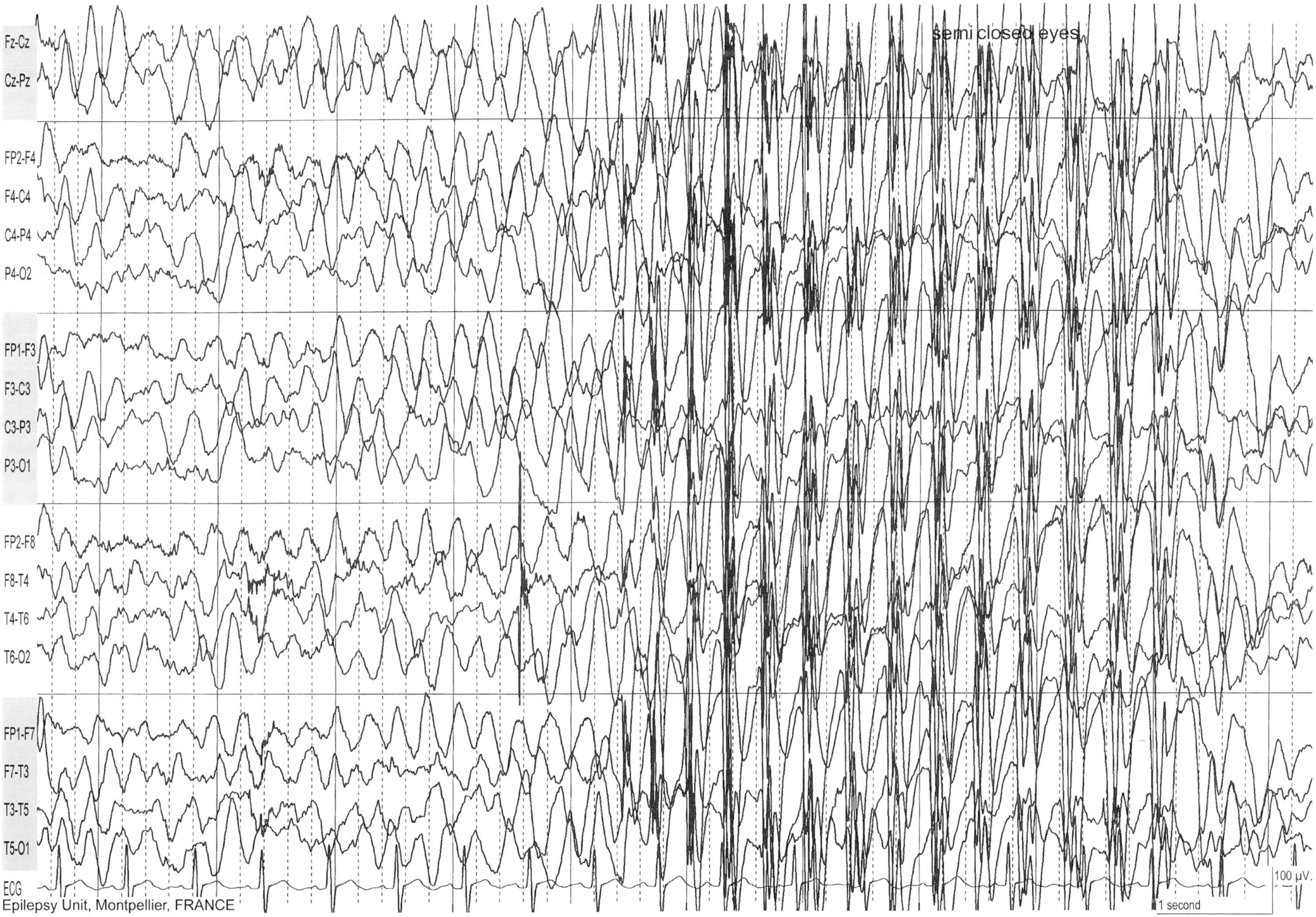
Fz-Cz
Cz-Pz
FP2-F4
F4-C4
C4-P4
P4-O2
FP1-F3
F3-C3
C3-P3
P3-O1
FP2-F8
F8-T4
T4-T6
T6-O2
FP1-F7
F7-T3
T3-T5
T5-O1
ECG
semi closed eyes
100 µV
1 second
Epilepsy Unit, Montpellier, FRANCE

• 7 Focal slow waves during hyperventilation

Context

37-year-old man with lateral temporal lobe epilepsy.

What to note

End of hyperventilation. Background activity with posterior alpha rhythm. Some focal slow theta over the left temporal region. This is not a physiological response. Before hyperventilation, no slow wave or spike had been observed. Rare spikes were only observed in NREM sleep stage 3 (see below).

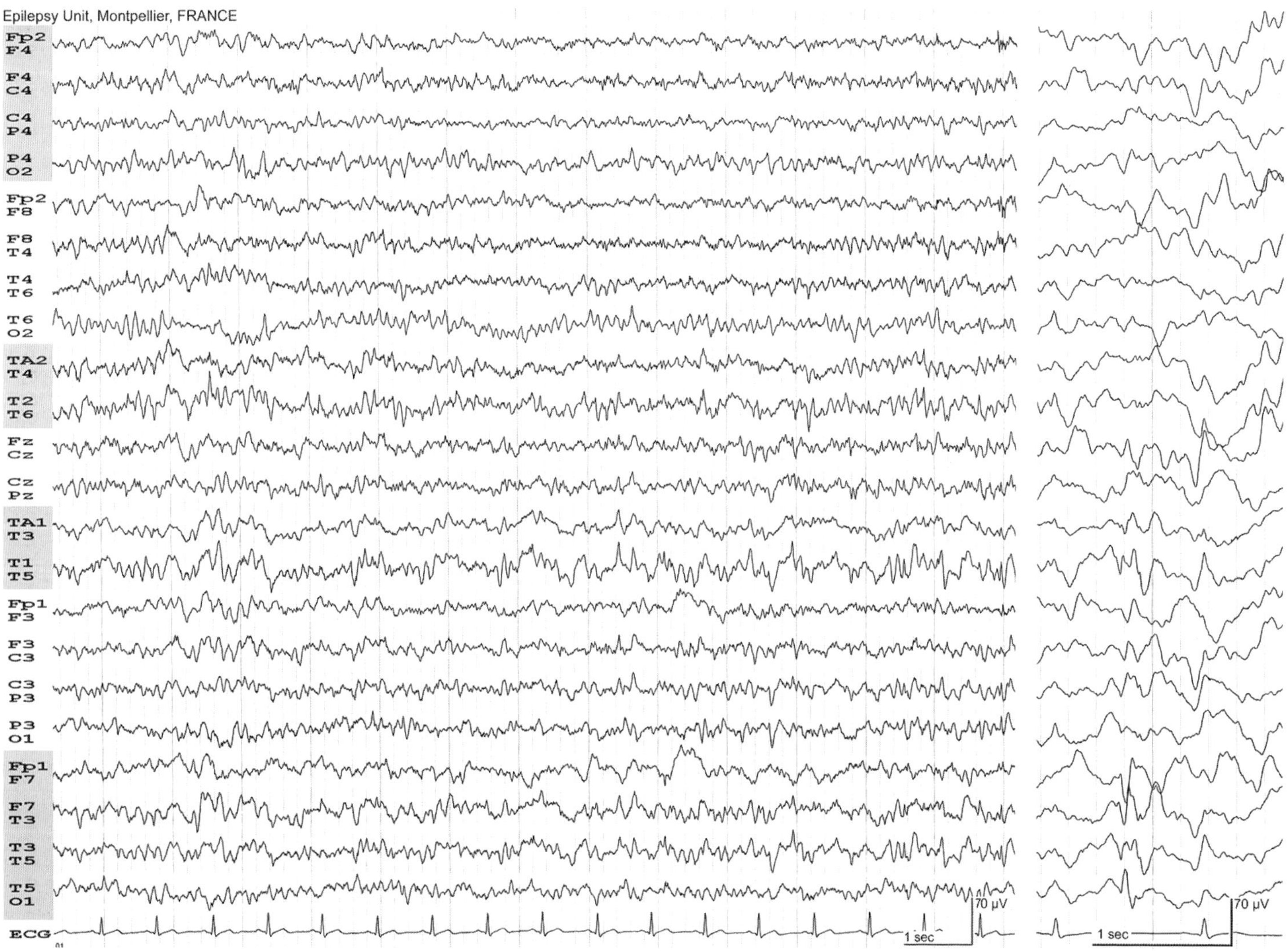

Figure a / On the left, recording at 15 mm/s. On the right, recording at 30 mm/s. Stage N3 sleep. Spike over the left temporal region.

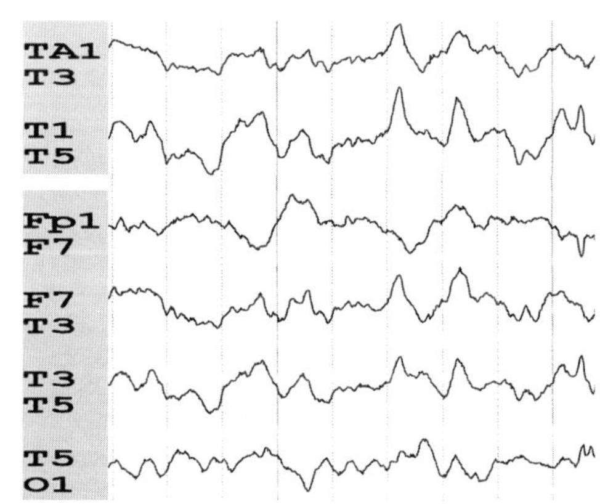

Figure b / Left temporal theta waves during hyperventilation.

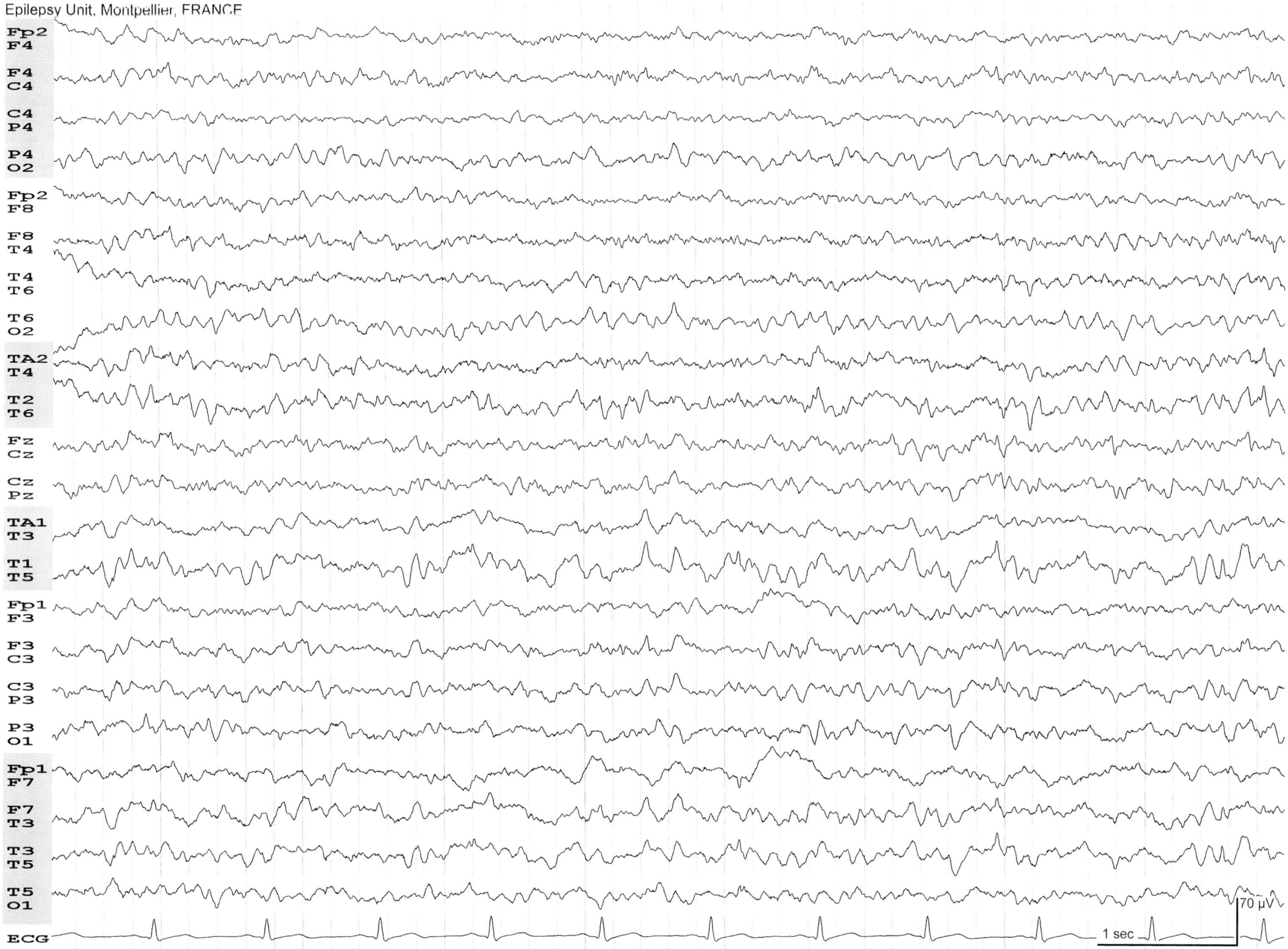
Epilepsy Unit, Montpellier, FRANCE
Fp2
F4
F4
C4
C4
P4
P4
O2
Fp2
F8
F8
T4
T4
T6
T6
O2
TA2
T4
T2
T6
Fz
Cz
Cz
Pz
TA1
T3
T1
T5
Fp1
F3
F3
C3
C3
P3
P3
O1
Fp1
F7
F7
T3
T3
T5
T5
O1
ECG
70 µV
1 sec

II • 8 Slow waves after hyperventilation (Moyamoya disease)

Context

8-year-old boy with moyamoya disease diagnosed after a stroke 2 years ago.

What to note

After three minutes of hyperventilation with physiological slowing, the EEG had gone back to normal. Anterior delta waves (0.5 to 1 Hz) occur one minute after cessation of hyperventilation. The slow waves continue for more than one minute. Delayed occurrence of high-voltage slow delta waves after cessation of hyperventilation is pathognomonic of moyamoya disease.

Comment

Hyperventilation must not be carried out if moyamoya disease has been diagnosed due to the risk of stroke.

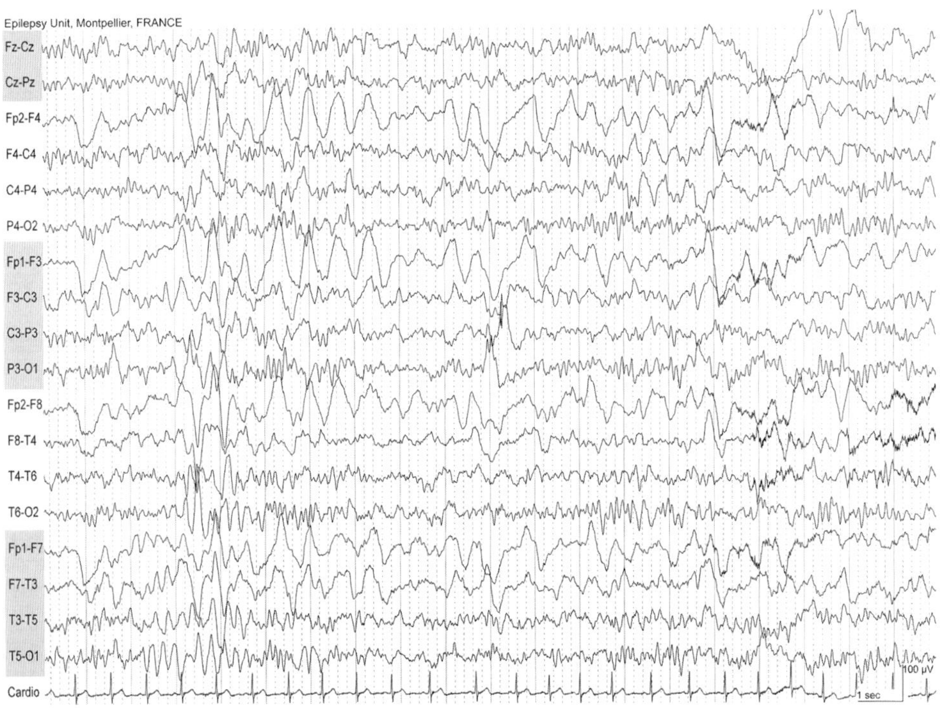

Figure a / Recording at 15 mm/s. Delayed high-voltage slow delta waves (one minute after cessation of hyperventilation).

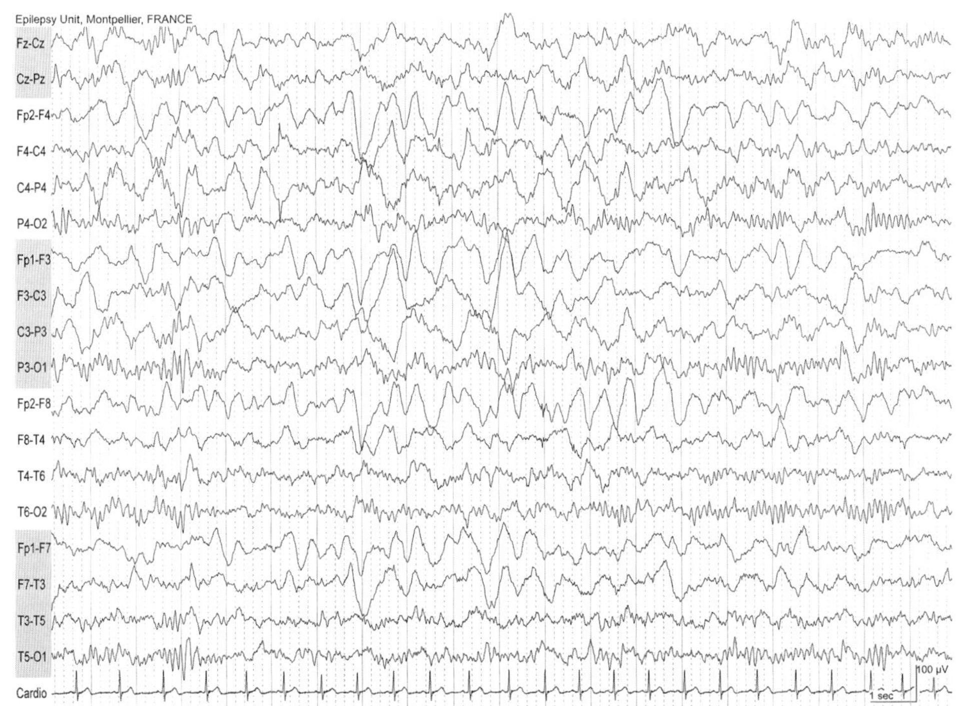

Figure b / Recording at 15 mm/s. High voltage delta waves continue.

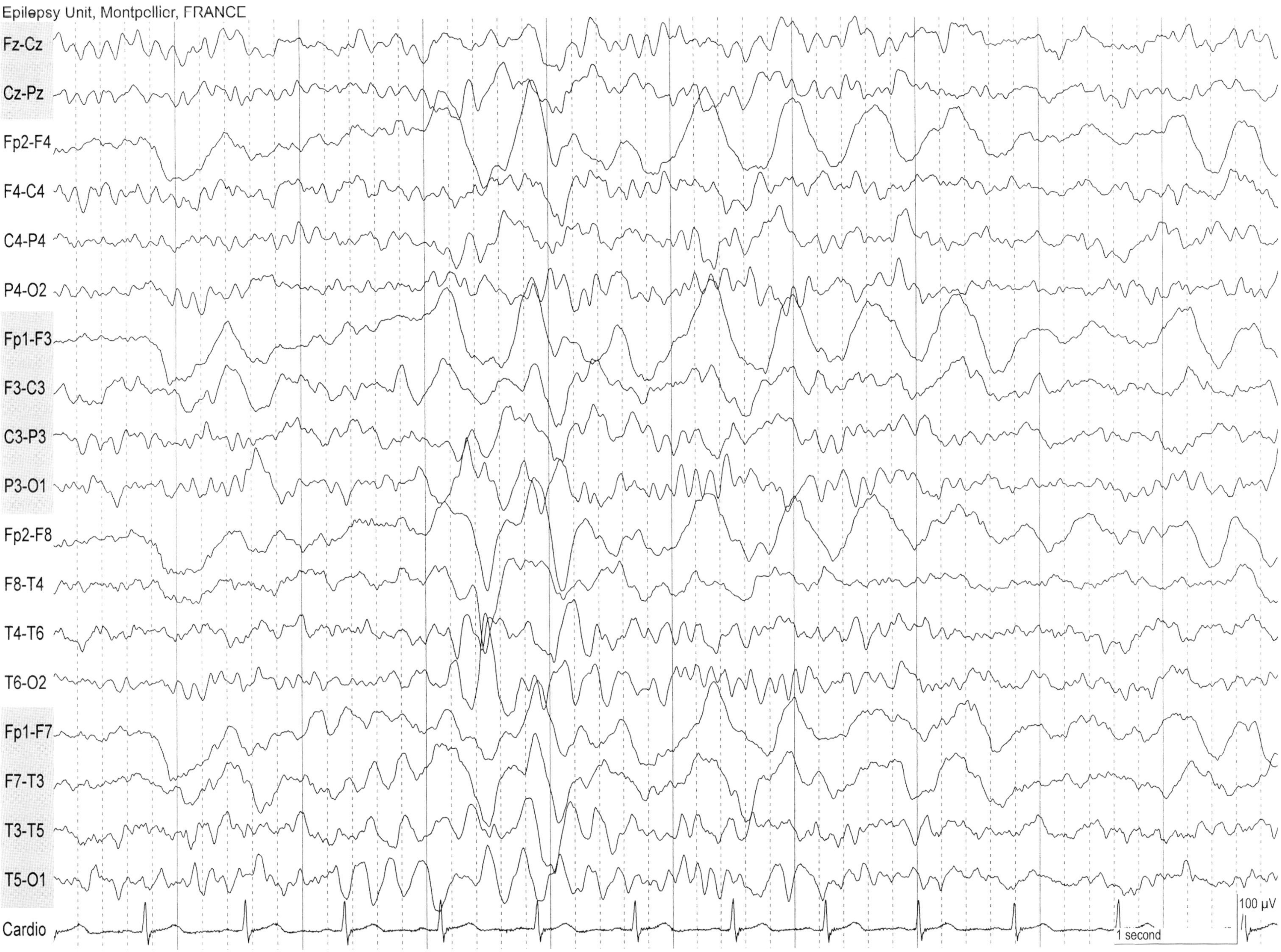
Epilepsy Unit, Montpellier, FRANCE
Fz-Cz
Cz-Pz
Fp2-F4
F4-C4
C4-P4
P4-O2
Fp1-F3
F3-C3
C3-P3
P3-O1
Fp2-F8
F8-T4
T4-T6
T6-O2
Fp1-F7
F7-T3
T3-T5
T5-O1
Cardio
100 µV
1 second

II • 9 Photic driving in an infant

Context

24-month-old infant referred for a seizure.

What to note

This plate only displays the right suprasylvian derivations with 3, 4, 8 and 12 Hz intermittent photic stimulation (IPS). Tracing amplitude was reduced to 15 µV/mm. Patient's eyes are open (muscular activities on the fronto-polar derivations). Photic driving is observed at low frequency but also at 8 and 12 Hz. It is unusual to observe photic driving at this age, but it can be seen more frequently in children around 6 years. In infants, IPS is often performed at the beginning of the recording, because its calming effect helps the infant fall asleep.

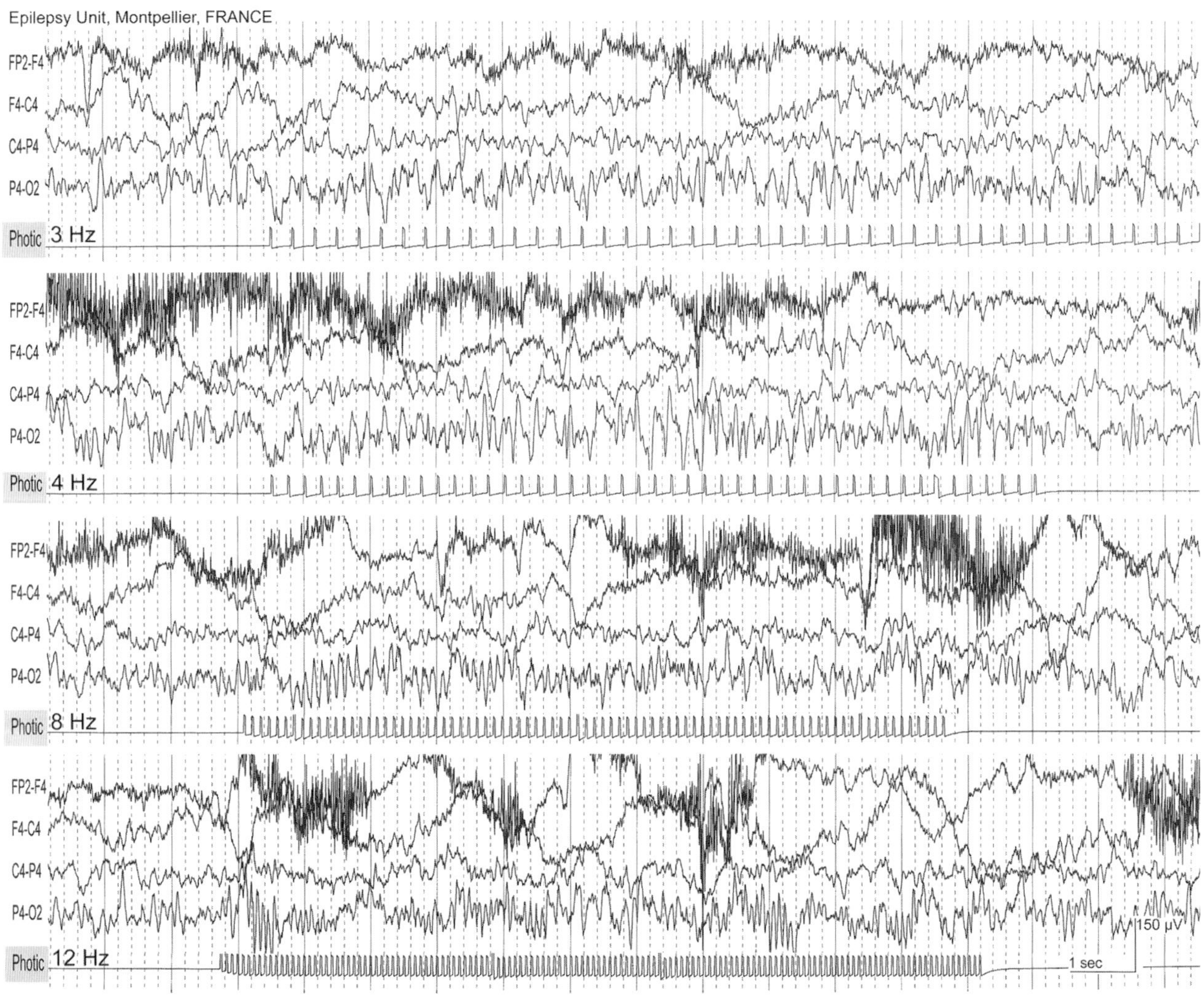

Figure a / Recording at 15 mm/s.

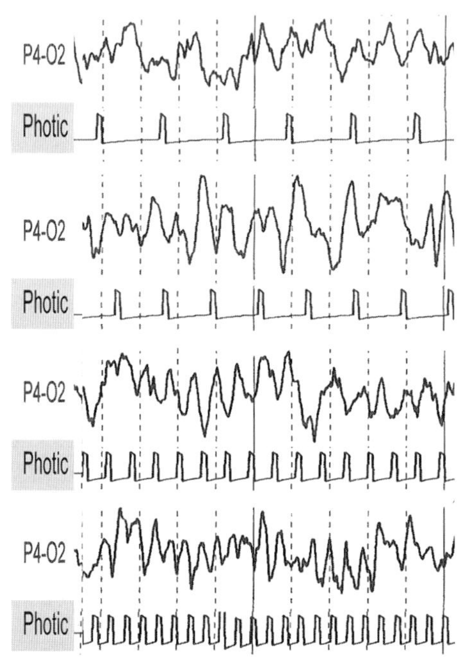

Figure b / Photic driving at 3, 4, 8 and 12 Hz.

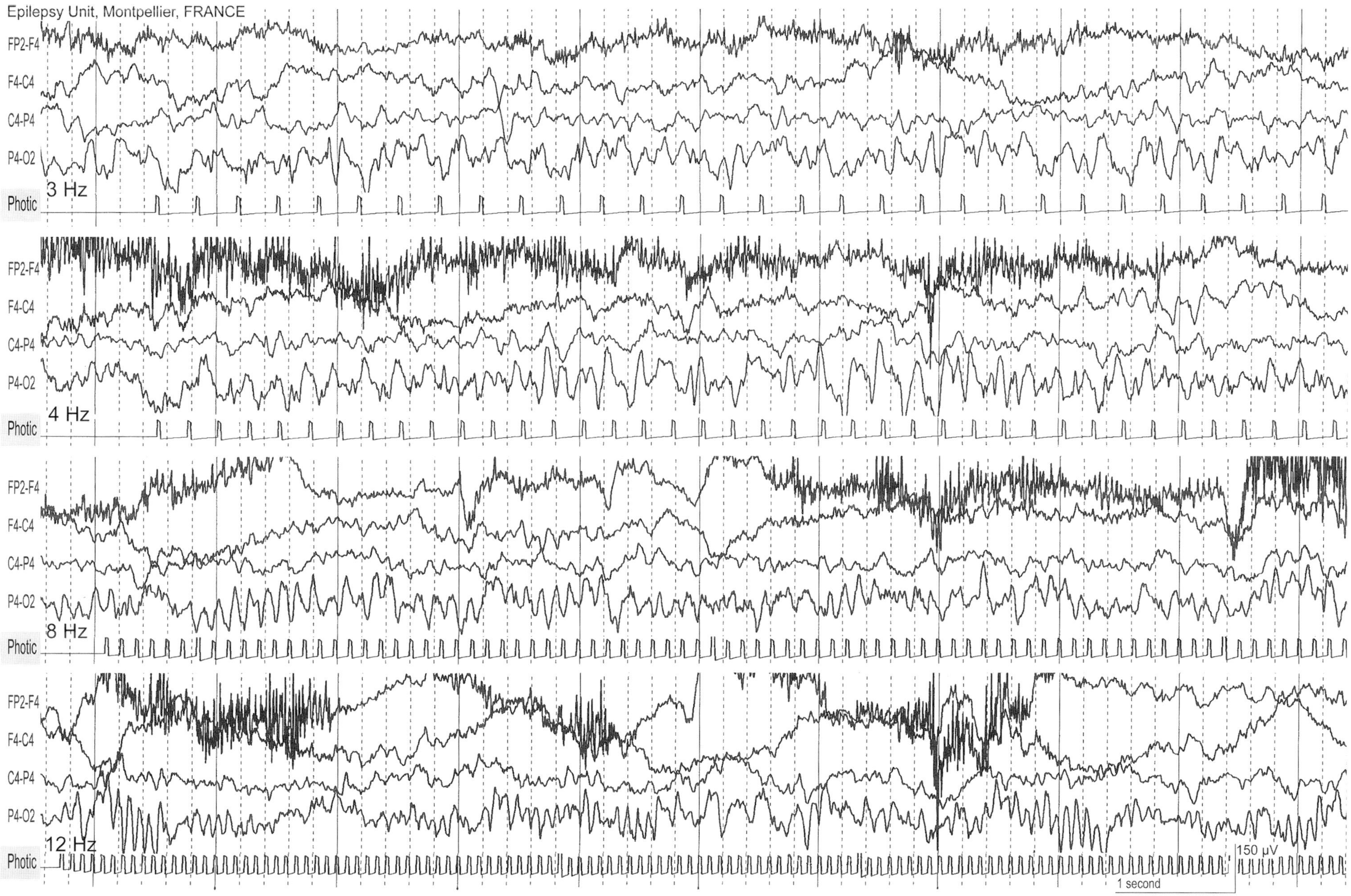
Epilepsy Unit, Montpellier, FRANCE
FP2-F4
F4-C4
C4-P4
P4-O2
3 Hz
Photic
4 Hz
8 Hz
12 Hz
150 µV
1 second

II • 10 Photic driving at low frequency in a child

Context

10-year-old girl with focal epilepsy and migraine.

What to note

Photic stimulation at 3 Hz, eye closed. Bilateral photic driving.

Comment

Photic driving at low frequency is not unusual in children. In children and adolescents, the reactivity is stronger than in adults. Patients with migraine have a higher incidence of photic driving. This response is also best elicited with eyes closed. Eyelids are a red filter and enhances photic driving.

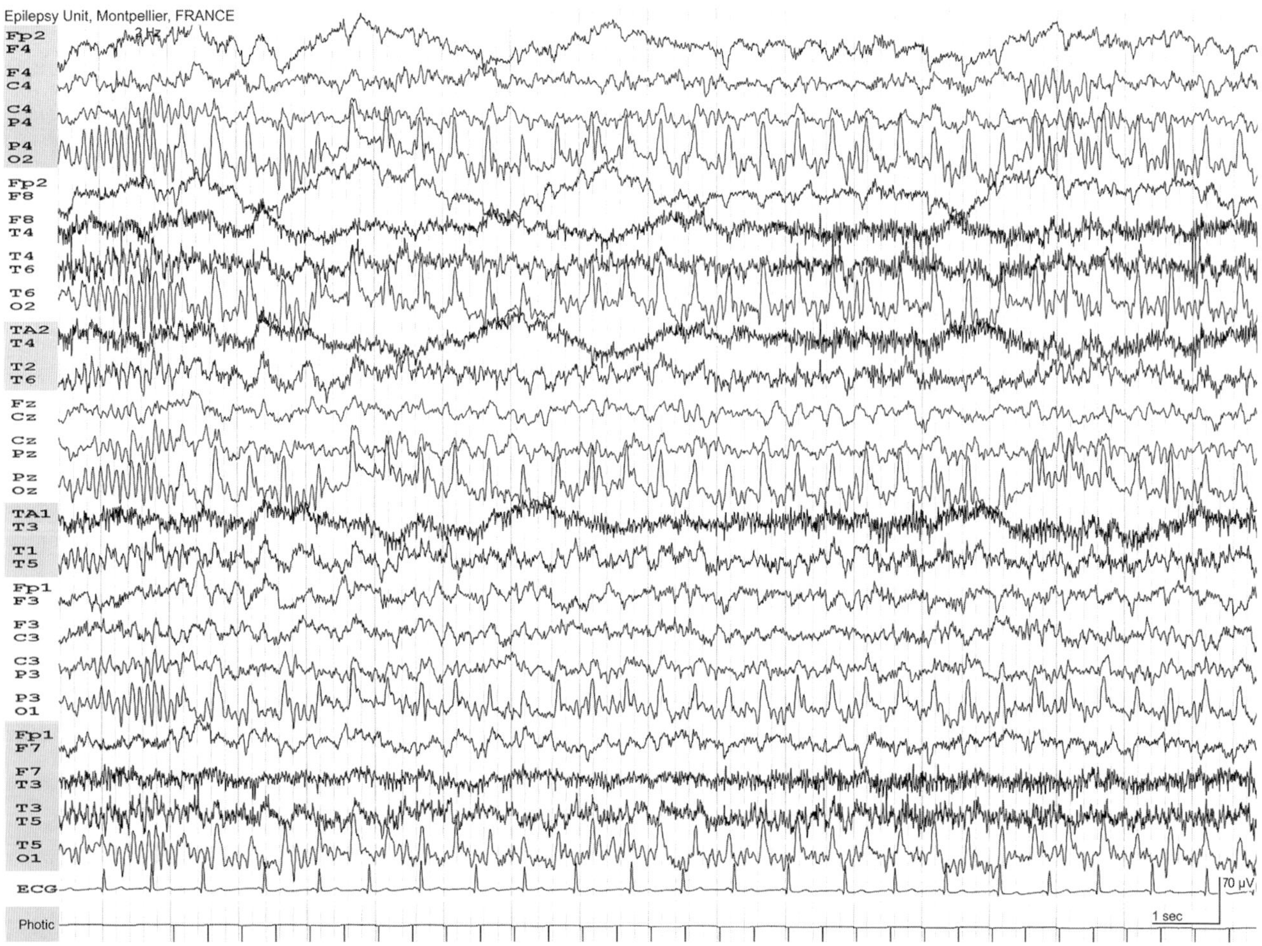

Figure a / Recording at 15 mm/s.

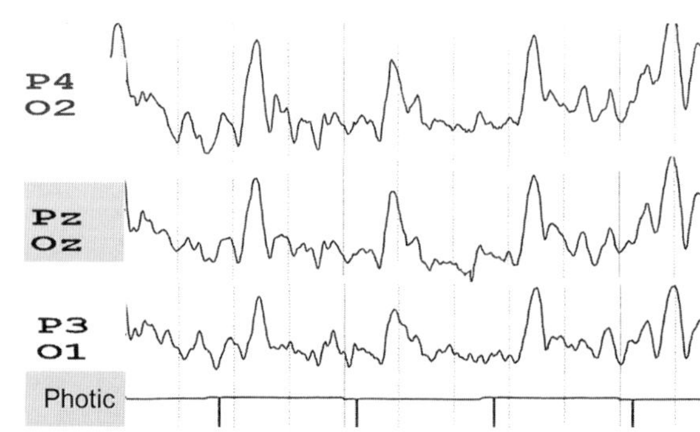

Figure b / Photic driving at low frequency. Note the interval between the flashes and the waves.

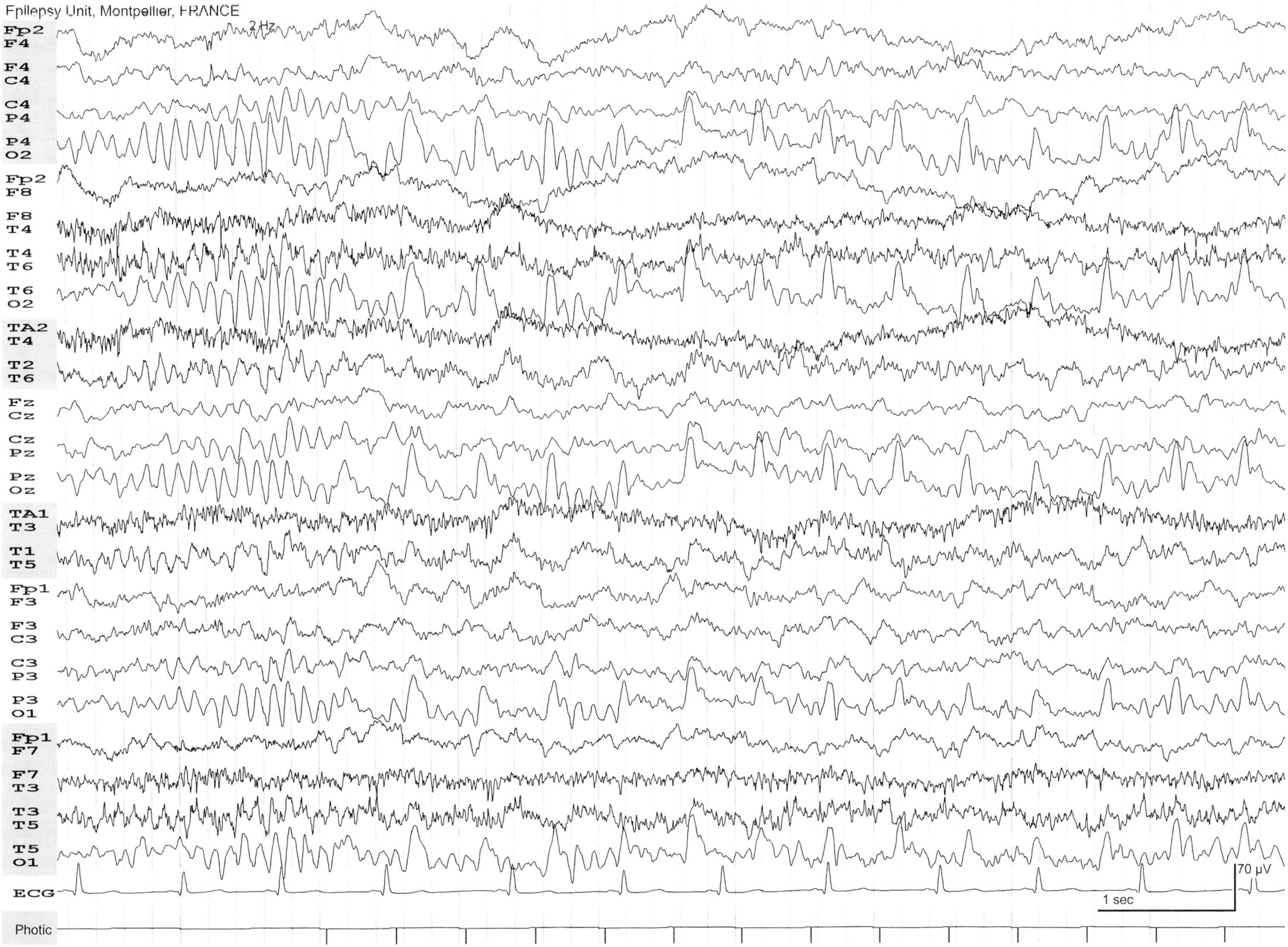
Epilepsy Unit, Montpellier, FRANCE
2 Hz
Fp2 F4
F4 C4
C4 P4
P4 O2
Fp2 F8
F8 T4
T4 T6
T6 O2
TA2 T4
T2 T6
Fz Cz
Cz Pz
Pz Oz
TA1 T3
T1 T5
Fp1 F3
F3 C3
C3 P3
P3 O1
Fp1 F7
F7 T3
T3 T5
T5 O1
ECG
Photic
70 µV
1 sec

II • 11 Photic driving in a child

Context

10-year-old girl, same patient as on the previous plate.

What to note

The patient closes her eyes (eyelid movement artifact). Photic stimulation is performed at 19 Hz. Bilateral photic driving can be seen with greater amplitude over P4-O2 and Pz-Oz. The photic driving is asymmetrical and corresponds to the physiological asymmetry of the background activity, with usually higher amplitude on the right (non-dominant) hemisphere. Note the presence of a mu rhythm at F4-C4 that spreads to P4-02.

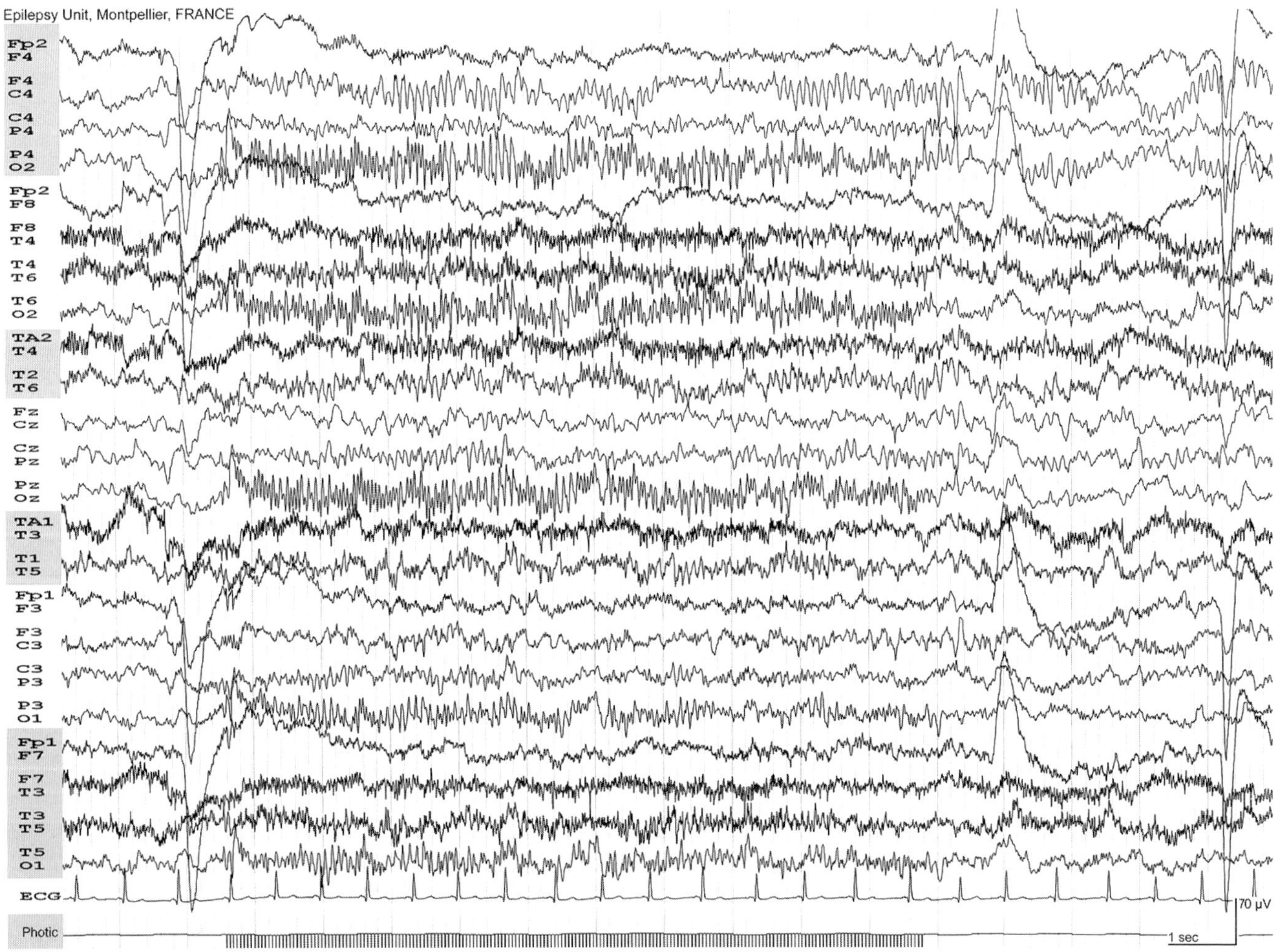

Figure a / Recording at 15 mm/s. Mu rhythm at F4-C4 continues after eyes opening.

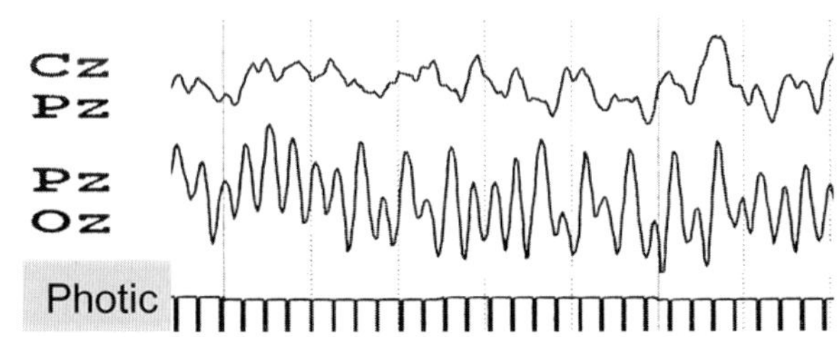

Figure b / Photic driving at 19 Hz.

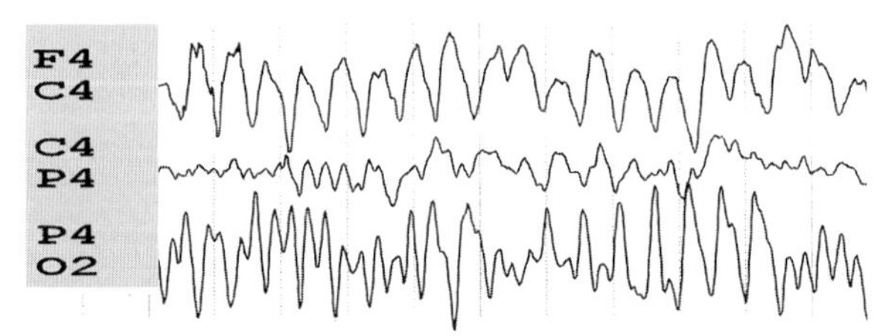

Figure c / Mu rhythm that spreads to P4-O2.

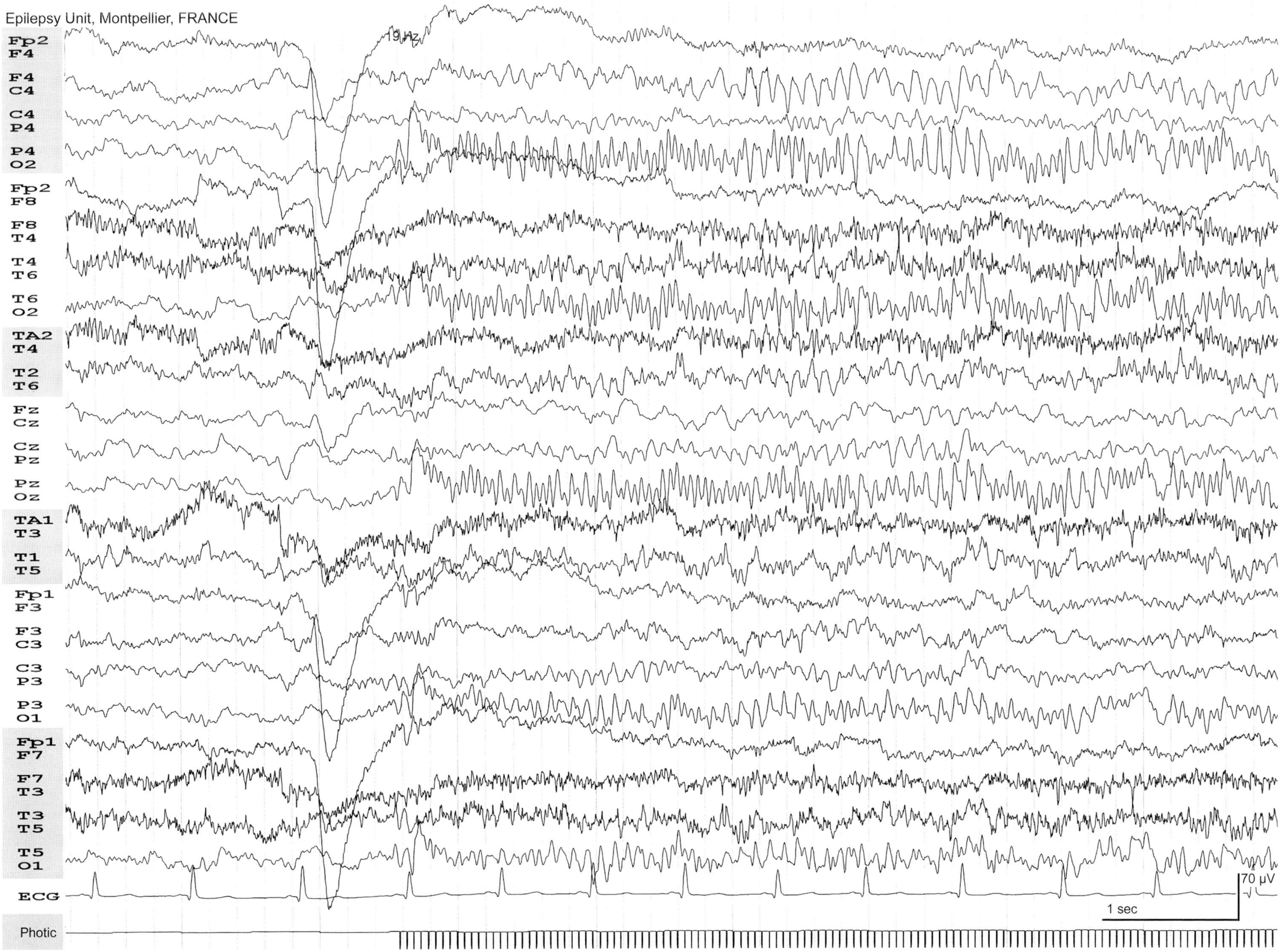
Epilepsy Unit, Montpellier, FRANCE
19 Hz
Fp2 F4
F4 C4
C4 P4
P4 O2
Fp2 F8
F8 T4
T4 T6
T6 O2
TA2 T4
T2 T6
Fz Cz
Cz Pz
Pz Oz
TA1 T3
T1 T5
Fp1 F3
F3 C3
C3 P3
P3 O1
Fp1 F7
F7 T3
T3 T5
T5 O1
ECG
Photic
70 µV
1 sec

II • 12 Photic driving in an adult (1): subharmonic

Context

18-year-old woman with migraine.

What to note

The patient's eyes are closed. Background activity with alpha rhythm at 10.5 Hz. At photic stimulation at 5 Hz, a division of the alpha rhythm occurs with appearance of a sub-harmonic at 5 Hz. Note the presence of a mu rhythm on F3-C3 and eye movements on the frontal polar derivations. The photic stimulation has no effect on mu rhythm.

Comment

A sub-harmonic during photic stimulation is defined as a division in the alpha rhythm that appears during photic stimulation at a frequency corresponding to half of the patient's alpha rhythm.

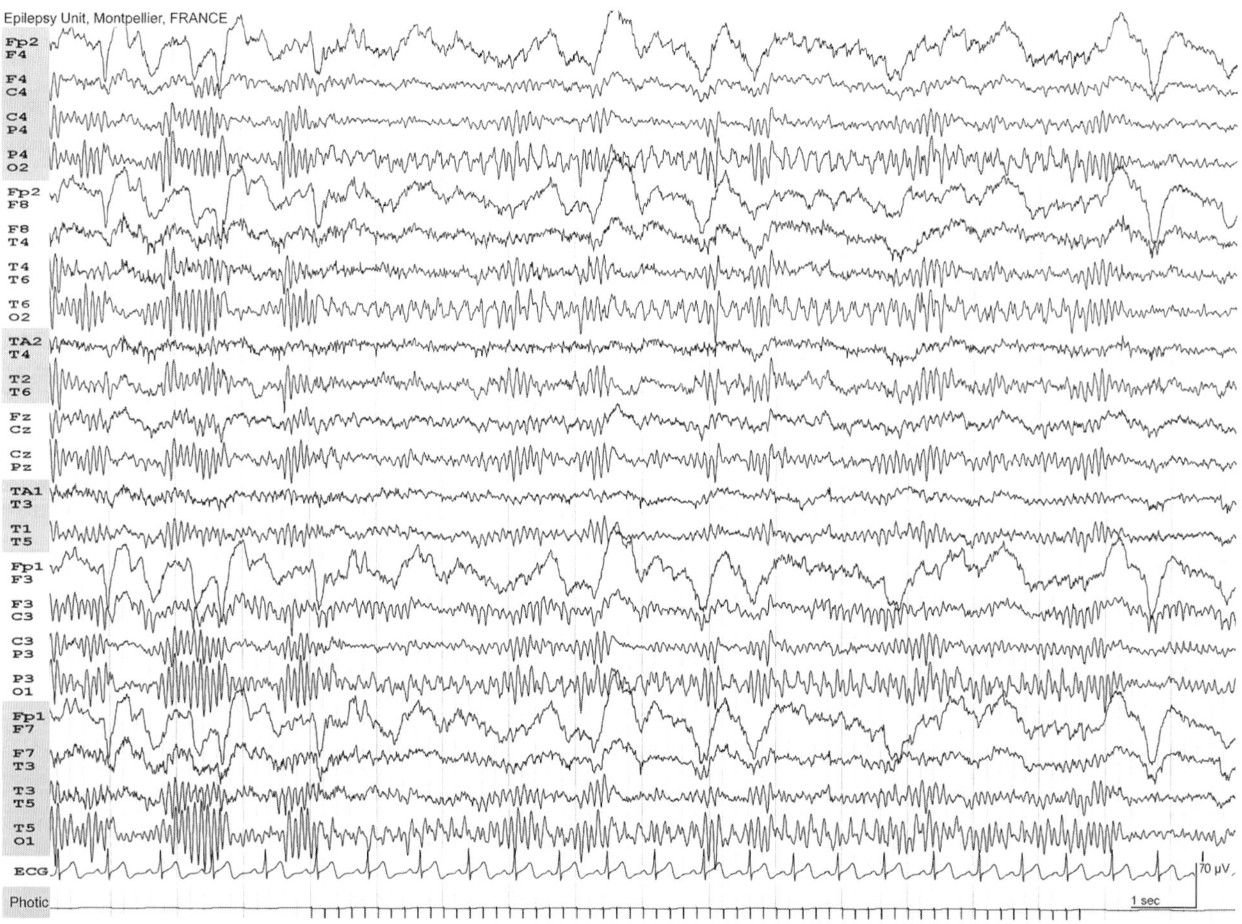

Figure a / Recording at 15 mm/s. As soon as photic stimulation ceases, the alpha rhythm reappears.

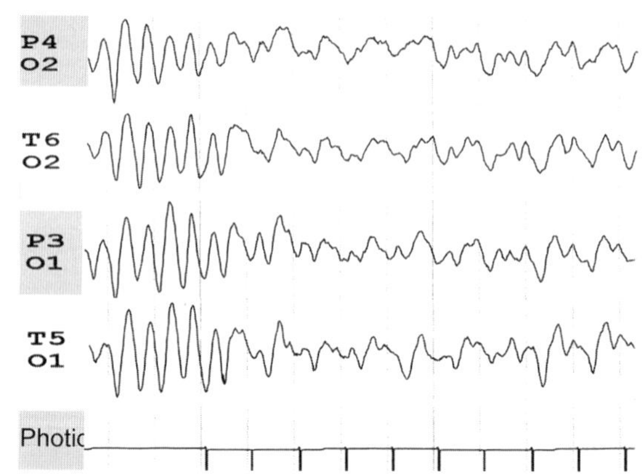

Figure b / Photic stimulation divides the alpha rhythm (10.5 Hz) at 5 Hz frequency.

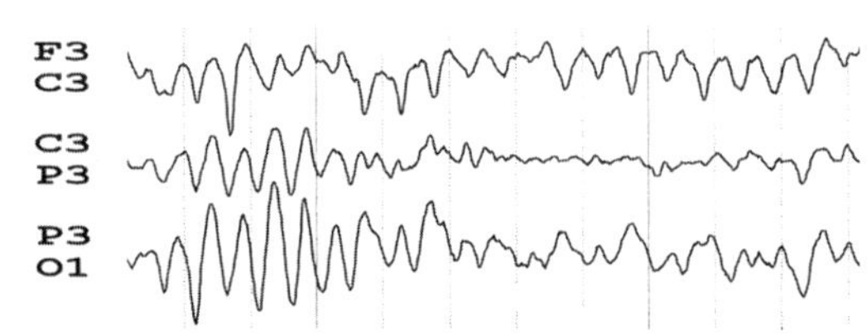

Figure c / Mu rhythm at F3-C3.

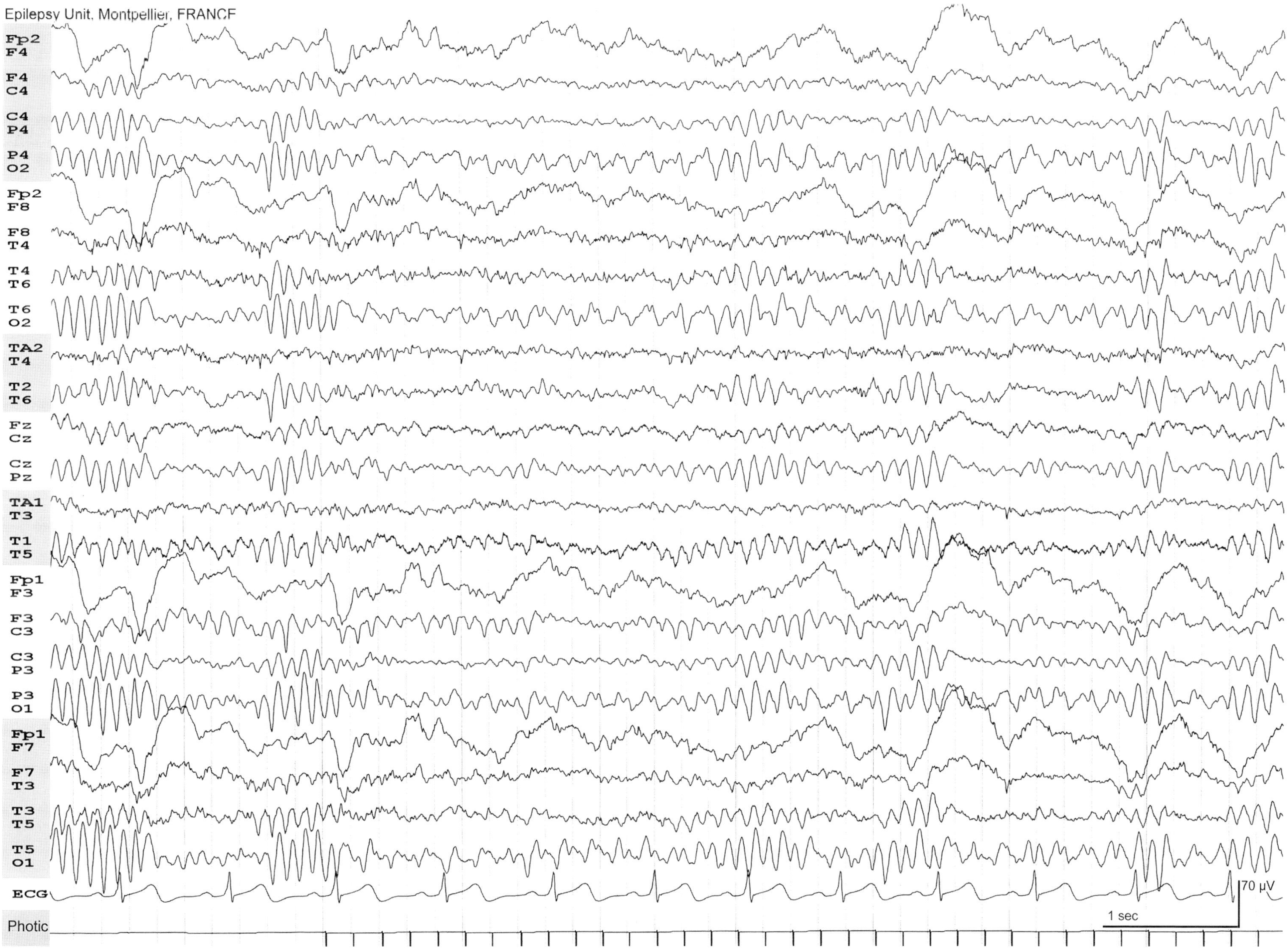
Epilepsy Unit, Montpellier, FRANCE
Fp2 F4
F4 C4
C4 P4
P4 O2
Fp2 F8
F8 T4
T4 T6
T6 O2
TA2 T4
T2 T6
Fz Cz
Cz Pz
TA1 T3
T1 T5
Fp1 F3
F3 C3
C3 P3
P3 O1
Fp1 F7
F7 T3
T3 T5
T5 O1
ECG
Photic
70 µV
1 sec

II • 13 Photic driving in an adult (2)

Context

18-year-old woman, same patient as on the previous plate.

What to note

The patient's eyes are closed. Background activity with posterior alpha rhythm (10 Hz). Photic driving at 20 Hz during 3 seconds. Then there is a fall-off. Alpha rhythm reappears. Note the presence of a mu rhythm of greater amplitude over F3-C3, detectable during photic driving. On close examination, it appears that the mu rhythm was already present at the beginning but it conveyed a false impression of anterior spread of the alpha rhythm. Photic stimulation has no effect on mu rhythm.

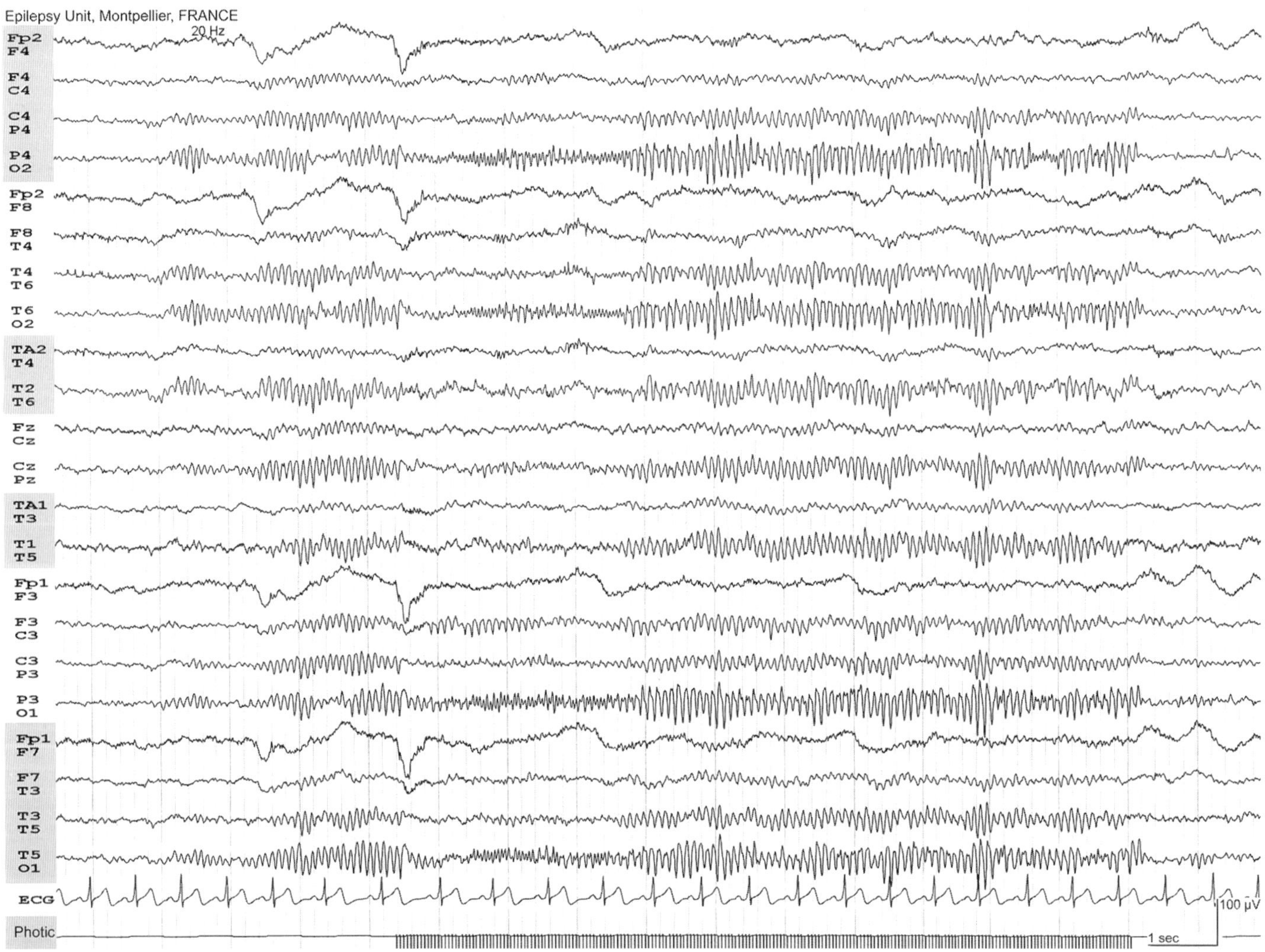

Figure a / Recording at 15 mm/s.

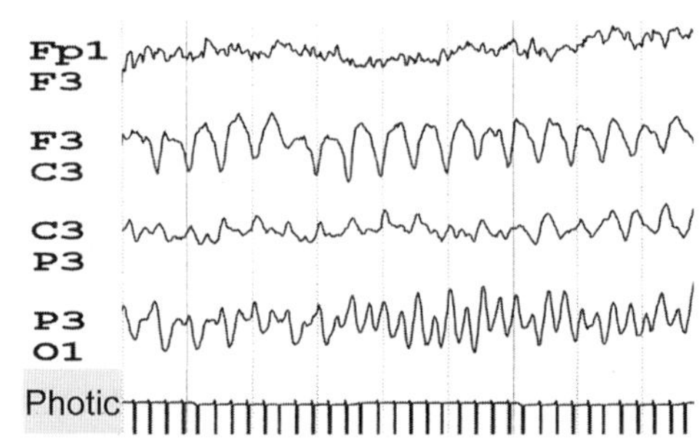

Figure b / Photic driving at 20 Hz (P3-O1); mu rhythm at F3-C3.

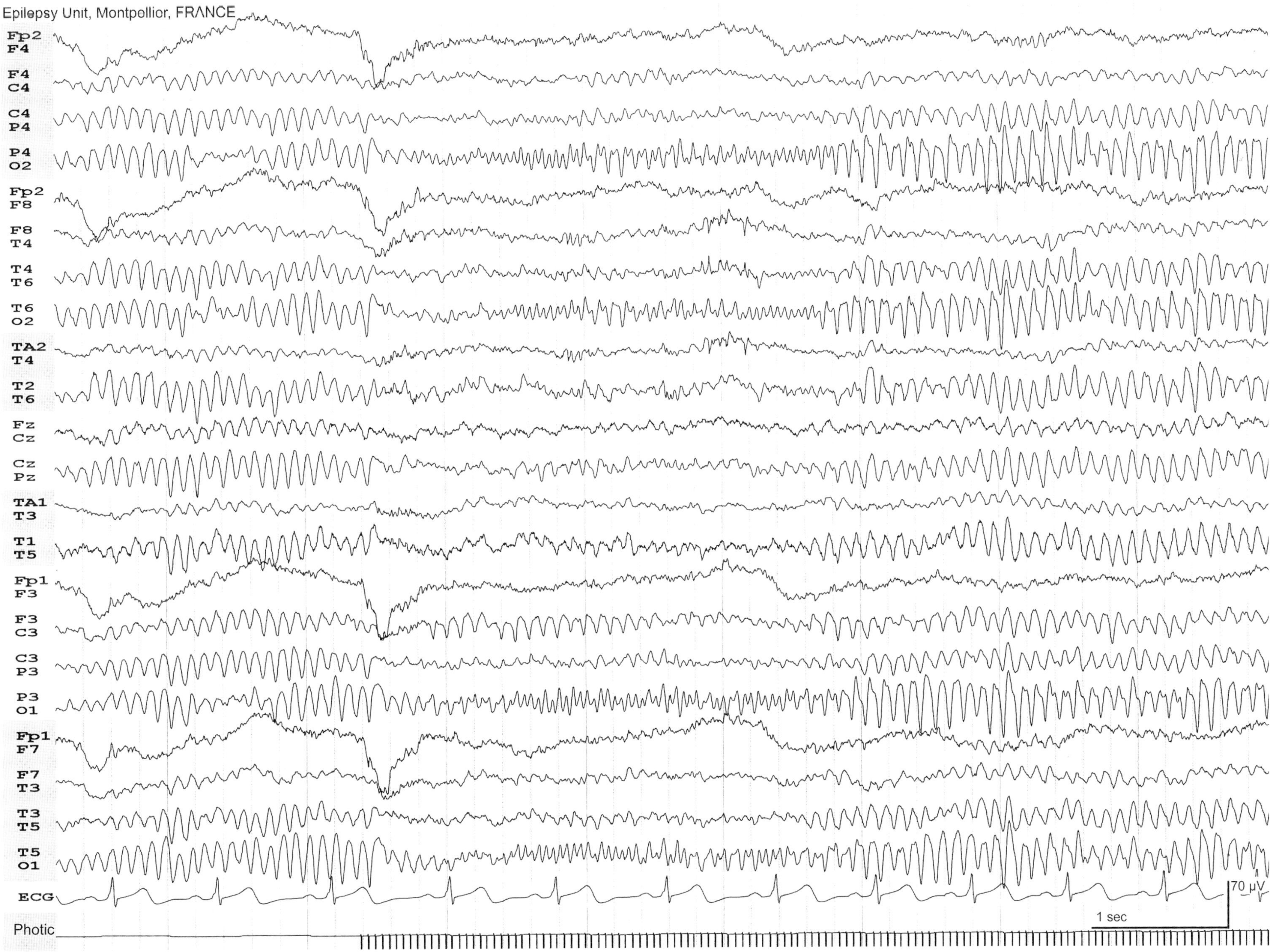
Epilepsy Unit, Montpellier, FRANCE
Fp2 F4
F4 C4
C4 P4
P4 O2
Fp2 F8
F8 T4
T4 T6
T6 O2
TA2 T4
T2 T6
Fz Cz
Cz Pz
TA1 T3
T1 T5
Fp1 F3
F3 C3
C3 P3
P3 O1
Fp1 F7
F7 T3
T3 T5
T5 O1
ECG
Photic
70 µV
1 sec

II • 14 Photic driving in an adult (3)

Context

22-year-old woman with migraine.

What to note

On the upper plate, the patient closes her eyes. Alpha background activity at 10 Hz. Other plates with photic stimulation at 3, 5 and 9 Hz. Patient closes her eyes just before the flashes. Alpha rhythm can be seen followed by photic driving. The waves are time locked to the flash frequency. Patients with migraine have a higher incidence of photic driving.

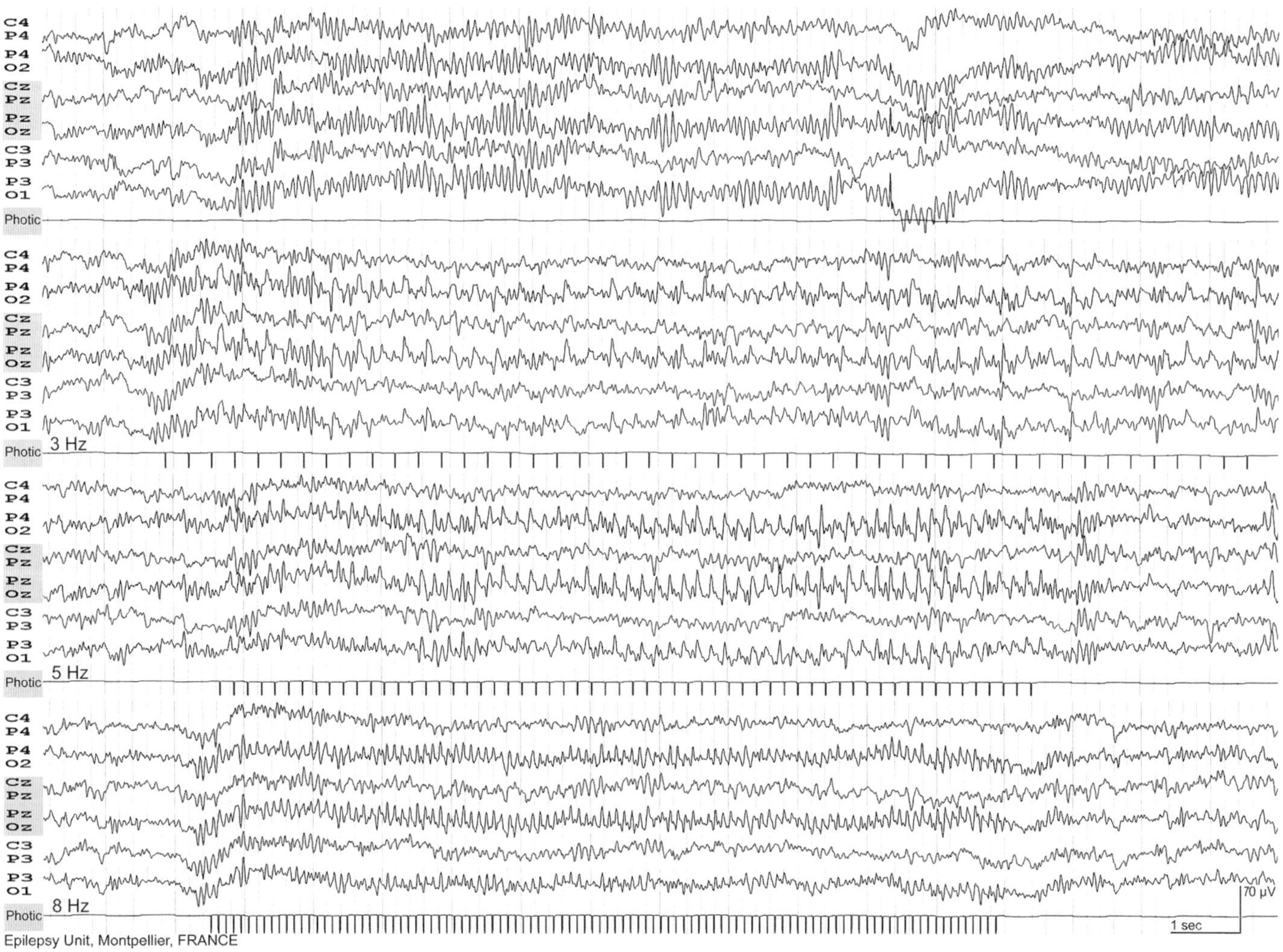

Figure a / Recording at 15 mm/s.

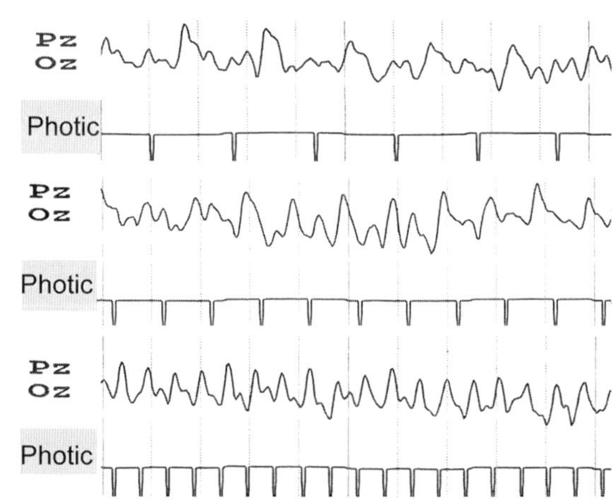

Figure b / Photic driving occurring at 3, 5 and 9 Hz.

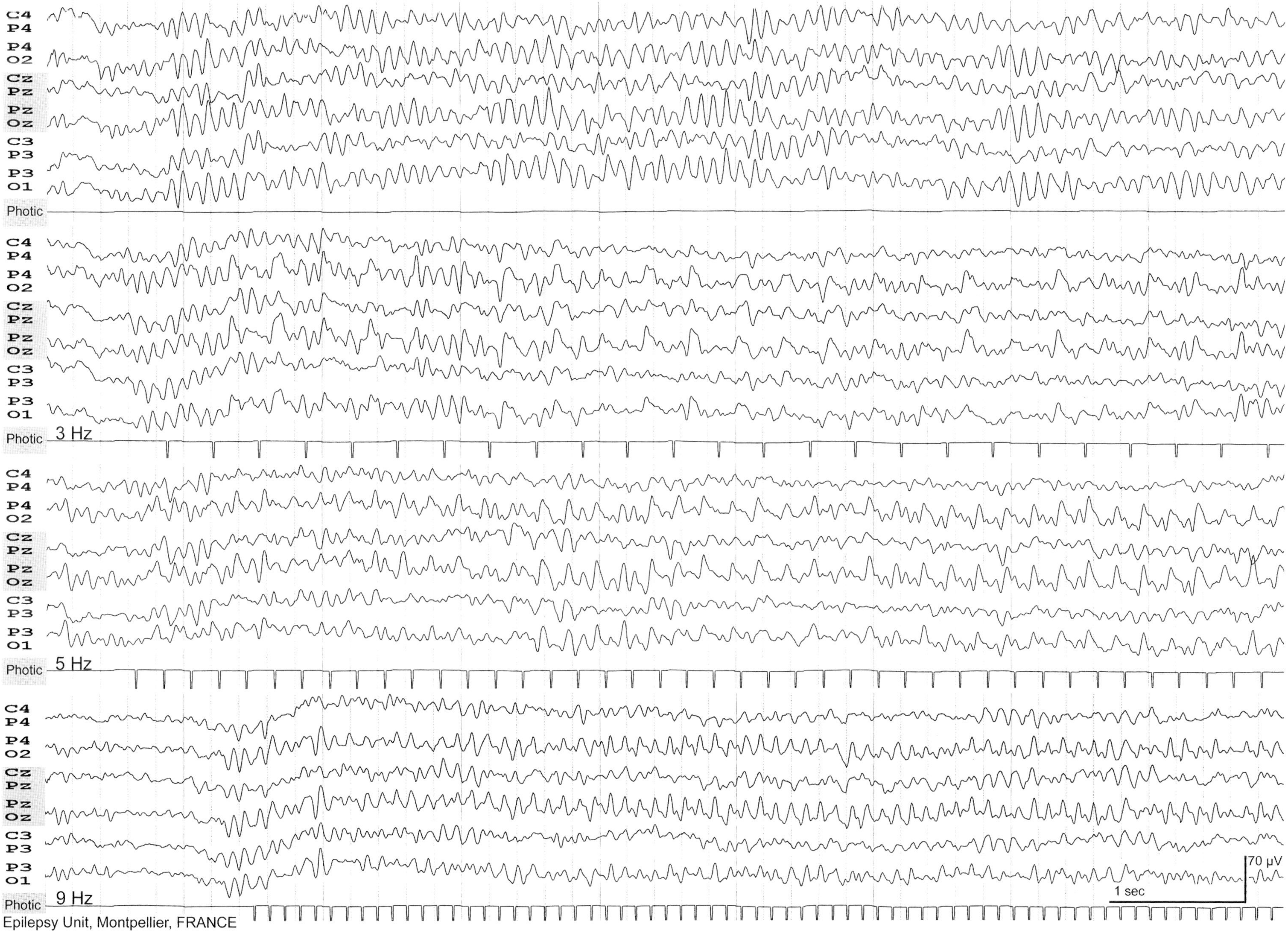
C4 P4
P4 O2
Cz Pz
Pz Oz
C3 P3
P3 O1
Photic
3 Hz
5 Hz
9 Hz
70 µV
1 sec
Epilepsy Unit, Montpellier, FRANCE

II • 15 Photic driving in an adult (4)

Context

41-year-old woman with gliomatosis cerebri.

What to note

On the upper plate, the patient's eyes are closed. Alpha background activity at 11 Hz. Other plates with photic stimulation at 12, 16, 18 and 21 Hz. The patient closes her eyes. Photic driving. At 16, 18 and 21 Hz, photic driving at the beginning of the flashes, then there is a fall-off.

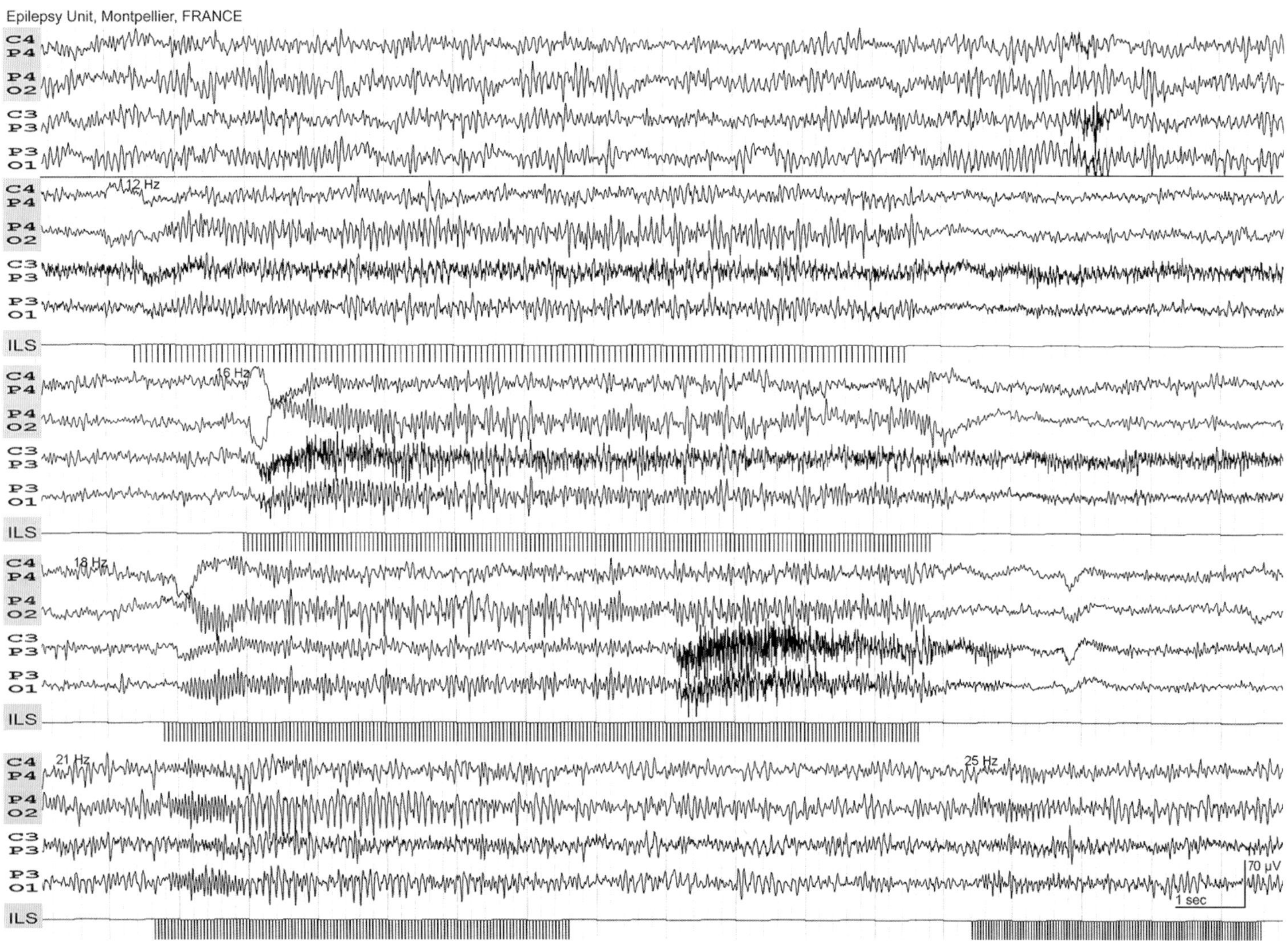

Figure a / Recording at 15 mm/s.

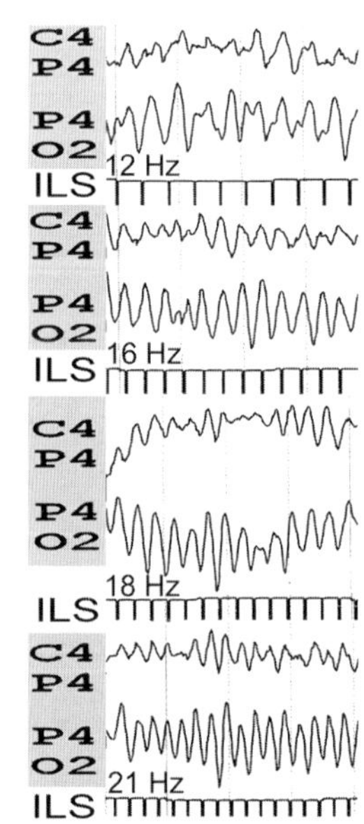

Figure b / The waves are time locked to the flash frequency

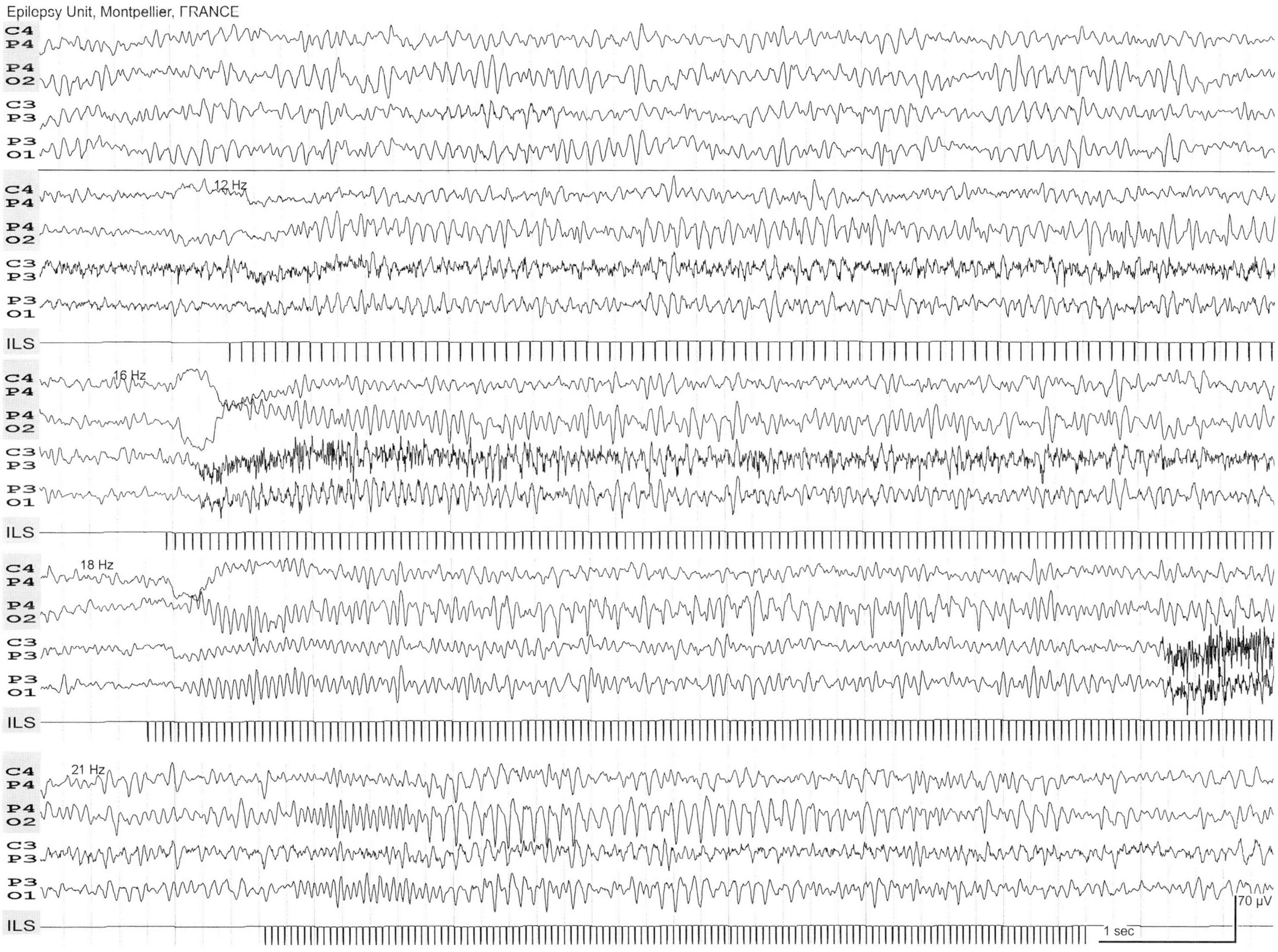
Epilepsy Unit, Montpellier, FRANCE
C4 P4
P4 O2
C3 P3
P3 O1
12 Hz
ILS
16 Hz
18 Hz
21 Hz
70 µV
1 sec

II • 16 Fast alpha variant appearing during photic stimulation

Context

58-year-old woman seen after a loss of consciousness.

What to note

Photic stimulation at 11 Hz triggers a posterior background activity at 20 Hz when all waves are counted. However, on closer examination, the waves are forked. This is a fast alpha variant of the alpha rhythm triggered by photic stimulation. For this individual, all the stimulation frequencies triggered a posterior rhythm at 20 Hz but the forked aspect was most clearly visible at 11 Hz.

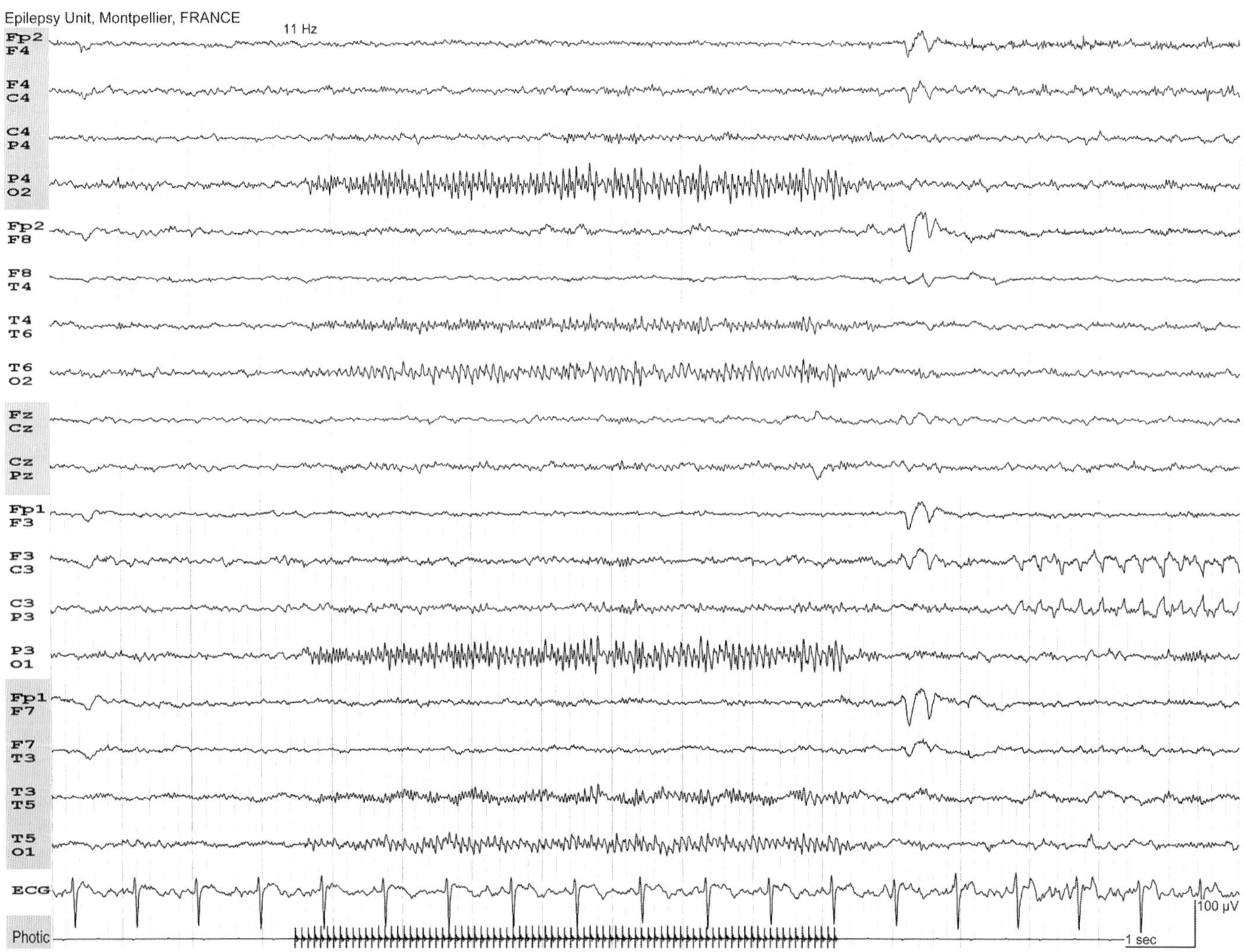

Figure a / Recording at 15 mm/s. Note at the end of the plate, the presence of an electrode artifact at C3.

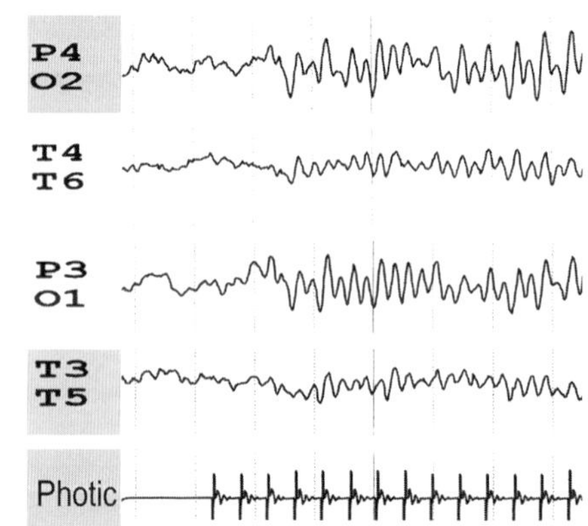

Figure b / Fast alpha variant.

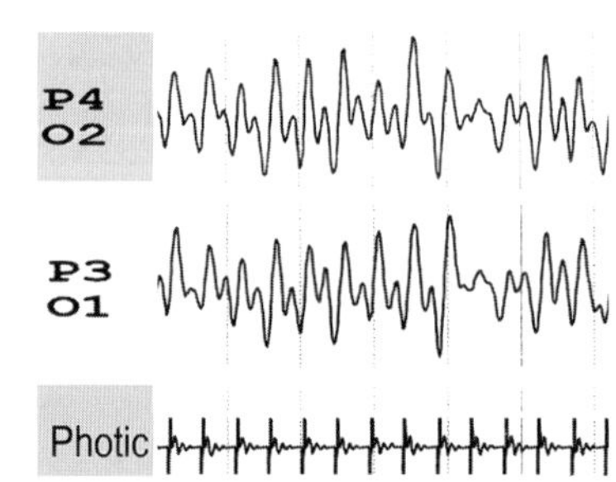

Figure c / The waves are forked.

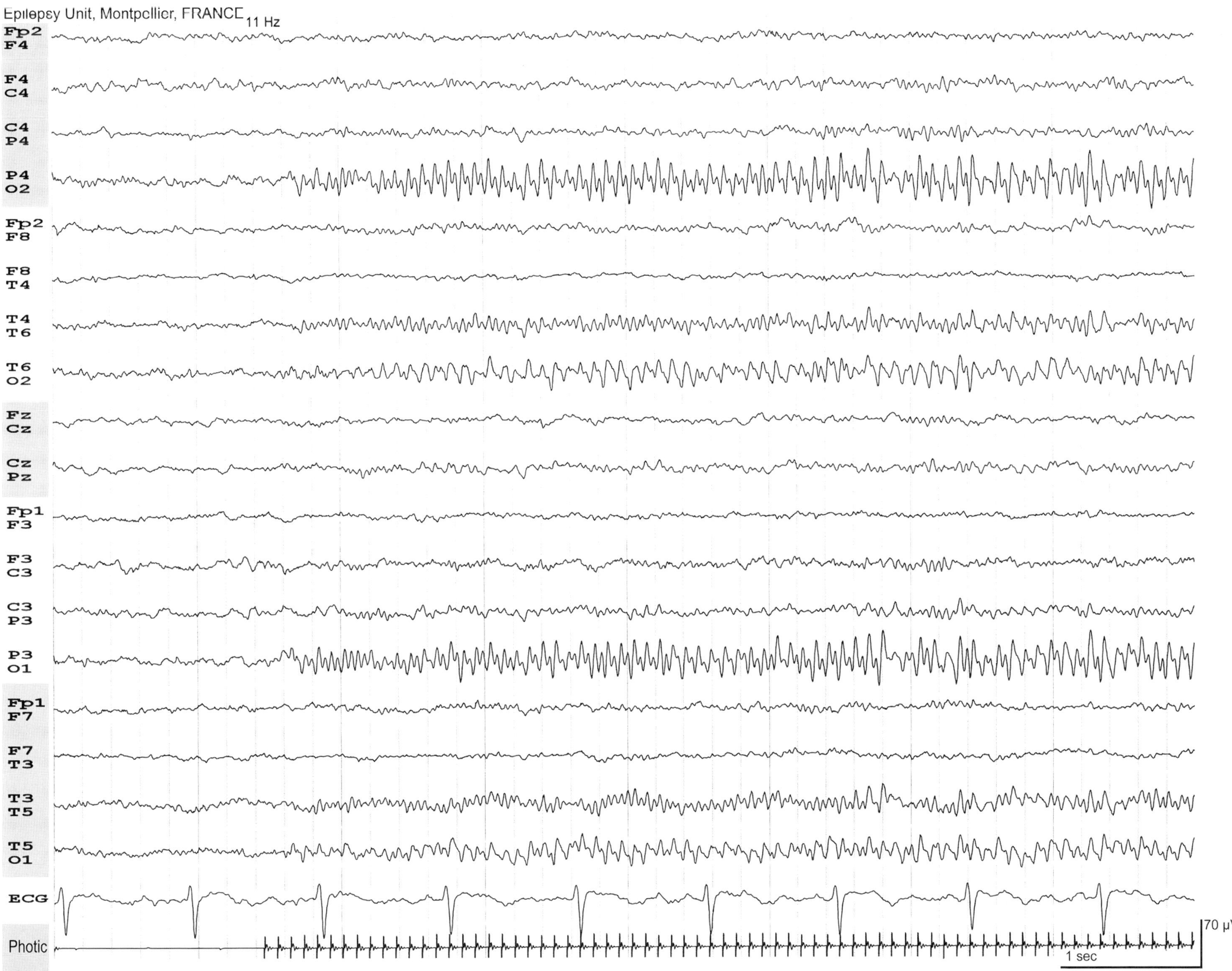
Epilepsy Unit, Montpellier, FRANCE
11 Hz
Fp2 F4
F4 C4
C4 P4
P4 O2
Fp2 F8
F8 T4
T4 T6
T6 O2
Fz Cz
Cz Pz
Fp1 F3
F3 C3
C3 P3
P3 O1
Fp1 F7
F7 T3
T3 T5
T5 O1
ECG
Photic
70 µV
1 sec

II • 17 Pathological photic driving

Context

91-year-old man referred after several epileptic seizures. Left posterior stroke on MRI.

What to note

The awake background activity is a well-developed alpha rhythm at 9 Hz (plate not shown). On this plate, a pathological photic response can be observed at 4 Hz, with the presence of a highly prominent photic driving with spikes that are clearly asymmetrically synchronous and time locked to the flash frequency (spikes of much higher amplitude on the side of the interictal epileptic abnormalities). This asymmetrical photic response was observed at all the frequencies but the amplitude was higher at low frequencies (see plate at 15 mm/s).

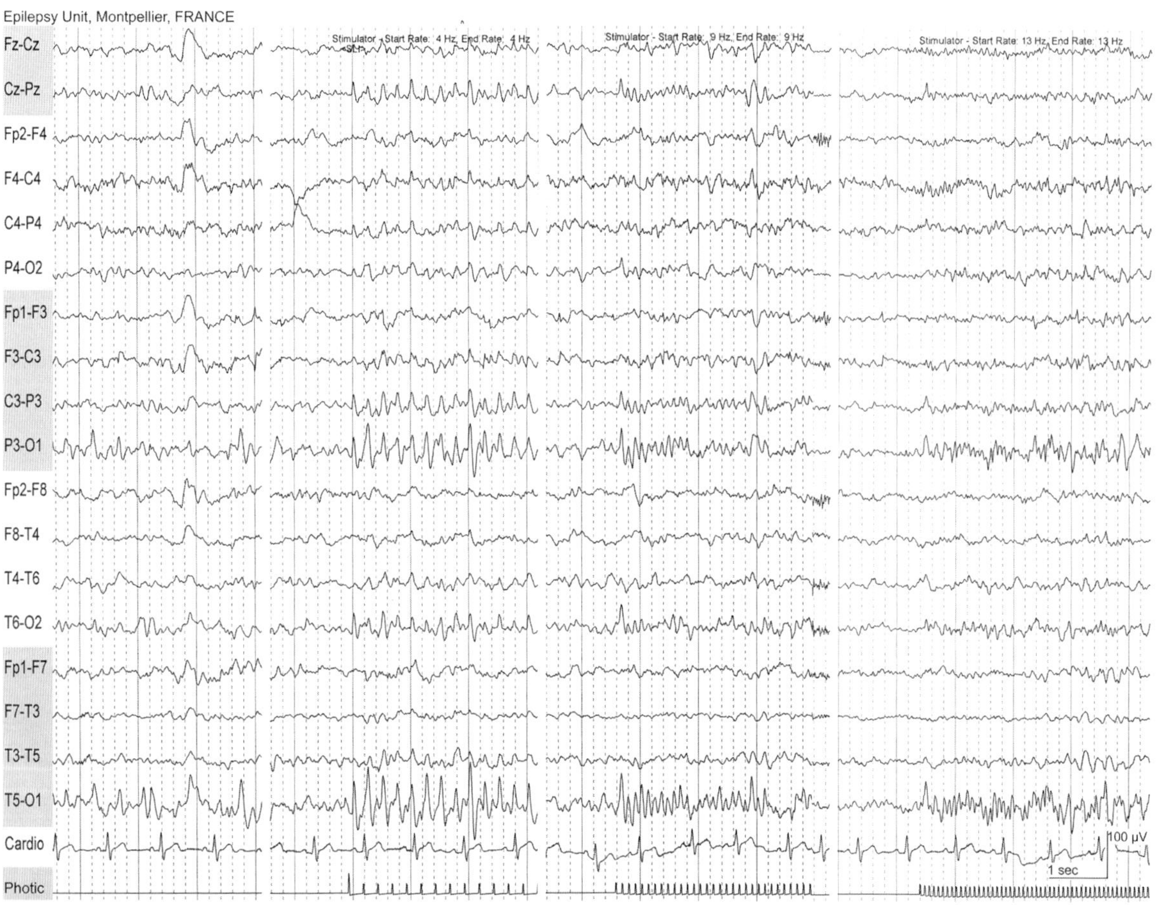

Figure a / Recording at 15 mm/s. On the left plate, patient asleep (anterior slow wave). Interictal spikes and slow waves on the left occipital region. Photic stimulations at 4, 9 and 13 Hz triggering asymmetrical photic driving.

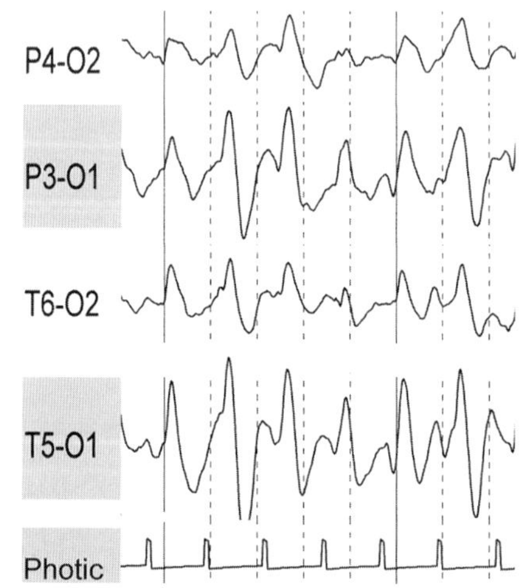

Figure b / During 4-Hz photic stimulation, a very prominent photic driving response resembling spikes with a significantly higher amplitude on the side of the epileptic focus. Note the interval between the flashes and the waves.

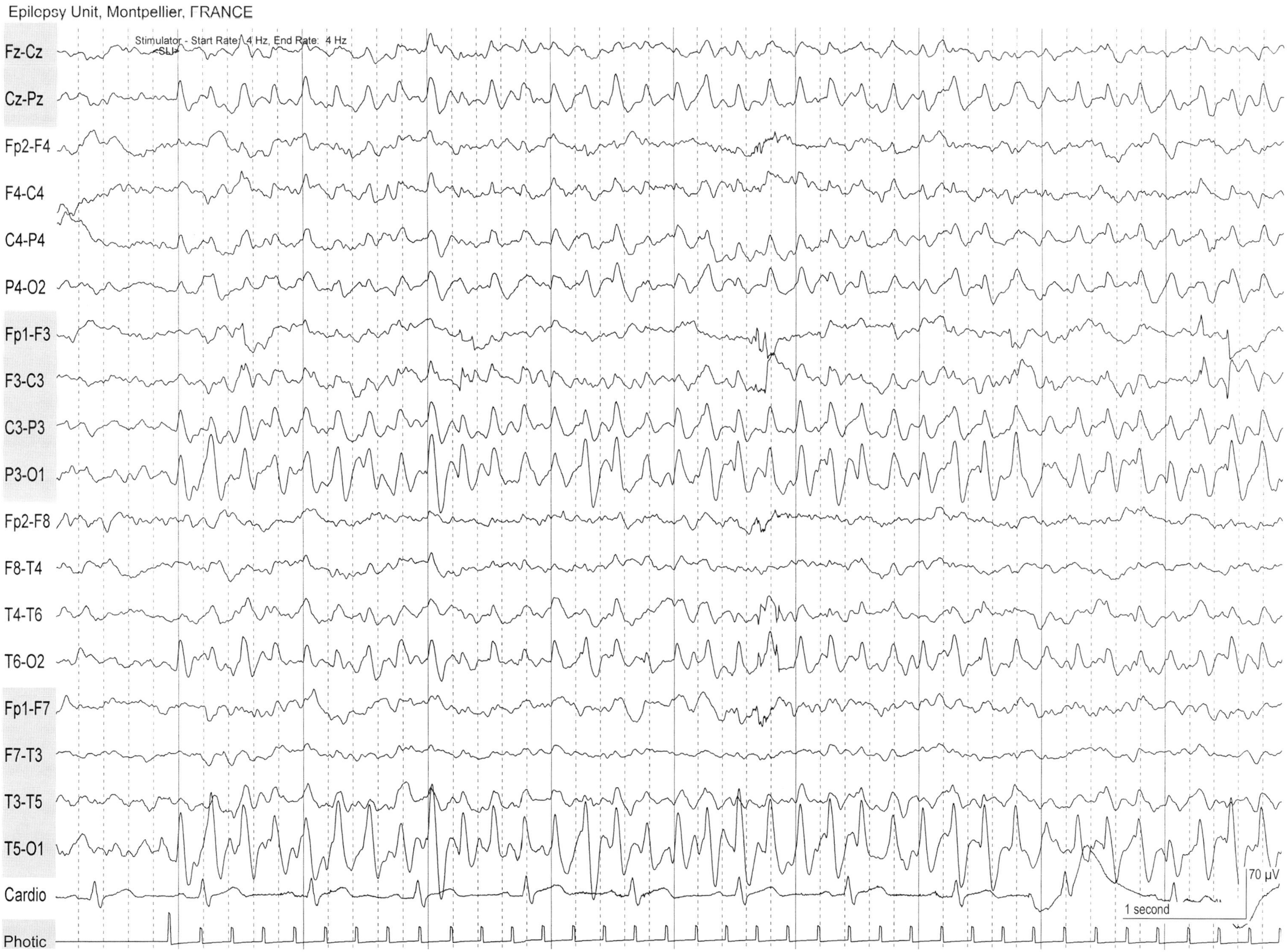
Epilepsy Unit, Montpellier, FRANCE
Stimulator - Start Rate: 4 Hz, End Rate: 4 Hz
Fz-Cz
Cz-Pz
Fp2-F4
F4-C4
C4-P4
P4-O2
Fp1-F3
F3-C3
C3-P3
P3-O1
Fp2-F8
F8-T4
T4-T6
T6-O2
Fp1-F7
F7-T3
T3-T5
T5-O1
Cardio
Photic
70 µV
1 second

• 18 Photomyogenic response (1)

Context

72-year-old woman with Parkinson disease.

What to note

The patient's eyes are closed. Slow background activity. Onset of photic stimulation at 12 Hz triggers contraction of periocular muscles with muscle artifacts on the anterior derivations.

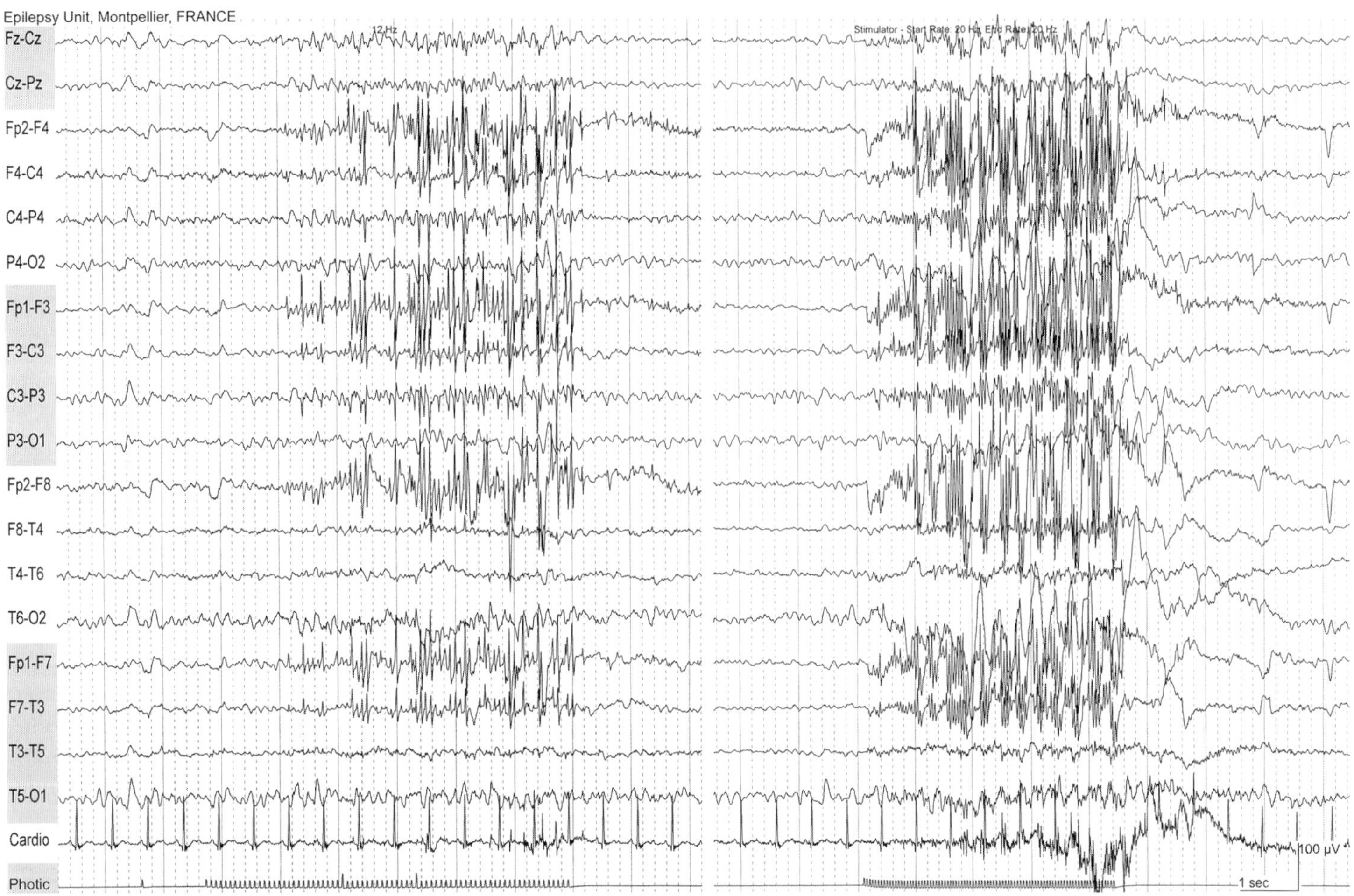

Figure a / Recording at 15 mm/s. On the left, photic stimulation at 12 Hz and, on the right, photic stimulation at 20 Hz. Muscle contraction is more intense at 20 Hz and spreads to neck muscles (muscle artifacts clearly detectable on the ECG derivation) because the patient moves his head.

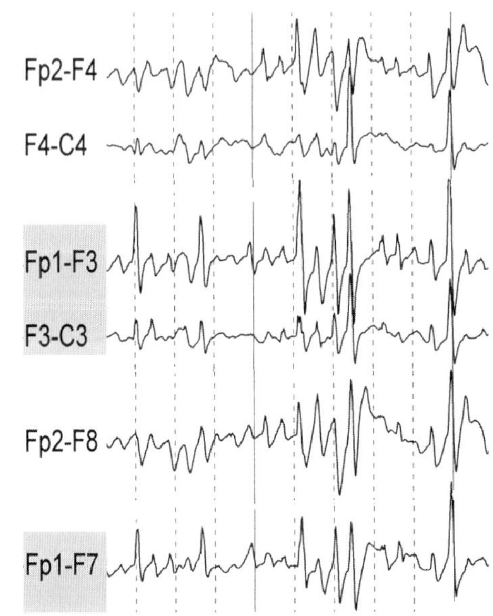

Figure b / Electromyographic potentials.

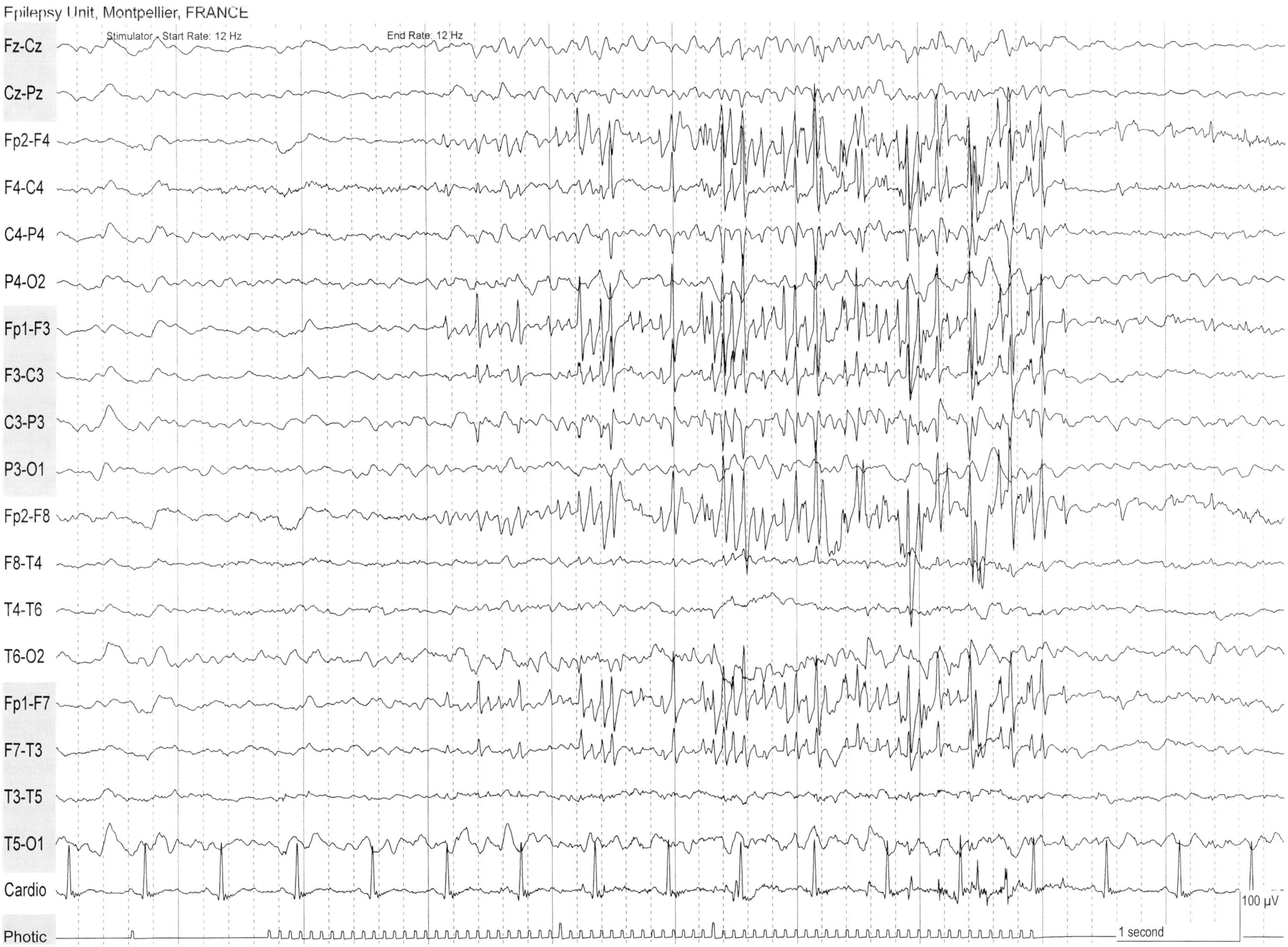
Epilepsy Unit, Montpellier, FRANCE
Stimulator - Start Rate: 12 Hz
End Rate: 12 Hz
Fz-Cz
Cz-Pz
Fp2-F4
F4-C4
C4-P4
P4-O2
Fp1-F3
F3-C3
C3-P3
P3-O1
Fp2-F8
F8-T4
T4-T6
T6-O2
Fp1-F7
F7-T3
T3-T5
T5-O1
Cardio
Photic
100 µV
1 second

• 19 Photomyogenic response (2)

Context

79-year-old man with a history of cerebrovacular accident.

What to note

Photic stimulation at 16 Hz triggering contractions of the periorbital muscles conveyed on the EEG by eyelid and muscle artifacts on the frontal derivations. The photomyogenic response ceases immediately with termination of stimulation.

Comment

Photomyogenic response is observed in particular in the elderly or in withdrawal syndromes (e.g. alcohol, psychotropics, barbiturates).

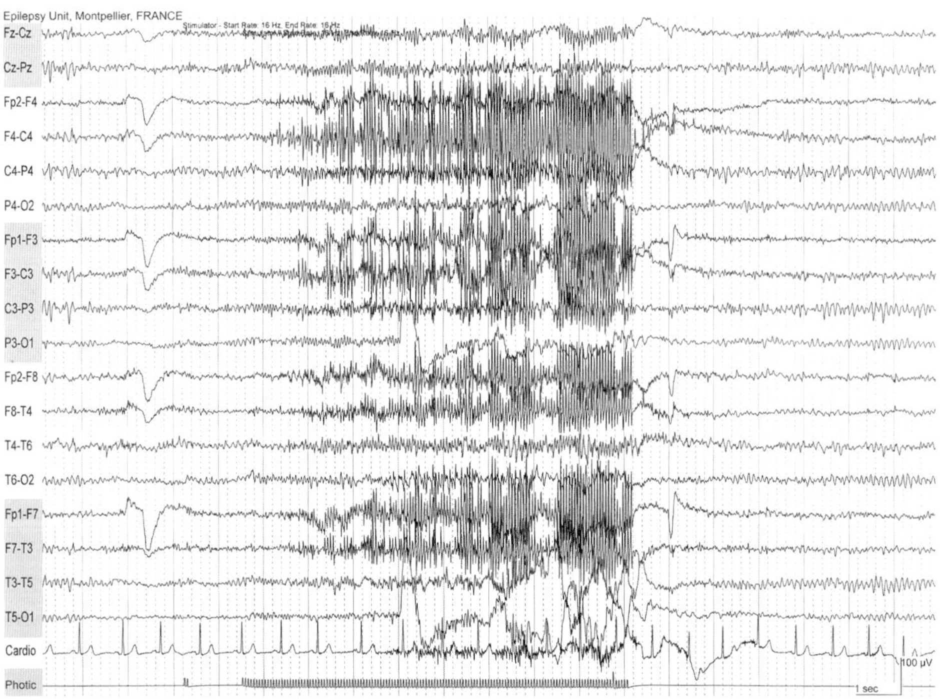

Figure a / Recording at 15 mm/s.

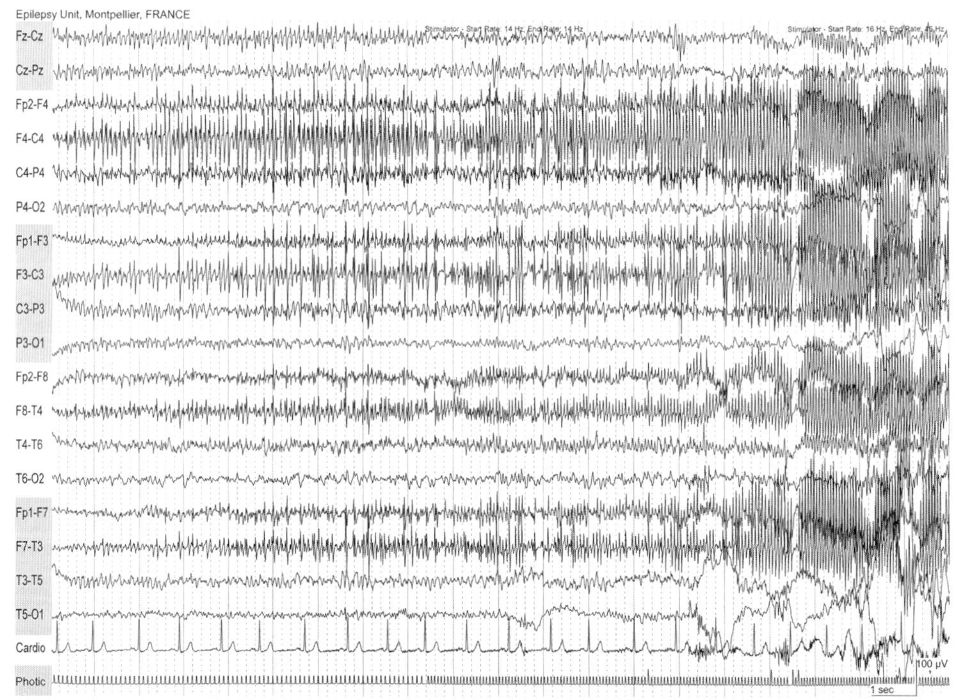

Figure b / Same patient (recording at 15 mm/s). The amplitude of the photic response gradually builds up with photic stimulation.

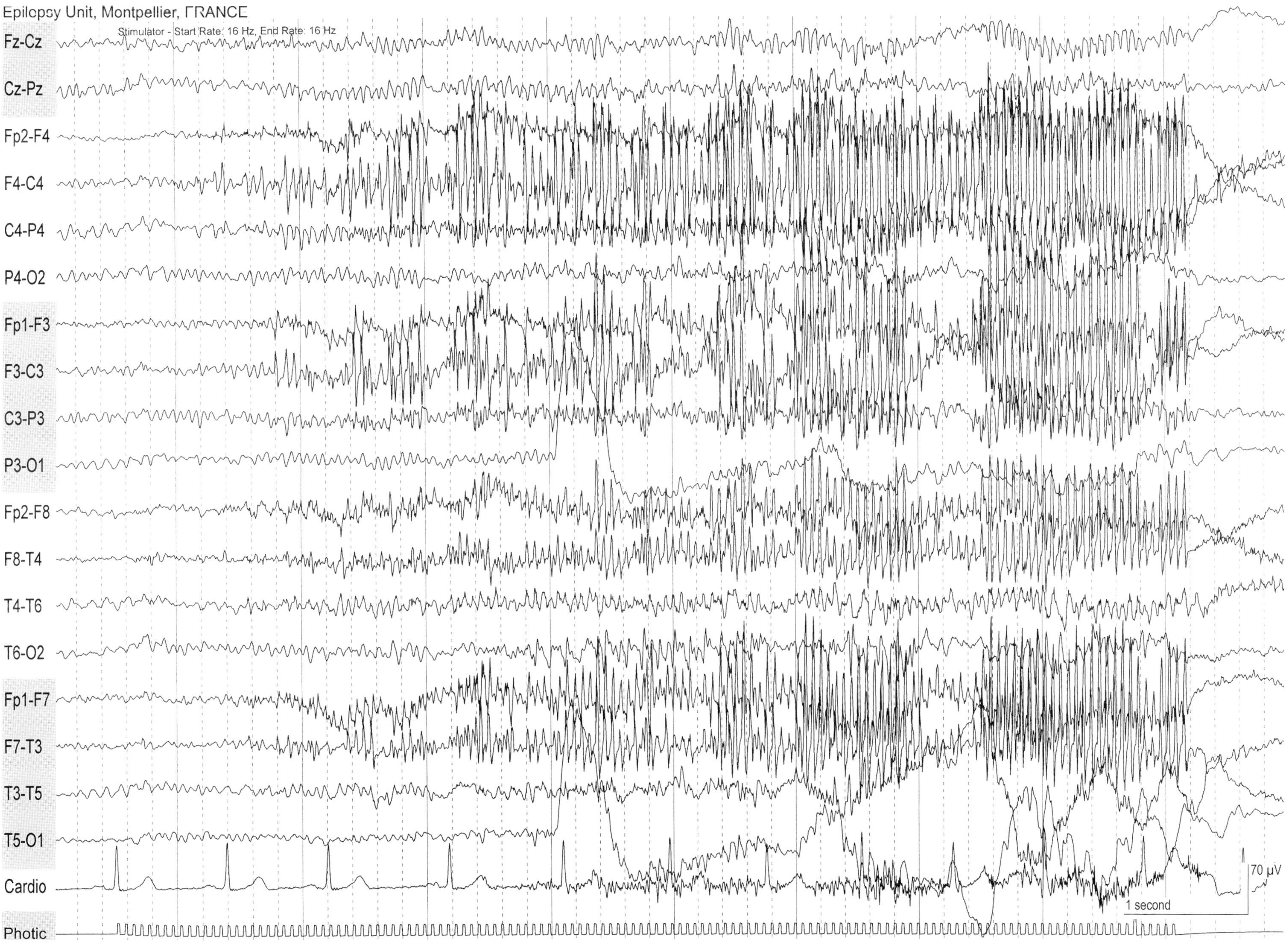
Epilepsy Unit, Montpellier, FRANCE
Stimulator - Start Rate: 16 Hz, End Rate: 16 Hz
Fz-Cz
Cz-Pz
Fp2-F4
F4-C4
C4-P4
P4-O2
Fp1-F3
F3-C3
C3-P3
P3-O1
Fp2-F8
F8-T4
T4-T6
T6-O2
Fp1-F7
F7-T3
T3-T5
T5-O1
Cardio
Photic
70 µV
1 second

• 20 Paroxysmal photosensitive response (photoparoxysmal response) (1)

Context

22-year-old woman with idiopathic generalized epilepsy.

What to note

First the patient's eyes are open, then she closes her eyes two seconds before stimulation at 19 Hz. Irregular spike-waves appear rapidly during 3 seconds but they are limited to the occipital regions, then the background alpha rhythm can be seen again. This is a subtle photoparoxysmal response.

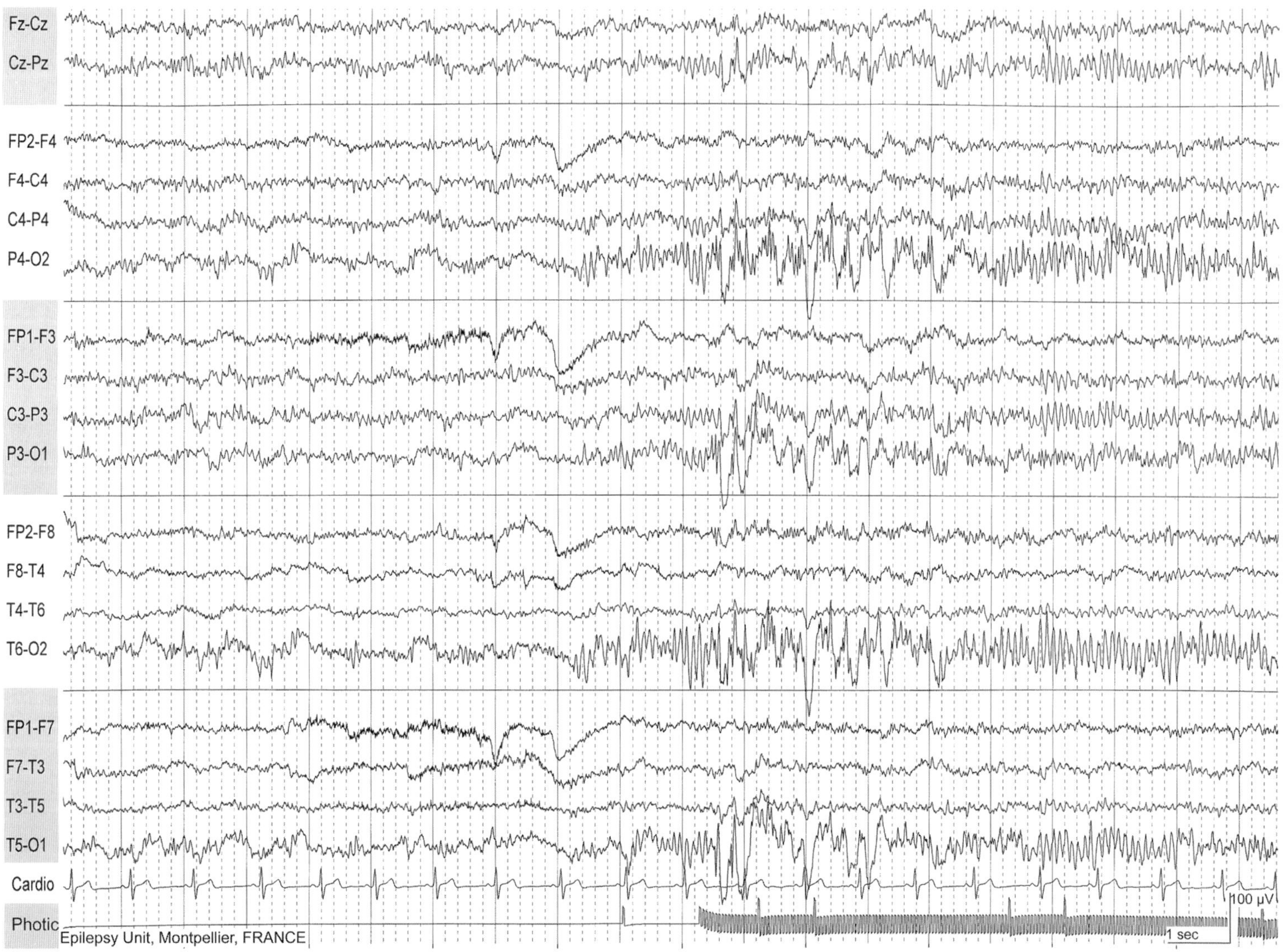

Figure a / Recording at 15 mm/s.

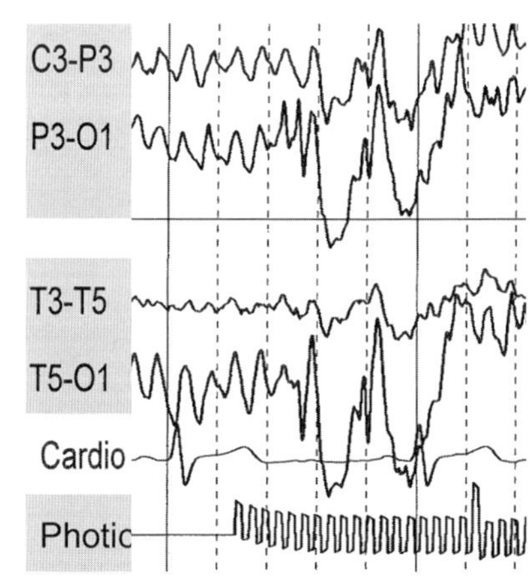

Figure b / Spike-waves.

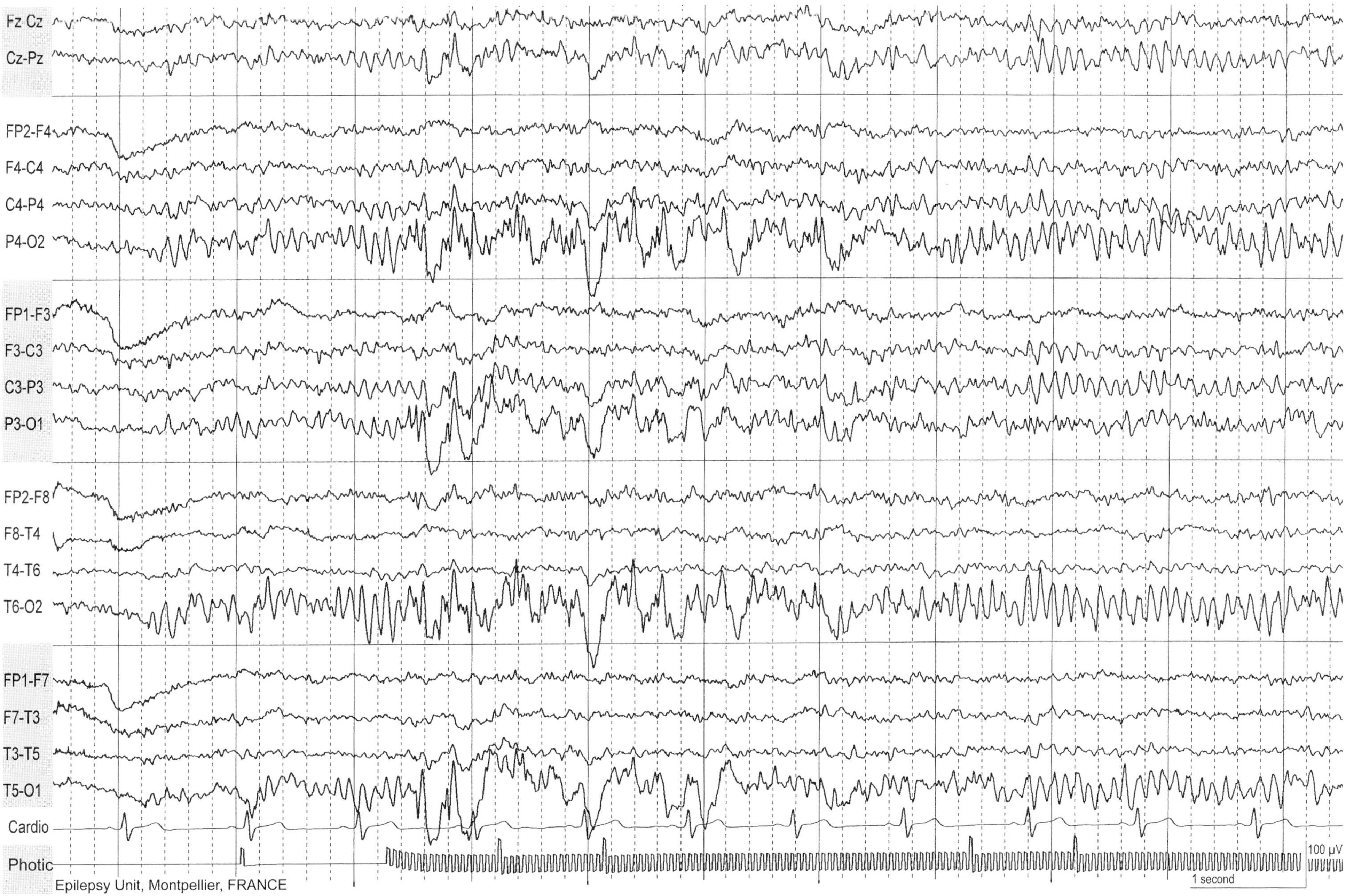
Fz Cz
Cz-Pz
FP2-F4
F4-C4
C4-P4
P4-O2
FP1-F3
F3-C3
C3-P3
P3-O1
FP2-F8
F8-T4
T4-T6
T6-O2
FP1-F7
F7-T3
T3-T5
T5-O1
Cardio
Photic
Epilepsy Unit, Montpellier, FRANCE
100 µV
1 second

II • 21 Paroxysmal photosensitive response (photoparoxysmal response) (2)

Context

20-year-old woman referred for idiopathic generalized epilepsy.

What to note

Symmetrical posterior alpha rhythm, closed eyes. On the left, photic stimulation at 11 Hz triggers a discharge of irregular diffuse fast spike-waves. On the right, with photic stimulation at 13 Hz, a more generalized discharge of irregular diffuse spike-waves that continues after termination of the stimulation.

Comment

It is not necessary to increase frequency to 13 Hz after obtaining a photoparoxysmal response at 11 Hz. When the lower photosensitivity threshold is determined, it is interesting to assess the photosensitivity range. To do so, photic stimulation is then performed at high frequencies (60 Hz) after which the frequencies are decreased gradually to determine the upper threshold. Repeating stimulations within the photosensitivity range is stressful for the patient and there is a risk of provoking a seizure.

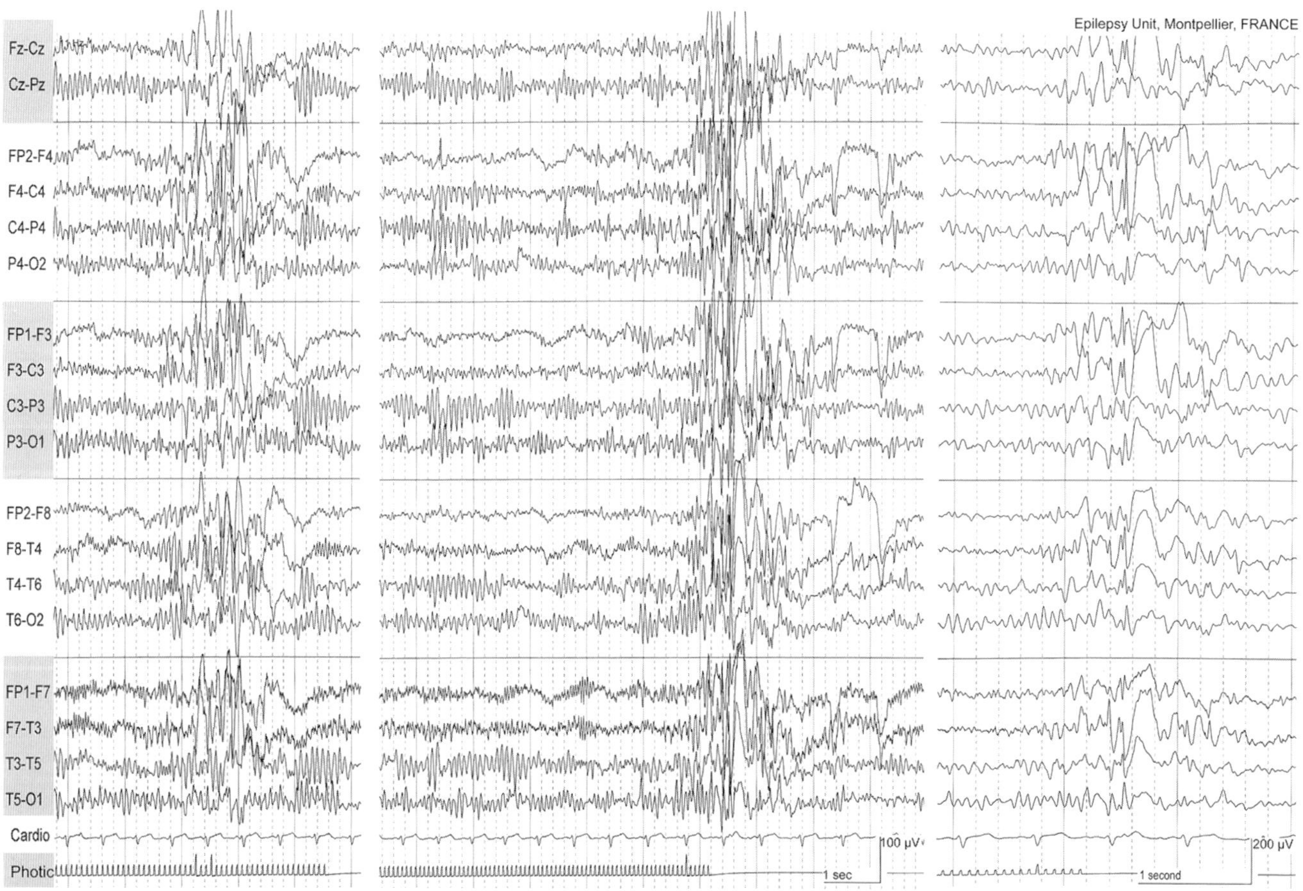

Figure a / On the left and in the middle, recording at 15 mm/s. On the right, when input is recalibrated (20 µV/mm and 30 mm/s), the spikes are clearly visible.

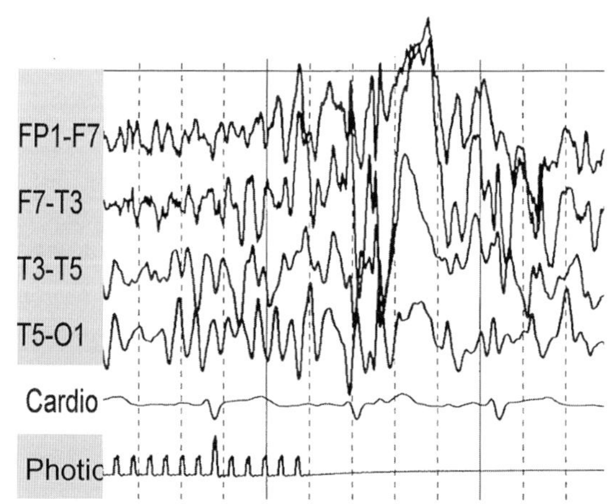

Figure b / Intermittent photic stimulation triggers a response at 13 Hz.

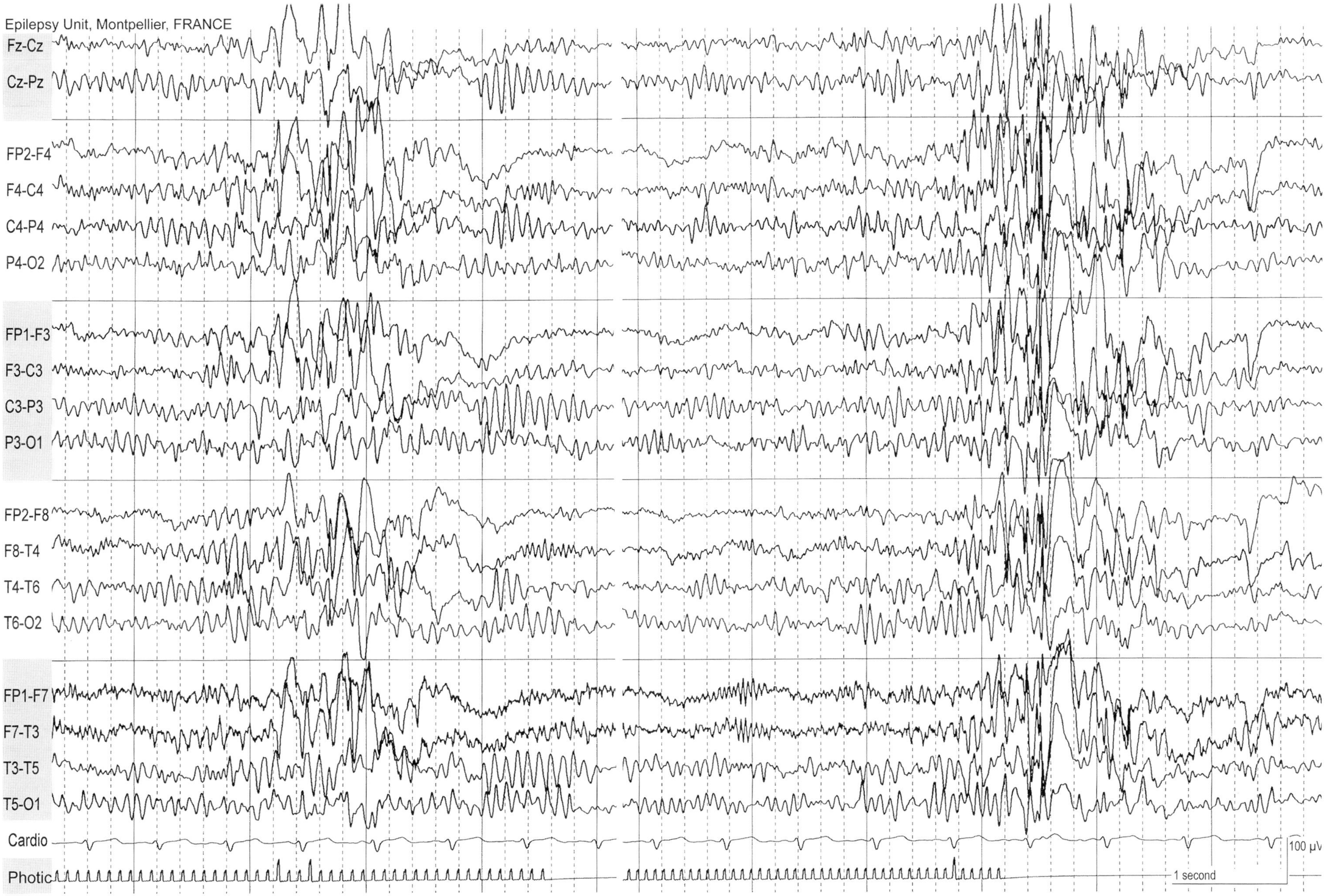
Epilepsy Unit, Montpellier, FRANCE
Fz-Cz
Cz-Pz
FP2-F4
F4-C4
C4-P4
P4-O2
FP1-F3
F3-C3
C3-P3
P3-O1
FP2-F8
F8-T4
T4-T6
T6-O2
FP1-F7
F7-T3
T3-T5
T5-O1
Cardio
Photic
100 µV
1 second

II • 22 Paroxysmal photosensitive response (photoparoxysmal response) (3)

Context

45-year-old woman with juvenile myoclonic epilepsy.

What to note

The patient's eyes are open. Photic stimulation flashing at 92 Hz. During stimulation, the background activity change indicates photosensitivity. At 4 seconds of stimulation, a burst of irregular diffuse spike-waves appears that continues after termination of the stimulation. This patient's photosensitivity ranges from 8 to 93 Hz (see below IPS at 93 Hz). A range as wide as this patient's is quite unusual.

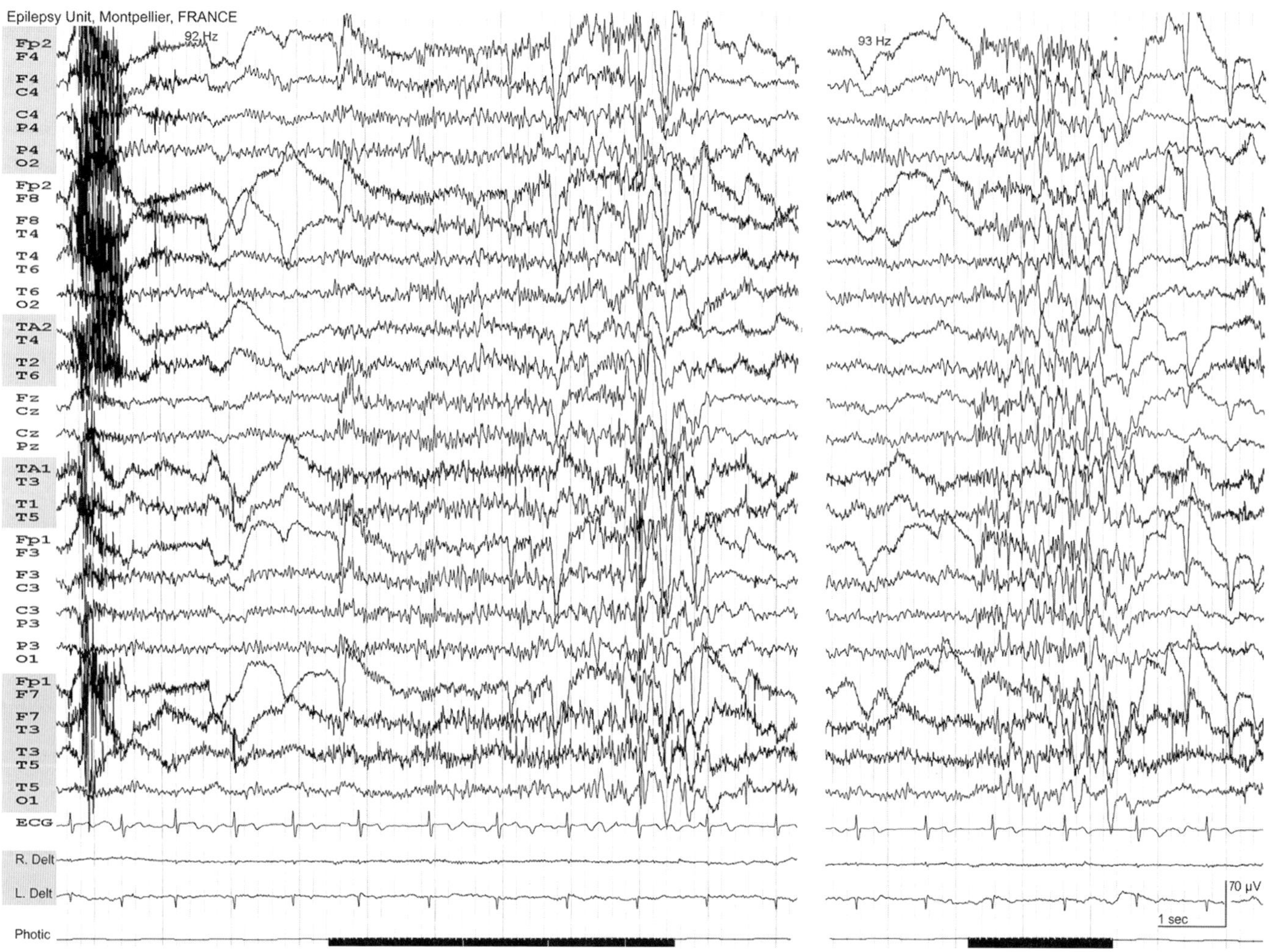

Figure a / Recording at 15 mm/s. Right segment, paroxysmal photosensitive response at 93 Hz.

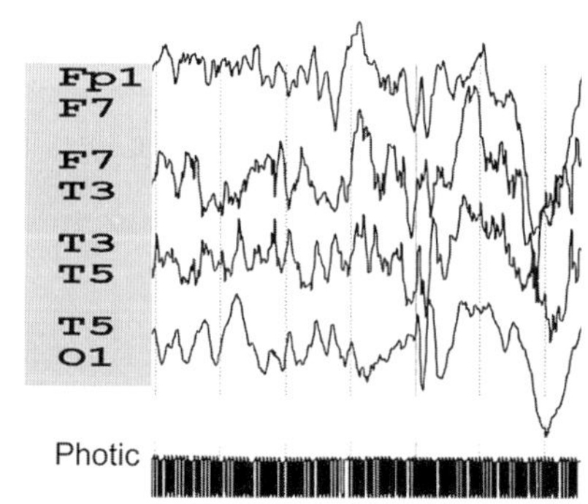

Figure b / Irregular spike-waves during intermittent photic stimulation at 92 Hz.

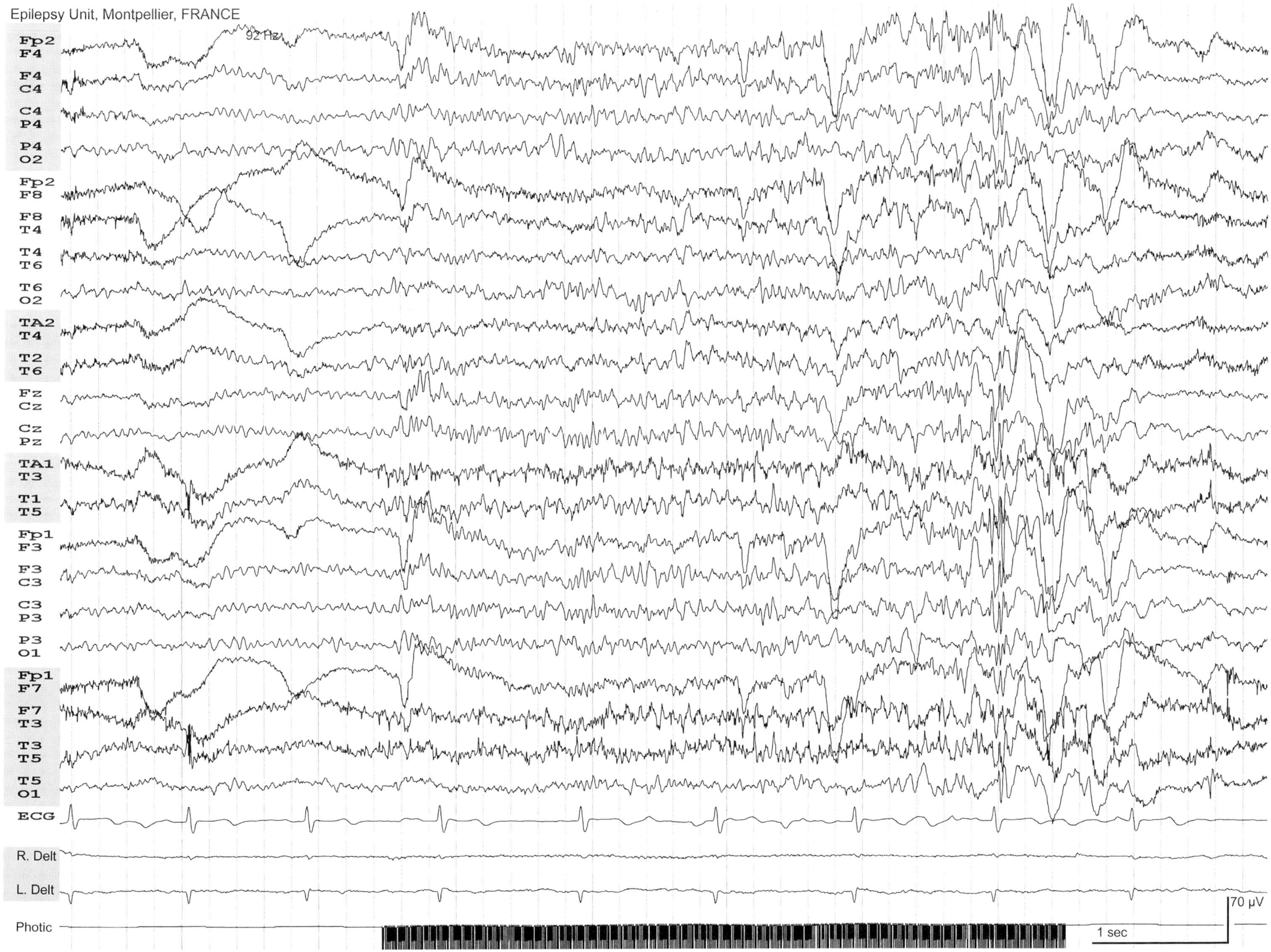
Epilepsy Unit, Montpellier, FRANCE
92 Hz
Fp2 F4
F4 C4
C4 P4
P4 O2
Fp2 F8
F8 T4
T4 T6
T6 O2
TA2 T4
T2 T6
Fz Cz
Cz Pz
TA1 T3
T1 T5
Fp1 F3
F3 C3
C3 P3
P3 O1
Fp1 F7
F7 T3
T3 T5
T5 O1
ECG
R. Delt
L. Delt
Photic
70 µV
1 sec

II • 23 Paroxysmal photosensitive response (photoparoxysmal response) at the same frequency as the flashes

Context

19-year-old woman referred for photogenic epilepsy (Jeavons syndrome).

What to note

The patient's eyes are closed. Left segment, photic stimulation at 10 Hz triggers alpha-like activity over the occipital regions. The amplitude of the photic response gradually builds up. Right segment, photoparoxysmal response at 18 Hz. There are spikes over the posterior regions at the same frequency of the flashes. This response is not a photic driving.

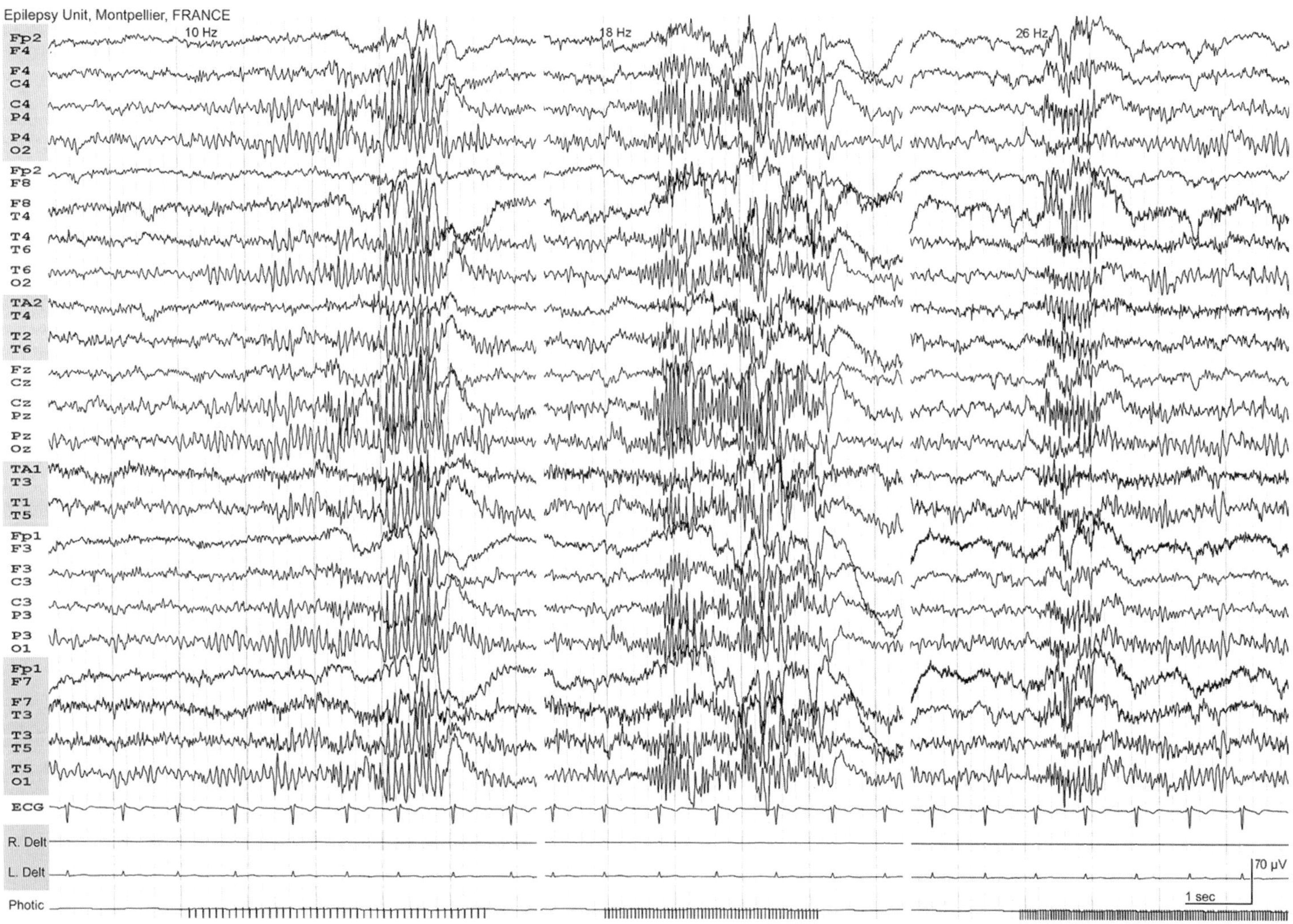

Figure a / Recording at 15 mm/s. Right segment, IPS at 26 Hz triggers spikes at 26 Hz during 0.5 second. Then there is a fall-off.

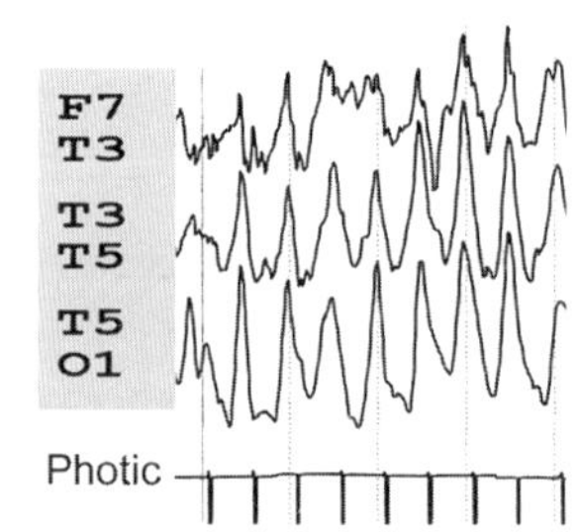

Figure b / The spikes are time-locked to the flash frequency at 10 Hz.

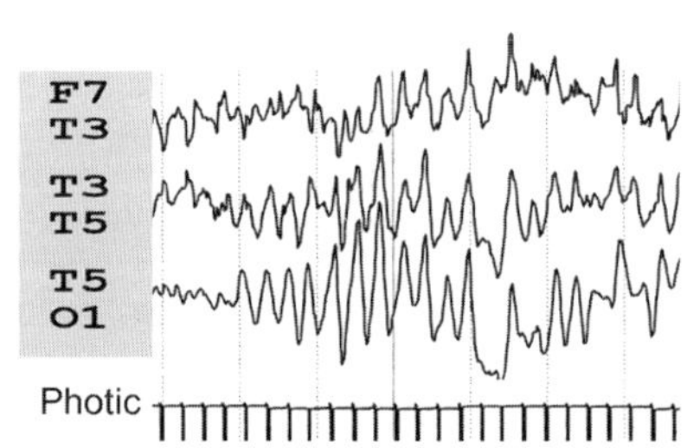

Figure c / The spikes are time-locked to the flash frequency at 18 Hz.

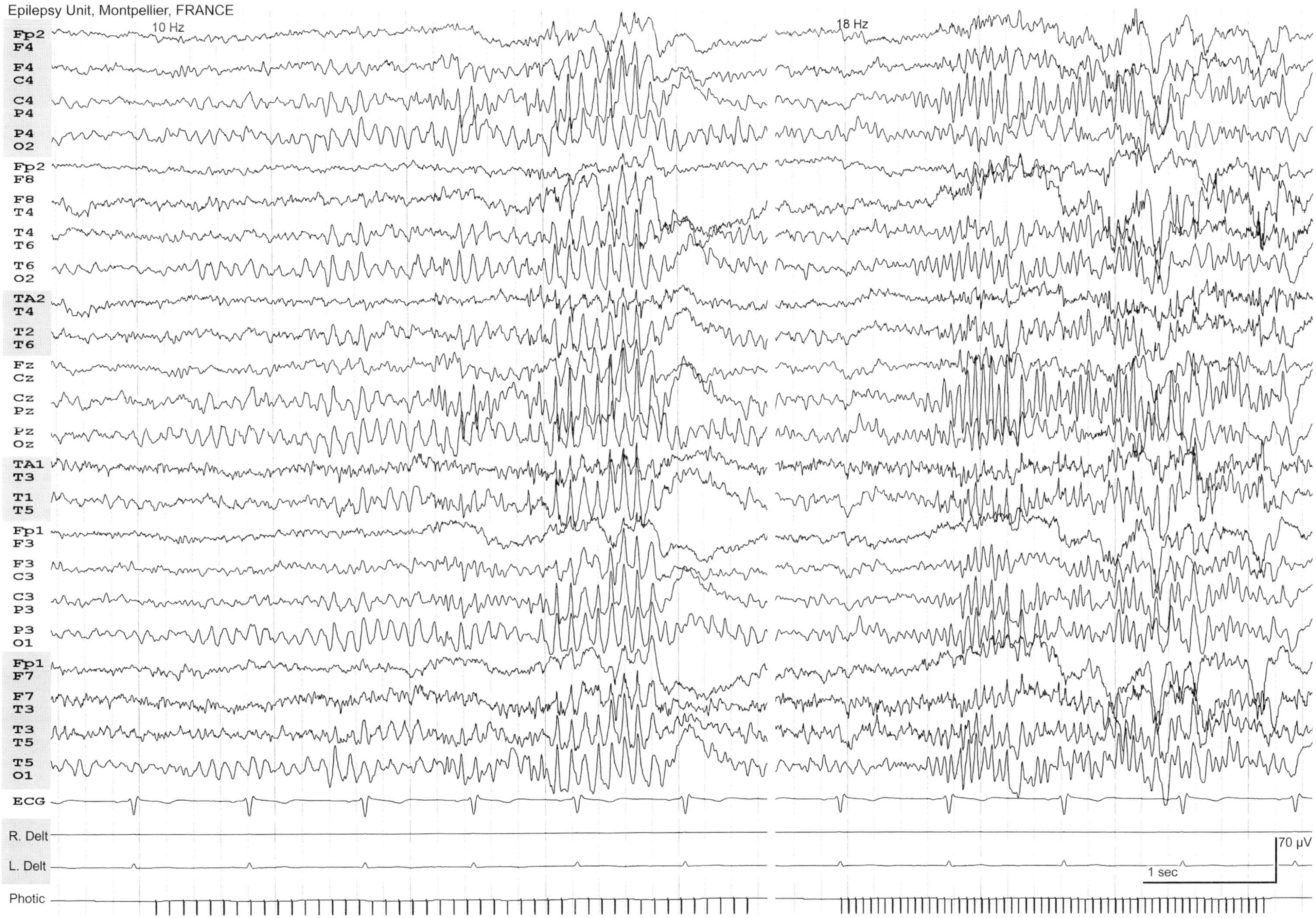
Epilepsy Unit, Montpellier, FRANCE
10 Hz
18 Hz
Fp2 F4
F4 C4
C4 P4
P4 O2
Fp2 F8
F8 T4
T4 T6
T6 O2
TA2 T4
T2 T6
Fz Cz
Cz Pz
Pz Oz
TA1 T3
T1 T5
Fp1 F3
F3 C3
C3 P3
P3 O1
Fp1 F7
F7 T3
T3 T5
T5 O1
ECG
R. Delt
L. Delt
Photic
70 µV
1 sec

II • 24 Asymmetrical paroxysmal photosensitive response (photoparoxysmal response)

Context

25-year-old man with frontal lobe epilepsy. Brain MRI is normal.

What to note

The patient's eyes are closed. Photic stimulation at 8 Hz triggers sharp waves at 8 Hz over the left occipital region and then spike-waves at 8 Hz over the left fronto-polar region. The delay (1.4 seconds) between the onset of photic stimulation to the appearance of the response is the same at 8 Hz and 12 Hz (see below).

Comment

A photoparoxysmal respone in extraoccipital epilepsy is very uncommon (Jukkarwala *et al.*, 2011), as is an asymmetrical response.

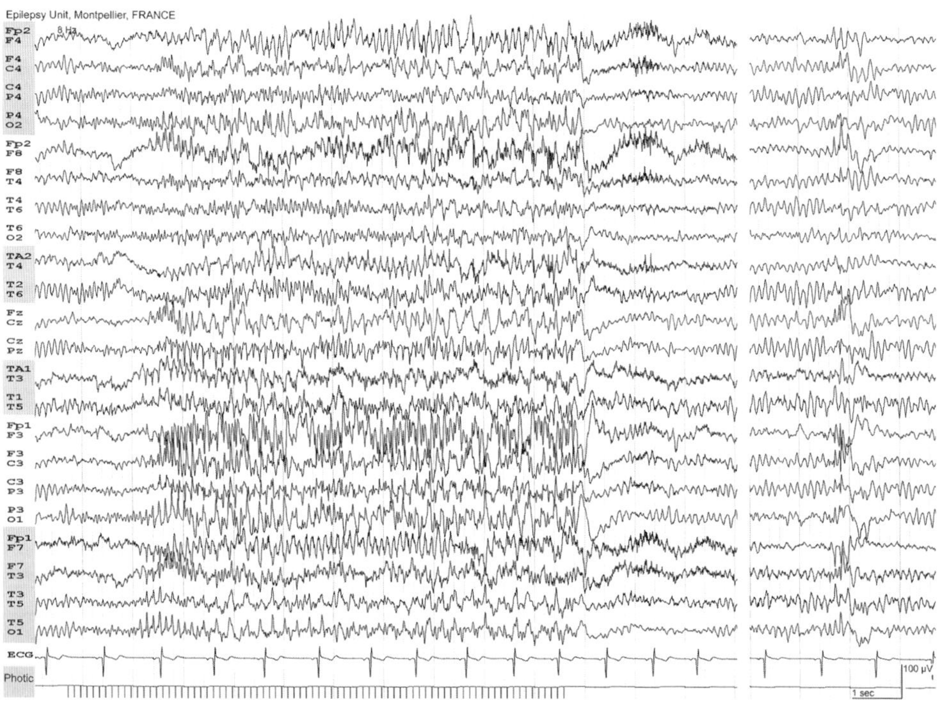

Figure a / Recording at 15 mm/s. Left segment, the photoparoxysmal response stops when the stimulation stops. Right segment, interictal fast spike-waves at the frontal derivations.

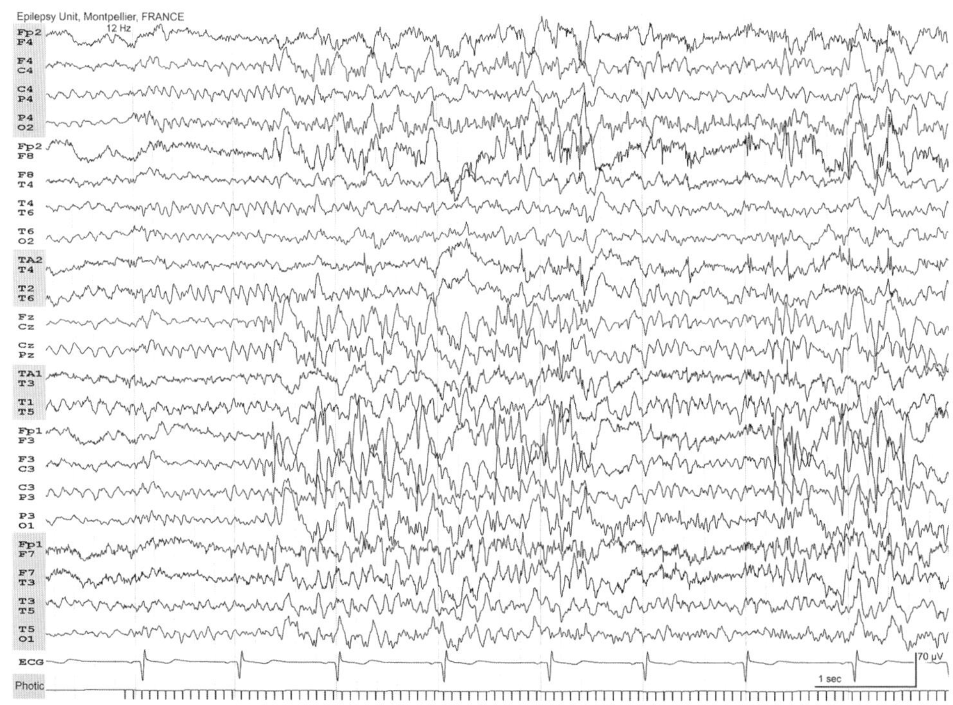

Figure b / Recording at 30 mm/s. Asymmetrical photoparoxysmal response on the left hemisphere at 12 Hz.

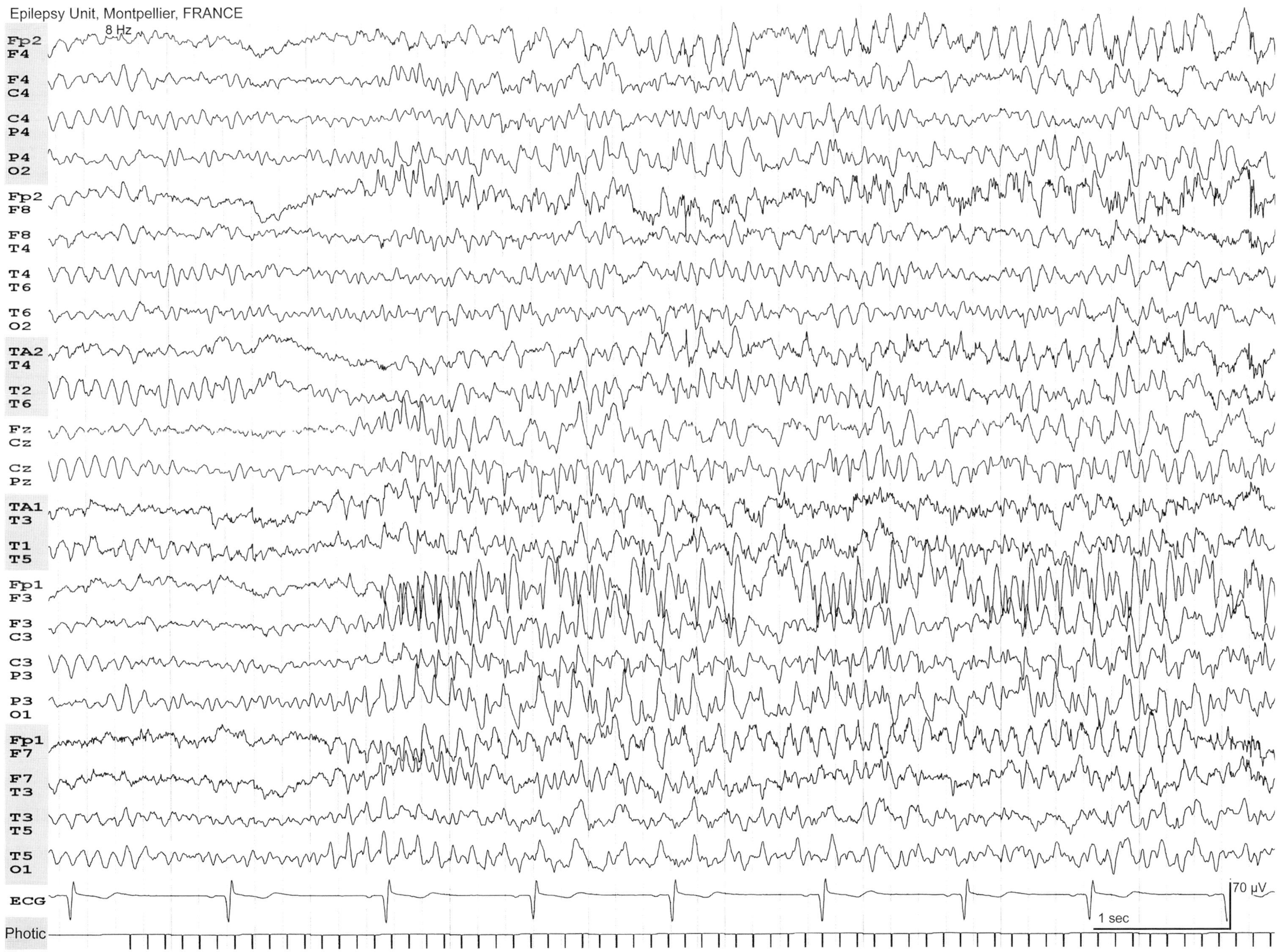

Epilepsy Unit, Montpellier, FRANCE
8 Hz
Fp2 F4
F4 C4
C4 P4
P4 O2
Fp2 F8
F8 T4
T4 T6
T6 O2
TA2 T4
T2 T6
Fz Cz
Cz Pz
TA1 T3
T1 T5
Fp1 F3
F3 C3
C3 P3
P3 O1
Fp1 F7
F7 T3
T3 T5
T5 O1
ECG
Photic
70 µV
1 sec

II • 25 Myoclonic jerks triggered by intermittent photic stimulation

Context

18-year-old woman with juvenile myoclonic epilepsy.

What to note

Photic stimulation at 15 Hz triggers a burst of irregular generalized spike-waves associated with a myoclonic jerk seen on the right deltoid muscle. The patient reported discomfort and myoclonic jerks when driving along roads lined with trees (alternating shade/sunlight).

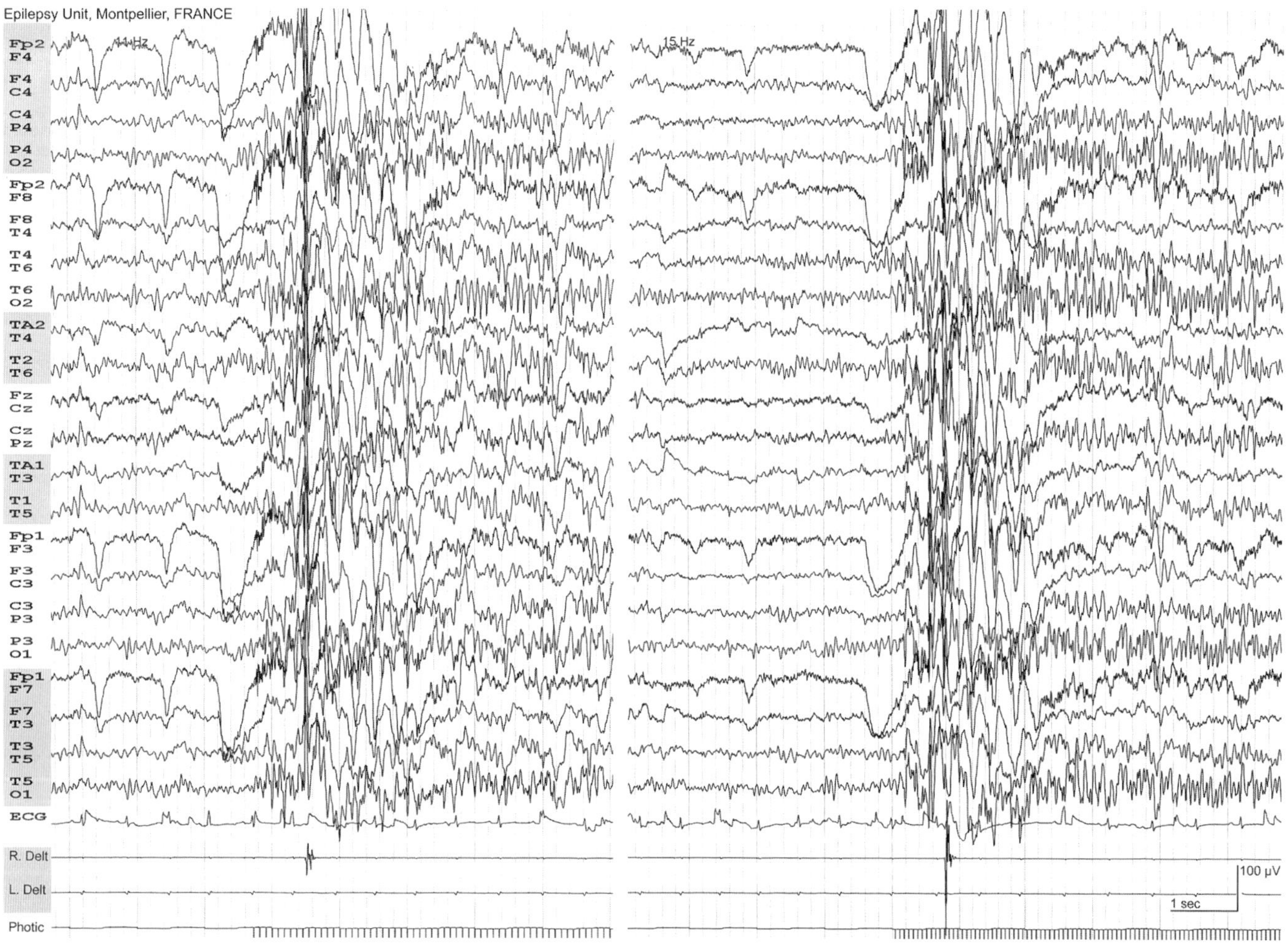

Figure a / Recording at 15 mm/s. IPS at 11 and 15 Hz. Burst of spike-waves with a myclonic jerk on the right deltoid muscle. It is not necessary to increase frequency to 15 Hz after obtaining a photoparoxysmal response at 11 Hz and the stimulation should be stopped immediately when a jerk occurs.

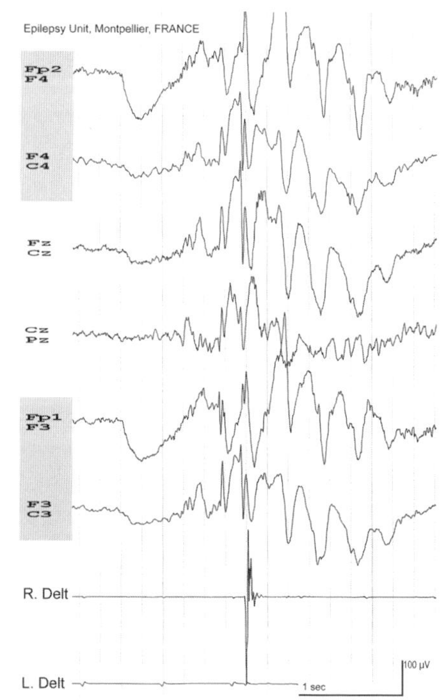

Figure b / Spike-waves discharge associated with myoclonic jerk seen on the right deltoid muscle.

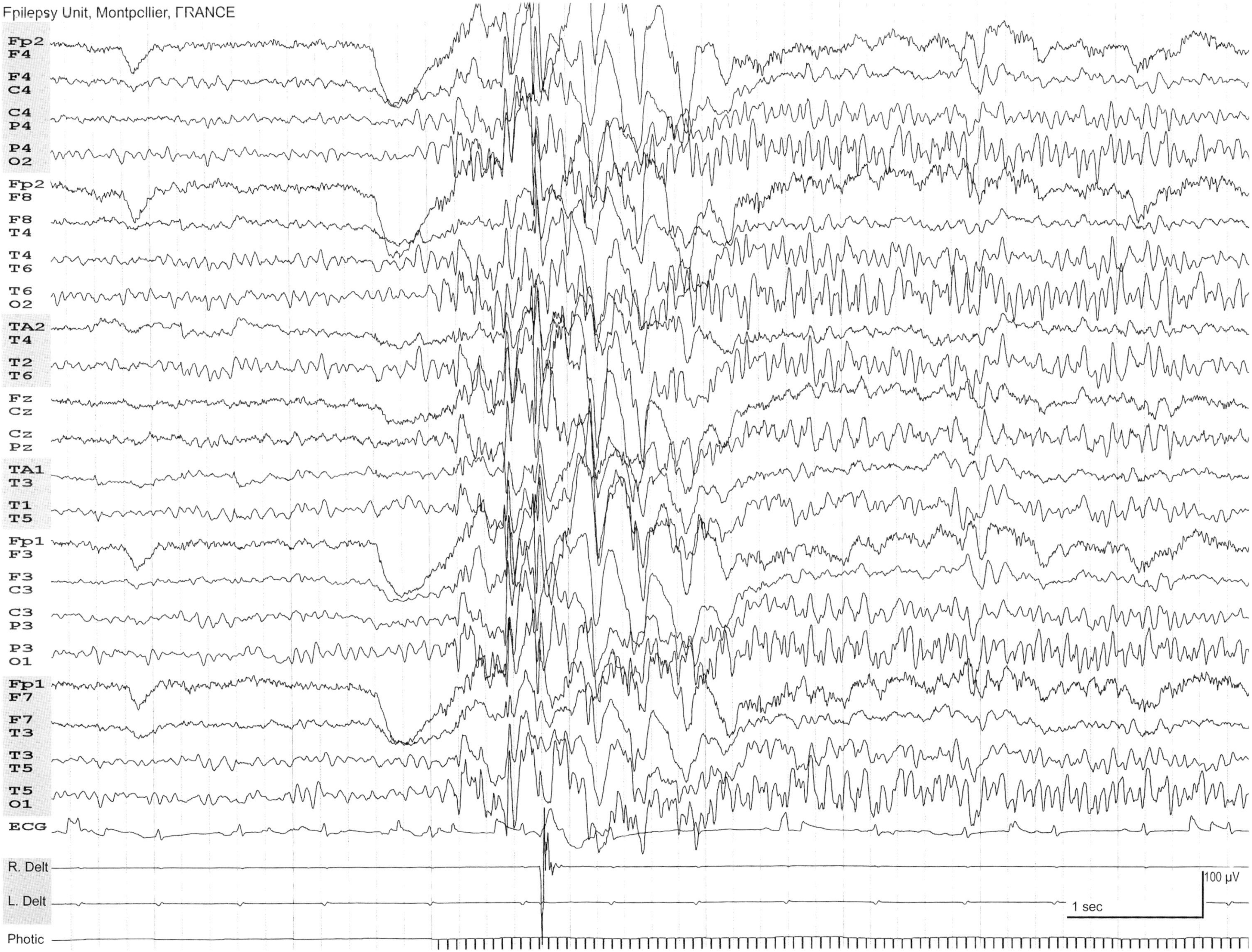
Epilepsy Unit, Montpellier, FRANCE
Fp2 F4
F4 C4
C4 P4
P4 O2
Fp2 F8
F8 T4
T4 T6
T6 O2
TA2 T4
T2 T6
Fz Cz
Cz Pz
TA1 T3
T1 T5
Fp1 F3
F3 C3
C3 P3
P3 O1
Fp1 F7
F7 T3
T3 T5
T5 O1
ECG
R. Delt
L. Delt
Photic
100 μV
1 sec

II • 26 Absence triggered by intermittent photic stimulation (1)

Context

15-year-old woman with idiopathic generalized epilepsy.

What to note

An intermittent photic stimulation (IPS) is performed at a 30 Hz frequency and triggers at 8 seconds (see plate at 15 mm/s) a polyspike-wave discharge followed by 3.5 Hz generalized spike-waves for more than 5 seconds after offset of this stimulation, which corresponds to a clinical absence.

Comment

When abnormal responses triggered by stimulation persist after offset of IPS, there is a high probability of epilepsy.

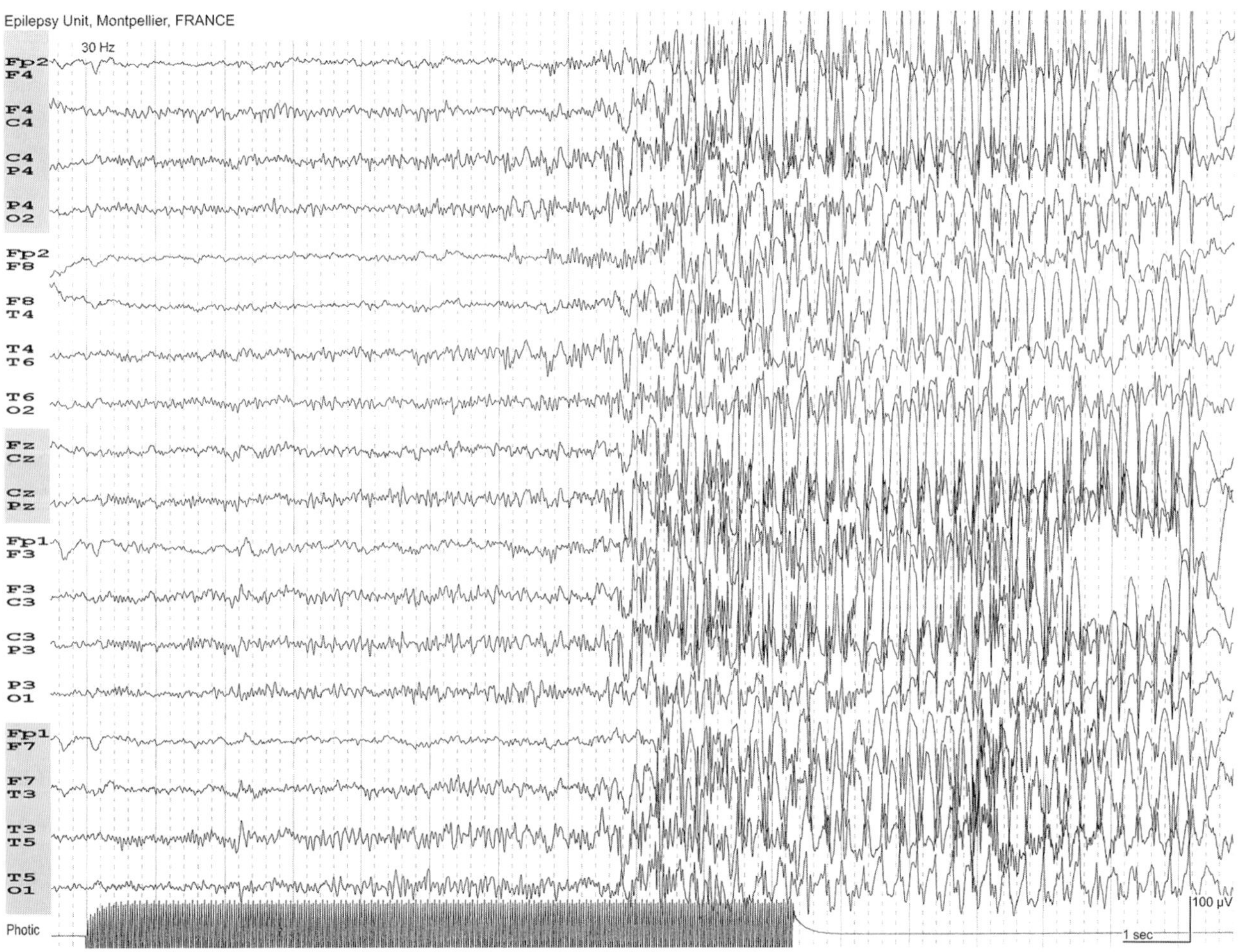

Figure a / Recording at 15 mm/s. Mu rhythm at F4-C4 at the beginning of the plate. An IPS triggers at 8 seconds a clinical absence.

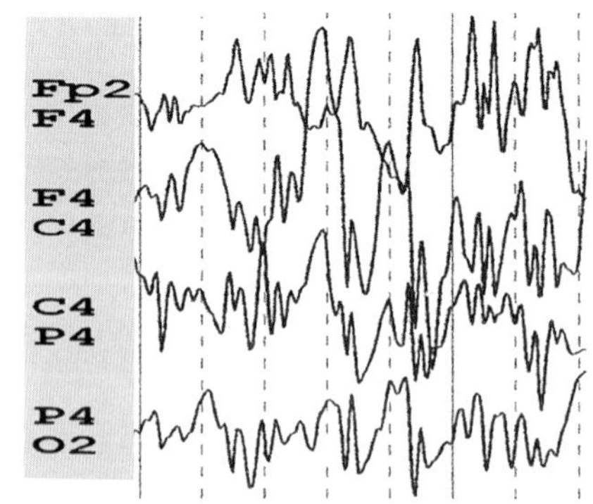

Figure b / Polyspike-waves.

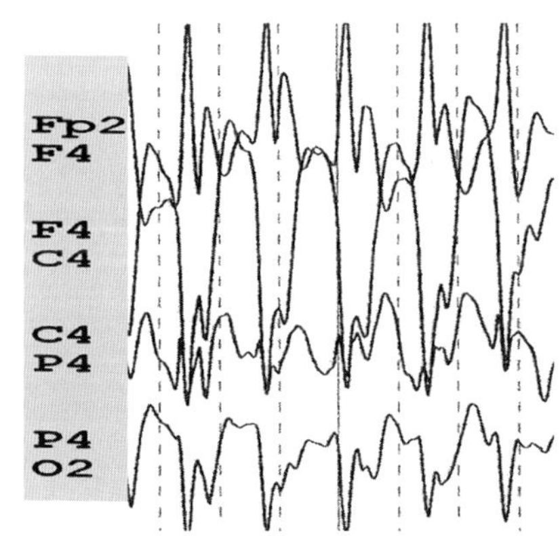

Figure c / 3.5 Hz generalized spike-waves.

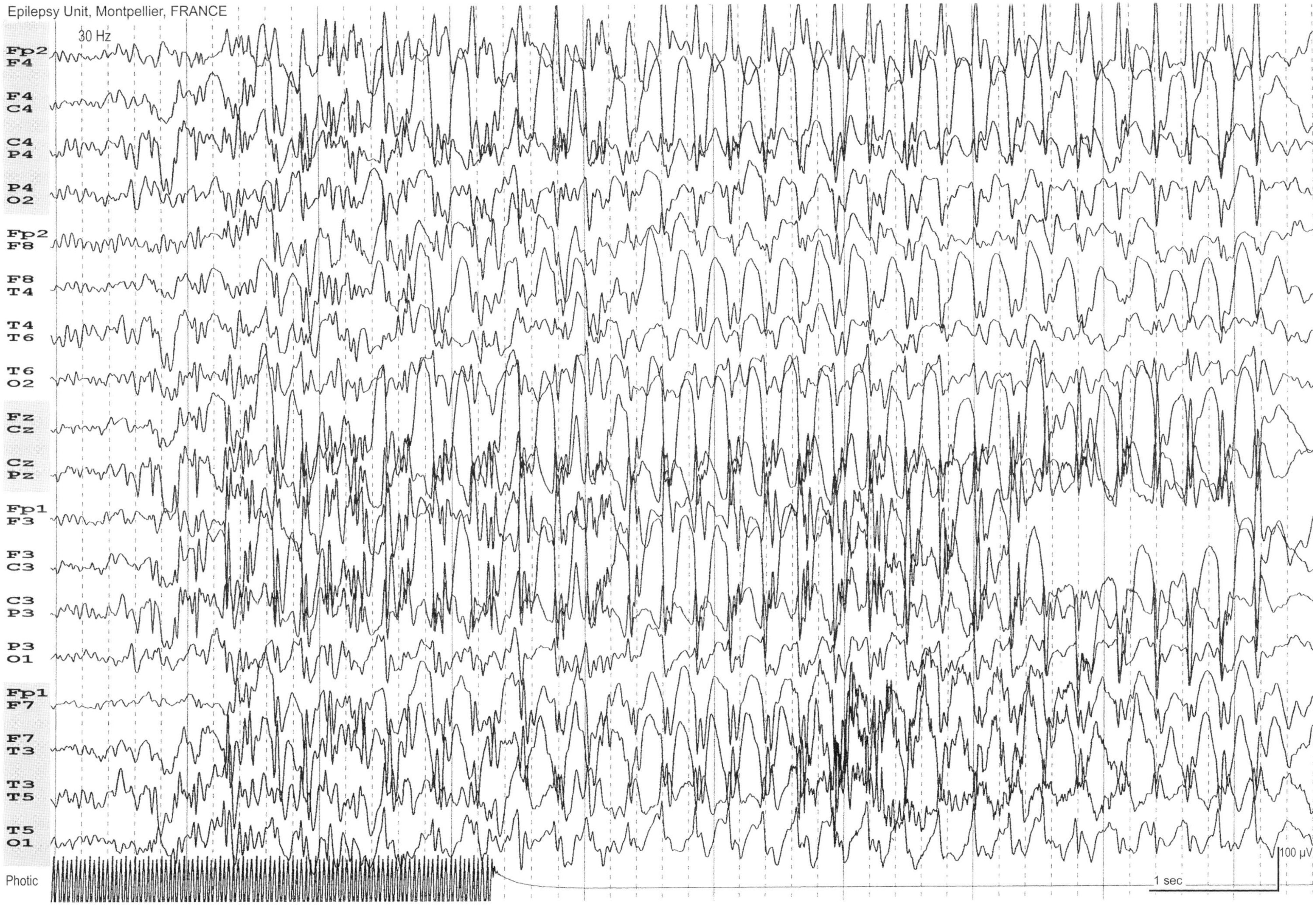
Epilepsy Unit, Montpellier, FRANCE
30 Hz
Fp2 F4
F4 C4
C4 P4
P4 O2
Fp2 F8
F8 T4
T4 T6
T6 O2
Fz Cz
Cz Pz
Fp1 F3
F3 C3
C3 P3
P3 O1
Fp1 F7
F7 T3
T3 T5
T5 O1
Photic
100 µV
1 sec

• 27 Absence triggered by intermittent photic stimulation (2)

Context

16-year-old woman with photosensitive idiopathic generalized epilepsy.

What to note

The patient's eyes are open and she is asked to close them at onset of the photic stimulation at 15 Hz. Half a second after onset of flashes, a discharge of regular generalized spike-waves occurs at 3 Hz during 3 seconds, corresponding to an absence. As soon as the technician notices the onset of the discharge, the stimulation is stopped and she speaks to the patient to check her state of consciousness.

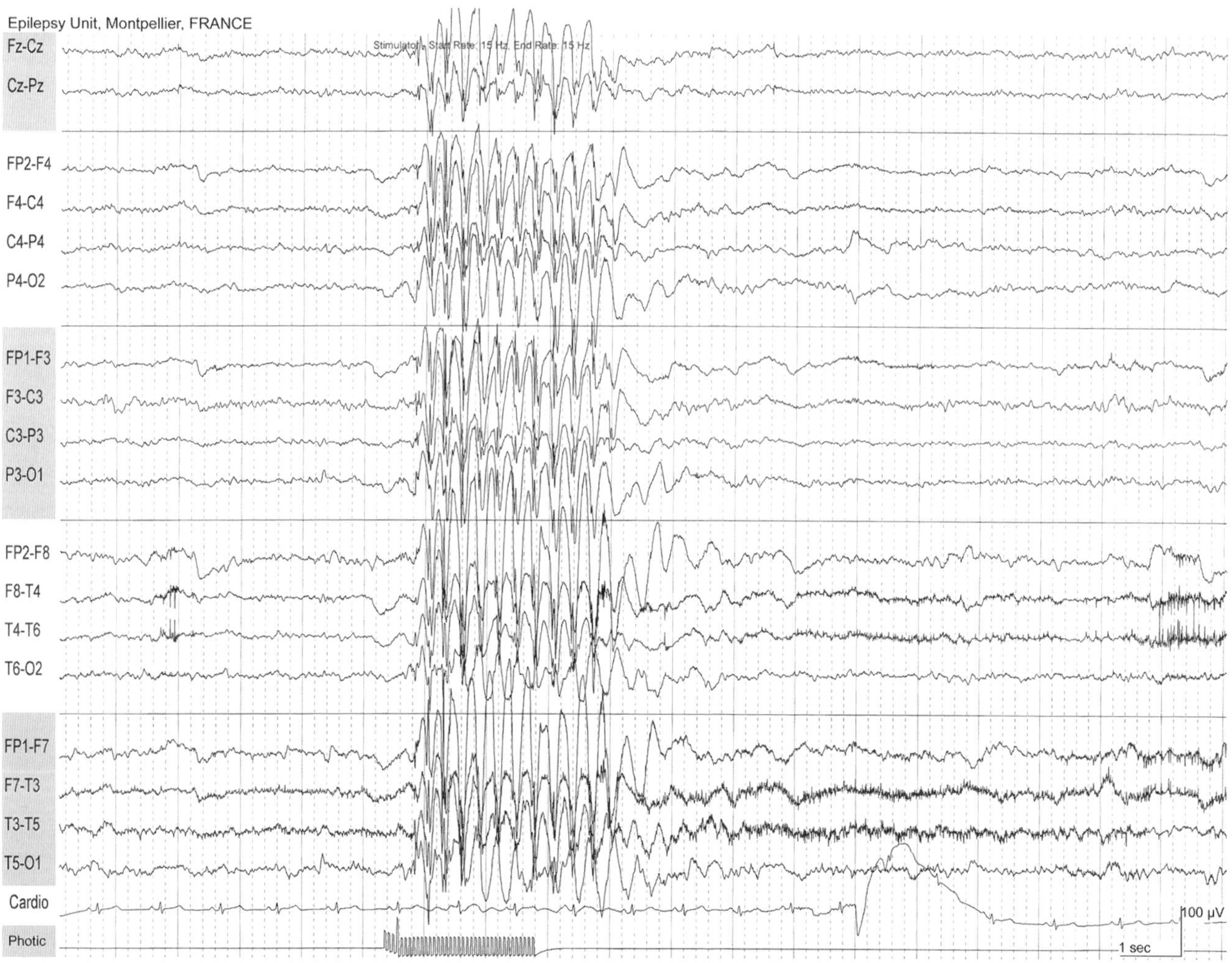

Figure a / Recorded at 15 mm/s.

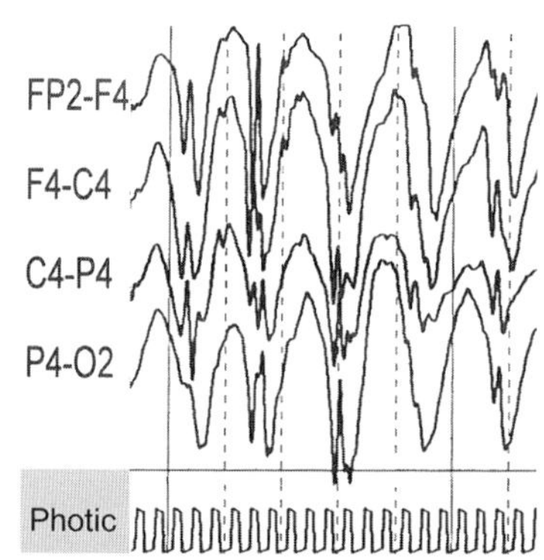

Figure b / Discharge of generalized spike-waves (absence triggered by the IPS).

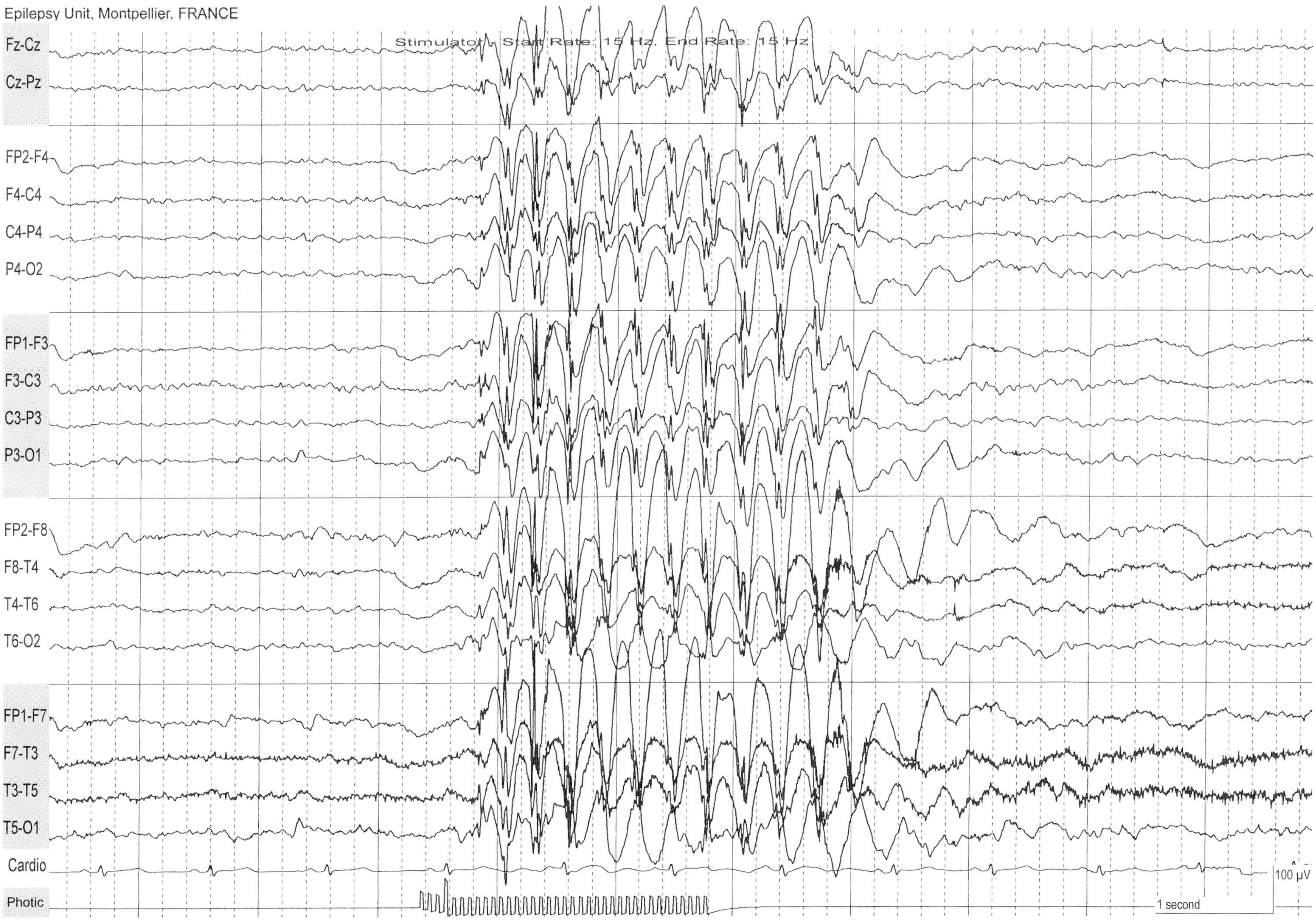
Epilepsy Unit, Montpellier, FRANCE
Stimulator, Start Rate: 15 Hz, End Rate: 15 Hz
Fz-Cz
Cz-Pz
FP2-F4
F4-C4
C4-P4
P4-O2
FP1-F3
F3-C3
C3-P3
P3-O1
FP2-F8
F8-T4
T4-T6
T6-O2
FP1-F7
F7-T3
T3-T5
T5-O1
Cardio
Photic
100 µV
1 second

II • 28 Focal seizure triggered by intermittent photic stimulation

Context

25-year-old woman referred for symptomatic occipital lobe epilepsy due to brain abscess at age 14 years (congenital hypogammaglobulinemia).

What to note

The patient closes her eyes when stimulation is at 19 Hz. Two seconds following onset of the intermittent photic stimulation, high-amplitude spike-waves appeared on the right temporal region and organized into an ictal discharge over the whole right hemisphere. A secondary tonic-clonic generalization was observed later.

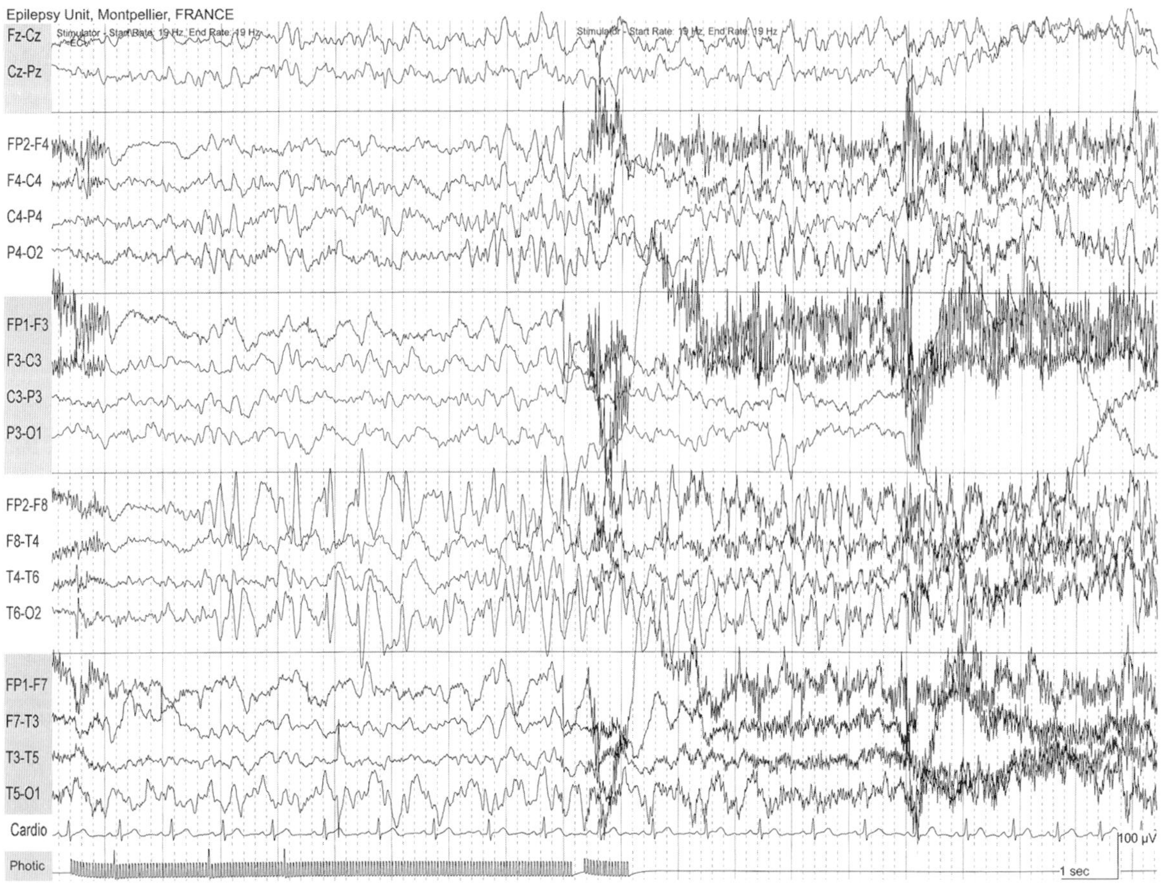

Figure a / Recording at 15 mm/s.

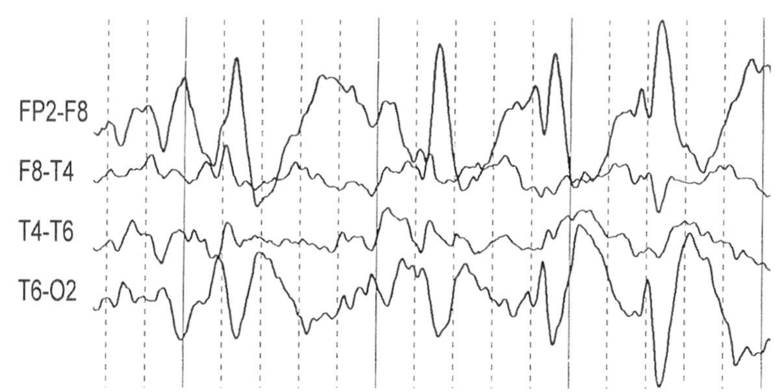

Figure b / High-amplitude spike-waves appear on the right temporal region during IPS.

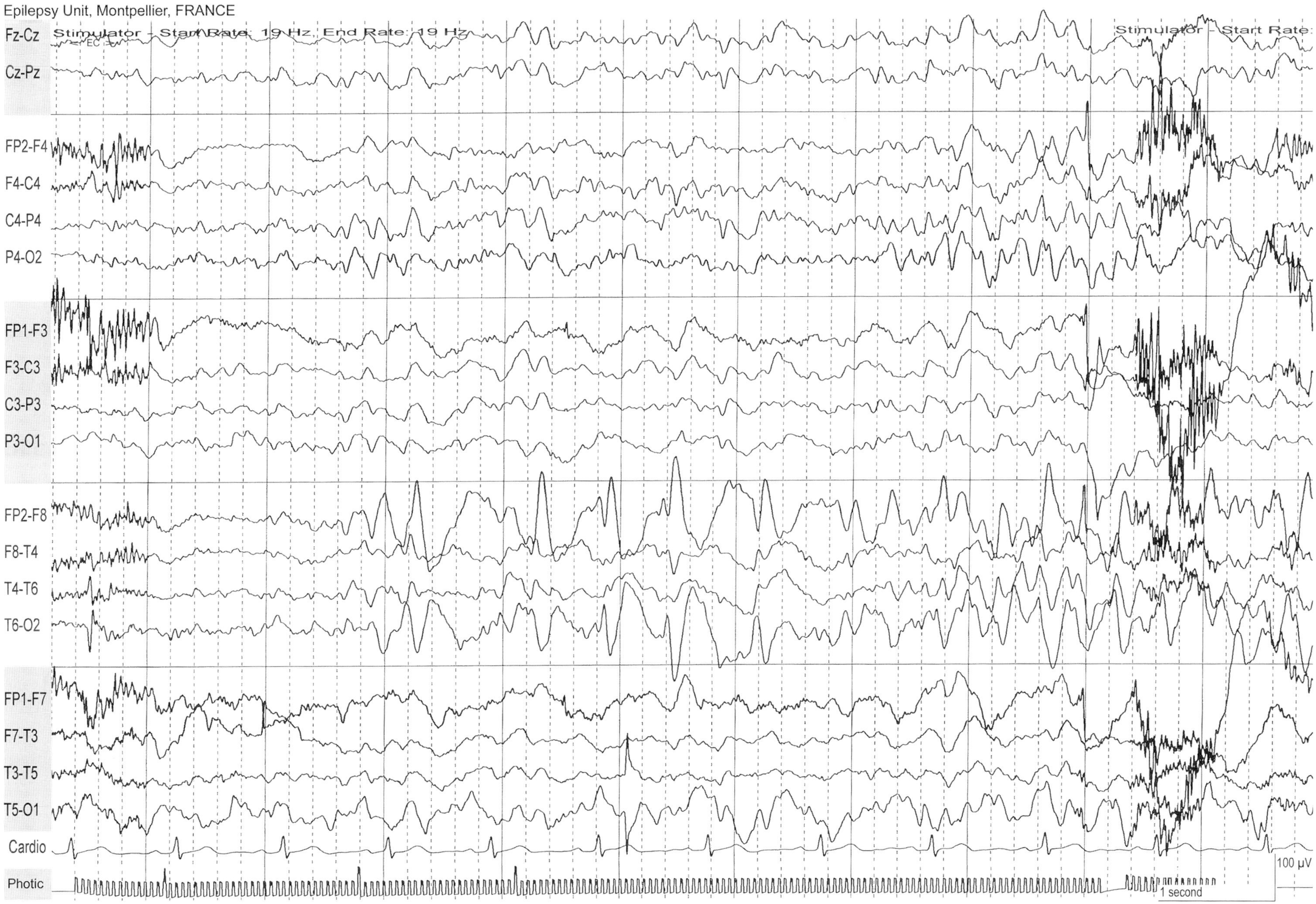
Epilepsy Unit, Montpellier, FRANCE
Stimulator - Start Rate: 19 Hz, End Rate: 19 Hz
Stimulator - Start Rate:
Fz-Cz
Cz-Pz
FP2-F4
F4-C4
C4-P4
P4-O2
FP1-F3
F3-C3
C3-P3
P3-O1
FP2-F8
F8-T4
T4-T6
T6-O2
FP1-F7
F7-T3
T3-T5
T5-O1
Cardio
Photic
100 µV
1 second

II • 29 Paroxysmal photosensitive response (photoparoxysmal response) triggered by television

Context

19-year-old girl referred for juvenile myoclonic epilepsy.

What to note

With this patient, watching a Japanese cartoon on cathodic television (red hued intermittent photic stimulation) triggers two bursts of irregular generalized polyspike-waves. Two myoclonic jerks are recorded on the deltoid muscles. The tracing is superimposed with an abundance of sharp potentials (electrodes O2 and T5) corresponding to an instrumental environmental artifact due to the presence of the television.

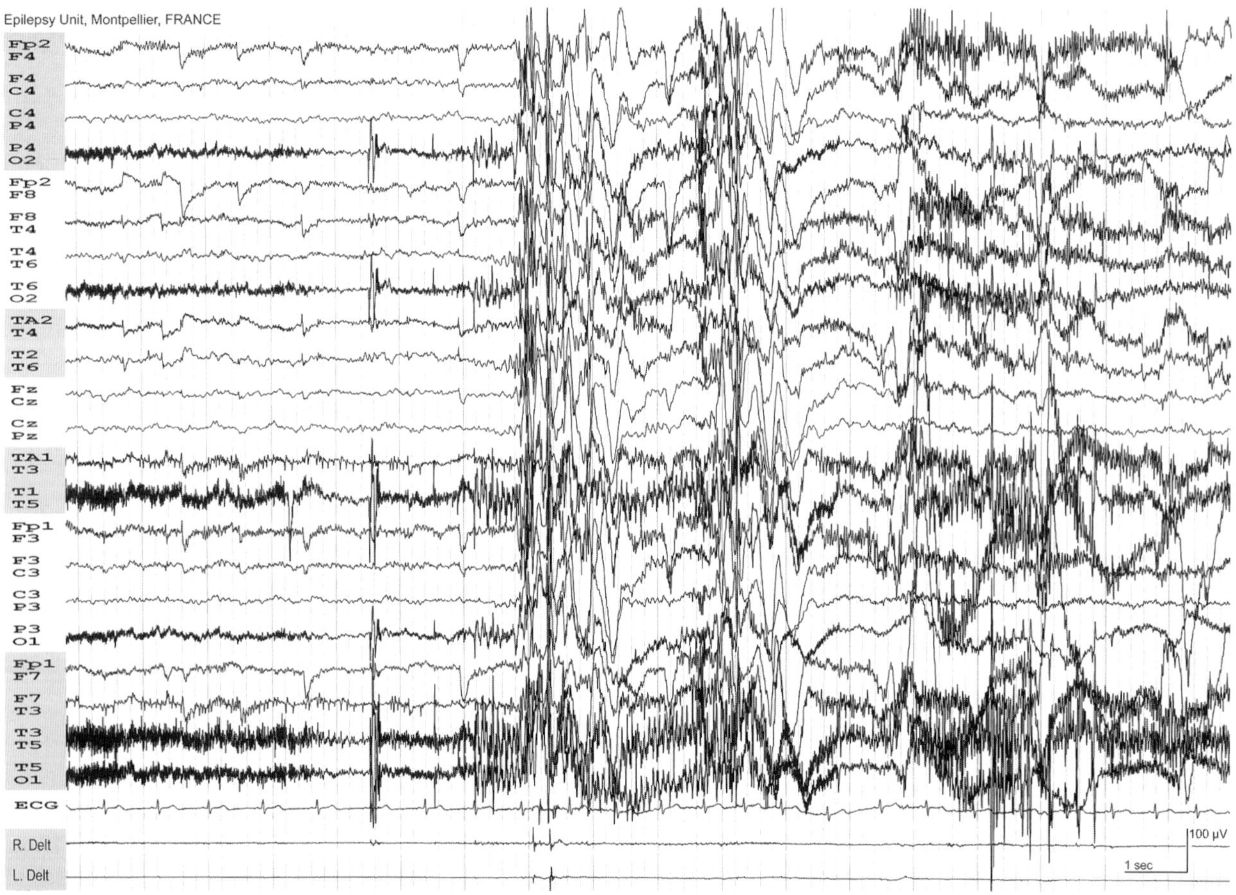

Figure a / Recording at 15 mm/s.

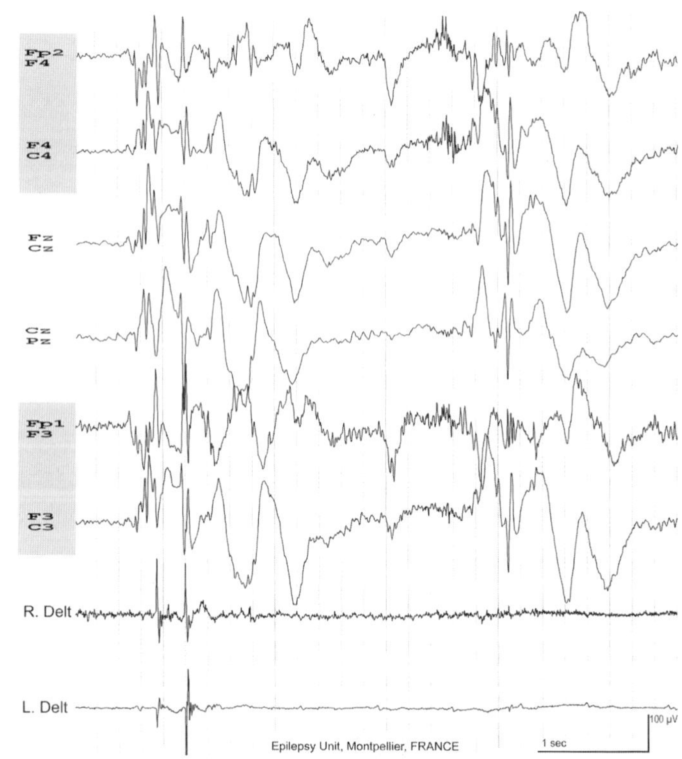

Figure b / Burst of polyspike-waves with two myoclonic jerks with a second burst two seconds later.

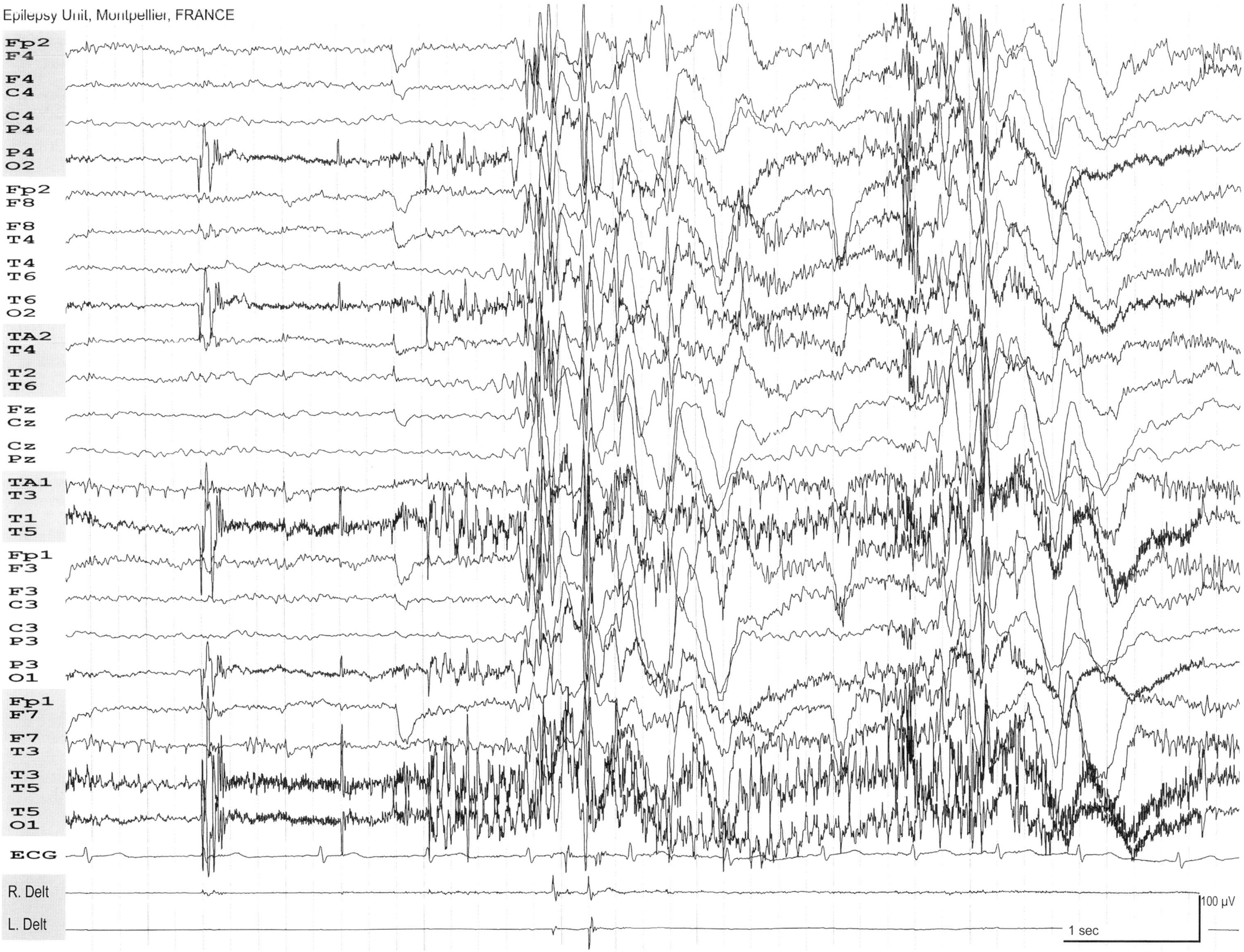
Epilepsy Unit, Montpellier, FRANCE
Fp2 F4
F4 C4
C4 P4
P4 O2
Fp2 F8
F8 T4
T4 T6
T6 O2
TA2 T4
T2 T6
Fz Cz
Cz Pz
TA1 T3
T1 T5
Fp1 F3
F3 C3
C3 P3
P3 O1
Fp1 F7
F7 T3
T3 T5
T5 O1
ECG
R. Delt
L. Delt
100 µV
1 sec

• 30 When the EEG complicates the situation! Paroxysmal photosensitive response (photoparoxysmal response) without epilepsy

Context

9-year-old girl with a history of febrile seizures referred for drug resistant epilepsy later diagnosed as psychogenic seizures in a context of divorce of her parents. The semiology was characterized by diffuse hypertonia during 5 to 15 minutes. She was nonreponsive, her eyes remained semiclosed, she also moved her abdomen. The seizures were precipitated by emotional factors.

What to note

Intermittent photic stimulation at 16 Hz. The amplitude of the photic response gradually builds up with high amplitude diffuse irregular spike-waves.

Comment

This patient had a genetic predisposition to idiopathic generalized epilepsy but no epilepsy at the time of this EEG. Antiepileptic drugs were stopped. She was advised to avoid sleep deprivation, intermittent photic stimulation and later alcohol abuse.

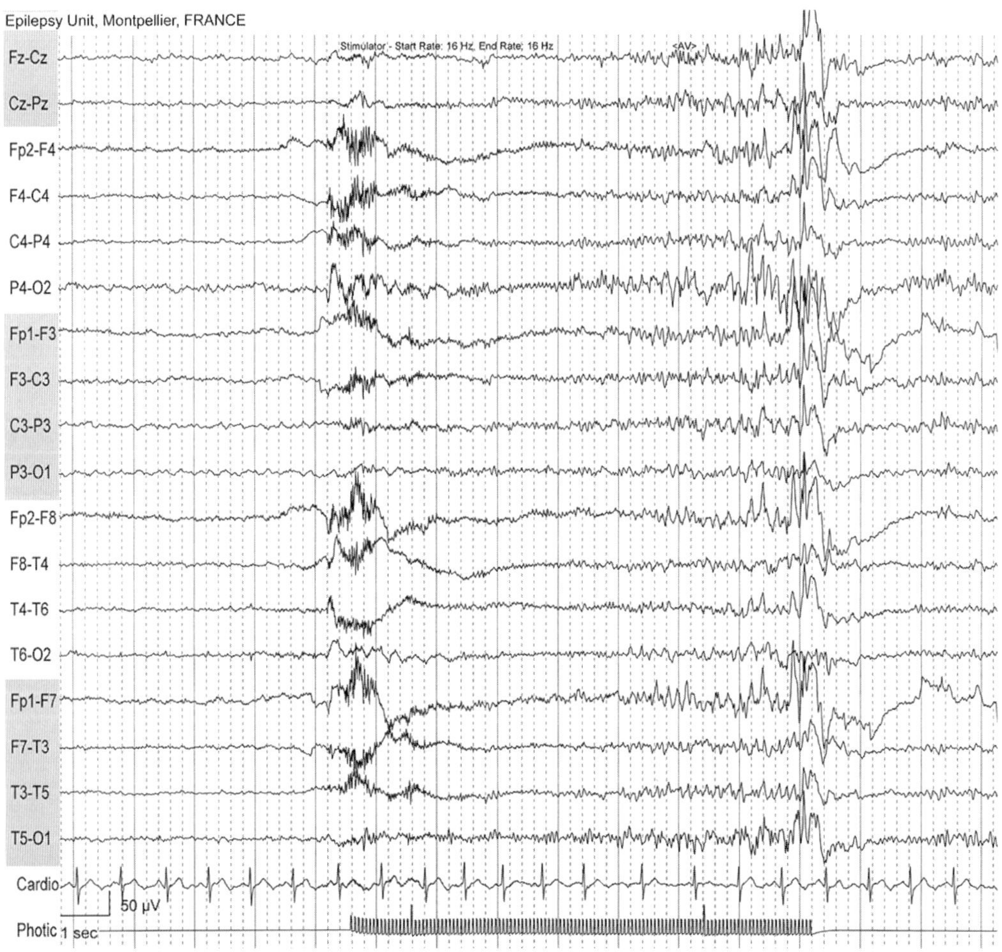

Figure a / Recording at 15 mm/s.

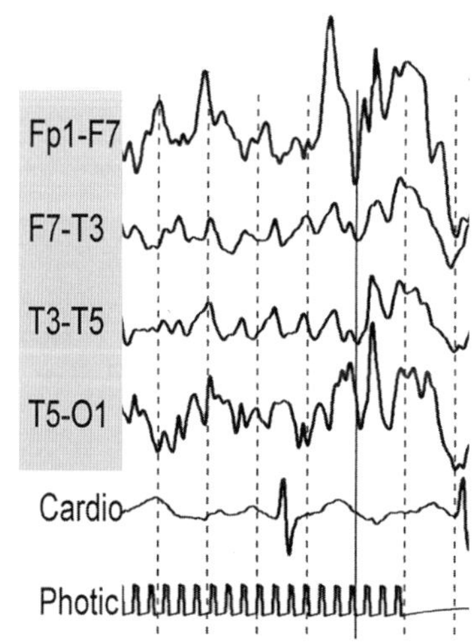

Figure b / Irregular spike-waves at the end of the flashes.

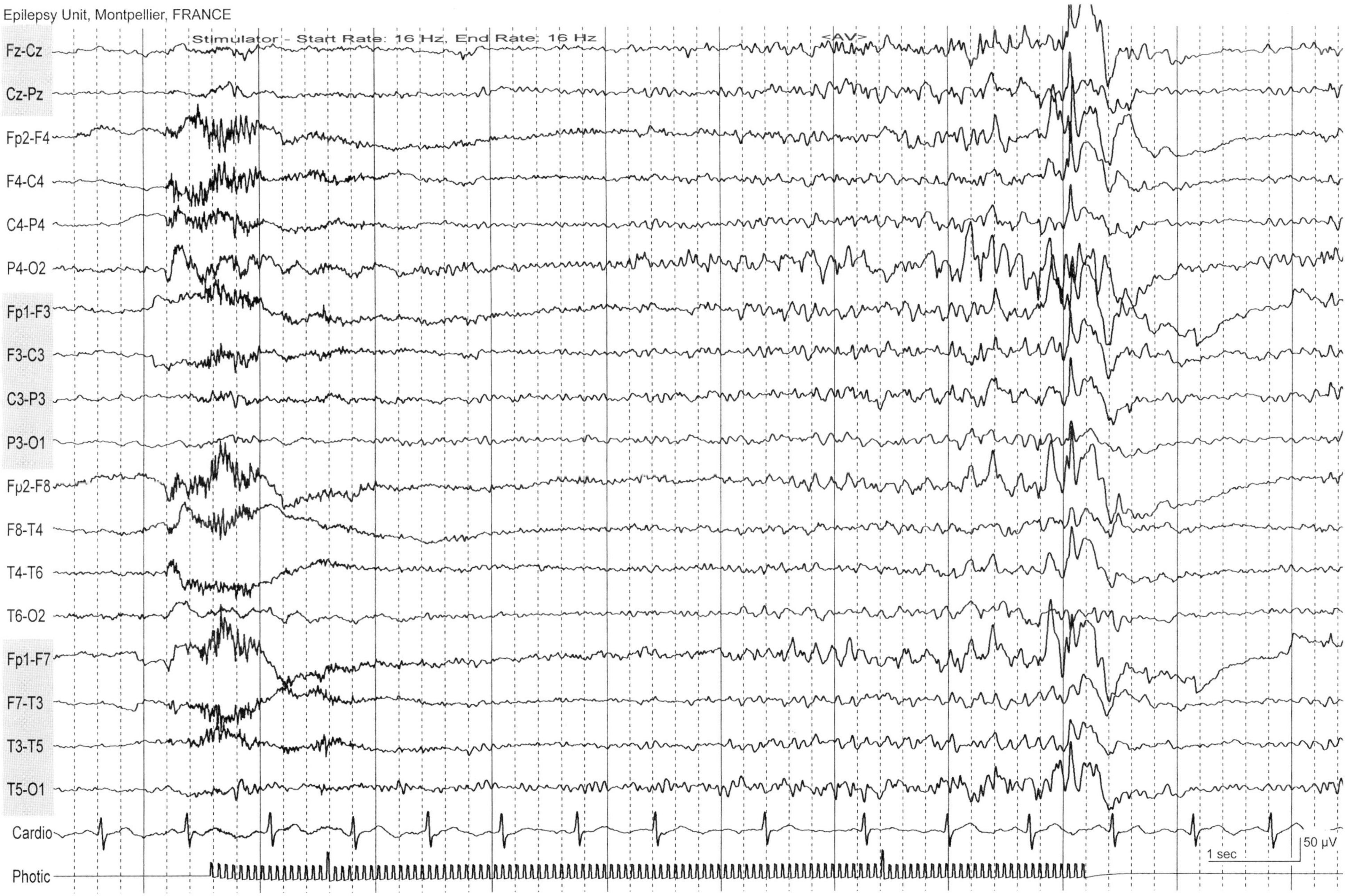
Epilepsy Unit, Montpellier, FRANCE
Stimulator - Start Rate: 16 Hz, End Rate: 16 Hz
<AV>
Fz-Cz
Cz-Pz
Fp2-F4
F4-C4
C4-P4
P4-O2
Fp1-F3
F3-C3
C3-P3
P3-O1
Fp2-F8
F8-T4
T4-T6
T6-O2
Fp1-F7
F7-T3
T3-T5
T5-O1
Cardio
Photic
1 sec
50 µV

II • 31 Heart arrest triggered by eye compression

Context

44-year-old man with drug-resistant epilepsy, later diagnosed as vagal syncopes.

What to note

The patient's eyes are closed. The physician presses firmly on the eyes (artifact on TA2-T4) then ceases after 7 seconds because the patient is unwell; bradycardia followed by a 4-second heart arrest. Note the presence of muscle activity at fronto-polar derivations during eye compression.

Comment

It is important to continue the recording even in absence of response during eye compression because bradycardia can be delayed after termination of eye compression.

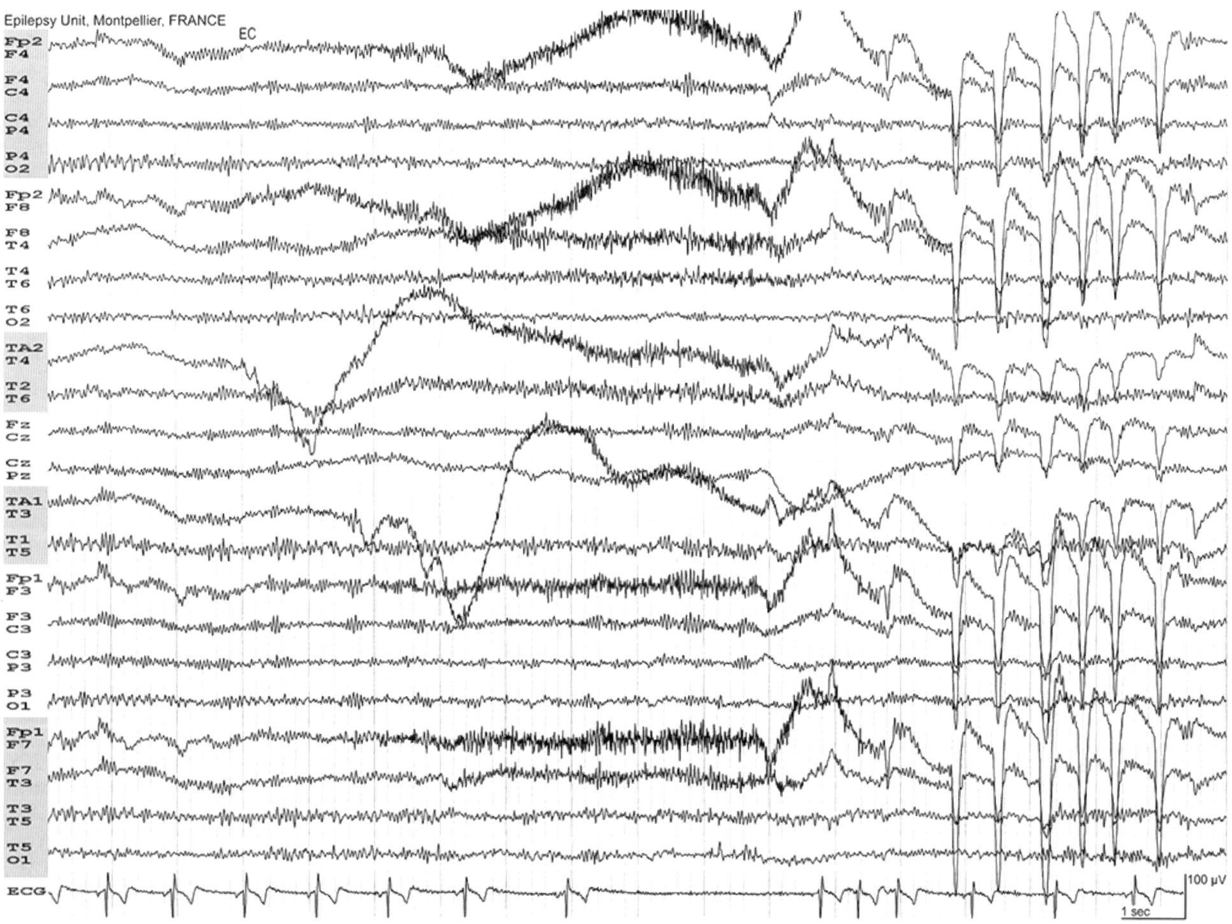

Figure a / Recording at 15 mm/s. Note progressive bradycardia before the cardiac arrest followed by tachycardia. EC: eye compression.

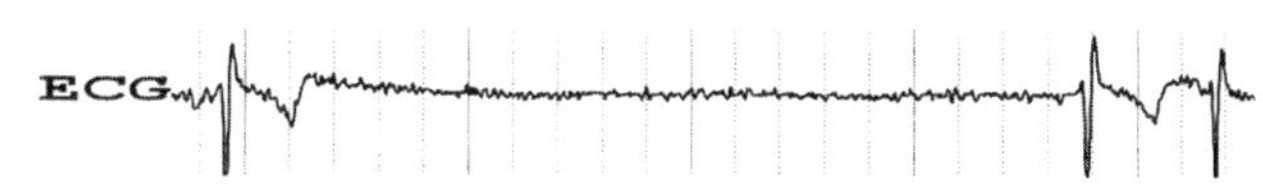

Figure b / Recording at 15 ms/s.
Occurrence of a 4-second heart arrest.

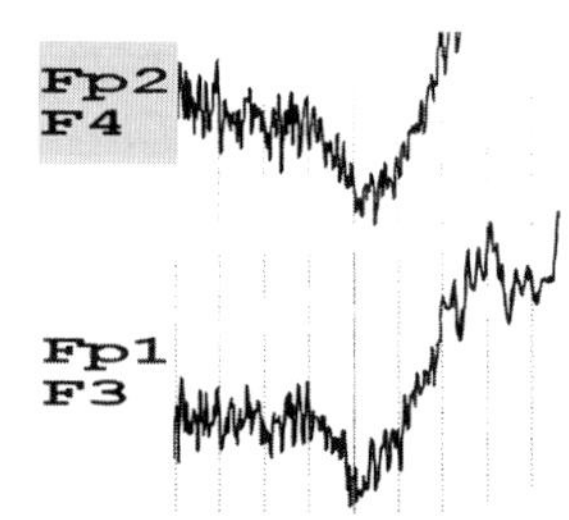

Figure c / Muscular artefacts
and artifact of eye decompression.

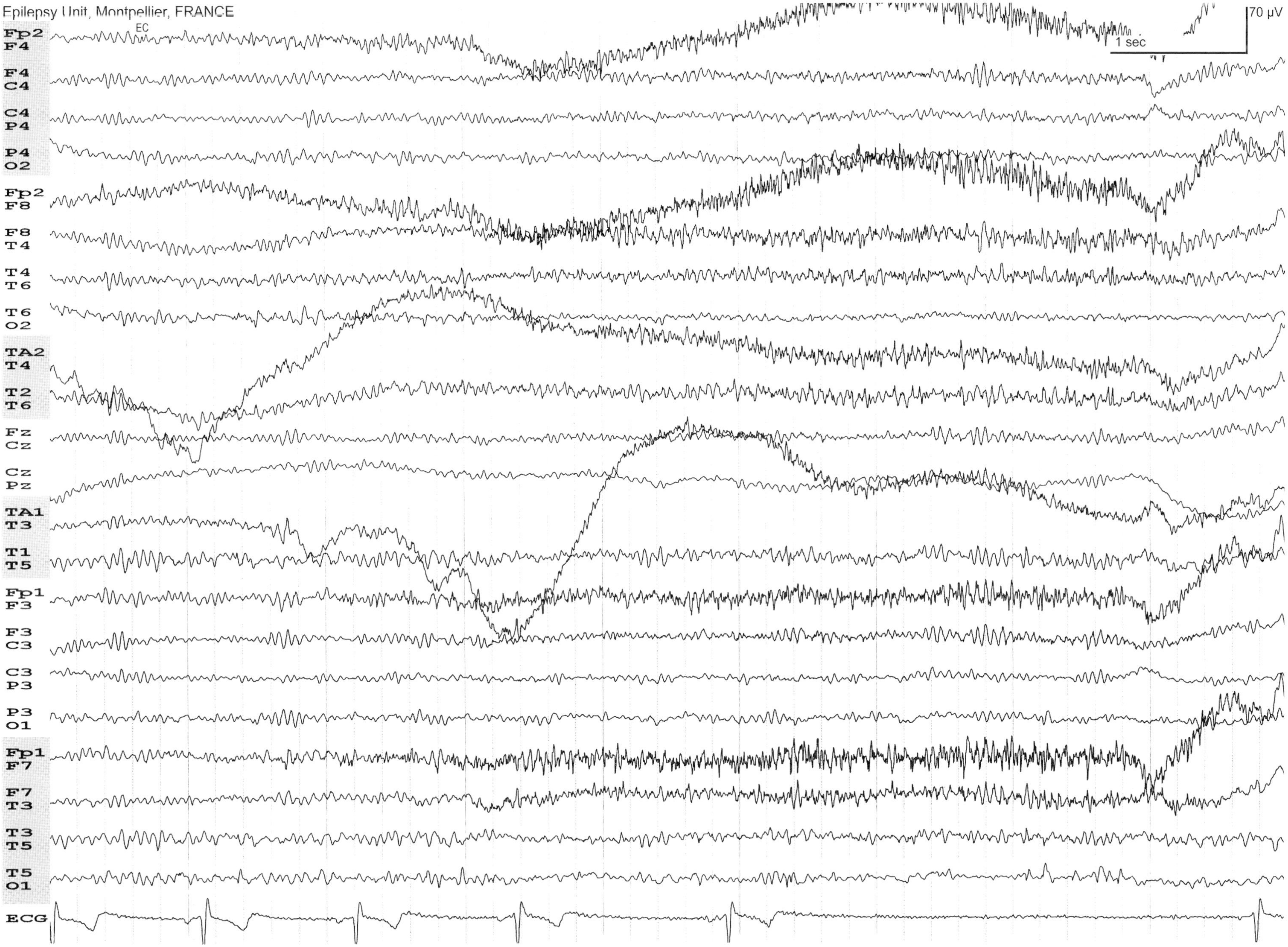
Epilepsy Unit, Montpellier, FRANCE
EC
70 µV
1 sec
Fp2 F4
F4 C4
C4 P4
P4 O2
Fp2 F8
F8 T4
T4 T6
T6 O2
TA2 T4
T2 T6
Fz Cz
Cz Pz
TA1 T3
T1 T5
Fp1 F3
F3 C3
C3 P3
P3 O1
Fp1 F7
F7 T3
T3 T5
T5 O1
ECG

II • 32 Syncope triggered by eye compression (1)

Context

14-year-old man with drug-resistant epilepsy, later diagnosed as vagal syncopes.

What to note

The patient's eyes are closed. The doctor presses firmly the eyes (A). Five second later, cardiac arrest. At this moment, eye compression should have been stopped but due to the lack of experience of the doctor and nurse, the procedure was continued.

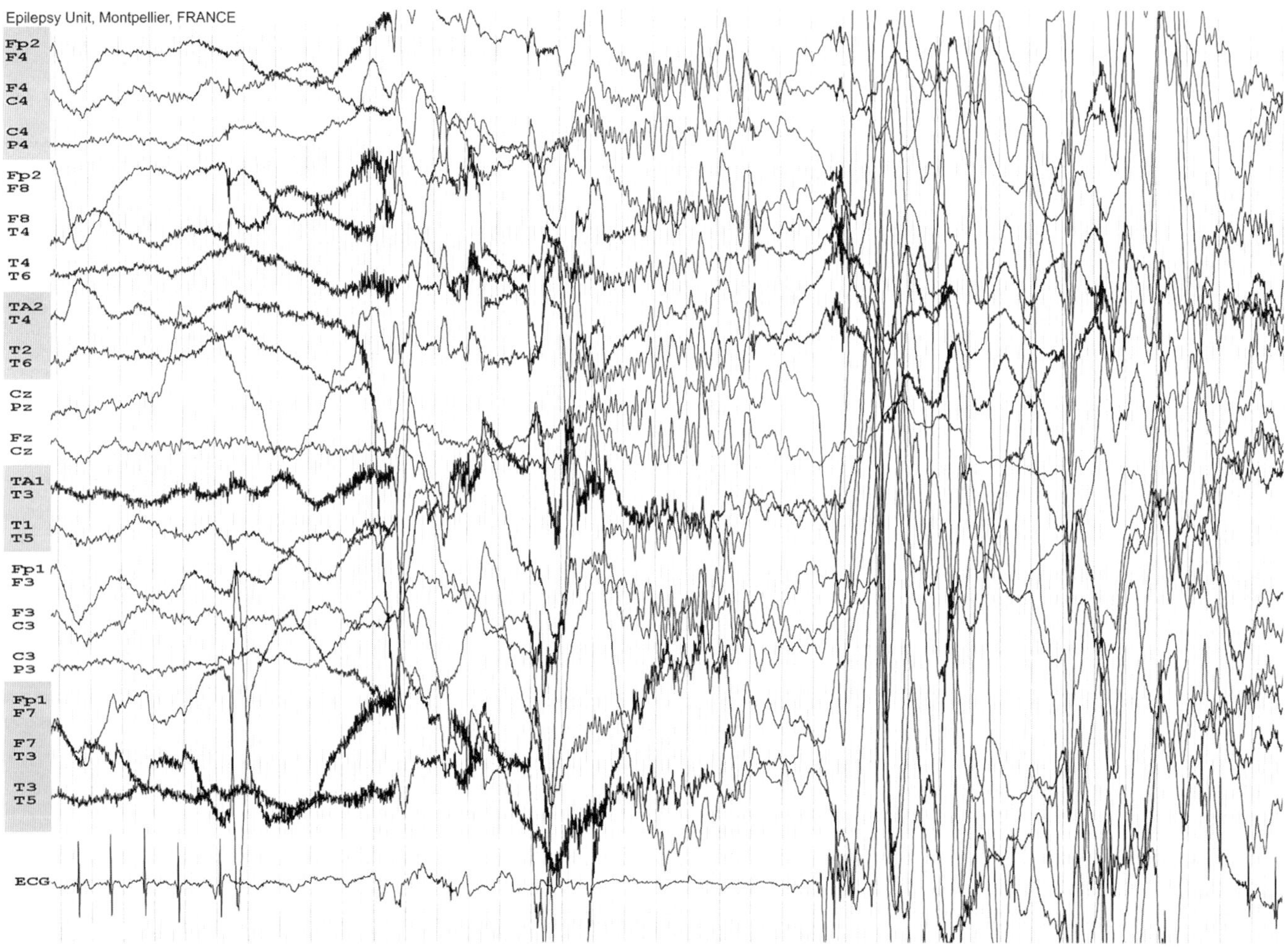

Figure a / Plate of 40 seconds. The ocular compression triggers a cardiac arrest that lasted 22.5 seconds. Note the sequence: until 9 seconds, the cardiac arrest has no effect on the EEG, then gradual slowing activity followed by EEG inactivity. At this moment, loss of consciousness. High amplitude slow waves corresponding to artifacts can be seen. Myoclonic jerks can occur during this phase. When the heart beat resumes, the EEG is still isoelectric. At the end of the plate, background activity reappears and the patient regains consciousness.

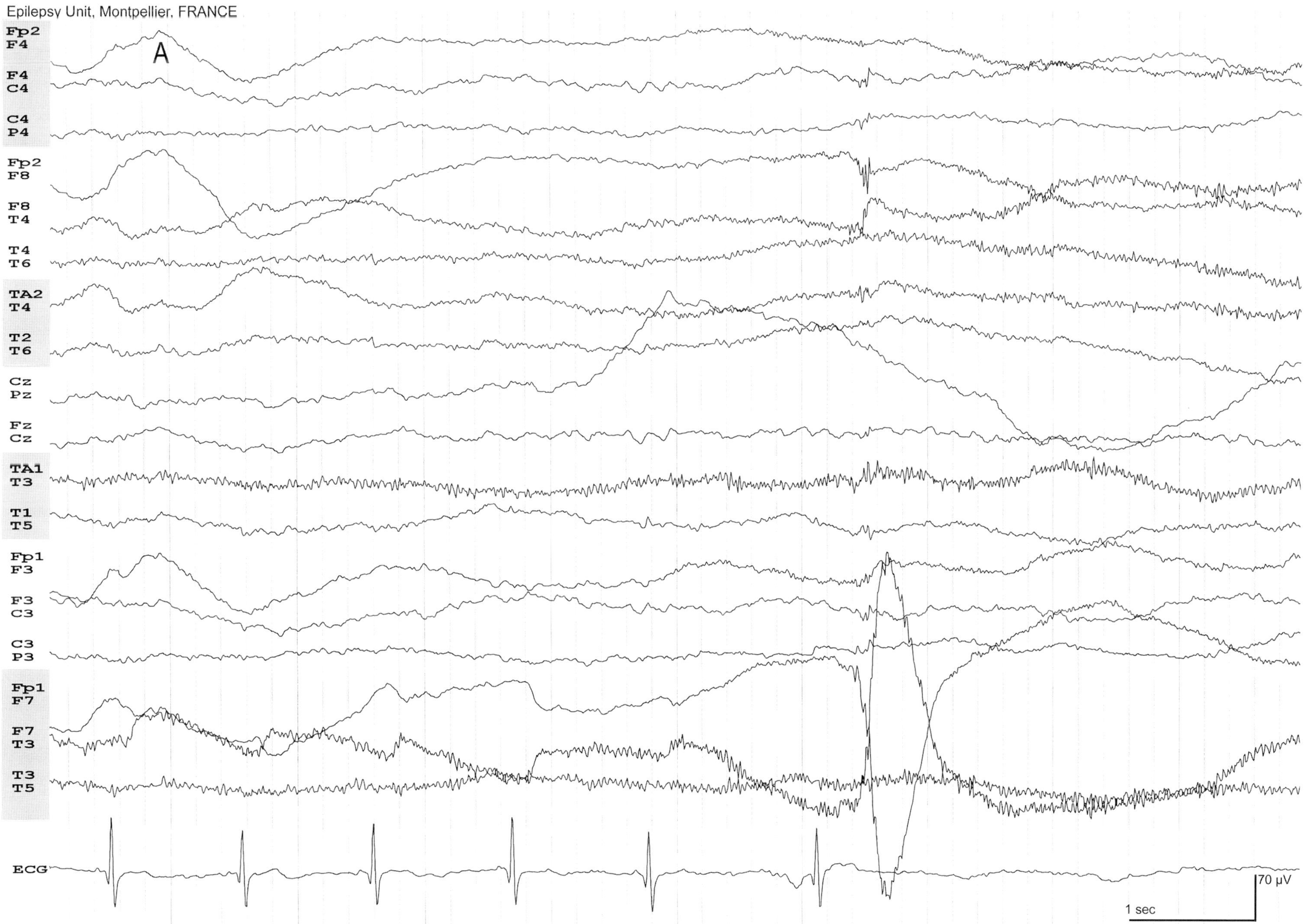
Epilepsy Unit, Montpellier, FRANCE
A
Fp2 F4
F4 C4
C4 P4
Fp2 F8
F8 T4
T4 T6
TA2 T4
T2 T6
Cz Pz
Fz Cz
TA1 T3
T1 T5
Fp1 F3
F3 C3
C3 P3
Fp1 F7
F7 T3
T3 T5
ECG
70 µV
1 sec

II • 33 Syncope triggered by eye compression (2)

Context

14-year-old man, from the previous plate, continued.

What to note

The compression is stopped, muscular activity disappears. Note the progressive slowing of the EEG with at the end of the plate diffuse slow waves. If the cardiac arrest does not exceed 8 to 10 seconds, the electroencephalography manifestations are limited to this "hypersynchrony" with a more or less severe obnubilation.

A: Stop compression; B: The doctor asks "How are you?". He answers "Yes".

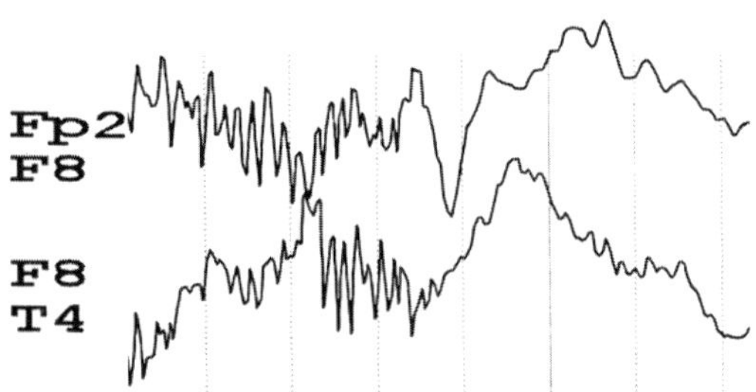

Figure a / Muscular activity disappears when the doctor stops eye compression.

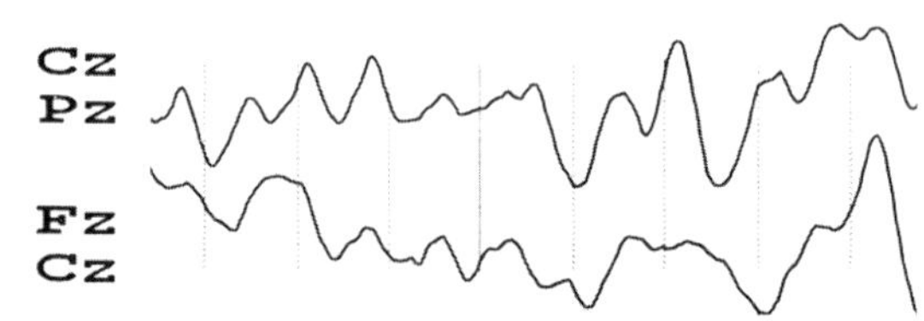

Figure b / Gradual slowing activity.

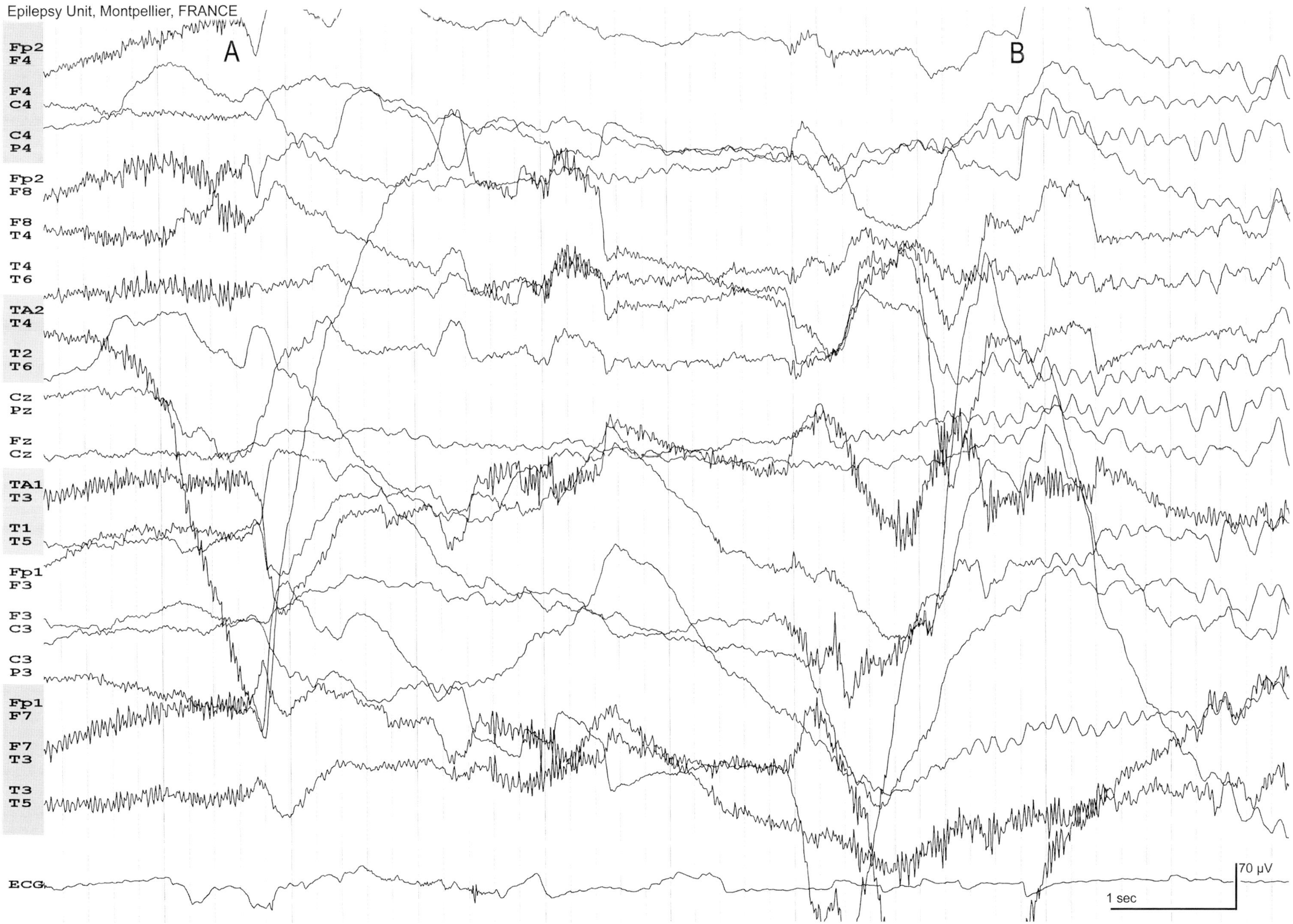
Epilepsy Unit, Montpellier, FRANCE
A
B
Fp2
F4
F4
C4
C4
P4
Fp2
F8
F8
T4
T4
T6
TA2
T4
T2
T6
Cz
Pz
Fz
Cz
TA1
T3
T1
T5
Fp1
F3
F3
C3
C3
P3
Fp1
F7
F7
T3
T3
T5
ECG
70 µV
1 sec

• 34 Syncope triggered by eye compression (3)

Context

14-year-old man, from the previous plate, continued.

What to note

Diffuse slow waves at the beginning of the plate. The patient is still conscious with normal breathing (A). Then, he loses consciousness with ocular revulsion (B) and at this moment the EEG demonstrates no cerebral activity. The head drops to the left side (D). The high-amplitude slow waves on the left hemisphere are artifacts. At this end of the plate, resumption of the EEG activity (E).

A: normal breathing; B: Ocular revulsion; C: Snorting; D: Head drops to the left; E: Resumption of the EEG activity.

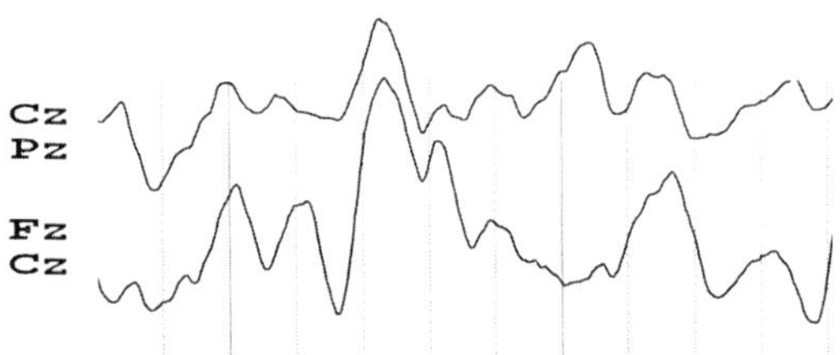

Figure a / Slow waves corresponding to "hypersynchrony".

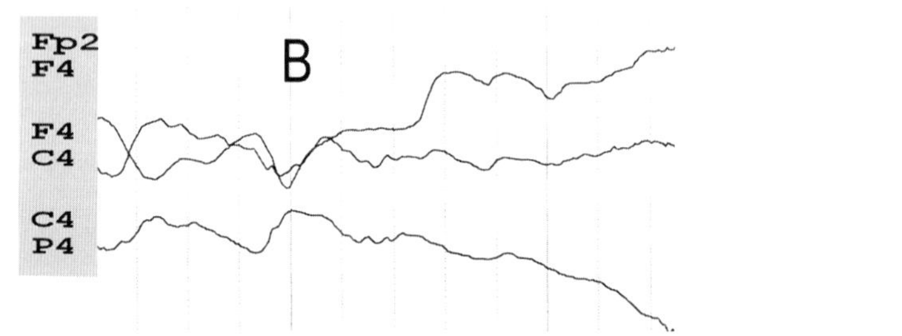

Figure b / Electrocerebral inactivity. The patient loses consciousness.

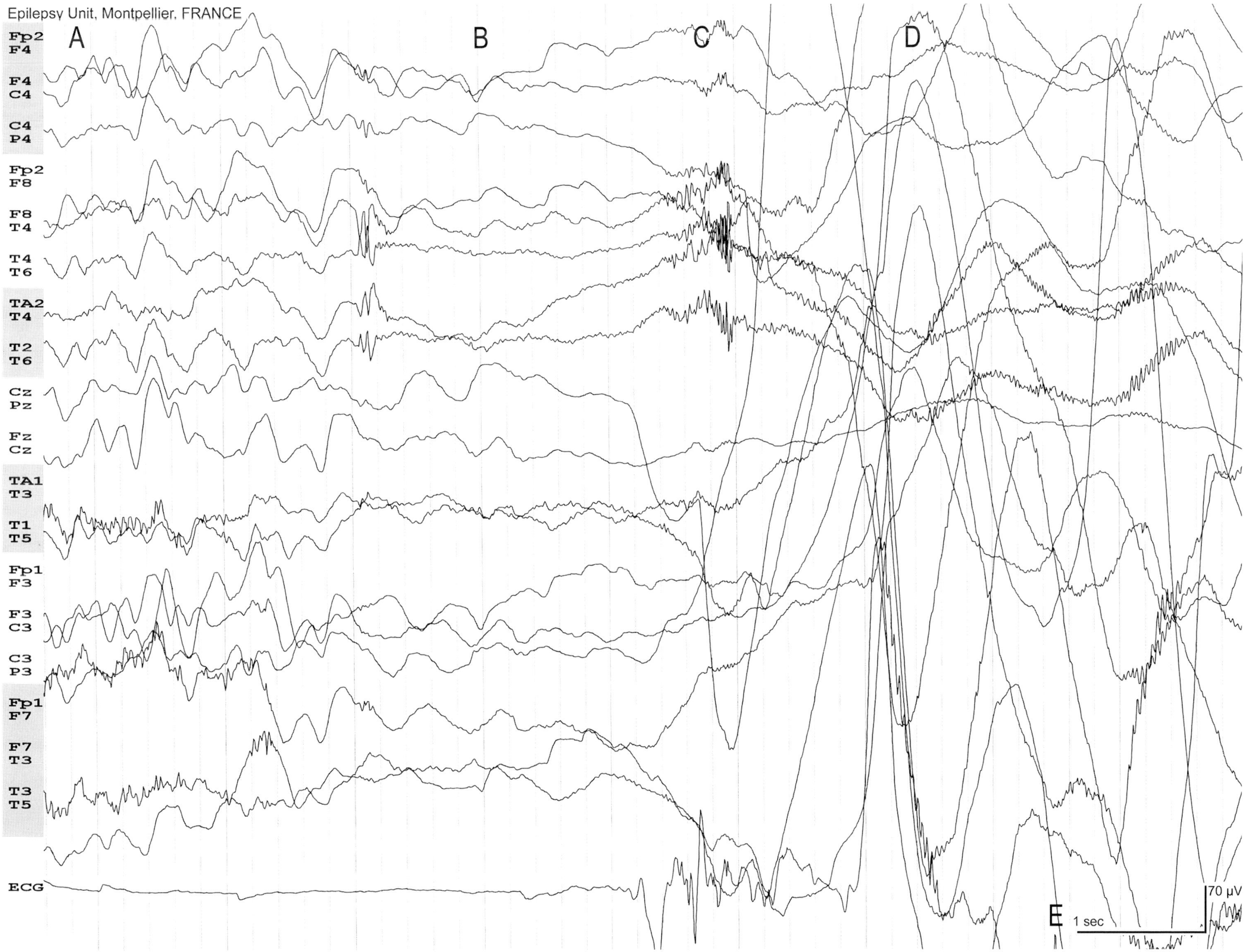
Epilepsy Unit, Montpellier, FRANCE
A
B
C
D
E
Fp2 F4
F4 C4
C4 P4
Fp2 F8
F8 T4
T4 T6
TA2 T4
T2 T6
Cz Pz
Fz Cz
TA1 T3
T1 T5
Fp1 F3
F3 C3
C3 P3
Fp1 F7
F7 T3
T3 T5
ECG
1 sec
70 µV

II • 35 Syncope triggered by eye compression (4)

Context

14-year-old man, from the previous plate, continued.

What to note

At the beginning of the plate, no cerebral activity despite resumption of the ECG activity. Deep breathing at the beginning of the plate (A). The isoelectric phase of the EEG is interrupted by a large downward positive deflection, which signals the return of the slow activity that normalizes within 4 seconds, coinciding with the return of consciousness.

A: Deep breathing; B: Moaning; C: Normal breathing.

Comment

Eye compression can confirm vasovagal hypersensitivity but should be performed with precautions. If there is a history of severe cardiac disorders, if eye compression is necessary, the procedure should be only performed by a cardiologist in a specialized unit. Atropine must be kept at hand. The doctor should have experience and needs to be aware of the risks. The doctor should have access to a monitor to control heartbeat. If a sinus arrest is obtained, eye compression must be stopped to avoid syncope.

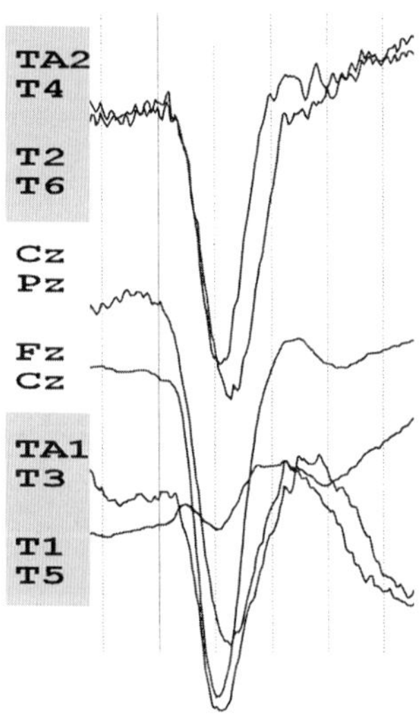

Figure a / Downward positive deflection.

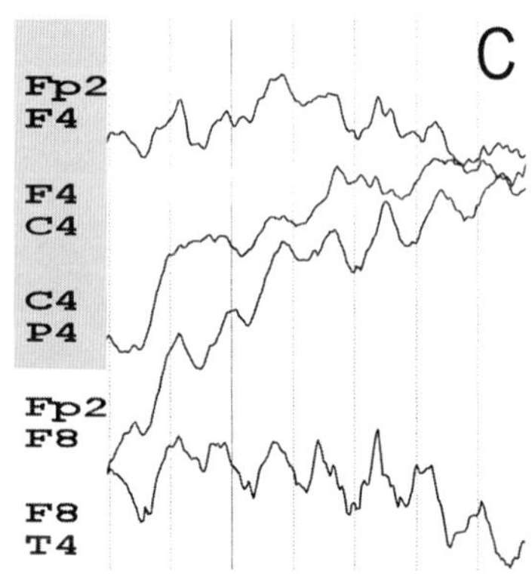

Figure b / Slow wave activity. The patient fully understands the doctor's question. There was no post-ictal confusion.

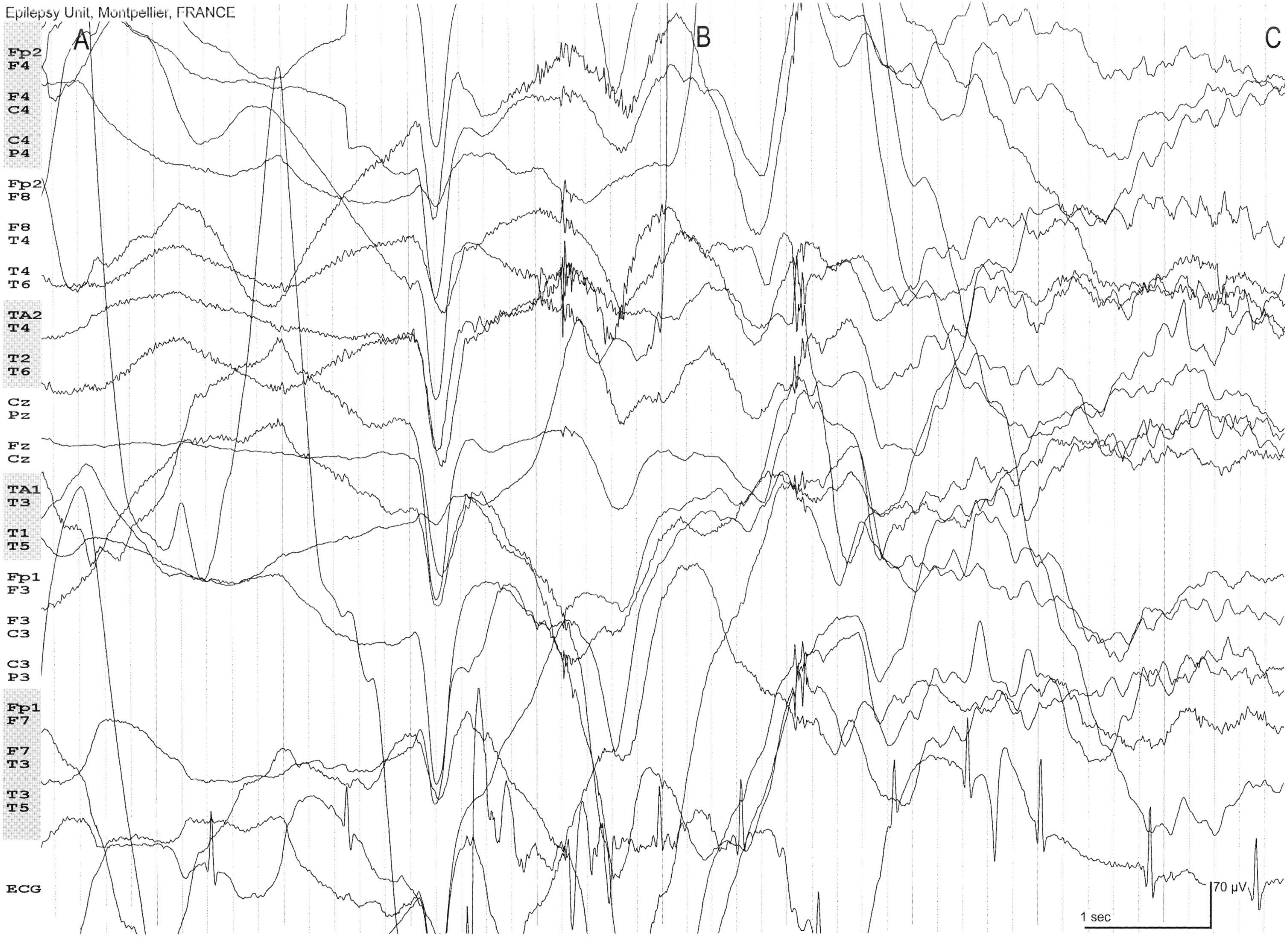
Epilepsy Unit, Montpellier, FRANCE
A
B
C
Fp2 F4
F4 C4
C4 P4
Fp2 F8
F8 T4
T4 T6
TA2 T4
T2 T6
Cz Pz
Fz Cz
TA1 T3
T1 T5
Fp1 F3
F3 C3
C3 P3
Fp1 F7
F7 T3
T3 T5
ECG
70 µV
1 sec

CHAPITRE III

EEG and sleep

INTRODUCTION

During an EEG, patients can become drowsy or even fall asleep spontaneously when they are requested to lie down, close their eyes, relax and hyperventilate. Given the difficulties of carrying out EEGs on young children, it is recommended to perform a sleep EEG in children under age 6 years whenever they fall asleep spontaneously. It is therefore necessary to be knowledgeable about sleep patterns and unusual physiological sleep patterns, often involving "sharp" waveforms which must be differentiated from genuine epileptic abnormalities.

There is a close link between sleep and epilepsy and thus prolonged EEGs are performed for this pathology, either during a nap or nightly sleep. This is particularly true in patients who experience sleep-related seizures. When a patient falls asleep during a standard EEG, he should not be woken up as sleep provides highly relevant information. Sleep can also be used to trigger epileptic abnormalities or to obtain a tracing without artifacts.

Unusual non-pathological activities can be observed during sleep, including fourteen-and six-Hz positive bursts, wicket spikes, rhythmic midtemporal discharges, positive occipital sharp transients (POSTs) of sleep and frontal arousal rhythms.

SLEEP DEPRIVATION PROCEDURE

A sleep EEG can be performed in the daytime after partial sleep deprivation the night before the EEG. Adults must sleep 5 hours at most. Children should shorten their usual night by 2 hours.

In absence of sleep deprivation in adults, it is recommended to perform sleep EEGs in the early afternoon, when they are more likely to fall asleep, rather than in the morning.

Most of the time, individuals manage to fall asleep so that it is not necessary to give sleep-inducing medication. Sleep-inducing medication is not recommended as it may alter the tracing.

However, sleep deprivation must not be too long because if the patient gets drowsy right from the onset of the recording session, the background activity can not be apprehended correctly. This disorganized tracing with overall slowing may, if not followed by sleep, convey an impression of a pathological background activity. If sleep deprivation lasts too long, the patient falls asleep very quickly, passing rapidly into deep sleep (stage N3). These stages are generally the least informative compared to the transitional periods and non-REM light sleep (for idiopathic generalized epilepsies, benign partial epilepsy of childhood with centro-temporal spikes, other focal epilepsies, Lennox-Gastaut syndrome and other encephalopathic epilepsies). Moreover, it is important to visualize the physiological elements present during non-REM light sleep (stages N1 and N2) in order to analyze the organization of the tracings.

DIFFERENT STAGES OF SLEEP

• Drowsiness

First the background activity (theta in children, alpha in adults) spreads towards the anterior regions, then it decreases gradually and disappears. Then bursts of monomorphic slow diffuse activity appear (theta in adults and delta in children), which can convey an impression of hypersychrony.

• Non-REM Sleep: light sleep (Stages N1-N2)

Stage N1: presence of slow lateral eye movements (SEMs) at 0.5 Hz and vertex sharp wave transients.

Stage N2: presence of K complexes and sleep spindles; less than 20% of an epoch is occupied by slow waves.

• Non-REM Sleep: deep sleep (Stage N3)

Stage N3 (formerly stage 3 and 4): more than 20% of an epoch are occupied by very high-voltage slow waves. K complexes and sleep spindles may persist throughout this stage.

• REM Sleep

REM sleep is characterized by low-voltage patterns with rhythms similar to those seen during wakefulness and drowsiness including fast beta rhythms over the anterior regions, but alpha activity is usually not prominent. REM sleep is also characterized by reduced muscle tone (atonia), rapid eye movements (REM), sawtooth waves and brief contraction (twitches) of facial muscles.

SLEEP ARCHITECTURE

Normal nightly sleep is organized in several consecutive sleep cycles during the night. Stage N1 represents 5 to 10% of total sleep time, stage N2 30 to 50%, stage N3 20 to 40%, and REM sleep around 25%.

The normal sleep features are vertex sharp wave transients (V waves), K complexes and sleep spindles. Their presence and abundance indicate a well-organized tracing, and therefore a good prognostic value. On the contrary, when a tracing is not well organized (e.g when they are asymmetrical or absent), it indicates a major alteration in children and sometimes a poor prognosis.

Deep sleep occurs predominate during the first and second cycles. Then REM sleep gradually increases, reaching its maximum proportion during the last third of nightly sleep.

In normal elderly individuals, the proportion of deep sleep may drop to less than 10%, and their sleep is more fragmented. The proportion of REM sleep also decreases to less than 20% of total sleep time and, contrary to normal young adults, REM sleep decreases during the second half of the night (Williamson *et al.*, 1990; Van Sweden *et al.*, 1999).

DROWSINESS

• Rhythms

First the alpha rhythm spreads over the anterior regions, then it starts to fluctuate, and a low-amplitude theta activity begins, lasting up to several minutes. Anterior fast beta activity becomes prominent, in particular when pharmacologically induced.

• Hypnagogic hypersynchrony

In young children, drowsiness is characterized by a diffuse rhythmic to sinusoidal theta or delta pattern. It is present from age 6 months (or even younger); remains frequent in young children, then declines in prominence after age 5 years.

• Intermittent temporal slow waves

Intermittent temporal slow waves are common in normal elderly individuals and are of no clinical importance. They occur either independently or in transient bursts, in particular during drowsiness. These slow theta waves, or more uncommonly slow delta waves, are monomorphic. Background activity is normal between the bursts. These intermittent slow waves can occur independently or asymmetrically predominating over the left hemisphere in more than two-thirds of individuals.

• Frontal slow delta waves of drowsiness

Frontal slow delta waves may occur in normal elderly individuals in drowsiness. They are intermittent and rhythmic. These slow waves (1.5-2.5 Hz) are bilateral and less well organized than those seen in intracranial hypertension (monomorphic high-voltage anterior delta activity) or in other pathological slowing referred to as FIRDA (frontal intermittent rhythmic delta activity). Several authors have used the term "FIRDA at sleep onset" to describe these physiological slow waves of drowsiness in elderly individuals (Katz et Horowitz, 1983). However, we prefer to use the less ambiguous term "frontal slow delta waves of drowsiness", thereby limiting the use of FIRDA for pathological abnormalities.

STAGE N1

• Slow eye movements

In drowsiness, there is a diffuse theta background activity with gradual onset of slow eye movements (SEMs) on the frontal polar and inferior frontal derivations. SEMs are characterized by 0.5 Hz frequency and are characteristically low-amplitude.

• Vertex sharp-wave transients

Vertex sharp-wave transients (vertex waves, V waves) may occur at onset of stage N1 and stage N2 sleep. V waves are mono- or diphasic slow spikes with negative and positive components over the vertex region (Cz). In children, these spikes often extend into frontal and parietal areas whereas in adults they remain more localized in the vertex region. They first appear at age 5-6 months and are broader than they are sharp. They take on a sharper appearance at age 3-4 years and, in young adolescents, they tend to be less "spike-like". In adults, V waves are less common, less characteristic and their morphology is less typical.

V waves are usually single. When they occur in bursts or in rhythmic trains, they may be mistaken for epileptiform discharges. These aspects are most commonly seen in children. Sometimes, when V waves recur at regular intervals, they form a spike-like theta rhythm of high amplitude over the vertex region.

In a routine EEG, V waves can be observed in normal children or adults during drowsiness and should not be misinterpreted as epileptiform abnormalities.

• Stage I transient arousal reactions

During transition to a lighter stage of sleep, fast rhythms can sometimes be observed in runs in the beta activity range. Compared to physiological beta rhythms which occur in shorter bursts, they are of higher amplitude, and their frequency and morphology tend to be more irregular.

STAGE N2

At this stage of sleep, K complexes and sleep spindles, both of which are typical physiological sleep components, are mixed with slow waves which represent less than 20% of the epoch.

• K complexes

Sleep architecture in stage N2 sleep is characterized by sleep spindles and K complexes. When K complexes are absent and less abundant, poor prognosis should be raised, in particular in children. K complexes are distributed over the frontal regions. They correspond to high-voltage diphasic deflections, with an initial wave that is sharper than the second one. K complexes last at least 0.5 s. They first appear at around age 6 months. It can be difficult to recognize K complexes in very young children because the waves are of higher amplitude and their morphology is less characteristic. Moreover, in children and adolescents, the first sharp wave is larger than the second one, which may lead to a mistaken diagnosis of spike-waves. In patients with epilepsy, K complexes can have a sharp configuration with an initial spike-like wave forming a pattern called the "epileptic K complex". When epileptic K complexes are isolated, a diagnosis of epilepsy should not be evoked. However, epileptic K complexes do indicate a modification of sleep architecture which can be observed in individuals with epilepsy.

• Sleep spindles

Sleep spindles are typically fusiform bursts of 12- to 16-Hz frequency. Their waveform and duration differ with age. Sleep spindles are dominant over the fronto-central regions in children over 5 years, in adolescents and in adults. In very young children, the distribution can be less localized. Sleep spindles first appear at age 2 months, then they become more visible at age 3 months. Between 6 months and 1 year, sleep spindles are abundant, occur in prolonged runs (2 to 3 seconds), and are commonly asynchronous. In a normal infant, several sleep spindles should occur in an epoch. Their absence between ages 3 and 8 months suggests a poor prognosis (Dreyfus & Curzi-Dascalova, 1975). After age 8 months, spindles become increasingly shorter and of higher amplitude. They become synchronous and symmetrical at around age 2 years. As with V waves and K complexes, their amplitude and abundance tend to decline in adults and elderly individuals.

Spindles can occur before or after a K complex, they may be partially superimposed on a K complex. Observation of a graphoelement in a spindle, even if it is spike-like, is most often an indication that this graphoelement is not pathological.

DEEP SLEEP

Stage N3 is characterized by the presence of mainly anterior high amplitude slow delta waves (> 75 µV). Stage N3 is defined by the presence of slow wave activity in more than 20% of an epoch. During this stage, sleep spindles and K complexes may still be observed.

In the elderly, sleep waves tend to be of lower amplitude, so that assessment based only on voltages of over 75 µV is no longer relevant.

Sometimes the slow waves in deep sleep are superimposed with theta (children) or alpha activities (adults). The topography of these is anterior.

REM SLEEP

REM sleep (REM = Rapid Eye Movement) resembles wakefulness or stage N1, except that the EEG tracing contains no V waves. The pattern can be of very low-voltage or else alpha-like. However, REM sleep differs from wakefulness insofar as it is more monomorphic and always slightly slower (by 1 to 2 Hz). Moreover, physiological or drug-induced beta rhythms reappear over the anterior regions in REM sleep.

REM sleep is typically characterized by reduced muscle activity (atonia), and often accompanied by muscle twitches, mostly facial. Thus, the EMG must be recorded with submental electrodes. Furthermore, REM sleep can also be identified by its characteristic graphoelements, i.e. sawtooth waves and rapid eye movements. Phasic REM sleep activity (presence of REMs) is opposed to tonic REM sleep activity (absence of REMs). Irregular non-pathological breathing and/or heart rates are frequent during REM sleep.

• Rapid eye movements (REMs)

REMs correspond to sharp deflections with fast initial components due to lateral shifting of the eyes. REMs are generally diphasic and last longer than one cycle per second. They often occur in bursts lasting a few seconds which are generally symmetrical but may be isolated. REMs are usually detected by the electrodes placed near the eyes, but with the 10-20 system, the frontal polar electrodes are also very reliable.

• Sawtooth waves

Sawtooth waves were first described by Passouant in 1975. They occur in brief runs of 4 to 6 Hz slow waves of low amplitude in the vertex region (Cz). Commonly said to occur with REMs, they are in fact quite frequently observed in the absence of REMs.

AROUSAL AND AWAKENING IN SLEEP

• Transient arousal reactions

Physiological awakenings may occur during non-REM sleep. They are characterized by the transition to a lighter stage of sleep and the reappearance of alpha (or faster) rhythms during several seconds. This aspect can be observed in particular during stage N2 after a K complex, referred to as a "K alpha" pattern. Transient arousal reactions are frequently observed during REM sleep, this stage being very close to wakefulness.

• Awakening/Postarousal hypersynchrony

In children, awakening (like drowsiness) is characterized by a rather diffuse rhythmic sinusoidal theta or delta activity. Postarousal hypersynchrony can first be seen at around age 6 months, is very common in young children, then declines from age 5 years on.

• Frontal arousal rhythms

Frontal arousal rhythms are very common in children over age 6 years and in adolescents, after which they become quite rare. Frontal arousal is evoked by rhythmic waves of intermixed frequencies conveying a sharply-contoured impression. Frontal arousal rhythms are predominant anteriorly with runs lasting up to 10 seconds. These rhythms disappear when the child is fully awake. They correspond to a transitional phase between non-REM sleep and waking, and are not pathological.

OTHER PHYSIOLOGICAL RHYTHMS AND UNUSUAL RHYTHMS IN SLEEP

The following sleep rhythms are not observed in all individuals or may be very unusual in some individuals. Nevertheless, it is important to be well acquainted with their morphology because they are often sharply contoured, and could therefore be mistaken for epileptiform activity.

• Positive occipital sharp transients of sleep (lambda/lambdoid waves during sleep)

First described by Gibbs and Gibbs in 1950, positive occipital sharp transients of sleep (POSTs) occur, either symmetrically or not, on the occipital areas. They are also sometimes called lambdoid waves. POSTs are frequent in adolescents and young adults, and have no pathological significance. They are monophasic or diphasic slow spikes, with a 3-to 6-Hz frequency. Their amplitude is usually below 50 µV. POSTs generally occur in stage N2 and they may persist in stage N3. They disappear during REM sleep. When abundant and ample, they may be confused with epileptiform abnormalities. However, thanks to their morphological specificities and their topography, this mistake can easily be avoided.

• Wicket spikes

First described by Reiher and Lebel (1977), wicket spikes are monophasic arciform waves with a 6-to 11-Hz frequency and a 60 to 200 µV amplitude. They occur over the temporal regions either bilaterally or independently, usually on the left (Van Sweden *et al.*, 1999). Background rhythms are not modified. Wicket spikes appear most often in 0.5 to 1 second bursts, but occasionally singly, in which case they resemble an epileptiform spike activity. They generally occur during drowsiness and light sleep (stage N1-N2) and disappear during deep sleep. In our experience, wicket spikes may also be seen during REM sleep with a similar morphology but with a slightly lower amplitude (Gélisse *et al.*, 2003, Serafini *et al.*, 2014).

Wicket spikes do not evoke epileptiform activity. Although they are considered para-physiological, some authors have suggested that wicket spikes may be linked to a certain degree of cerebrovascular dysfunction due to their predominance in individuals over 50 years (Asokan *et al.*, 1987). However, they can also be observed in young adults presenting no cognitive or vascular damage.

• Small Sharp Spikes (SSS)/Benign sporadic sleep spikes (BSSS)/Benign epileptiform transients of sleep (BETS)

Small sharp spikes (SSS), also called Benign sporadic sleep spikes (BSSS) or benign epileptiform transients of sleep (BETS), are low-voltage diphasic spikes which occur singly and predominantly over the anterior or mid-temporal regions. SSS generally occur as a unilateral waveform, but can occur bisynchronously or independently. They are mainly seen during drowsiness and at the onset of light sleep. It has been pointed out by several authors that SSS are most often observed in patients with a psychiatric, epileptic, or cardio-vascular history. The incidence of SSS is low (< 1.5%) with a predominance in adults between ages 30 and 40 years. They have not been observed in children under age 10 years (Niedermeyer, 1999).

• Fourteen- and Six-Hertz Positive Bursts

As indicated, these bursts occur at a rate of 6 Hz and/or 14 Hz. They consist of short trains of low-voltage arch-shaped waveforms lasting less than one second. They occur during drowsiness and light sleep, although occurrence during REM sleep has been reported by some authors (Okuma *et al.*, 1968; Tsuzuki, 1967 then Tassinari *et al.*, 1977; Velizarova *et al.*, 2011). Their topography is parieto-temporal and they usually occur symmetrically, even though their predominance can shift from side to side. They appear in children after 3-4 years, are maximally expressed in the adolescents and young adults, and then progressively decrease in adulthood (Velizarova *et al.*, 2011).

It has been reported that the fourteen- and six-Hertz positive bursts occur in 0.5% of 35,249 patients who underwent routine EEG recordings (Santoshkumar *et al.*, 2009) but in our series of 783 consecutive patients who underwent long-term video-EEG lasting 24 hours or more, we found this pattern in 50 (6.4%). Compared to other age groups, patients aged 15-25 years were more likely to have this activity (62%). Their identification depends mainly of the recording techniques and the duration of the sleep portion. Based on our experience, 14- and 6-Hz positive bursts are mainly seen during REM sleep. The application of a lower temporal line that explores the inferior part of the temporal lobe increases significantly the detection of the 14- and 6-Hertz positive bursts. They have the highest amplitude over the temporal leads, formed with the additional temporal electrodes (T1, TA1, T2, TA2) especially with the bipolar derivations T2-T6 and T1-T5 (Velizarova *et al.*, 2011).

This pattern has no pathological significance. In fact, fourteen- and six-Hz positive bursts resemble mu rhythms or sleep spindles but with a different distribution. Moreover, they do not always occur at precisely 6 Hz or 14 Hz and can vary by a few cycles per second.

• Rhythmic midtemporal discharge or rhythmic temporal theta burst of drowsiness

This unusual activity, present mainly in adolescents and young adults, has no correlation with clinical seizures. Initially described in 1952 by Gibbs and Gibbs with the term "psychomotor variant pattern", it was later called "rhythmic midtemporal discharge" by Lipman and Hughes (1969). In the literature, the preferred term is "rhythmic theta burst of drowsiness". The theta bursts, ranging from 5 to 6.5 Hz, occur predominantly over the mid-temporal regions. However, there can be some spread to adjacent regions (anterior or posterior temporal regions). They are mostly seen during drowsiness and usually cease in deeper sleep. They can be observed in relaxed wakefulness. Nevertheless, this activity can persist during non-REM sleep and above all during REM sleep, which is why we still prefer the name rhythmic midtemporal discharge (Gélisse & Crespel, 2014). The REM sleep pattern is identical to the one seen in wakefulness. The bursts can occur bilaterally and simultaneously or independently with a shifting emphasis from side to side. The bursts present a rhythmic pattern, i.e. their frequency remains stable throughout the discharge. The bursts last between a few seconds and more than one minute. Some authors have described this type of discharge in patients presenting personality disorders or some degree of dysautonomia and have suggested a possibility of autosomal dominant transmission (Eeg-Olofsson et Petersen, 1982). However, this pattern is considered non-specific with regard to epilepsy.

• Six-Hertz Spike-and-Wave Burst/ Phantom spike-and-wave bursts

Phantom spike-and-wave bursts, or 6 Hz spike-and-wave bursts, consist of brief bursts of spikes in very low amplitude with a repetition range of 5 to 7 Hz but usually occurring with a rate of 6 Hz. They are said to be "phantom" because of the low amplitude of the spike in contrast to the slow-wave component that follows and the more widespread distribution of the slow wave. Phantom spike-and-wave bursts can be seen in adolescents but their incidence is higher in adults. This pattern usually occurs bilaterally and it is generally synchronous during relaxed wakefulness, drowsiness or light sleep. They disappear during deeper levels of sleep but can reappear in REM sleep (Gelisse & Crespel, 2008). There remains some controversy about their pathological significance. They appear to be more often associated with epilepsy when they are predominant over the anterior regions than when they predominate over the posterior regions. Hughes (1980) distinguished two types of phantom spike-and-wave bursts in function of their topography, the individual's gender and the pathological significance of the bursts. FOLDs (female occipital predominant low amplitude and drowsiness) correspond to the benign variant whereas WHAMs (wake high amplitude anterior predominance in males) are more often associated with epilepsy.

• Breach rhythm

The breach rhythm, described in Chapter 1 on activities during wakefulness, can be seen during all stages of sleep. The amplitude of this pattern is slightly higher during light sleep. During REM sleep, it resembles the rhythm during wakefulness.

• Occipital spikes of blindness or needle-like occipital spikes of the blind

Needle-like occipital spikes are present in children who have congenital blindness then disappear in adolescence. They are located over the occipital or parietal regions, unilateral, bilateral but sometimes they can occur independently over the two occipital lobes (Lairy *et al.*, 1964). They are not related to an epileptic activity. They occur mainly during NREM sleep.

III • 1 Hypnagogic hypersynchrony (1)

Context

2-year-old child referred for generalized tonic-clonic seizure.

What to note

The child is starting to fall asleep. Theta background with a 3-second burst of slow sharp waves.

Comment

In children under age 4 years, it is relatively frequent to observe bursts of slow sharp waves in drowsiness, not to be confused with spike-waves.

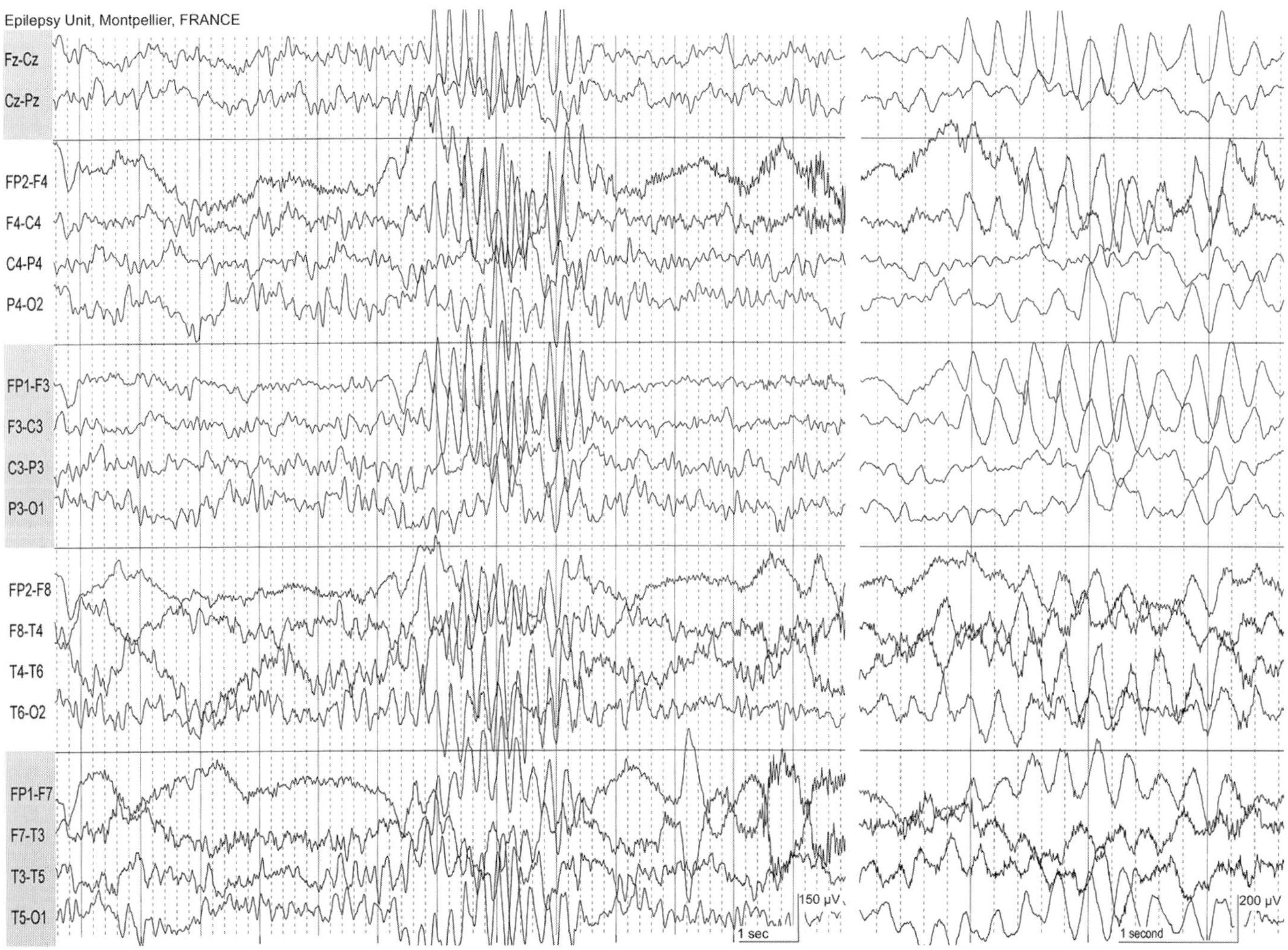

Figure a / Recording at 15 mm/s. With decreased amplitude, their non pathological significance becomes clear.

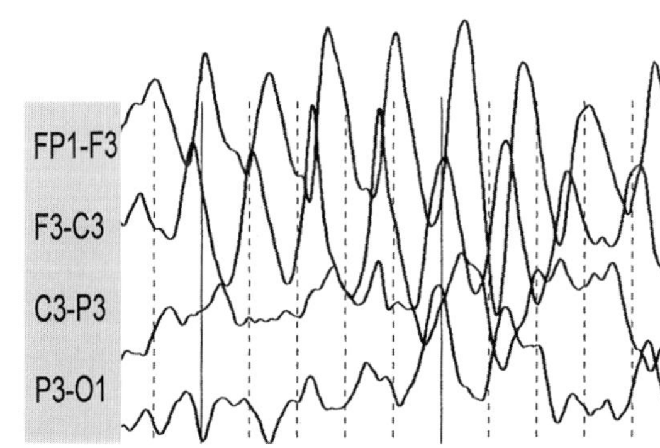

Figure b / Burst of slow waves.

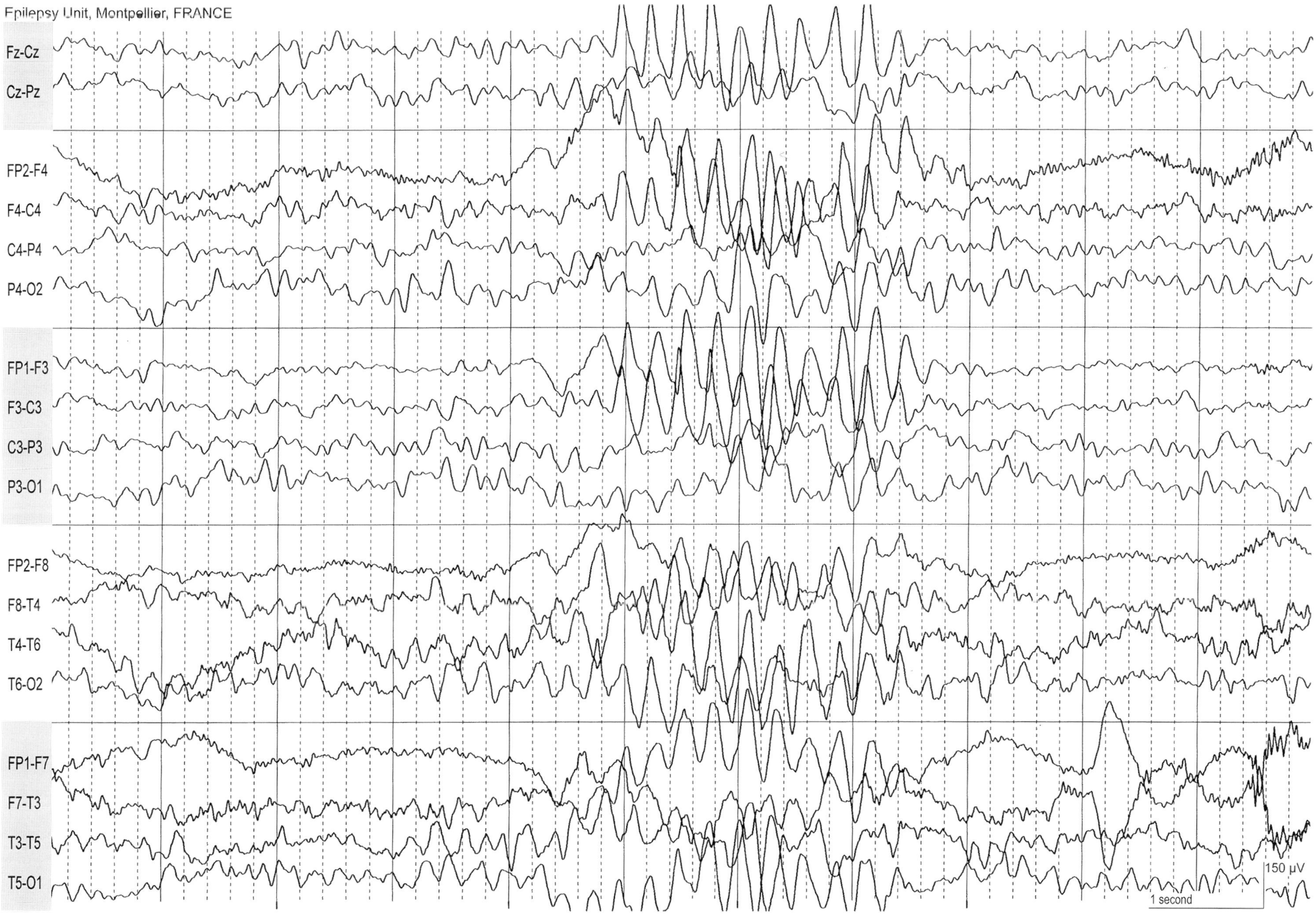
Epilepsy Unit, Montpellier, FRANCE
Fz-Cz
Cz-Pz
FP2-F4
F4-C4
C4-P4
P4-O2
FP1-F3
F3-C3
C3-P3
P3-O1
FP2-F8
F8-T4
T4-T6
T6-O2
FP1-F7
F7-T3
T3-T5
T5-O1
150 µV
1 second

III • 2 Hypnagogic hypersynchrony (2)

Context

3-year-old child seen after a fainting episode.

What to note

Recording with sensitivity set at 15 μV/mm. The child falls asleep in hypersynchrony. Slow background with bursts of ample diffuse sinusoidal 4 Hz theta-delta waves. These bursts are sometimes more prominent anteriorly or posteriorly, which is typical of hypnagogic hypersynchrony. On the EKG and at the frontal polar derivations, some fluctuation on the tracings corresponding to an electrodermogram (perspiration-related artifacts).

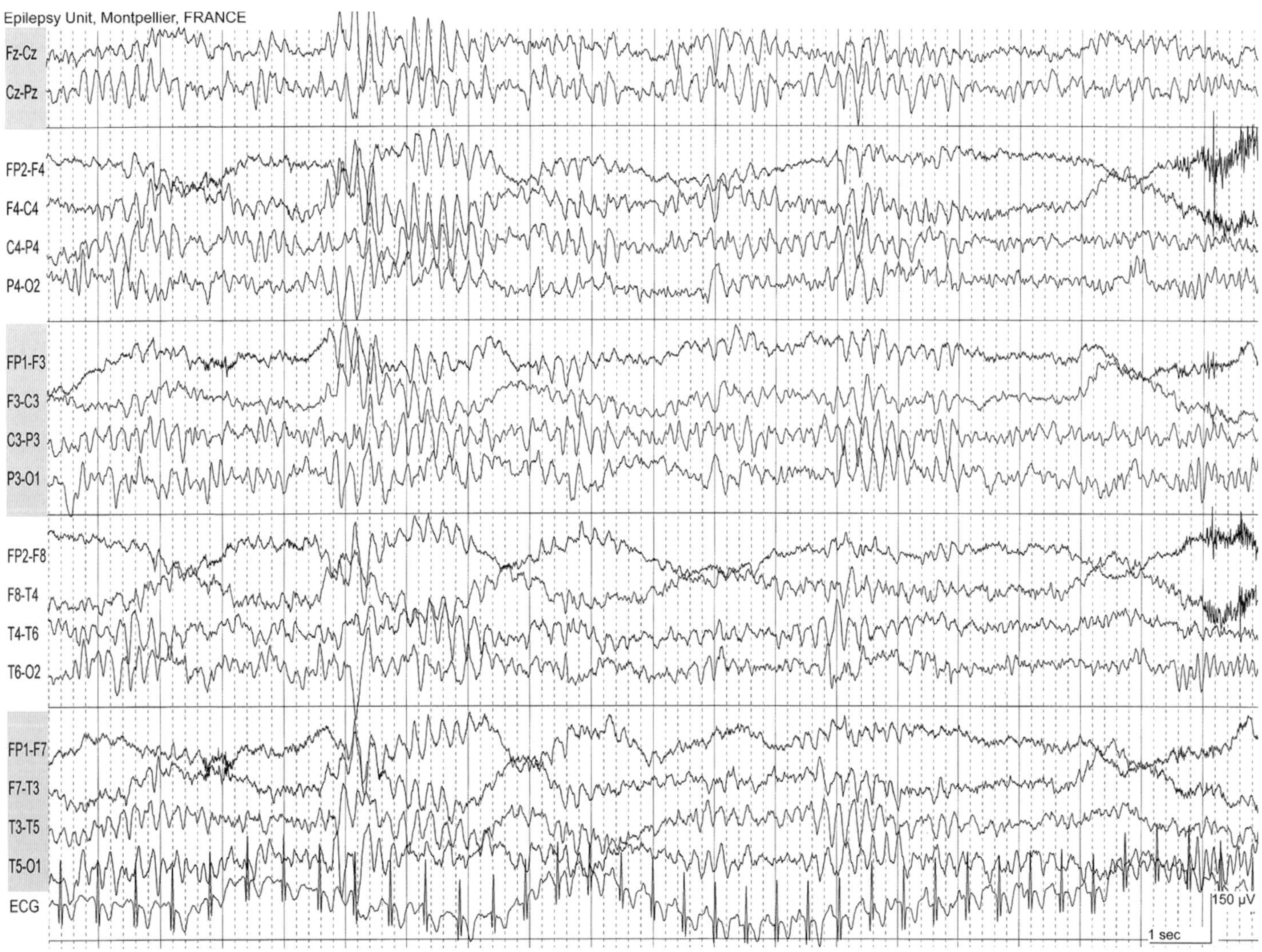

Figure a / Recording at 15 mm/s.

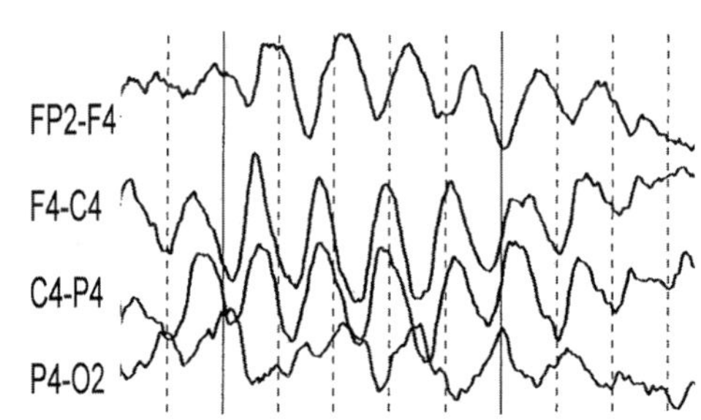

Figure b / Burst of sinusoidal slow waves.

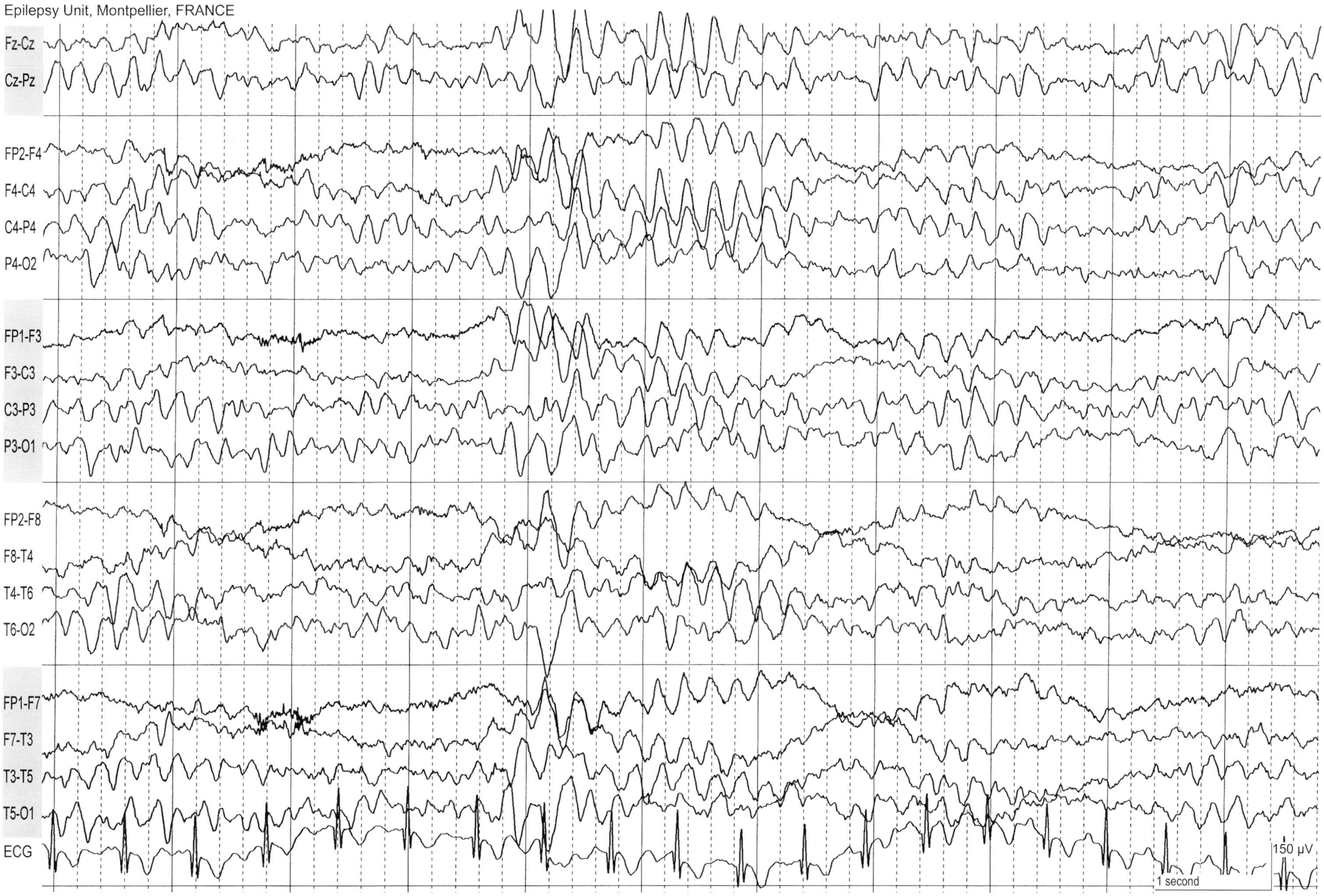
Epilepsy Unit, Montpellier, FRANCE
Fz-Cz
Cz-Pz
FP2-F4
F4-C4
C4-P4
P4-O2
FP1-F3
F3-C3
C3-P3
P3-O1
FP2-F8
F8-T4
T4-T6
T6-O2
FP1-F7
F7-T3
T3-T5
T5-O1
ECG
150 µV
1 second

III • 3 Hypnagogic hypersynchrony (3)

Context

3-year-old child with vertigo.

What to note

Recording with sensitivity set at 15 μV/mm.. As the child falls asleep, slow waves of hypersynchrony can be seen on the EEG. In the center, a burst of slow sharp waves lasting less than one second can be noted. These very-high-voltage elements cause blocking at this gain and convey the false impression of a spike-wave discharge. When in doubt amplitude should be decreased (see below). There are no spikes. This is typical of hypersynchrony in children under age 4 years.

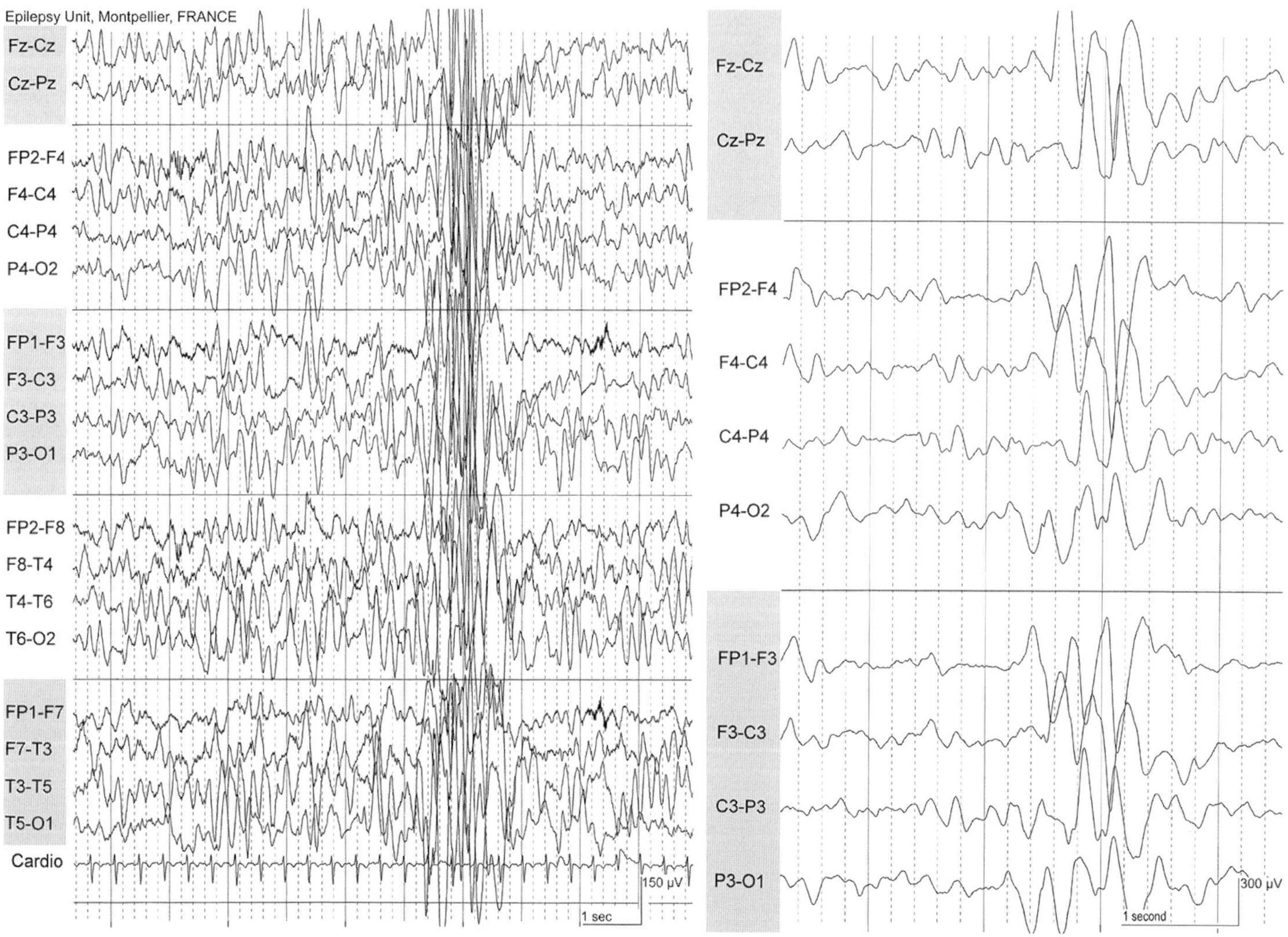

Figure a / On the left, recording at 15 mm/s. On the right, at 30 mm/s. Same burst with decreased amplitude showing the absence of pathological patterns.

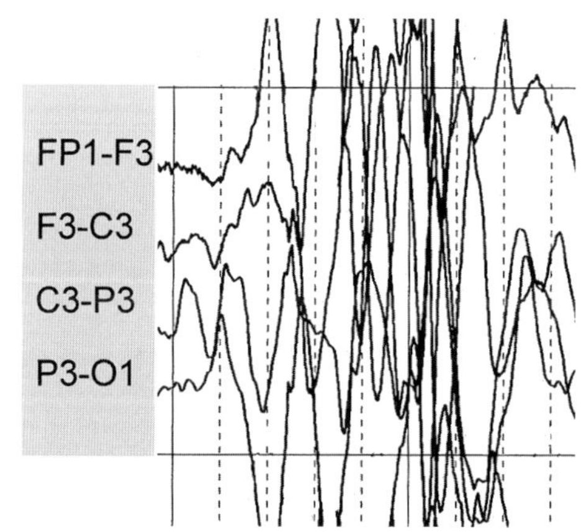

Figure b / Hypersynchrony with a burst of sharply-contoured waves.

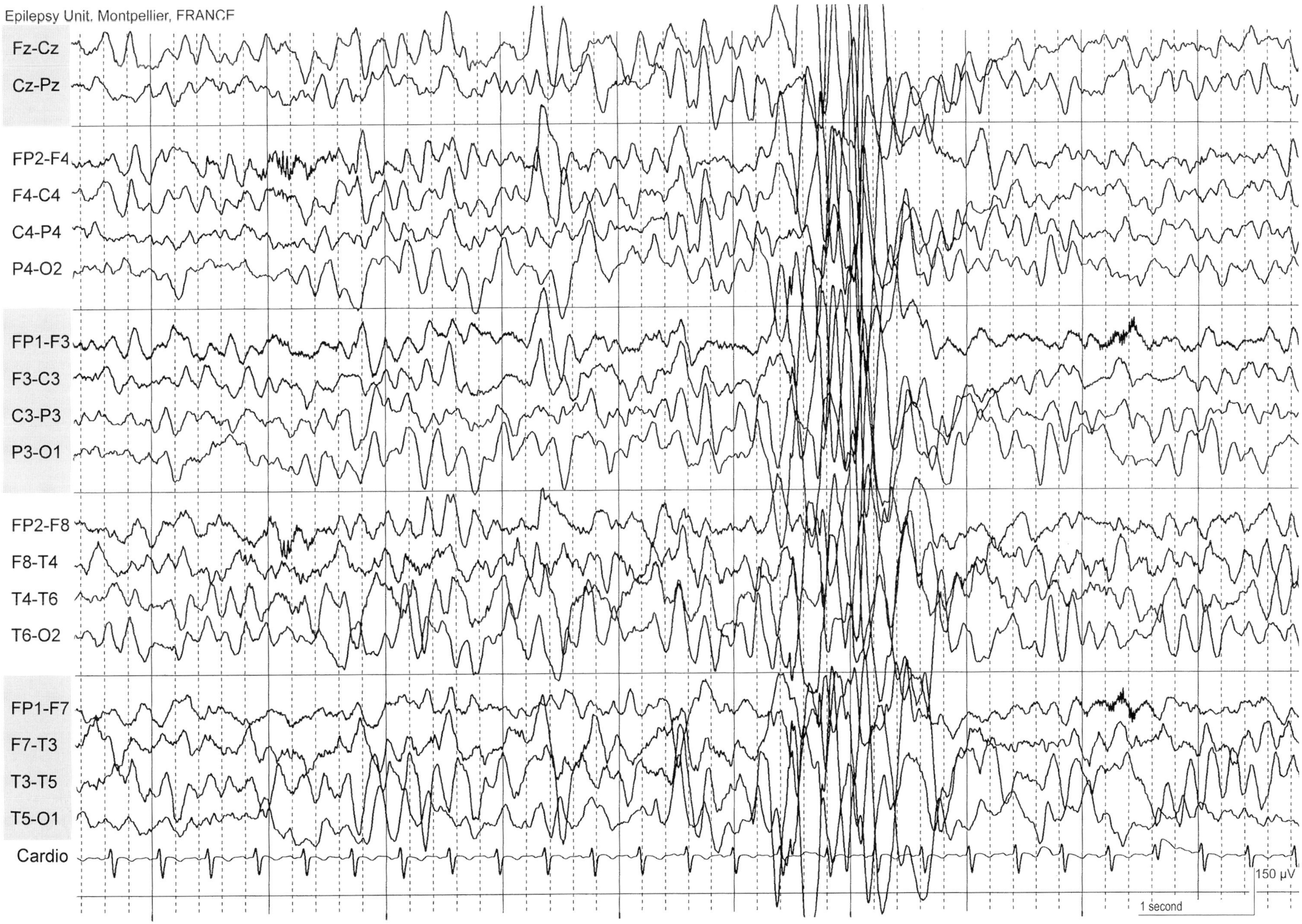
Epilepsy Unit, Montpellier, FRANCE
Fz-Cz
Cz-Pz
FP2-F4
F4-C4
C4-P4
P4-O2
FP1-F3
F3-C3
C3-P3
P3-O1
FP2-F8
F8-T4
T4-T6
T6-O2
FP1-F7
F7-T3
T3-T5
T5-O1
Cardio
150 µV
1 second

III • 4 Drowsiness in a child (1)

Context

5-year-old child seen after several episodes of loss of consciousness.

What to note

Posterior background alpha at onset of the tracing recorded at 15 mm/s (see below). Then offset of this rhythm and onset of low-voltage theta activity. Occurrence of theta waves at 5 Hz over the frontal regions and the vertex corresponding to hypnagogic hypersynchony but the amplitude is lower than on the previous plates. Note an irregularity of tracings at F8, TA2, TA1, T1 and F7, which corresponds to slow eye movements indicating onset of NREM sleep stage I.

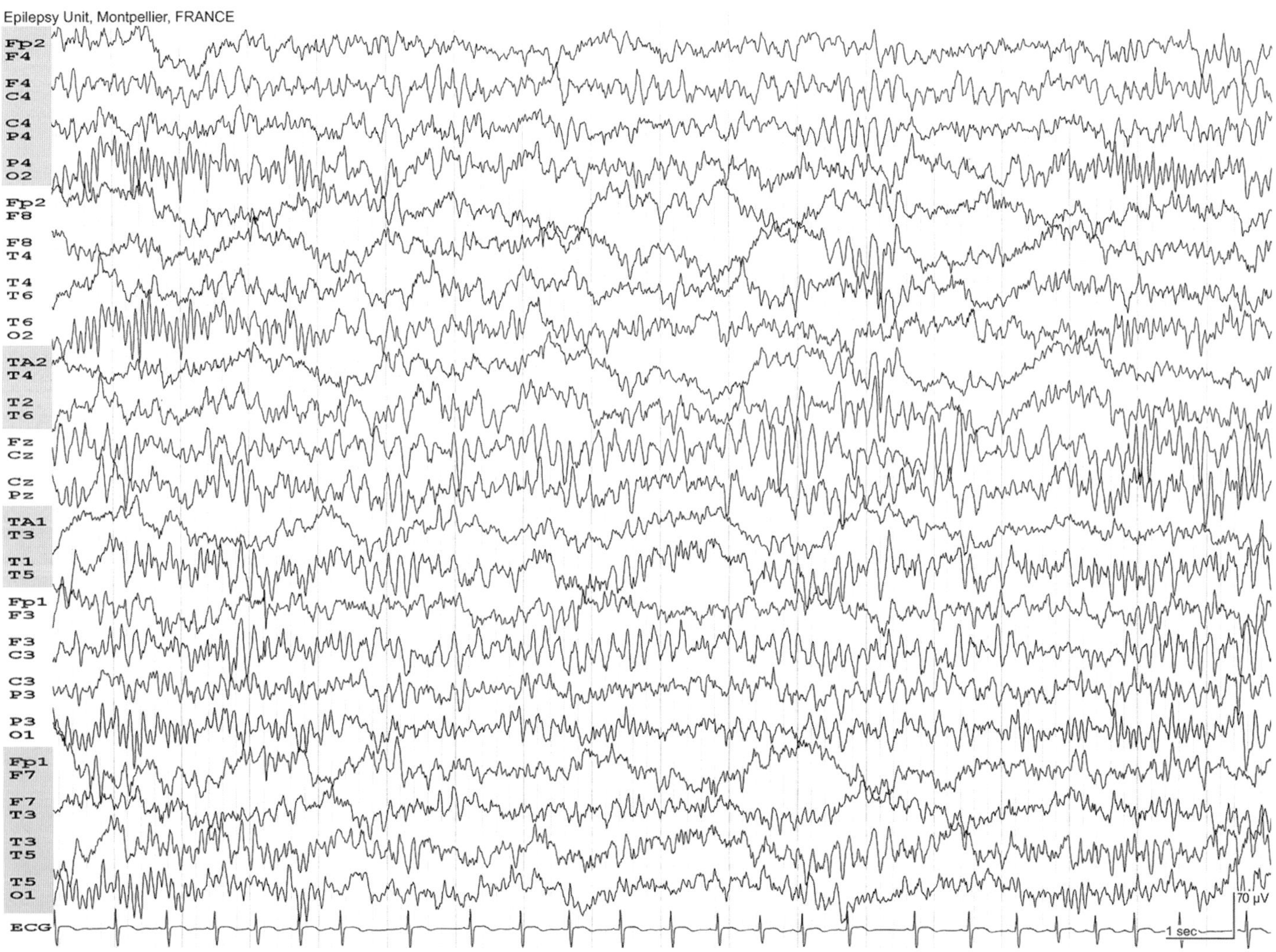

Figure a / Recording at 15 mm/s. Alpha rhythm at the beginning of the plate. It reappears at the end.

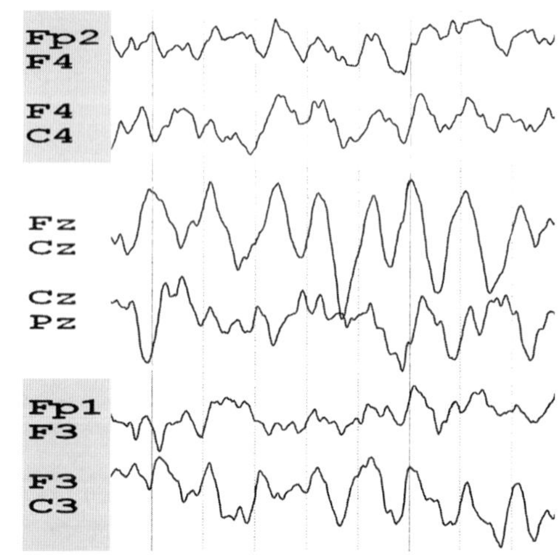

Figure b / Theta waves at 5 Hz.

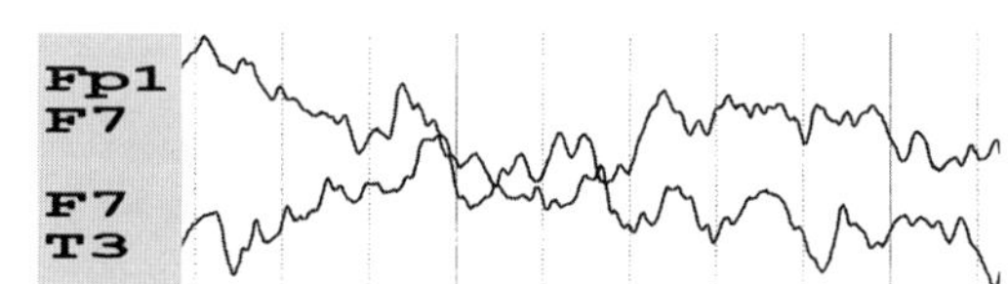

Figure c / Fluctuation of the tracing corresponding to slow eye movements.

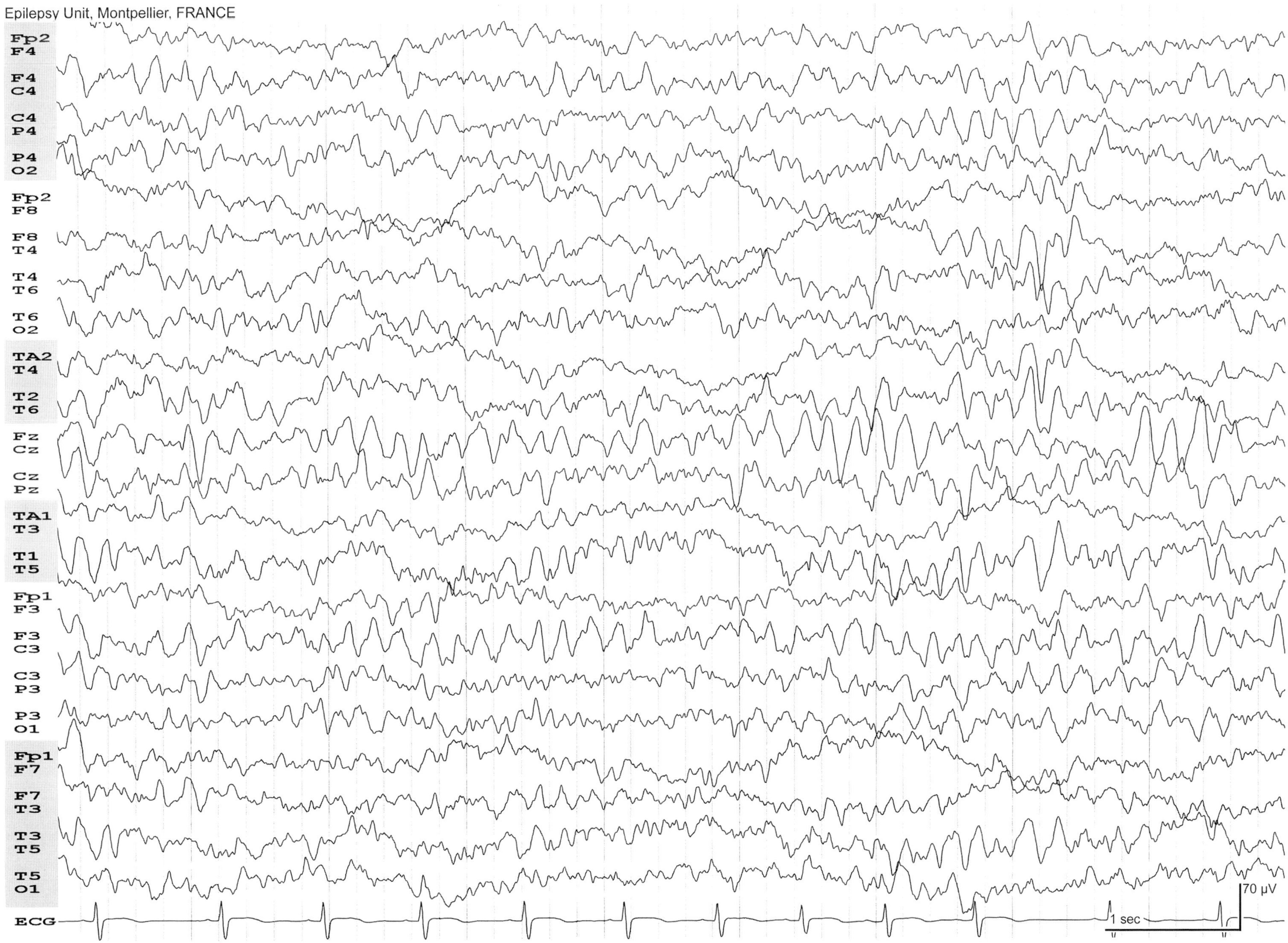
Epilepsy Unit, Montpellier, FRANCE
Fp2 F4
F4 C4
C4 P4
P4 O2
Fp2 F8
F8 T4
T4 T6
T6 O2
TA2 T4
T2 T6
Fz Cz
Cz Pz
TA1 T3
T1 T5
Fp1 F3
F3 C3
C3 P3
P3 O1
Fp1 F7
F7 T3
T3 T5
T5 O1
ECG
70 µV
1 sec

III • 5 Drowsiness in a child (2)

Context

9-year-old child with cryptogenic focal epilepsy.

What to note

Well-developed posterior alpha background, with some physiological posterior slow waves of youth. After the 4th second, offset of the alpha and occurrence of a burst of diffuse theta waves followed by a theta background. Fast pharmacological rhythms (due to benzodiazepines) are clearly reinforced over the frontal polar regions in drowsiness.

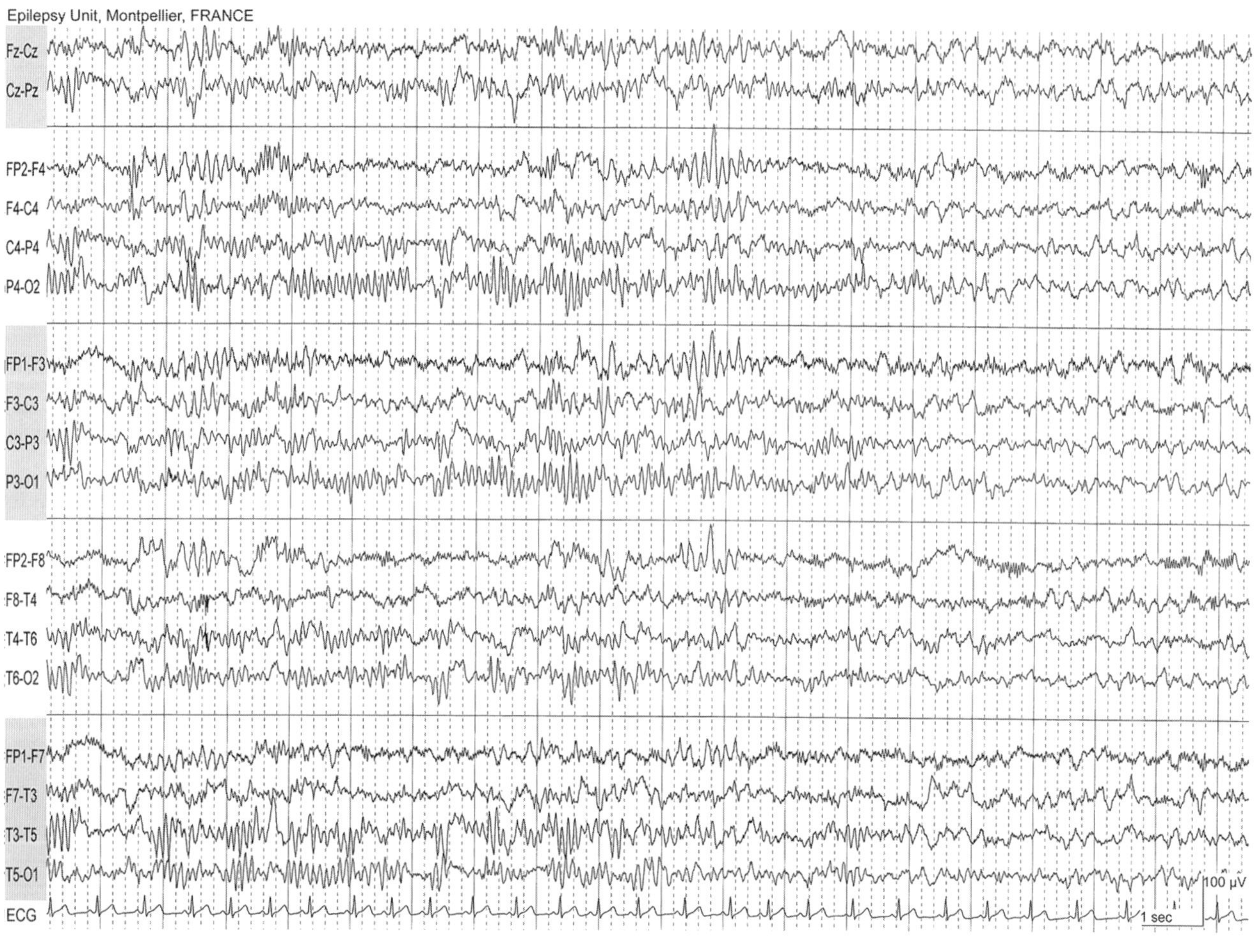

Figure a / Recording at 15 mm/s.

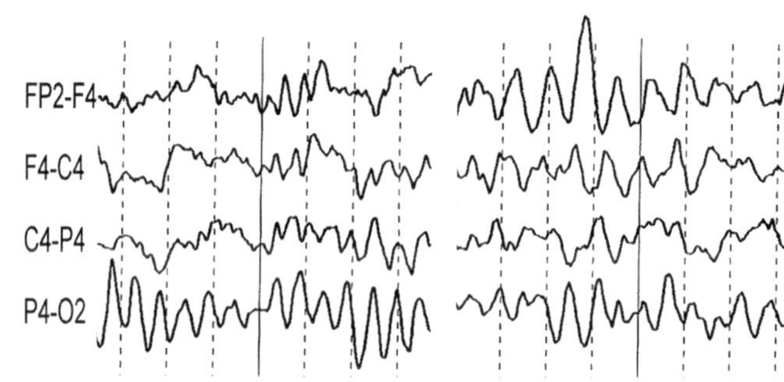

Figure b / Posterior alpha background rhythm. As the child falls asleep, offset of the alpha rhythms, onset of a diffuse theta rhythm.

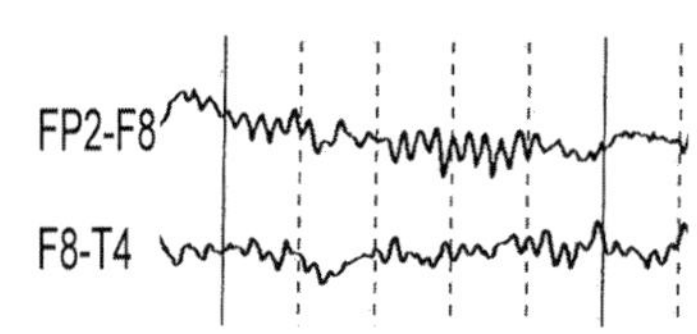

Figure c / Fast pharmacological beta rhythms at Fp2-F8.

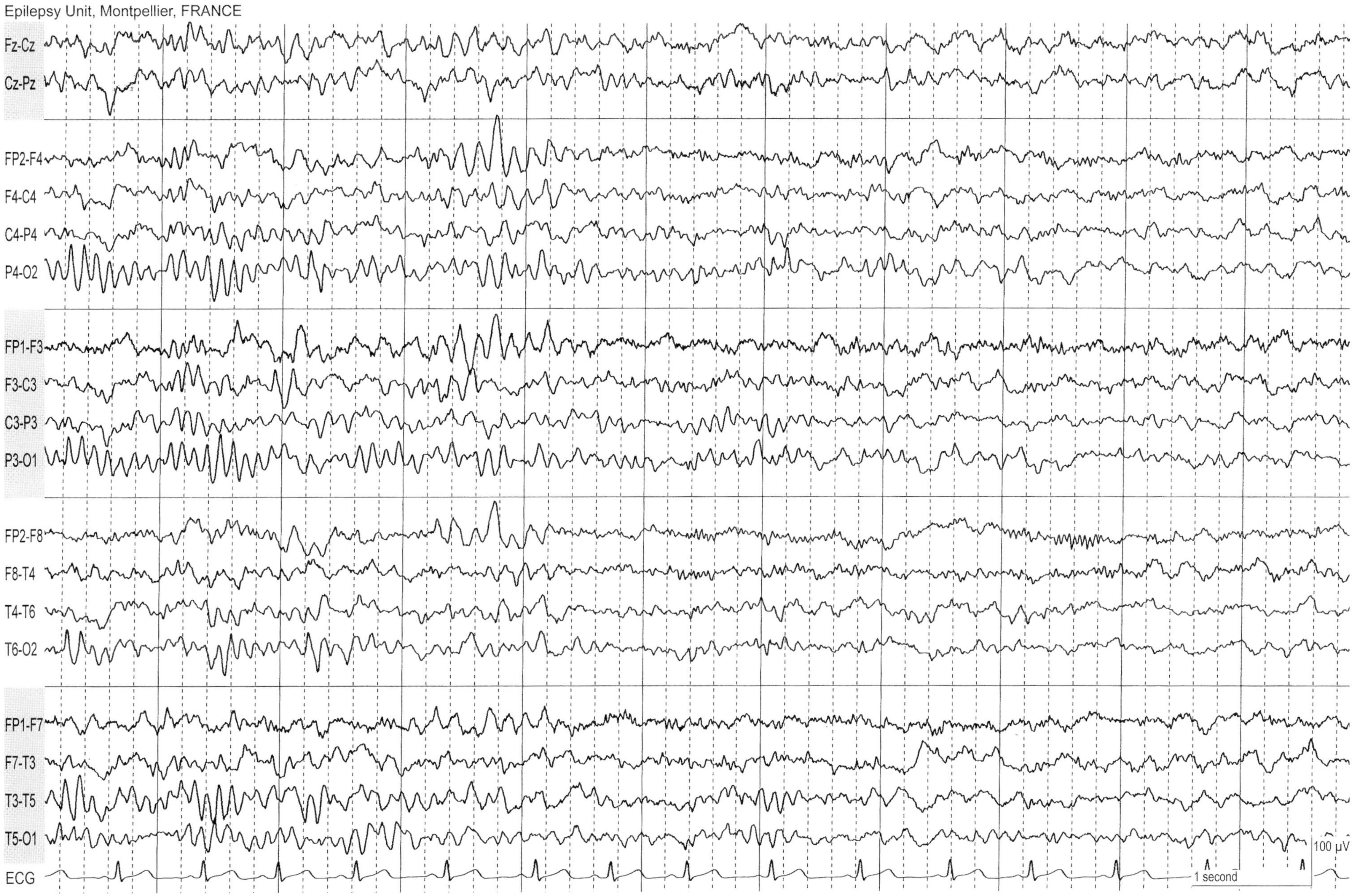
Epilepsy Unit, Montpellier, FRANCE
Fz-Cz
Cz-Pz
FP2-F4
F4-C4
C4-P4
P4-O2
FP1-F3
F3-C3
C3-P3
P3-O1
FP2-F8
F8-T4
T4-T6
T6-O2
FP1-F7
F7-T3
T3-T5
T5-O1
ECG
100 µV
1 second

III • 6 Drowsiness in an adolescent

Context

16-year-old man with psychogenic seizures.

What to note

Posterior background alpha. Then offset of this rhythm and onset of low-voltage theta activity. Note an irregularity of tracings at frontopolar and antero-inferior temporal derivations, which corresponds to slow eye movements indicating onset of NREM sleep stage I.

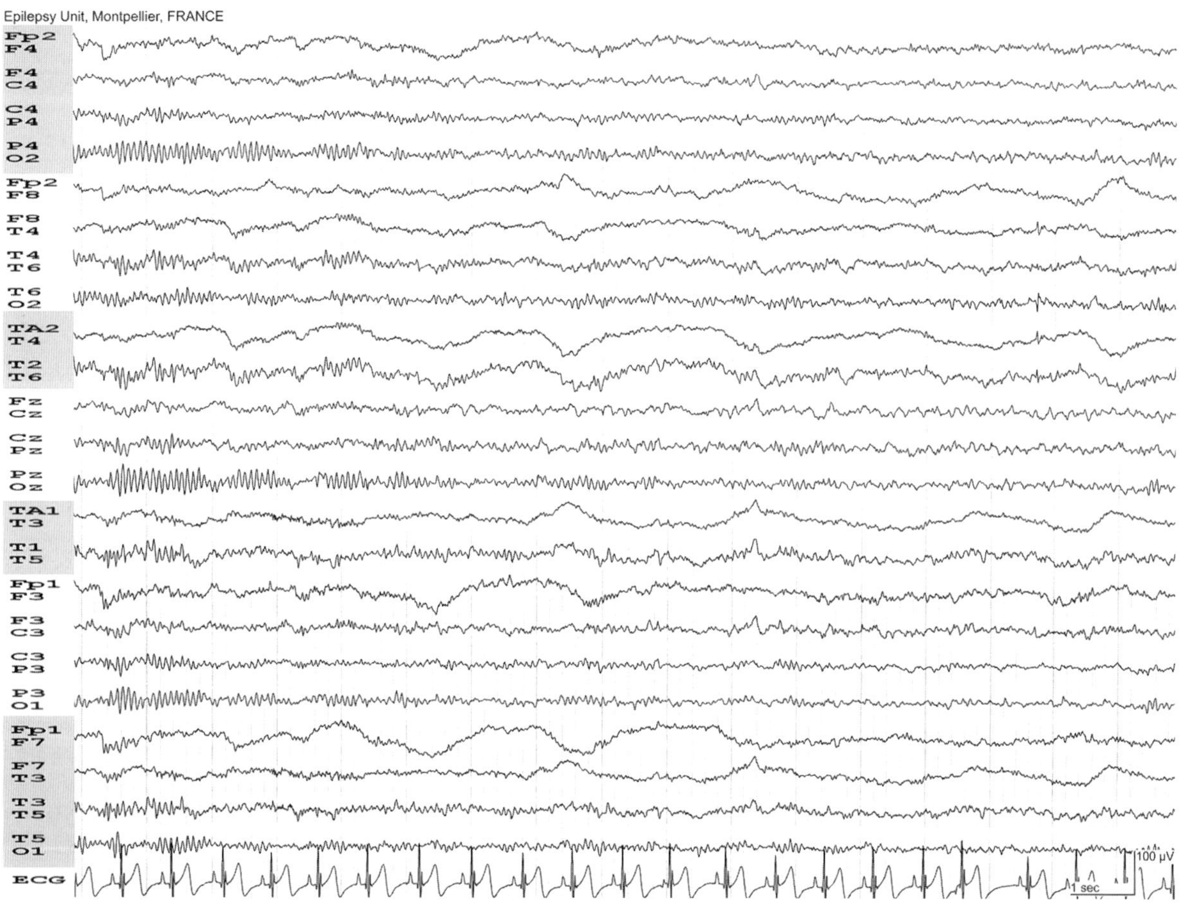

Figure a / Recording at 15 mm/s.

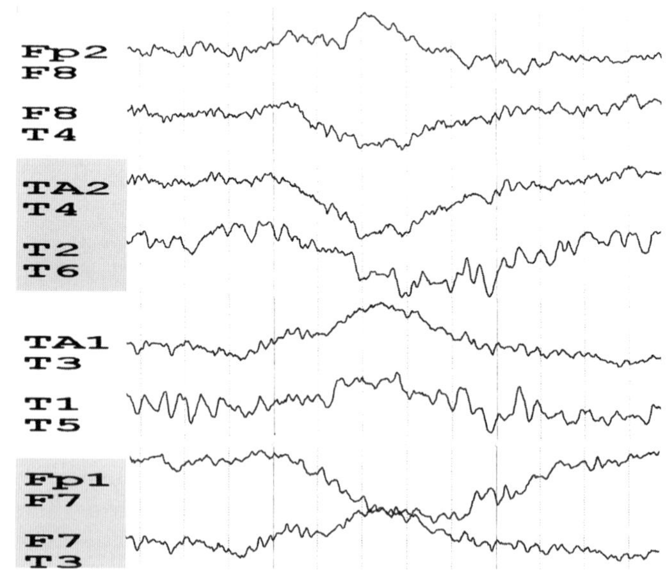

Figure b / Slow eye movements.

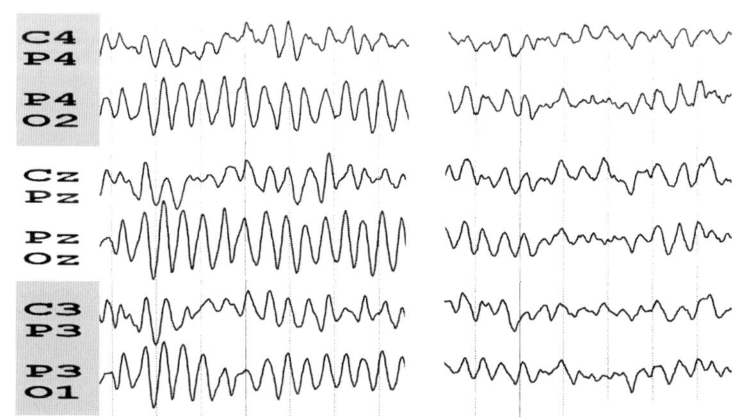

Figure c / Alpha rhythm disappears.

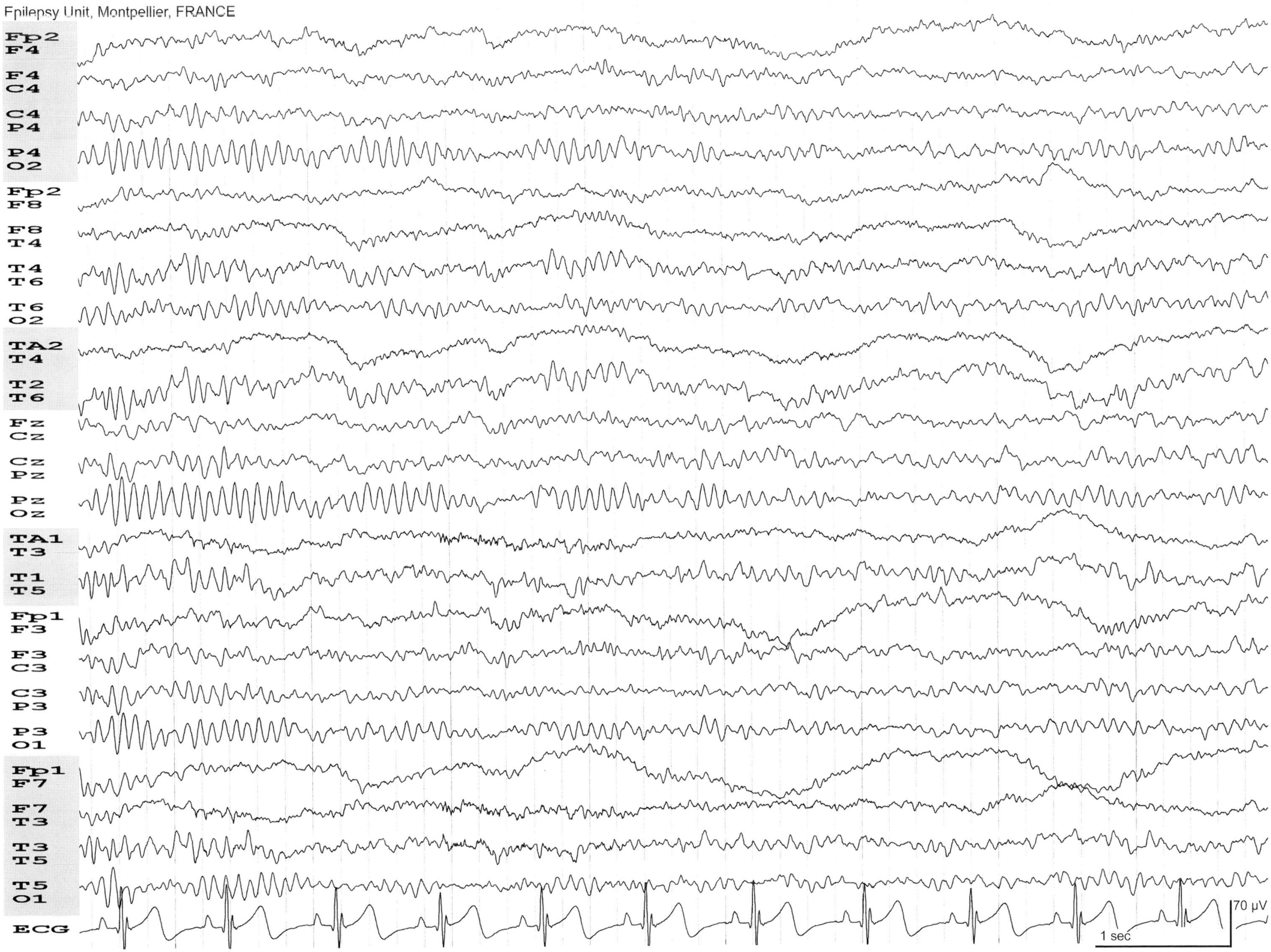
Epilepsy Unit, Montpellier, FRANCE
Fp2 F4
F4 C4
C4 P4
P4 O2
Fp2 F8
F8 T4
T4 T6
T6 O2
TA2 T4
T2 T6
Fz Cz
Cz Pz
Pz Oz
TA1 T3
T1 T5
Fp1 F3
F3 C3
C3 P3
P3 O1
Fp1 F7
F7 T3
T3 T5
T5 O1
ECG
70 µV
1 sec

III • 7 Fluctuation of level of consciousness in an elderly person

Context

96-year-old woman seen after an episode of loss of consciousness.

What to note

The left and right segments correspond to drowsiness. Offset of the alpha background rhythm and onset of low-voltage theta activity. Bursts of bilateral monomorphic high-voltage anterior delta waves can be observed at 1.5 Hz. This pattern expresses a fluctuation of the level of consciousness and corresponds to the frontal slow delta waves of drowsiness. This is a physiological activity in elderly individuals.

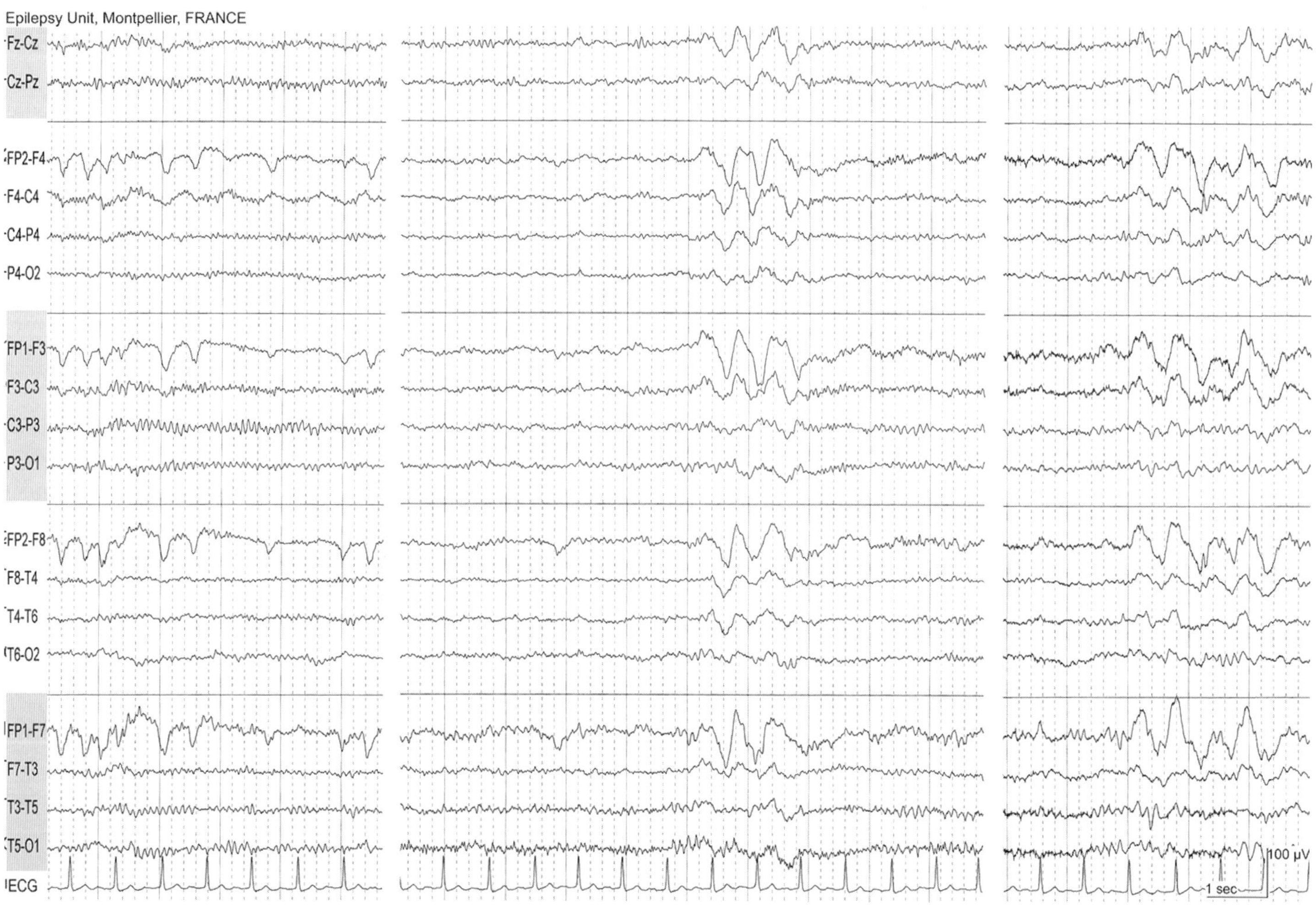

Figure a / Recording at 15 mm/s. In the left segment, alpha background rhythm at 9 Hz with a slight spread to the central region. It is better developed on the left than on the right hemisphere. Eye and eyelid movement artifacts at the frontal polar derivations.

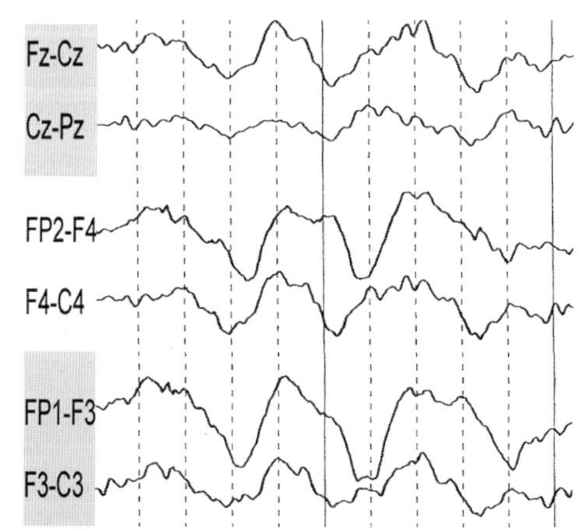

Figure b / Onset of anterior slow waves, fluctuating level of consciousness.

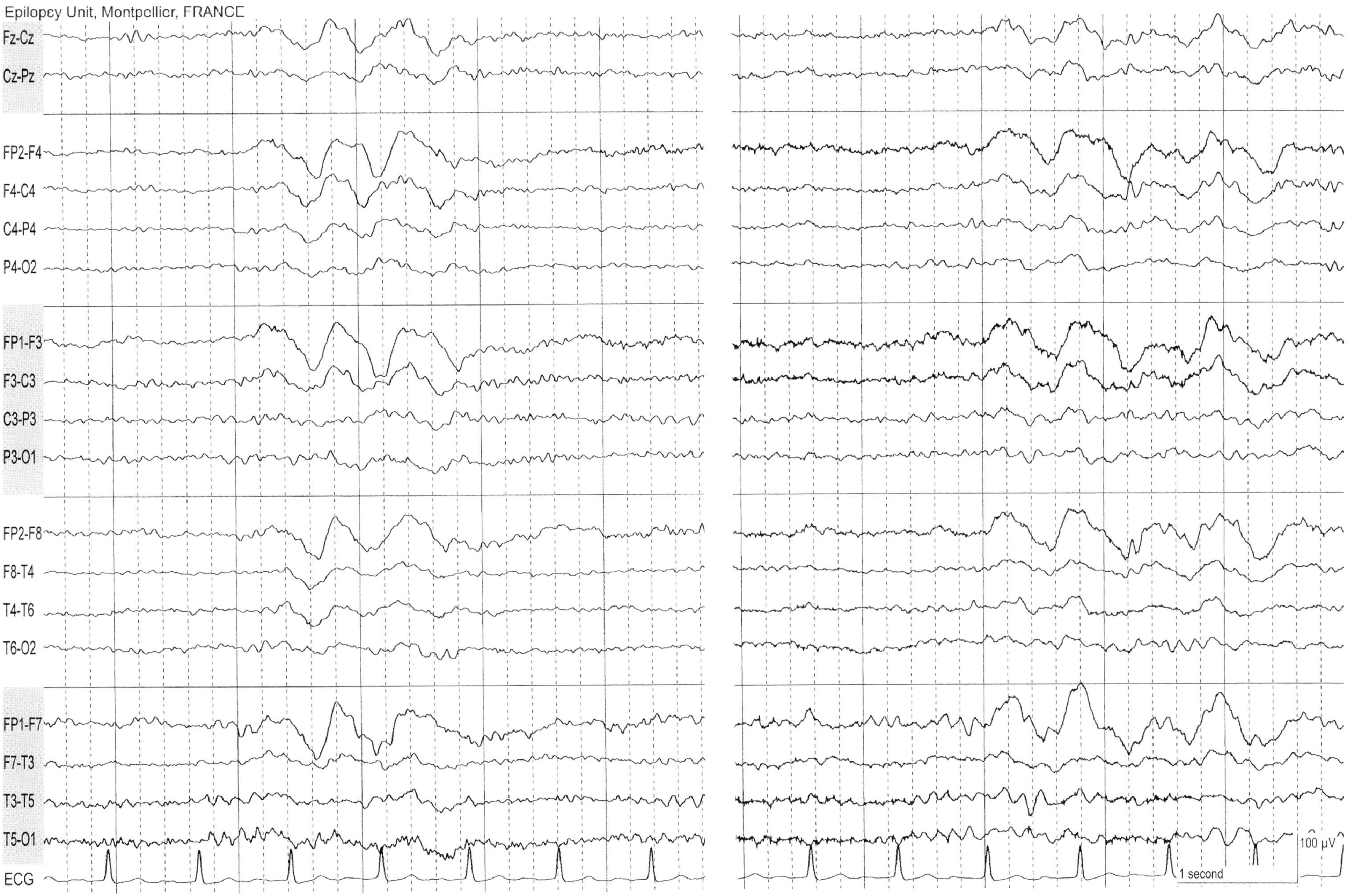
Epilepsy Unit, Montpellier, FRANCE
Fz-Cz
Cz-Pz
FP2-F4
F4-C4
C4-P4
P4-O2
FP1-F3
F3-C3
C3-P3
P3-O1
FP2-F8
F8-T4
T4-T6
T6-O2
FP1-F7
F7-T3
T3-T5
T5-O1
ECG
100 µV
1 second

III • 8 Beta rhythm

Context

25-year-old man with idiopathic generalized epilepsy.

What to note

Eyes closed. Drowsiness with disappearance of alpha rhythm and slow eye movements on the inferior frontal derivations, see plate recorded at 15 mm/s. With drowsiness, increased anterior beta rhythm. Onset of NREM sleep stage 1 at the end of the plate with V waves over the vertex.

Comment

Beta rhythms over the anterior regions are observed during drowsiness, NREM stage 1. They disappear in NREM stage 2 and 3 but reappear in REM sleep (see below).

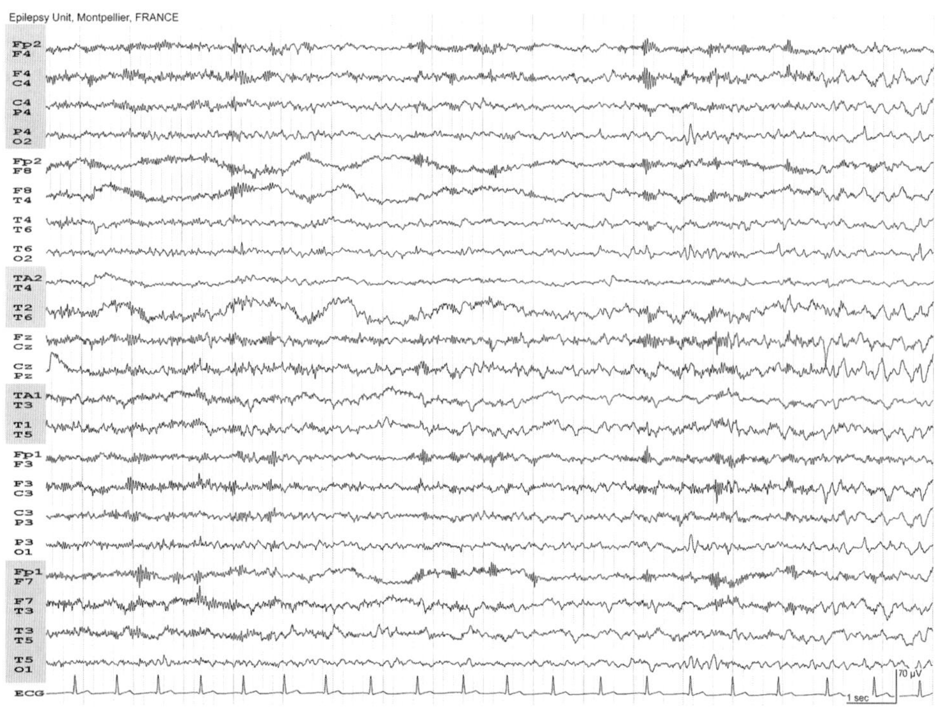

Figure a / Recording at 15 mm/s. Eye movement is sometimes easier to detect visually at F8 and F7.

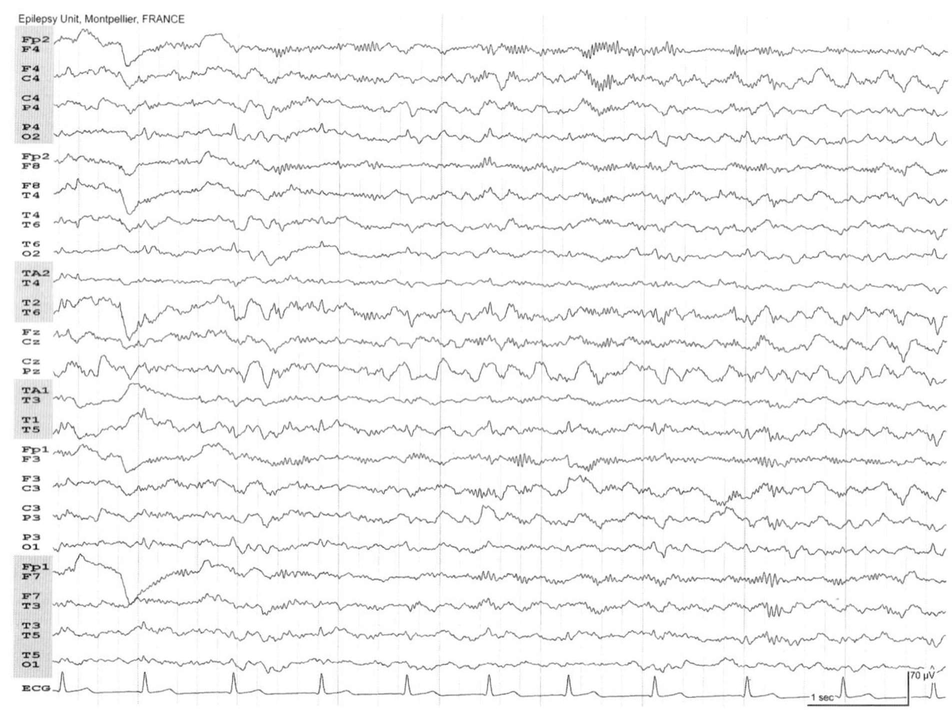

Figure b / Recording at 30 mm/s. REM sleep. The tracing includes rapid eye movements, sawtooth waves on the vertex and beta rhythms over the anterior regions.

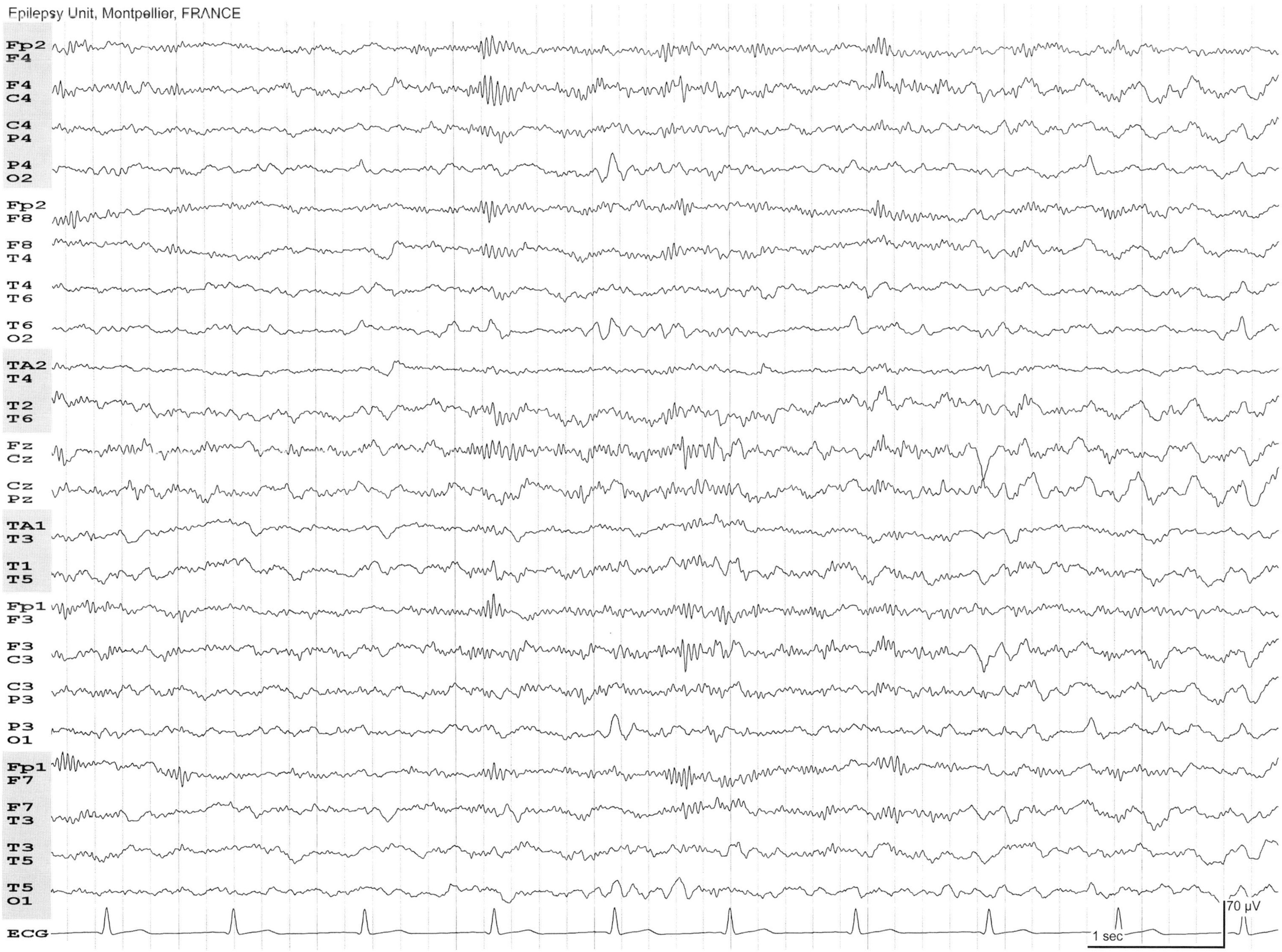
Epilepsy Unit, Montpellier, FRANCE
Fp2 F4
F4 C4
C4 P4
P4 O2
Fp2 F8
F8 T4
T4 T6
T6 O2
TA2 T4
T2 T6
Fz Cz
Cz Pz
TA1 T3
T1 T5
Fp1 F3
F3 C3
C3 P3
P3 O1
Fp1 F7
F7 T3
T3 T5
T5 O1
ECG
70 µV
1 sec

III • 9 NREM 1: Vertex waves in a child

Context

6-year-old girl seen after an episode of loss of consciousness.

What to note

Stage N1 sleep. Theta background activity with high-voltage slow spikes on the vertex and over the central regions. In children, V waves are sharply contoured and often occur in runs of bursts, not to be confused with epileptiform discharges. Note the presence of an artifact at Fp1 corresponding to a problem of impedance (Fp1-F3 and Fp1-F7 derivations). There is also an artifact of electrode at T4.

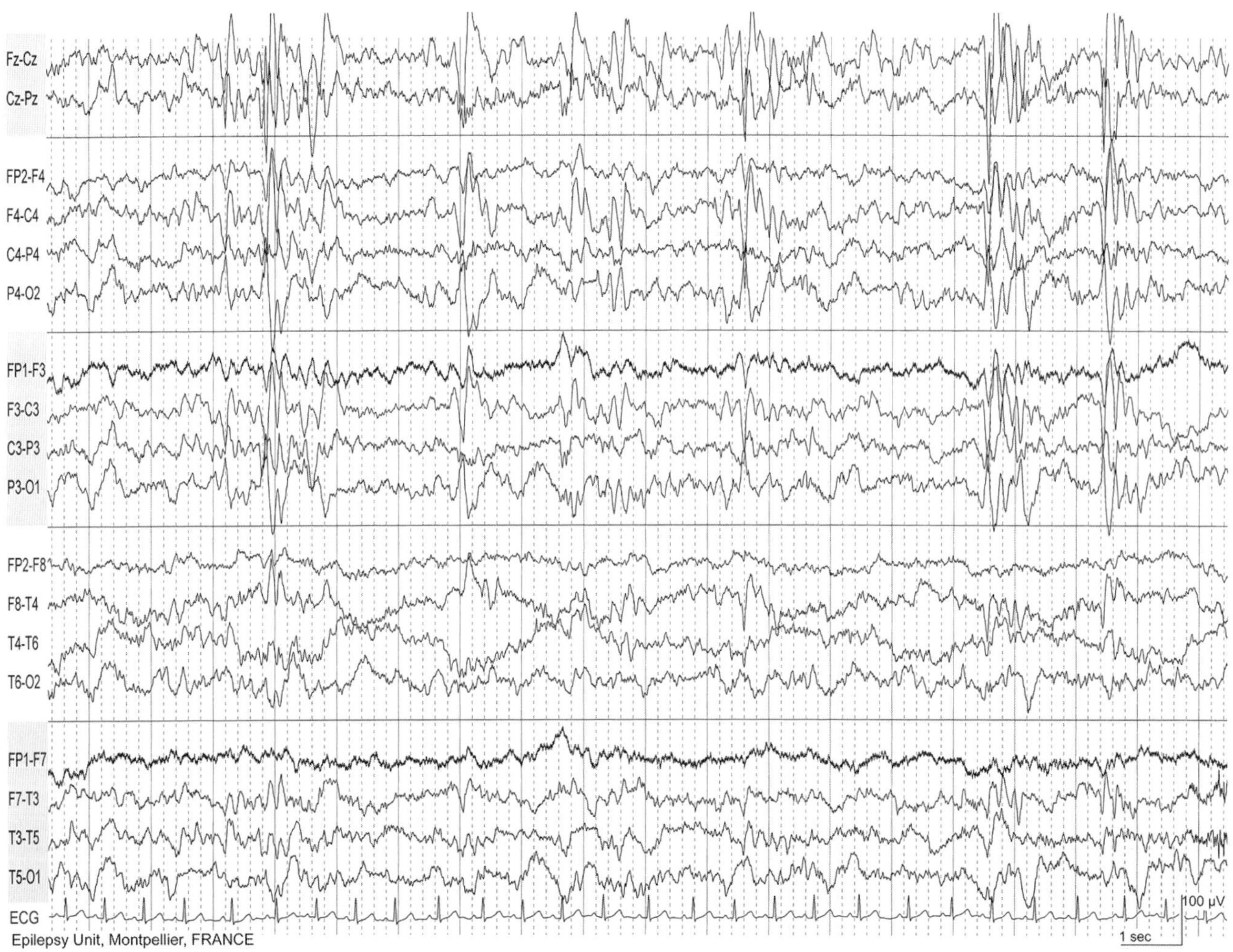

Figure a / Recording at 15 mm/s.

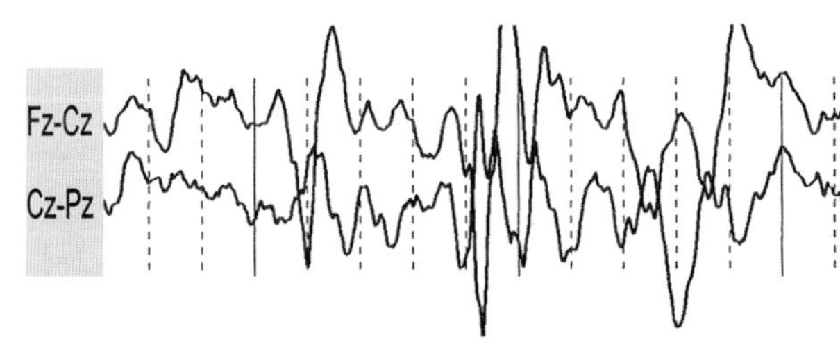

Figure b / High-voltage slow spikes corresponding to V waves.

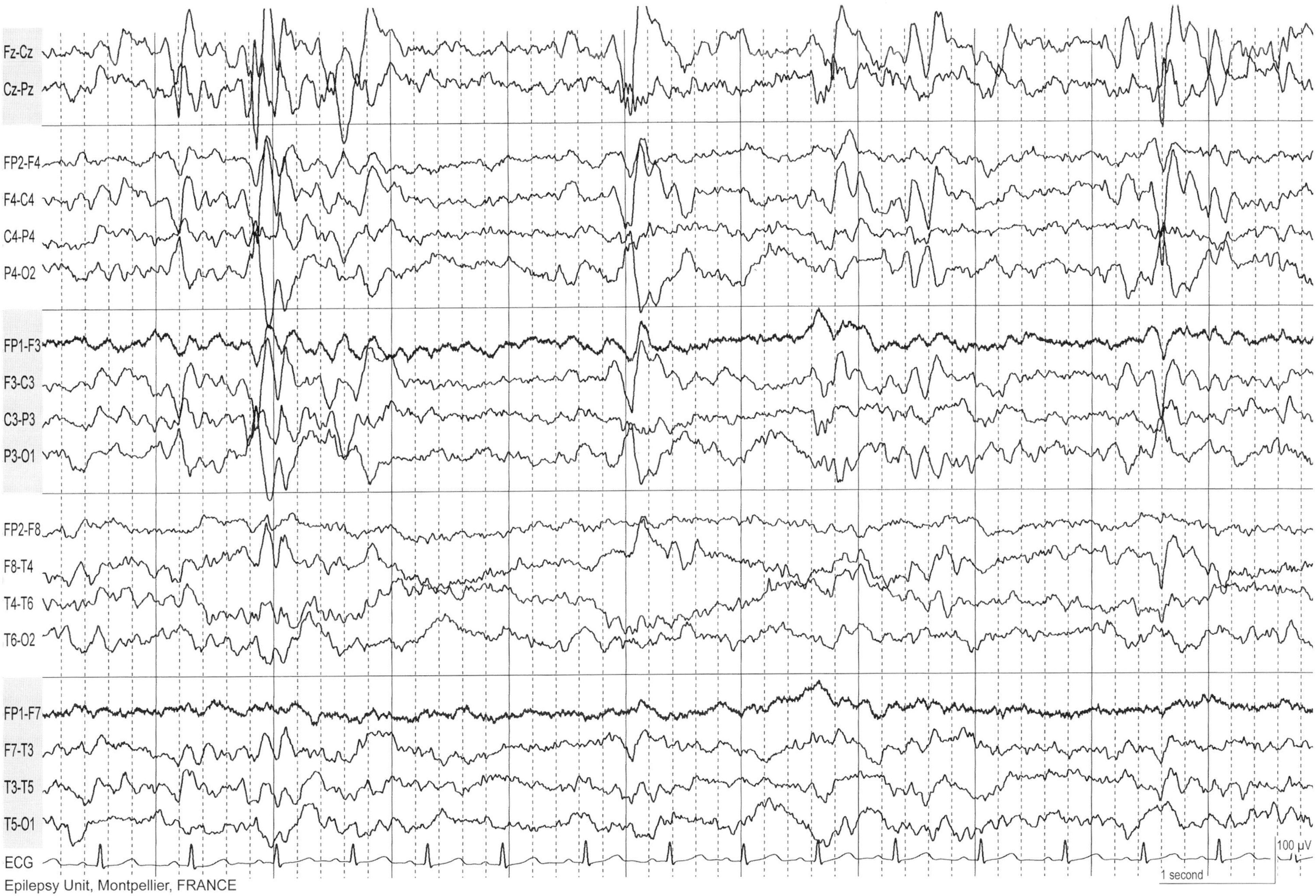
Fz-Cz
Cz-Pz
FP2-F4
F4-C4
C4-P4
P4-O2
FP1-F3
F3-C3
C3-P3
P3-O1
FP2-F8
F8-T4
T4-T6
T6-O2
FP1-F7
F7-T3
T3-T5
T5-O1
ECG
100 µV
1 second
Epilepsy Unit, Montpellier, FRANCE

III • 10 NREM 1: A train of vertex waves in a child

Context

9-year-old girl with learning difficulties.

What to note

Stage N1 sleep. V waves develop into a rhythmic 5 to 6-Hz theta activity over the vertex region for 7 seconds. This aspect is frequent in children under age 10 years. This pattern is a V wave continuum as usually described. As we can see on this plate, V waves can sometimes appear in rhythmic trains. This characteristic must be known and differentiate from an epileptic discharge. Fast beta rhythms are also clearly detectable on this plate over the inferior frontal regions (F8, F7). A pulse artifact can be observed on electrode T6.

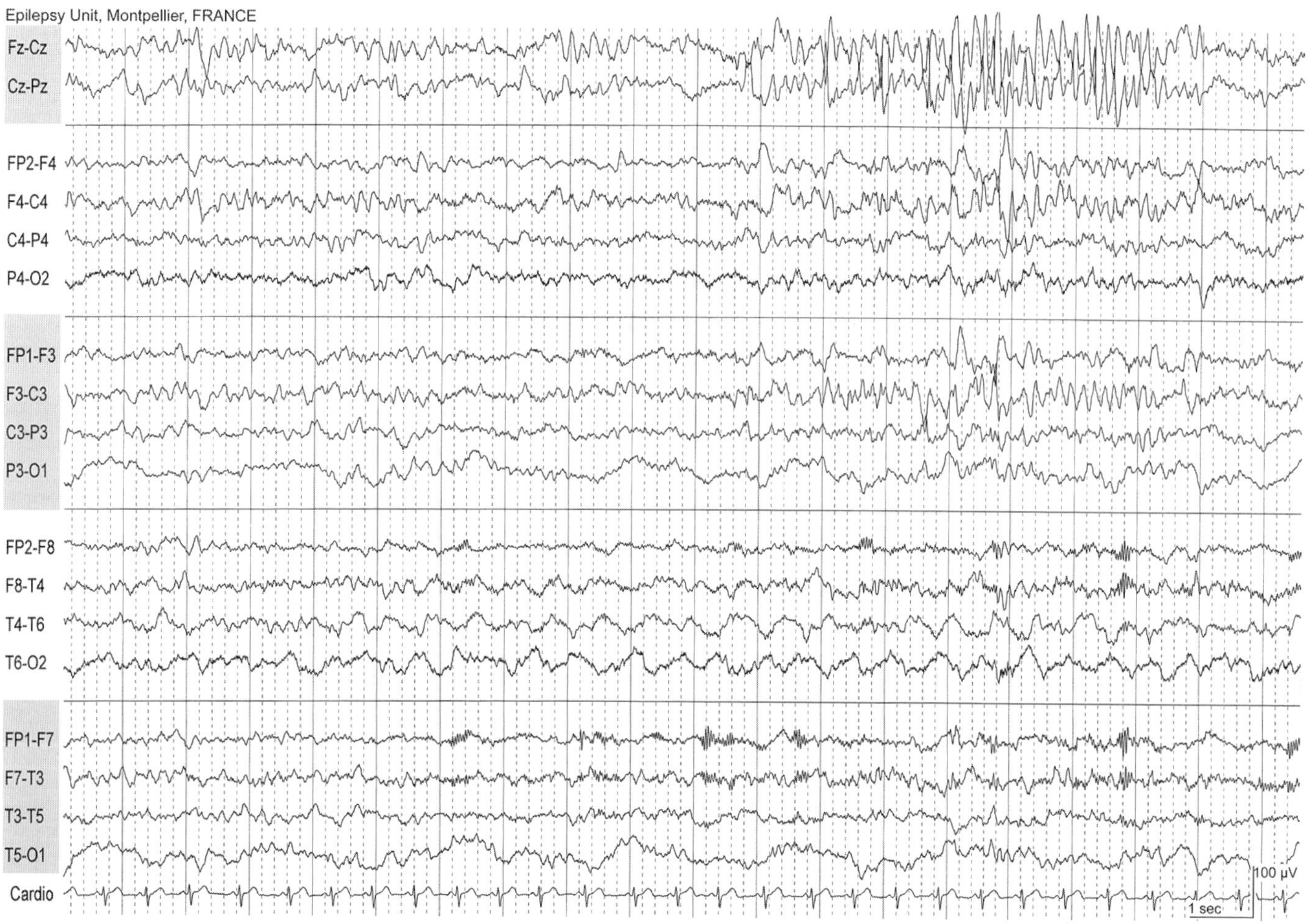

Figure a / Recording at 15 mm/s.

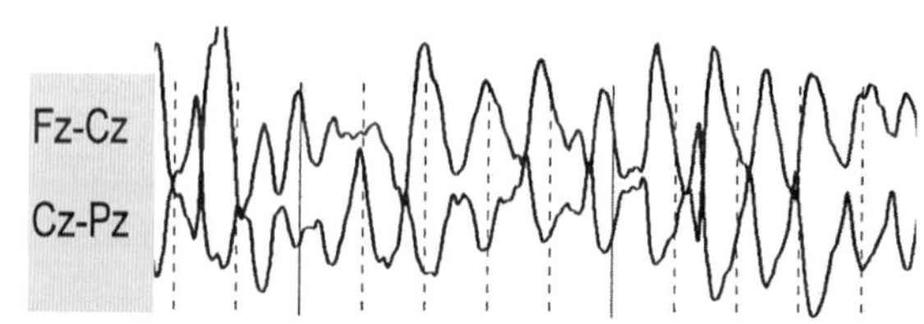

Figure b / V waves developing into 5 to 6-Hz rhytmic theta activity.

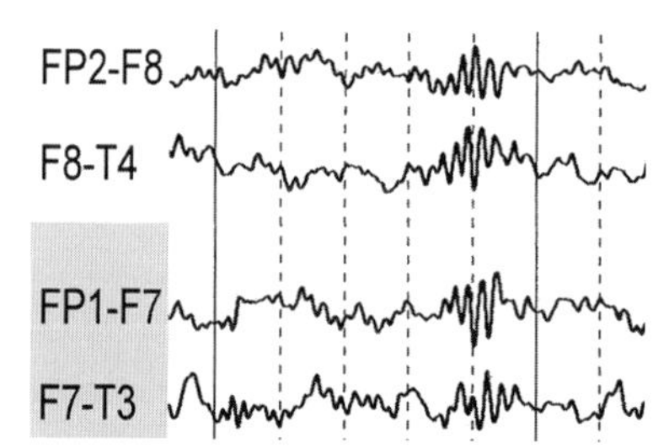

Figure c / Fast beta rhythms at Fp2-F8 and F8-T4.

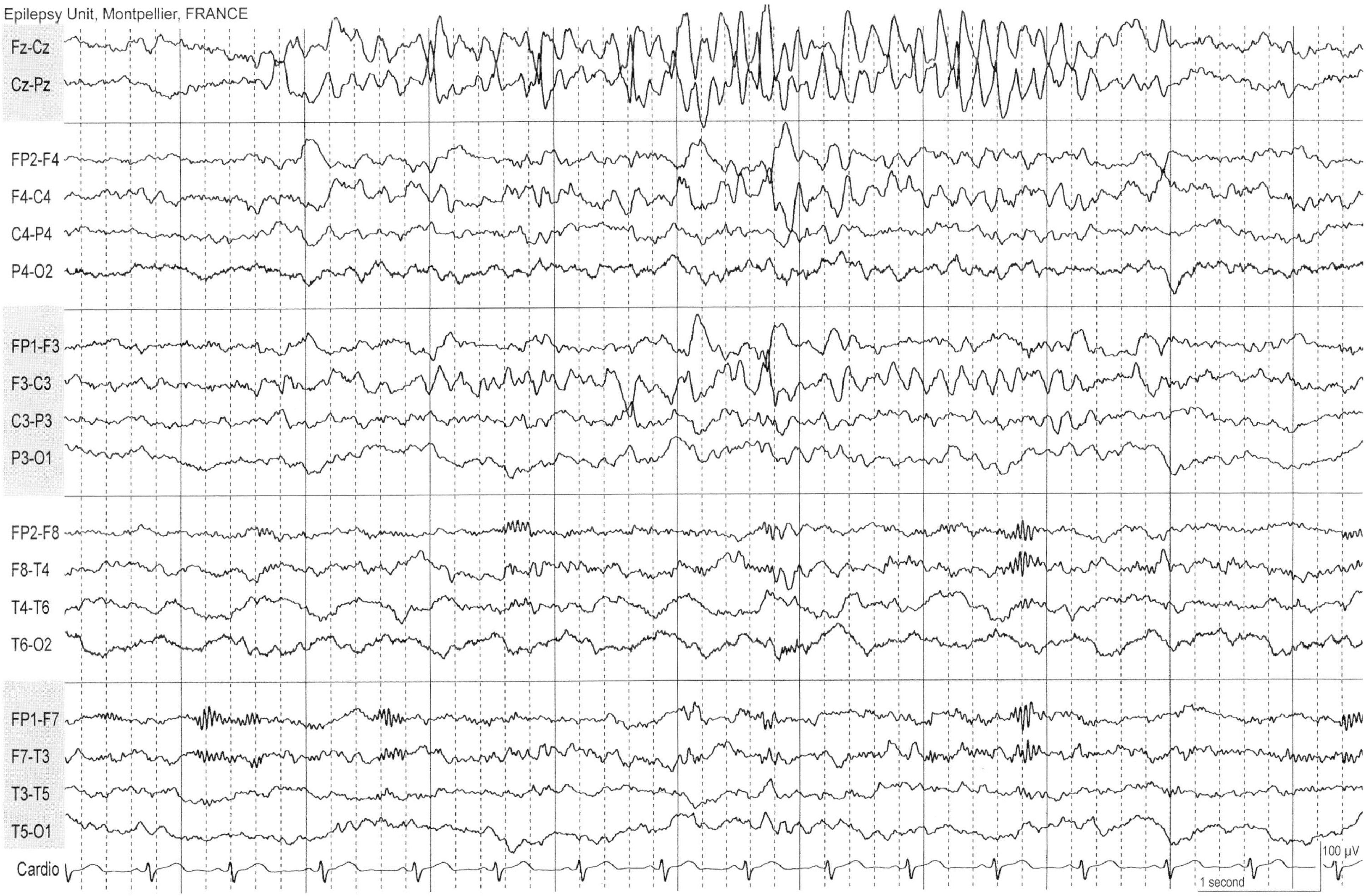
Epilepsy Unit, Montpellier, FRANCE
Fz-Cz
Cz-Pz
FP2-F4
F4-C4
C4-P4
P4-O2
FP1-F3
F3-C3
C3-P3
P3-O1
FP2-F8
F8-T4
T4-T6
T6-O2
FP1-F7
F7-T3
T3-T5
T5-O1
Cardio
100 µV
1 second

• 11 NREM 1: Vertex waves in an adolescent

Context

13-year-old girl with idiopathic generalized epilepsy.

What to note

The patient has fallen asleep. Sharp waves over the vertex and the right and left central regions. They correspond to V waves. At the beginning and in the middle of the plate, hypnagogic myoclonic jerks are recorded over the left deltoid muscle. Hypnic jerks usually happen in the beginnings of sleep and are normal. These jerks are often described as an electric shock after a falling sensation.

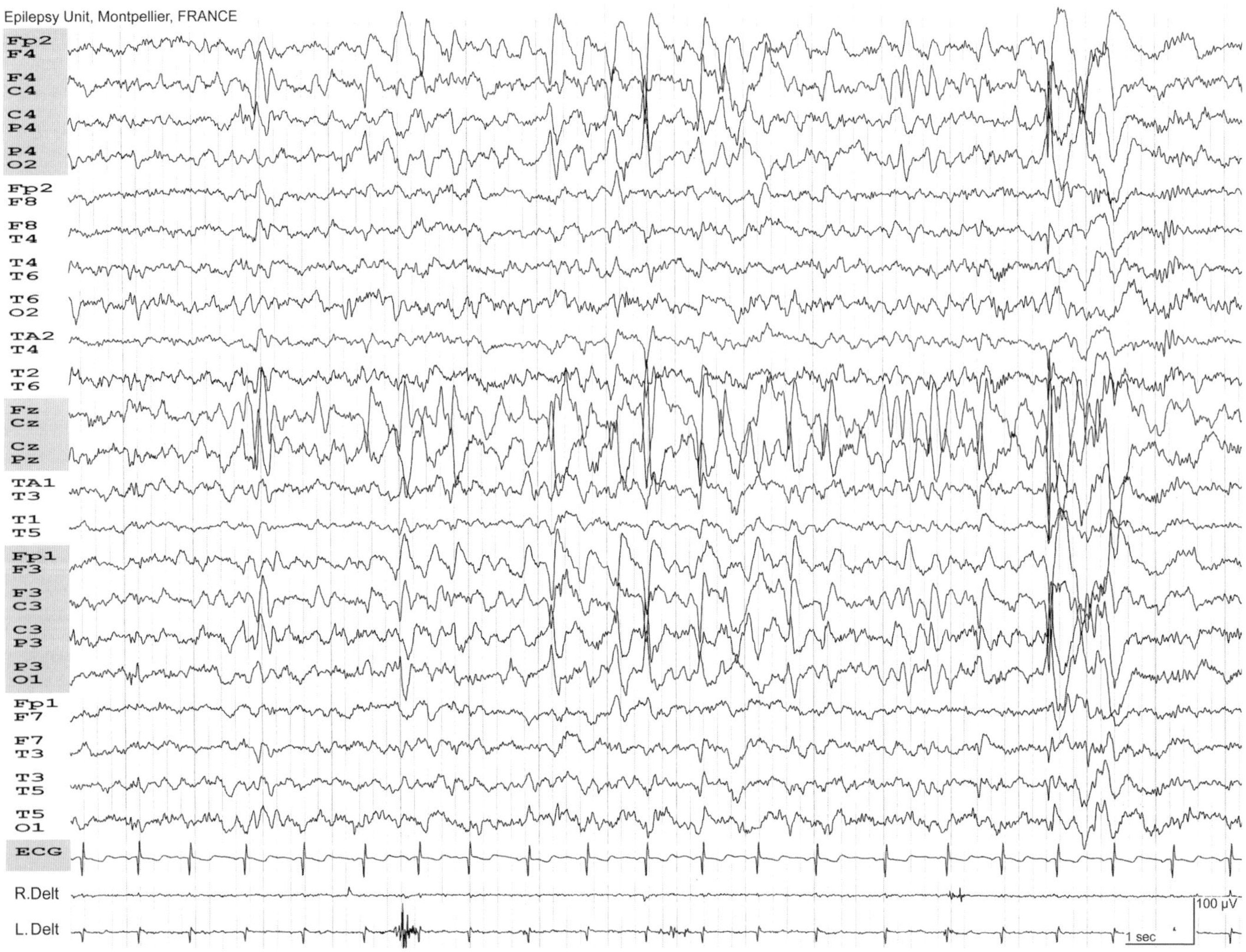

Figure a / Recording at 15 mm/s. Several myoclonic jerks, the two first ones are on the left deltoid, the last one is higher on the right deltoid.

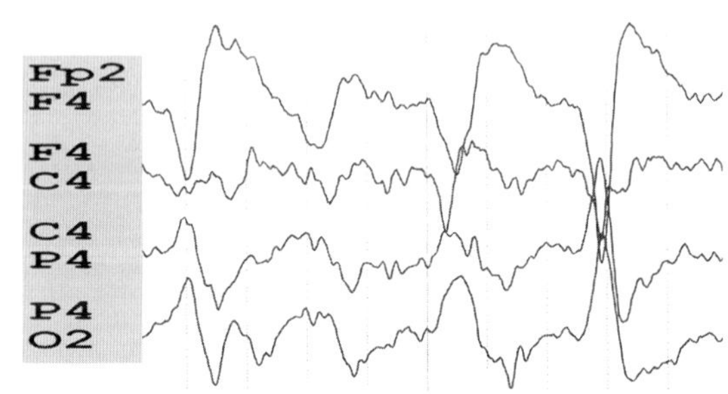

Figure b / Sharp waves in phase reversals over C4 corresponding to V waves.

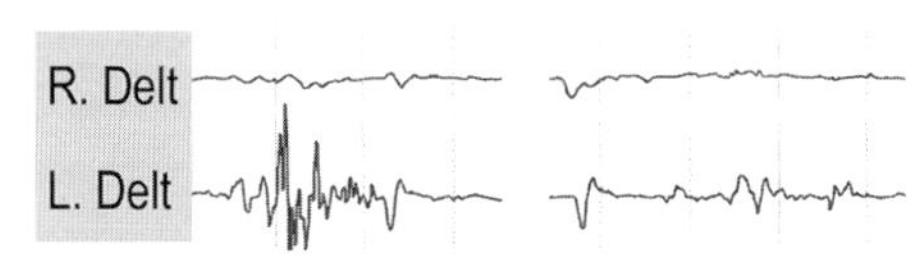

Figure c / Hypnic jerks on the left deltoid muscle. ECG artifact.

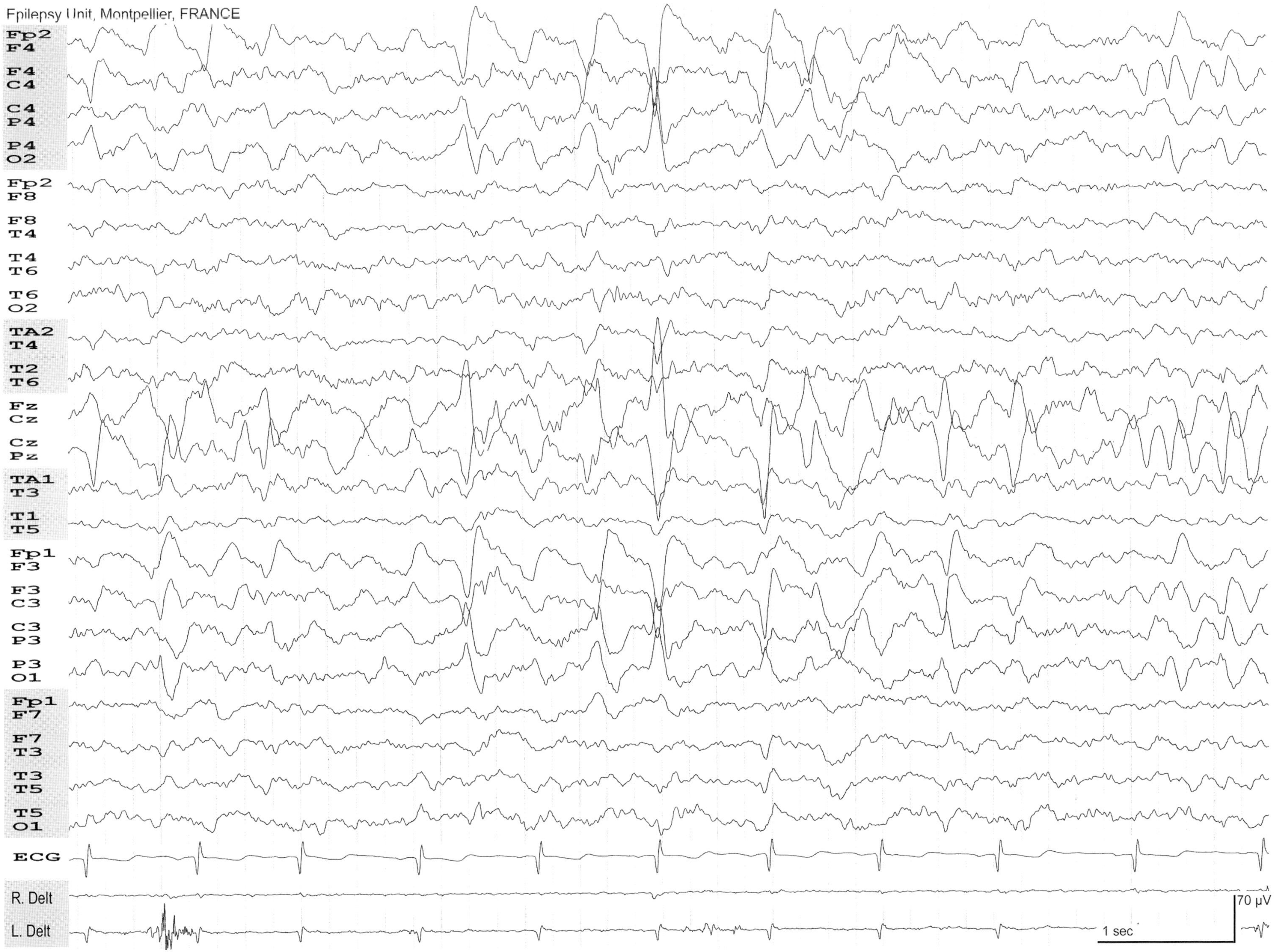
Epilepsy Unit, Montpellier, FRANCE
Fp2 F4
F4 C4
C4 P4
P4 O2
Fp2 F8
F8 T4
T4 T6
T6 O2
TA2 T4
T2 T6
Fz Cz
Cz Pz
TA1 T3
T1 T5
Fp1 F3
F3 C3
C3 P3
P3 O1
Fp1 F7
F7 T3
T3 T5
T5 O1
ECG
R. Delt
L. Delt
70 µV
1 sec

III • 12 NREM 1: Vertex waves in an adult (1)

Context

28-year-old woman seen after several episodes of loss of consciousness.

What to note

Spontaneous sleep onset in a routine EEG. First, the posterior alpha background develops into theta. Then occurrence of V waves, asymmetrical and better developed over the right hemisphere at Fp2-F4 and F4-C4. Asymmetry in one epoch has no clinical significance. However, constant asymmetry of physiological elements throughout a sleep recording (V waves, sleep spindles, K complexes) indicates altered organization in the hemisphere. An electrode "pop" artifact can be observed at F4, Fp1, O1 and P3. The morphology of V waves must not be confused with pathological patterns. V waves tend to become less typical as adults grow older.

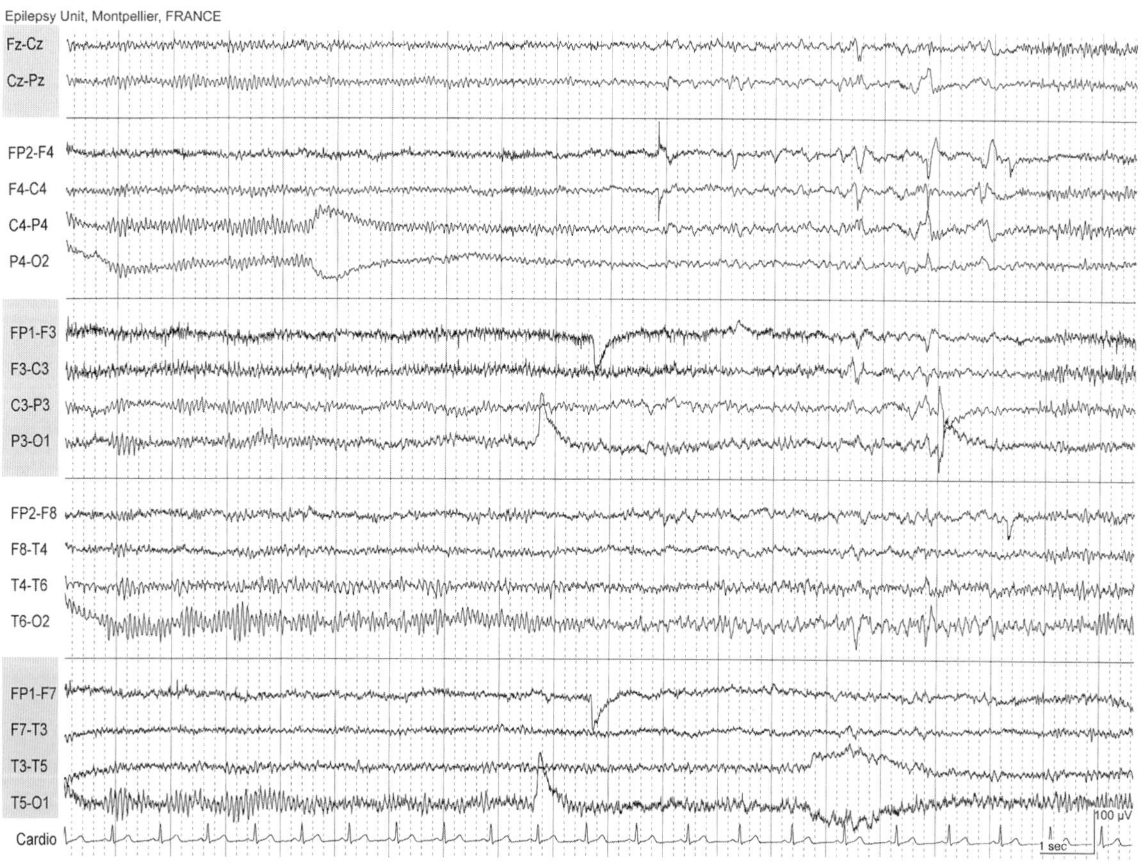

Figure a / Recording at 15 mm/s.

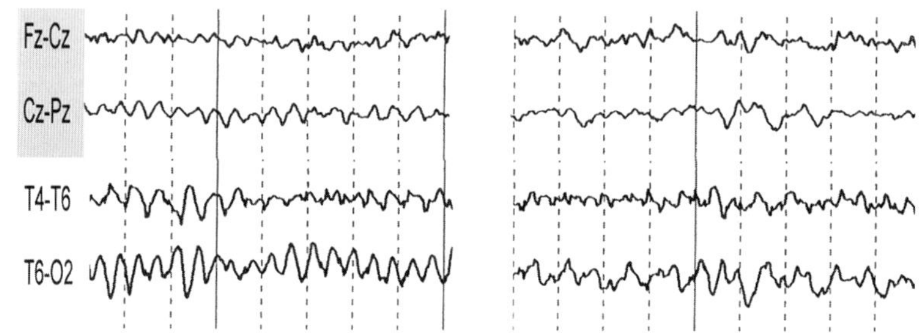

Figure b / The background activity goes from alpha to theta.

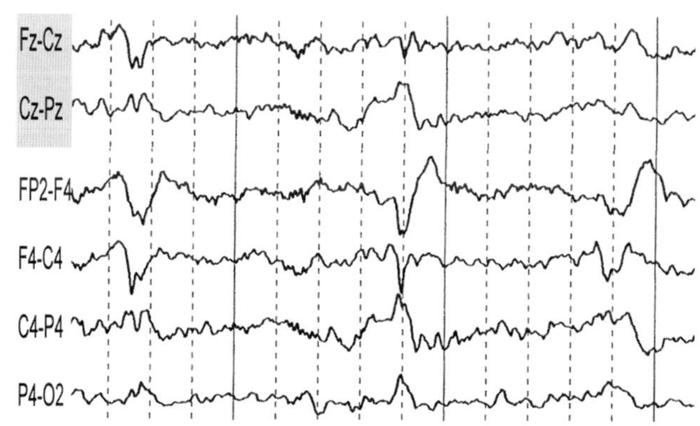

Figure c / V waves are more visible over the right central region.

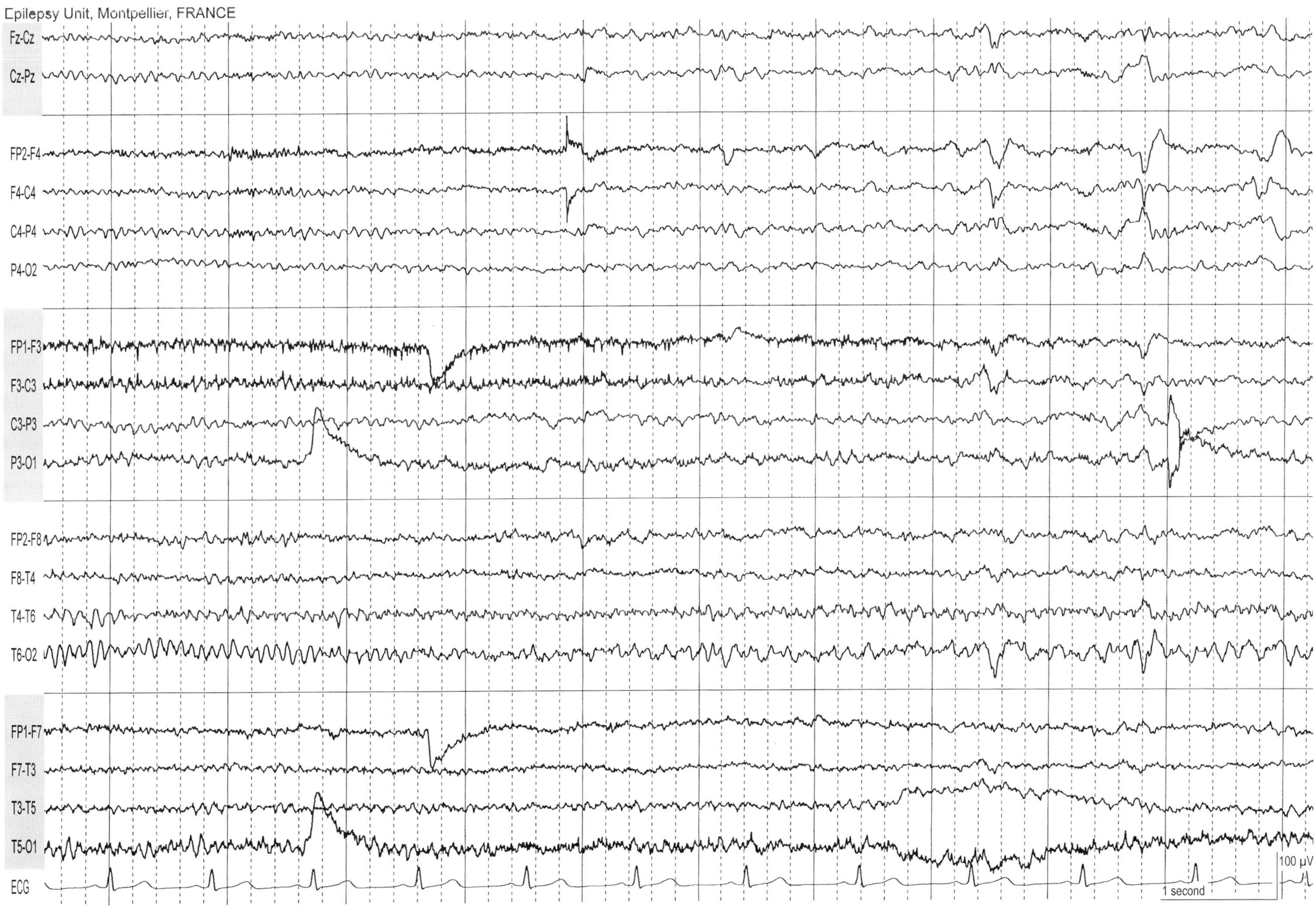
Epilepsy Unit, Montpellier, FRANCE
Fz-Cz
Cz-Pz
FP2-F4
F4-C4
C4-P4
P4-O2
FP1-F3
F3-C3
C3-P3
P3-O1
FP2-F8
F8-T4
T4-T6
T6-O2
FP1-F7
F7-T3
T3-T5
T5-O1
ECG
100 µV
1 second

III • 13 NREM 1: Vertex waves in an adult (2)

Context

23-year-old man with idiopathic generalized epilepsy.

What to note

Stage N1 sleep. V waves in phase reversal on Cz. Their morphology varies in sharpness and they spread to the left and right fronto-central regions.

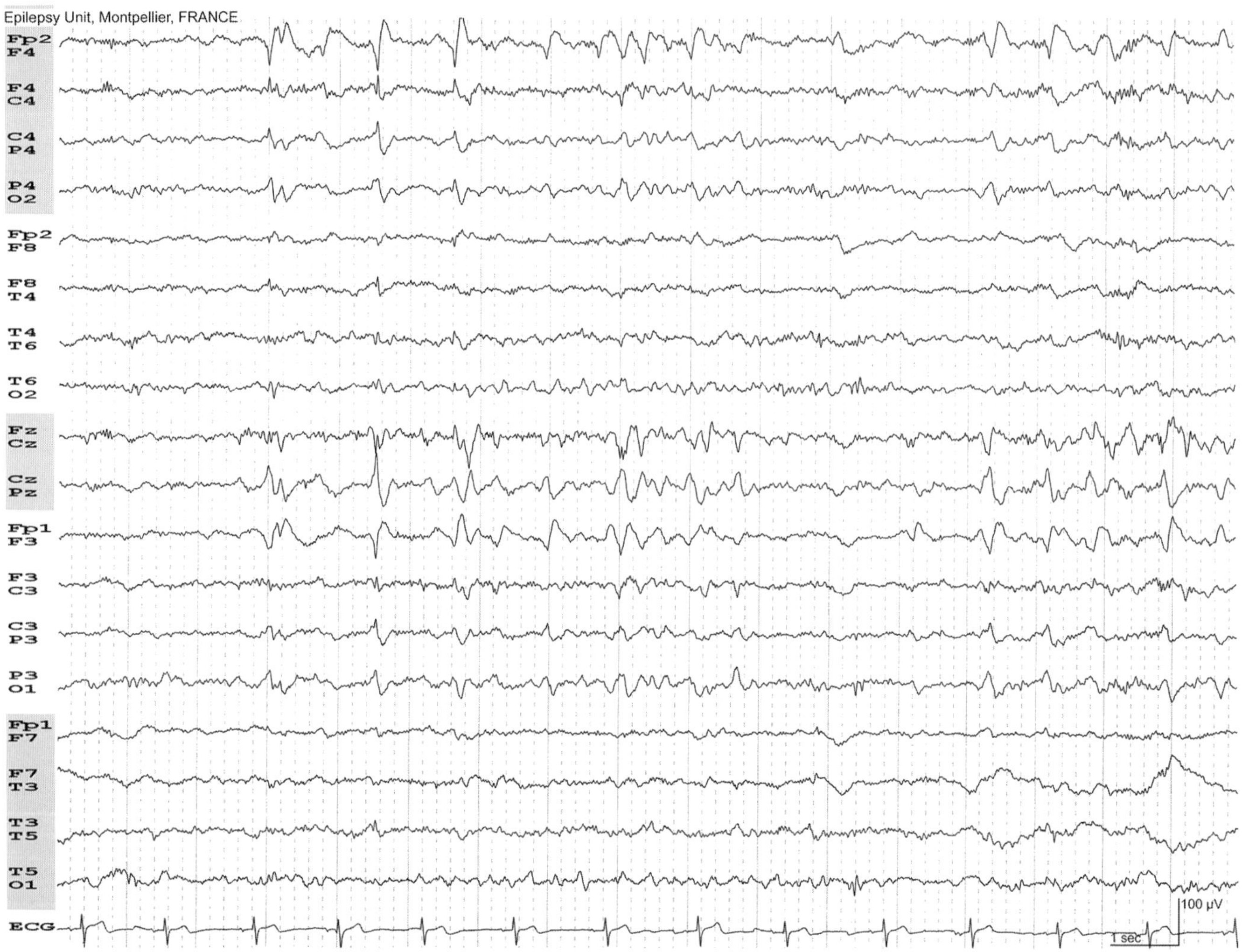

Figure a / Recording at 15 mm/s.

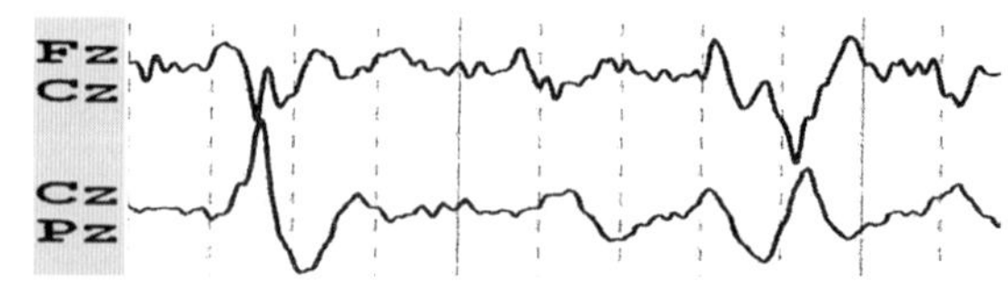

Figure b / V waves in phase reversal on Cz.

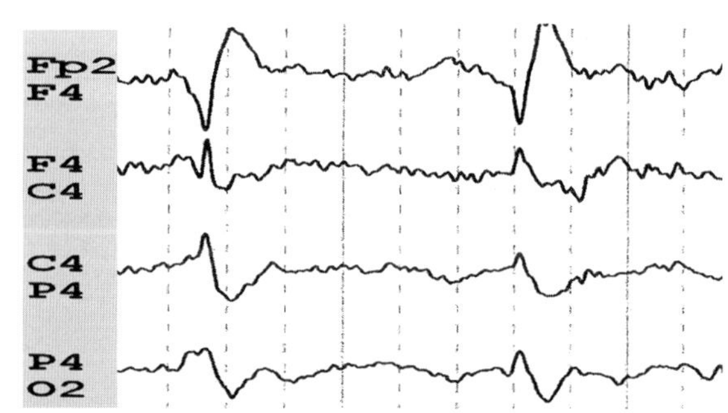

Figure c / V waves are also visible over the right fronto-central region.

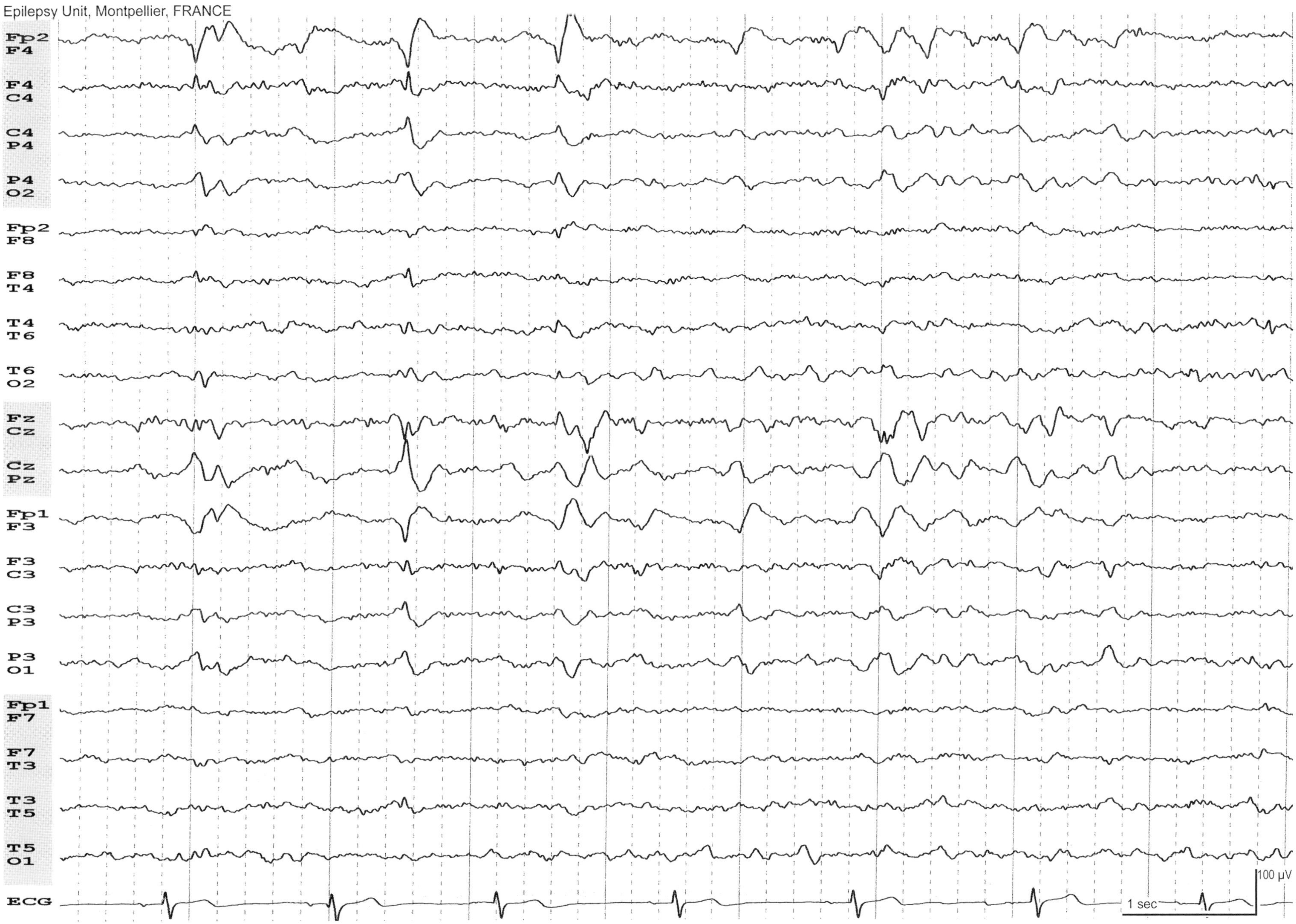
Epilepsy Unit, Montpellier, FRANCE
Fp2 F4
F4 C4
C4 P4
P4 O2
Fp2 F8
F8 T4
T4 T6
T6 O2
Fz Cz
Cz Pz
Fp1 F3
F3 C3
C3 P3
P3 O1
Fp1 F7
F7 T3
T3 T5
T5 O1
ECG
100 µV
1 sec

• 14 NREM 2: Physiological elements in an infant (1)

Context

6-month-old infant seen after a febrile seizure.

What to note

Stage N2 sleep. Amplitude is reduced to 15 μV/mm. Two asynchronous sleep spindles can be seen, first on the right then on the left. Duration of 2 to 3 seconds of sleep spindles is typical in infants.

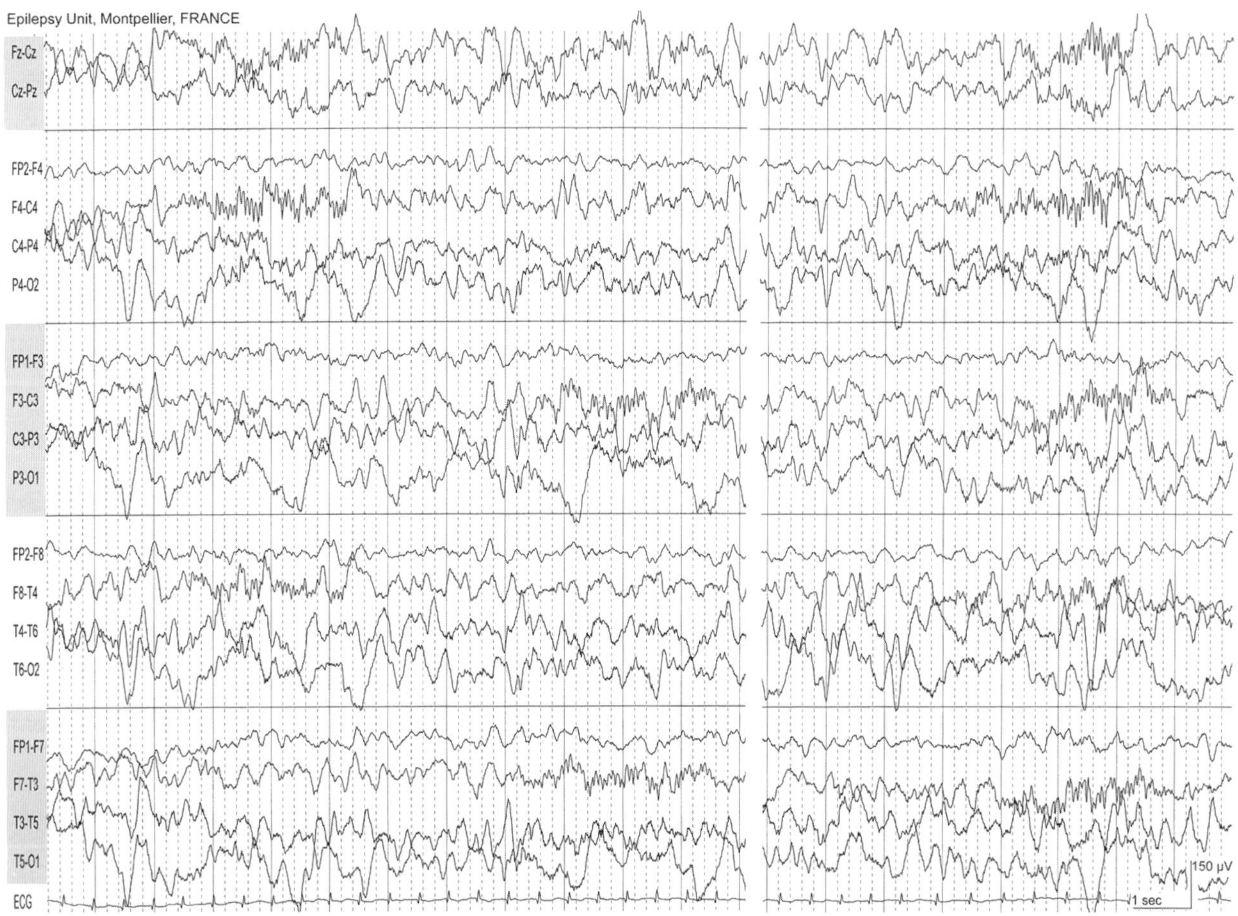

Figure a / Recording at 15 mm/s. On the right plate (same patient), synchronous spindles.

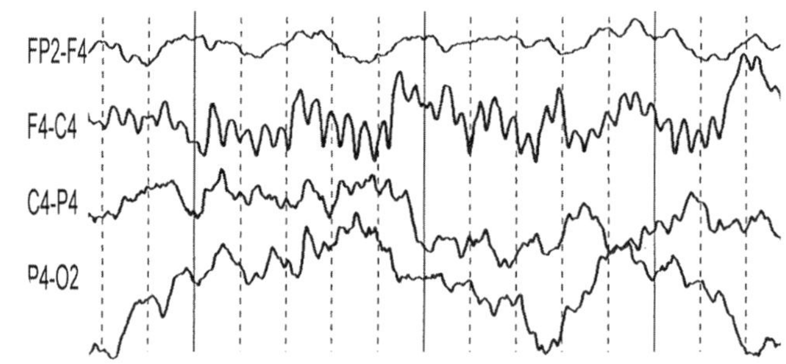

Figure b / Spindle on the right at F4-C4.

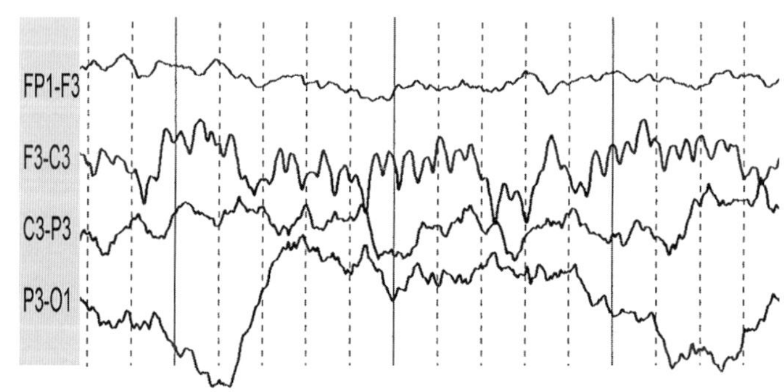

Figure c / Spindle on the left at F3-C3.

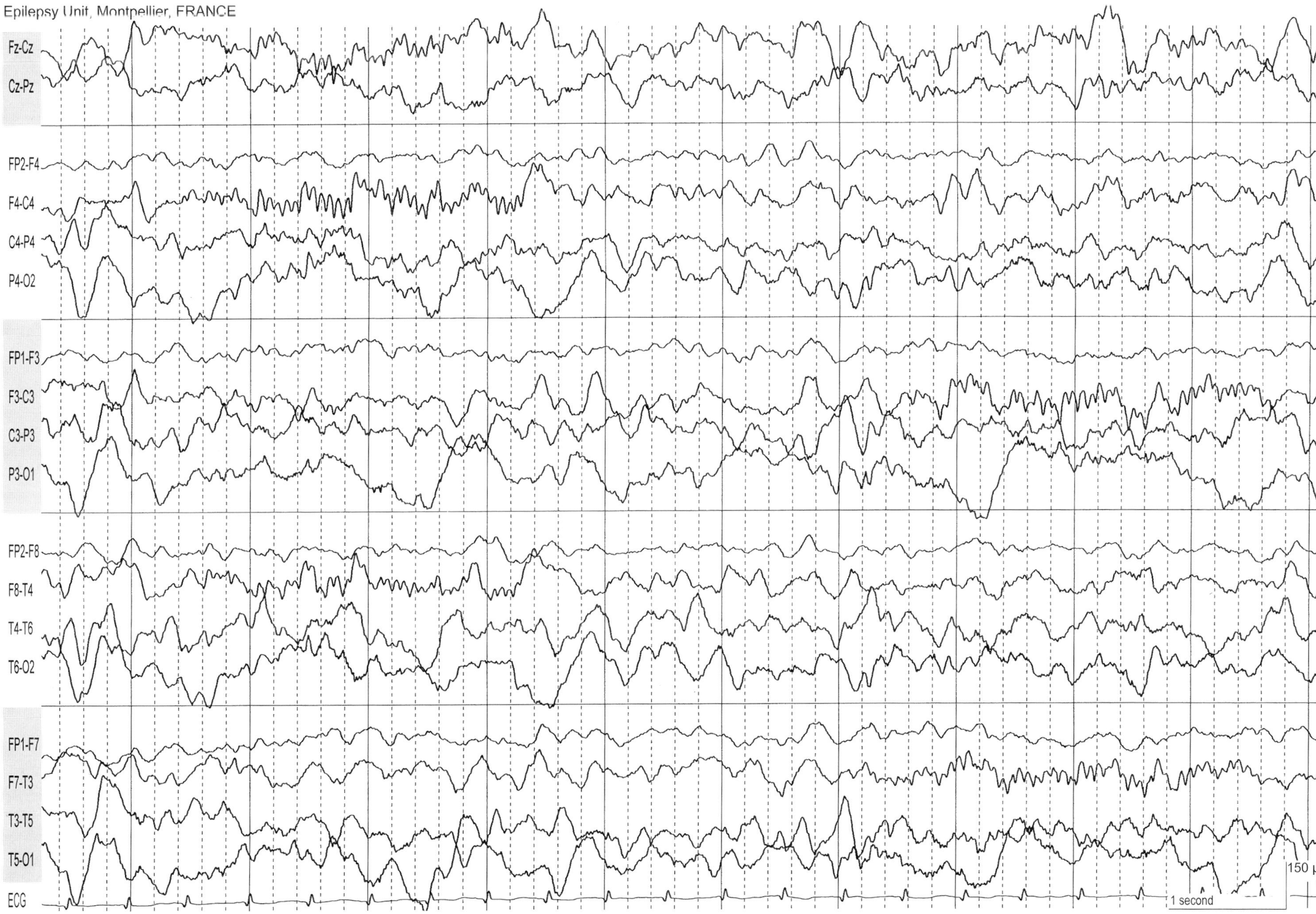
Epilepsy Unit, Montpellier, FRANCE
Fz-Cz
Cz-Pz
FP2-F4
F4-C4
C4-P4
P4-O2
FP1-F3
F3-C3
C3-P3
P3-O1
FP2-F8
F8-T4
T4-T6
T6-O2
FP1-F7
F7-T3
T3-T5
T5-O1
ECG
150 µV
1 second

• 15 NREM 2: Physiological elements in an infant (2)

Context

14-month-old infant with benign myoclonic epilepsy of infancy.

What to note

Stage N2 sleep. Three successive sleep spindles over the central regions. Duration of the spindles is shorter (1 second) than in the previous infant. Note a superimposition of spindle and theta waves conveying an impression of sharp waves.

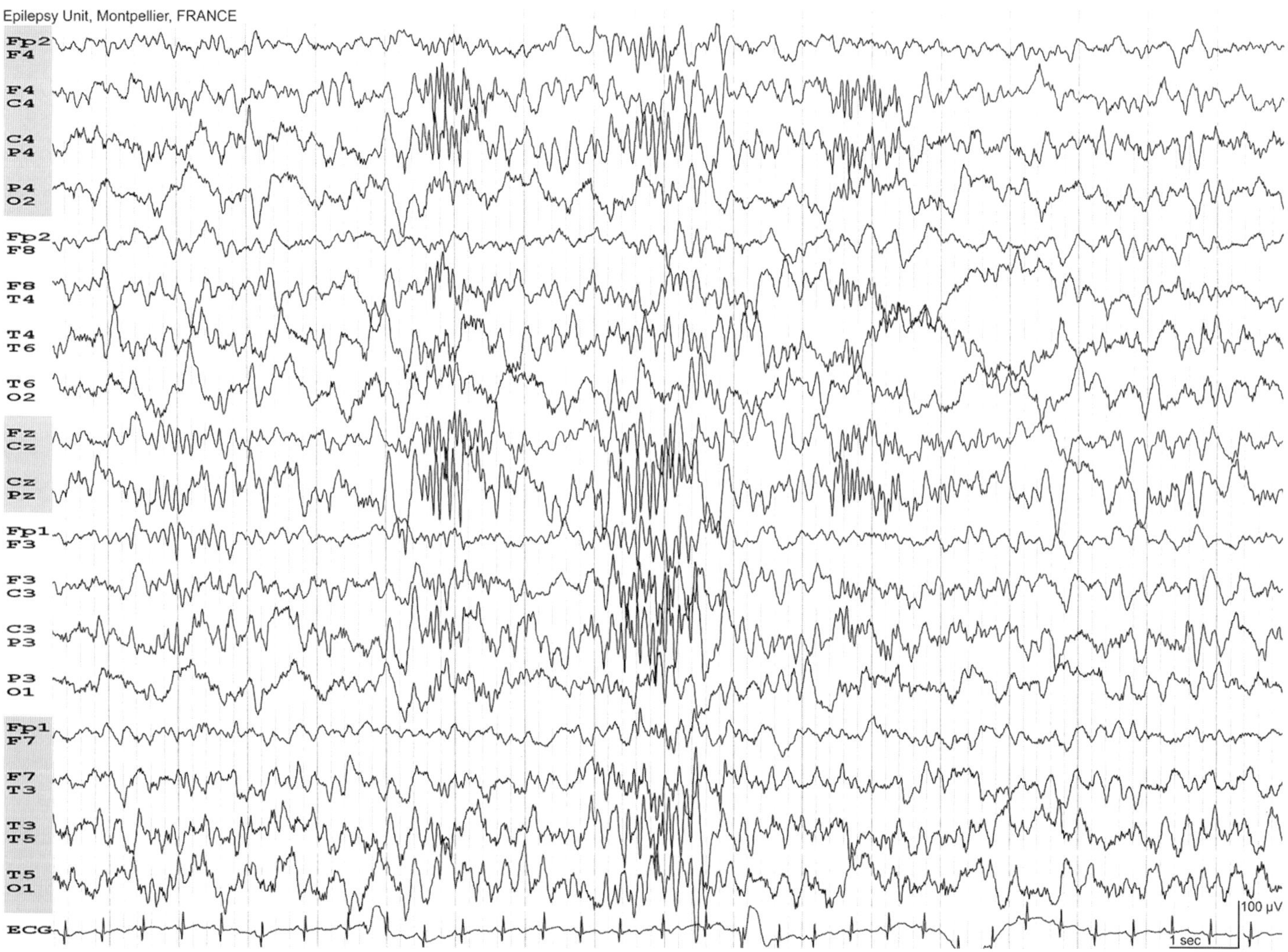

Figure a / Recording at 15 mm/s.

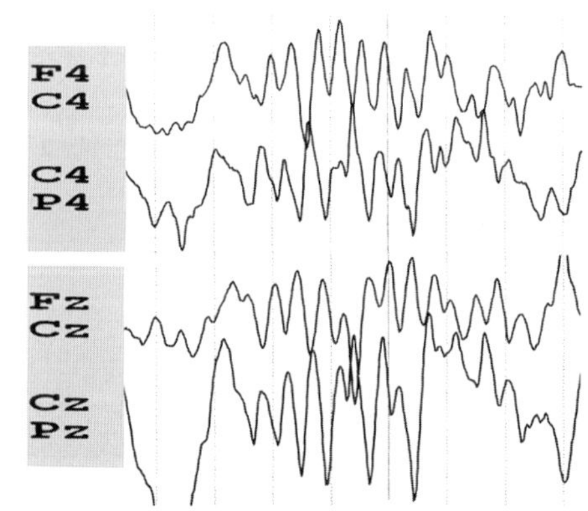

Figure b / Superimposition of spindle and theta waves conveying an impression of sharp waves.

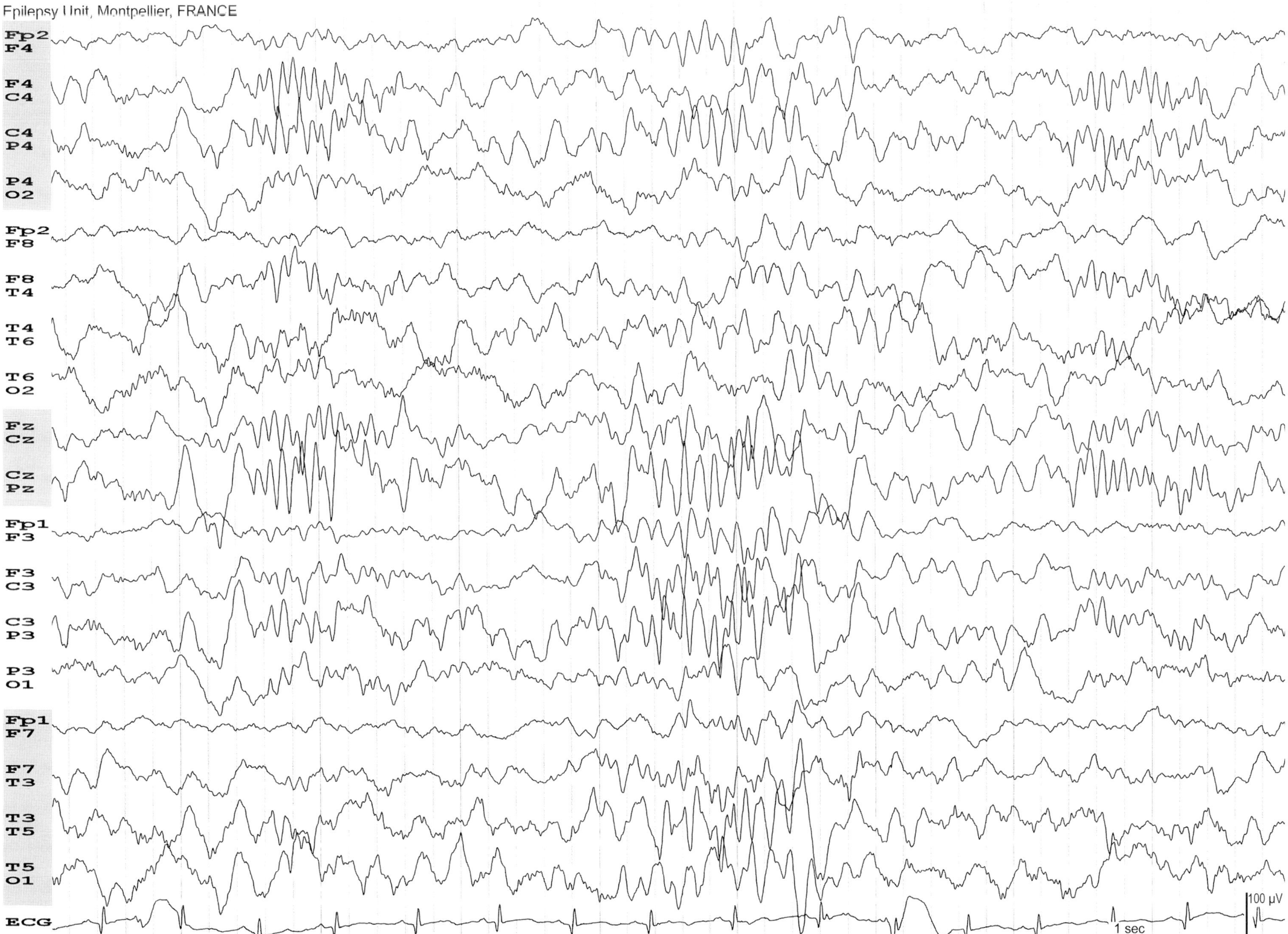
Epilepsy Unit, Montpellier, FRANCE
Fp2 F4
F4 C4
C4 P4
P4 O2
Fp2 F8
F8 T4
T4 T6
T6 O2
Fz Cz
Cz Pz
Fp1 F3
F3 C3
C3 P3
P3 O1
Fp1 F7
F7 T3
T3 T5
T5 O1
ECG
100 µV
1 sec

III • 16 NREM 2: Physiological elements in a young child

Context

3.5 year-old child seen after a febrile seizure. Same patient as plate III-29.

What to note

Amplitude reduced to 15 µV/mm. Stage N2 sleep. Firstly, a high-voltage sleep spindle can be seen over the right hemisphere. It spreads to the parietal regions. This diffusion to posterior regions is usual in children. A K complex can be observed blended with a spindle in a burst of ample, irregular and angular waveforms. This physiological element must not be confused with pathological element. In young children, the K complexes do not exhibit the strong diphasic deflection seen in older children or adolescents.

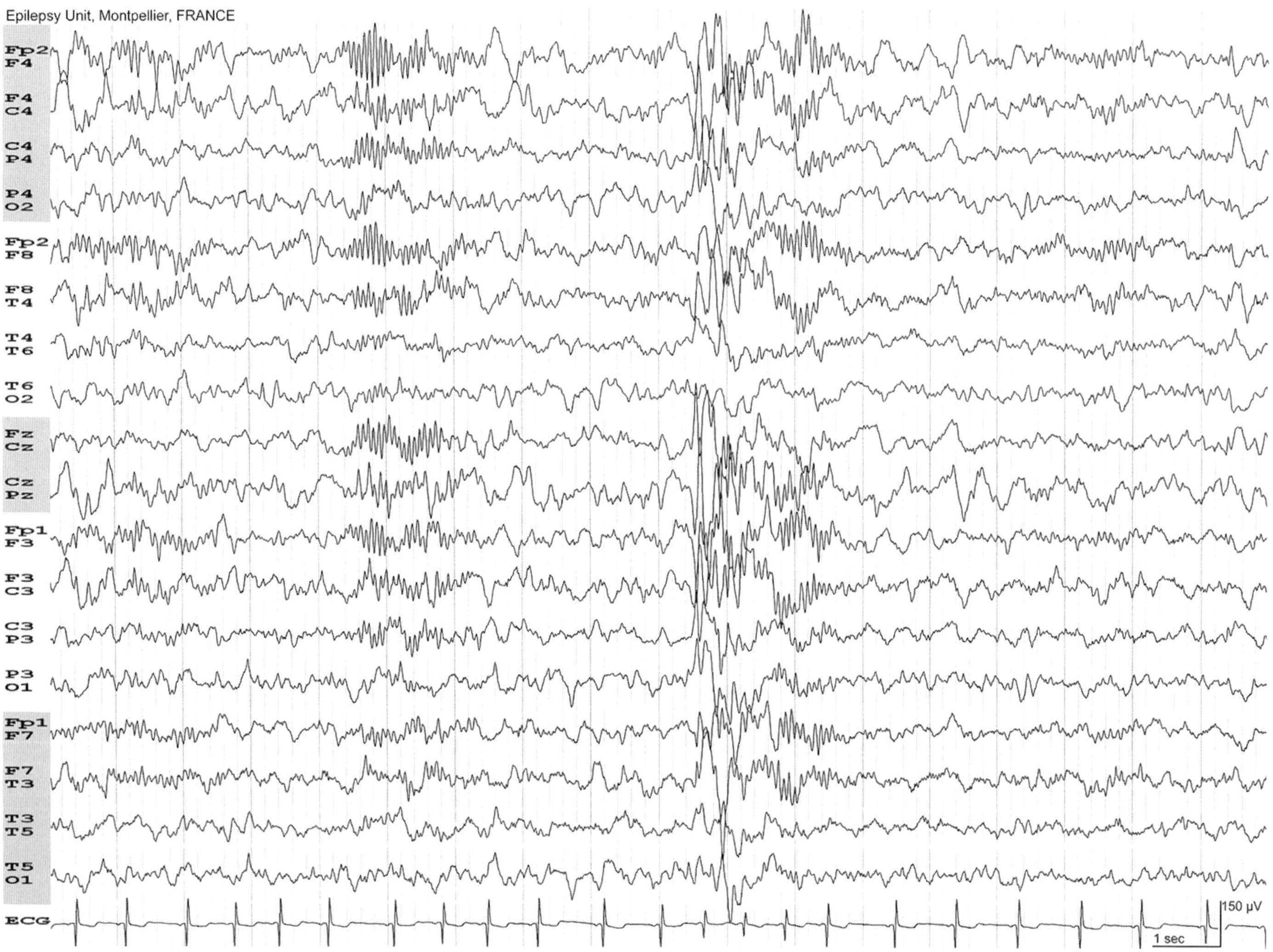

Figure a / Recording at 15 mm/s. At the beginning of the plate, a sleep spindle with sharply contoured waveforms.

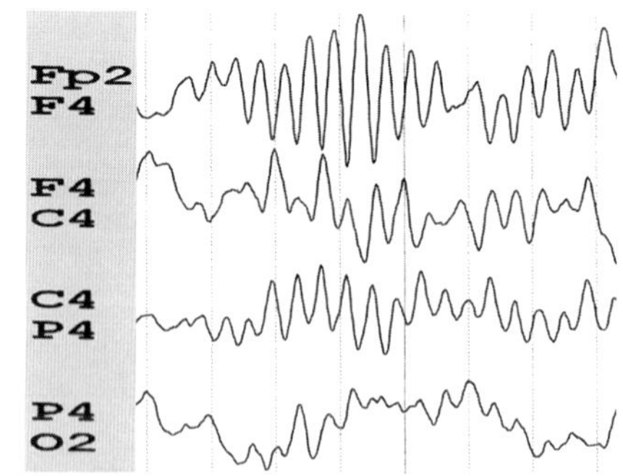

Figure b / High-voltage spindle that spreads to the parietal region.

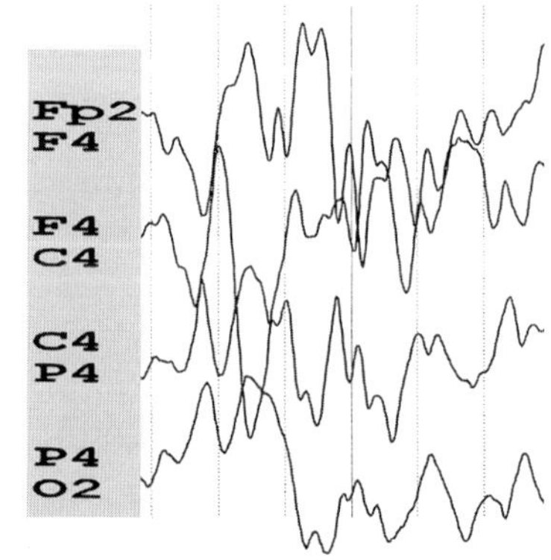

Figure c / Irregular K complex.

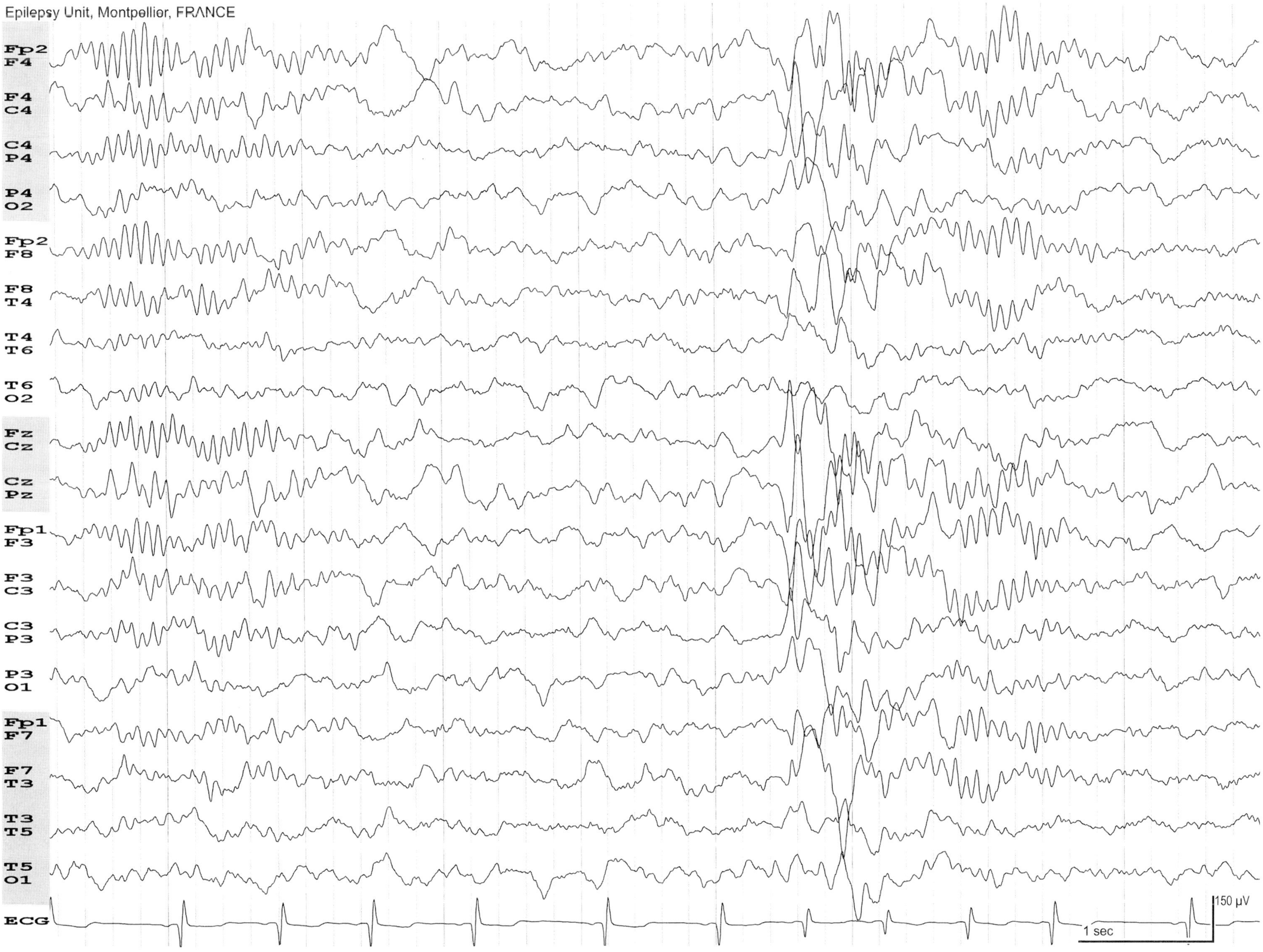
Epilepsy Unit, Montpellier, FRANCE
Fp2 F4
F4 C4
C4 P4
P4 O2
Fp2 F8
F8 T4
T4 T6
T6 O2
Fz Cz
Cz Pz
Fp1 F3
F3 C3
C3 P3
P3 O1
Fp1 F7
F7 T3
T3 T5
T5 O1
ECG
150 µV
1 sec

III • 17 NREM 2: Physiological elements in a child

Context

8-year-old boy seen after a first generalized tonic-clonic seizure.

What to note

Stage N2 sleep. K complexes are admixed with V waves, conveying the impression of a paroxysmal burst of ample, irregular and angular waveforms. Sleep spindles with anterior fusiform activity (fronto-central and inferior frontal) at 13 Hz can also be observed on this plate. The K complex and V wave admixture is rather frequent in children. These physiological elements must not be confused with pathological waves.

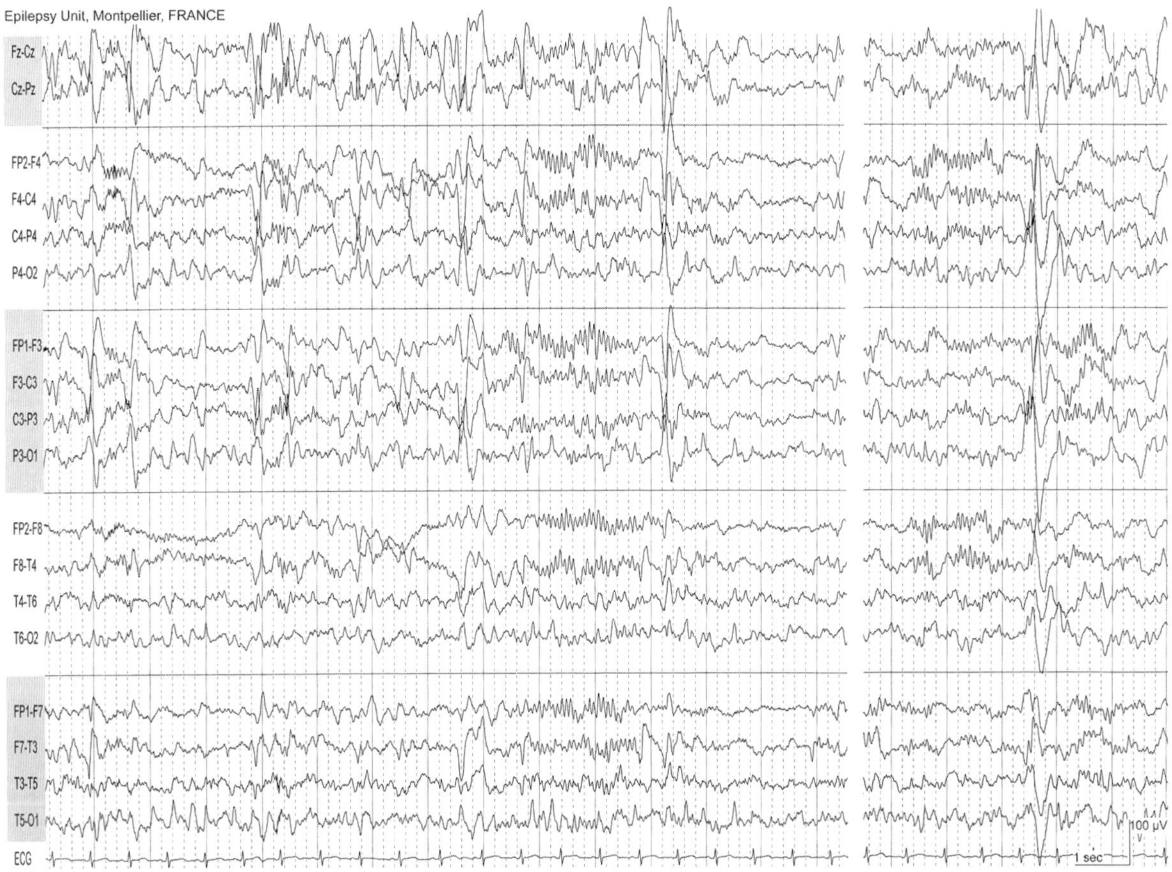

Figure a / Recording at 15 mm/s. Second segment, an asymmetrical spindle with a much higher amplitude on the right can be observed prior to a K complex with its characteristic strong diphasic deflection. On the left derivations, a spindle occurs after the K complex.

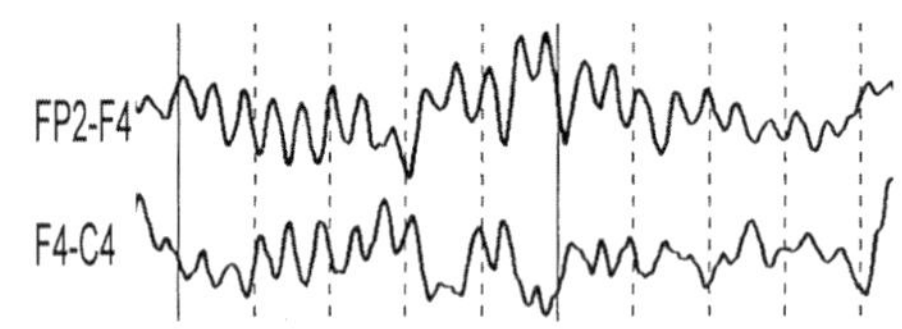

Figure b / Sleep spindle.

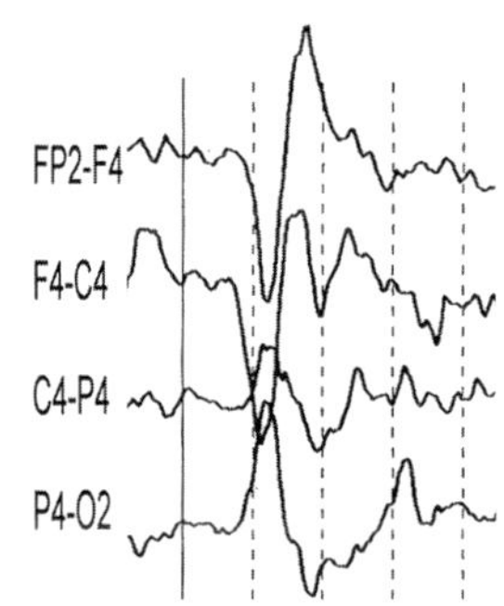

Figure c / K complex.

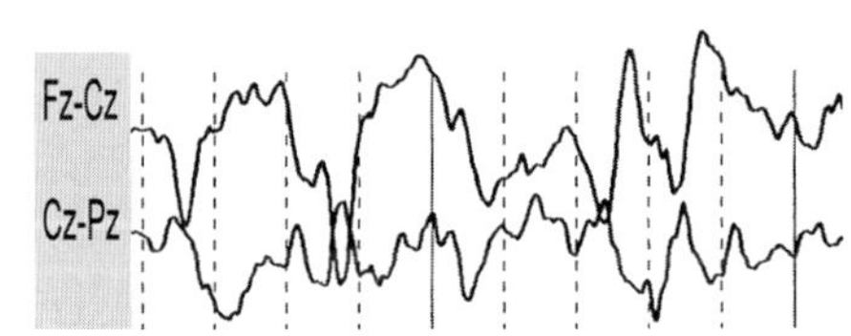

Figure d / V waves.

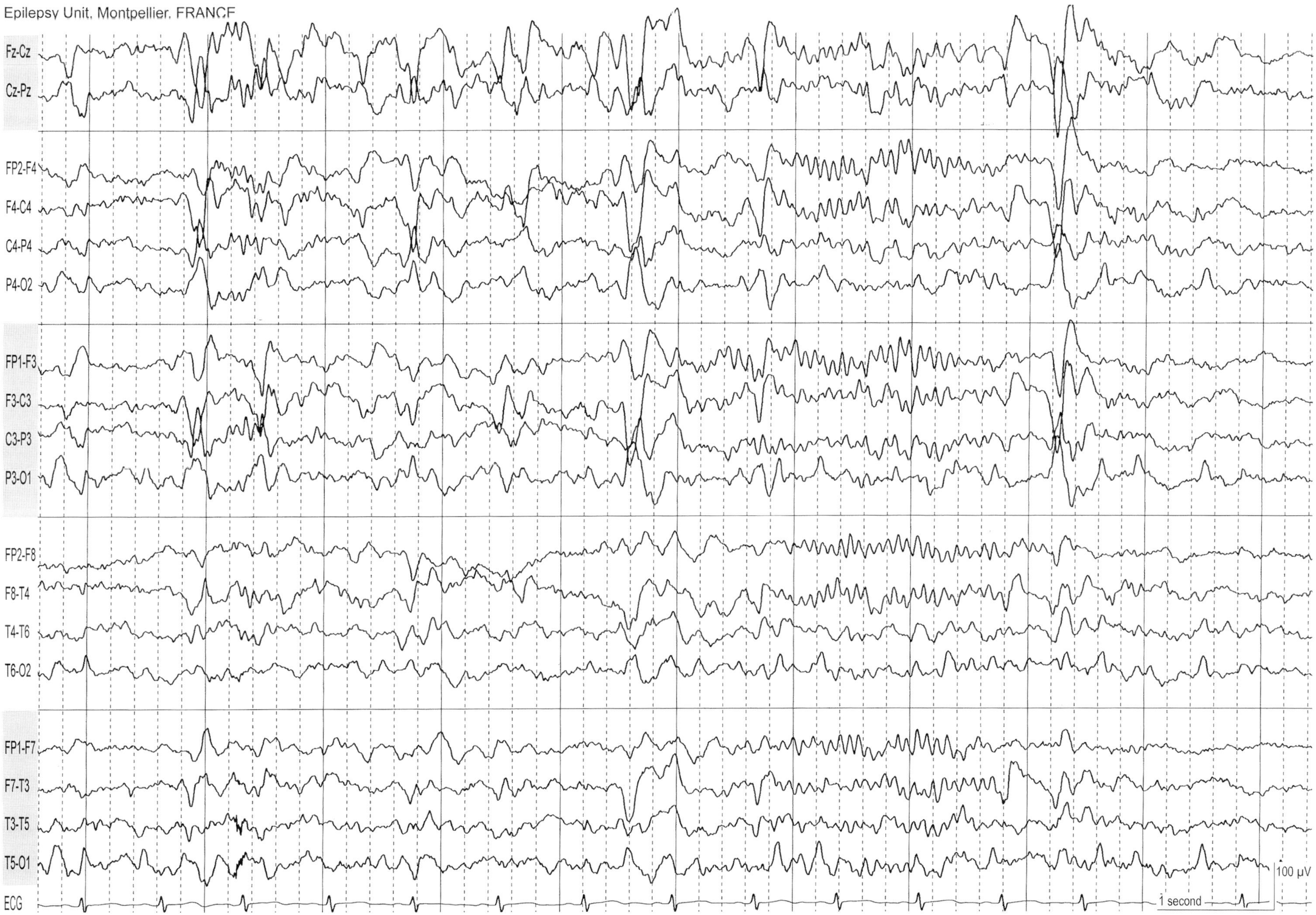
Epilepsy Unit, Montpellier, FRANCE
Fz-Cz
Cz-Pz
FP2-F4
F4-C4
C4-P4
P4-O2
FP1-F3
F3-C3
C3-P3
P3-O1
FP2-F8
F8-T4
T4-T6
T6-O2
FP1-F7
F7-T3
T3-T5
T5-O1
ECG
100 µV
1 second

III • 18 NREM 2: Physiological elements in an adolescent

Context

16-year-old man with a history of childhood absences epilepsy.

What to note

The patient is in stage N1-N2 sleep with occurrence of V waves. Some positive occipital sharp transients of sleep can be seen over the occipital regions. Note the presence of independent myoclonic jerks over the deltoid muscles. These jerks are physiological.

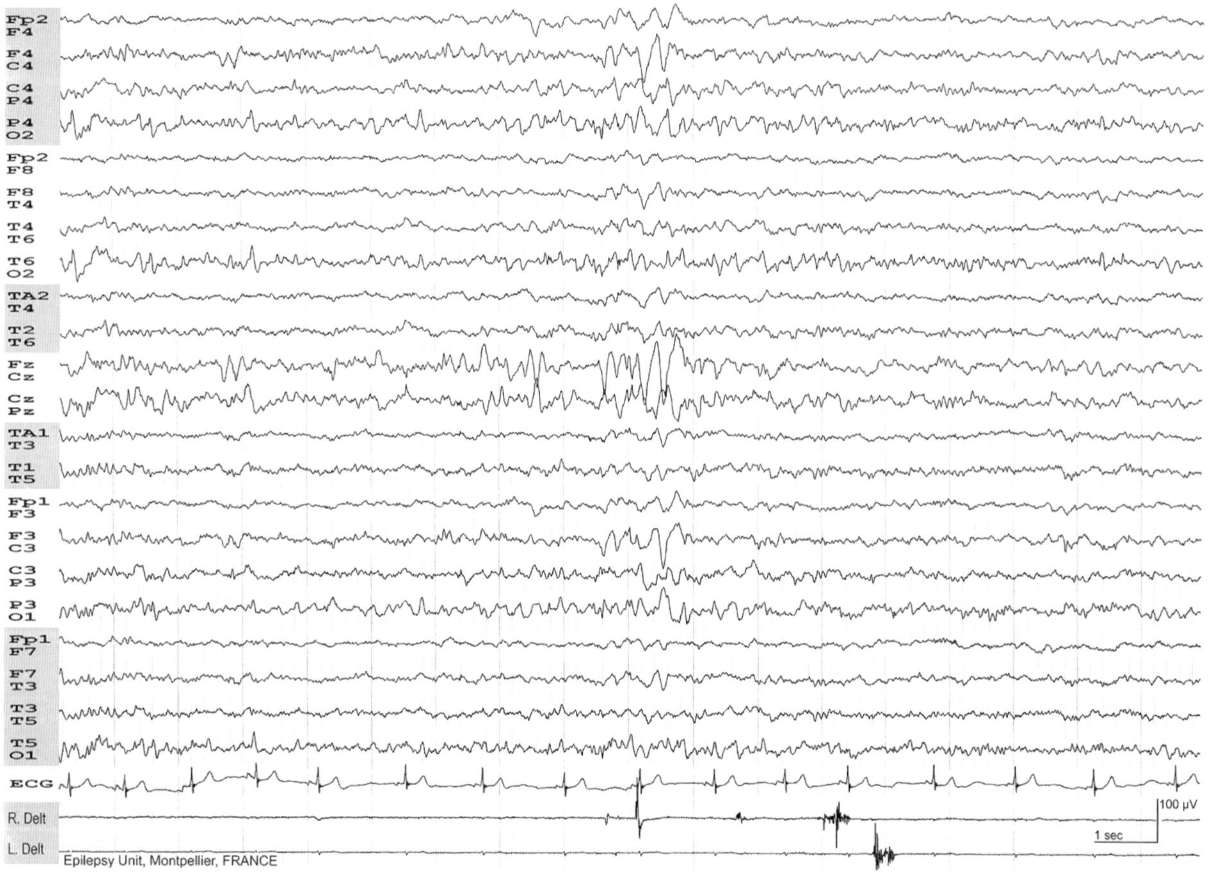

Figure a / Recording at 15 mm/s.

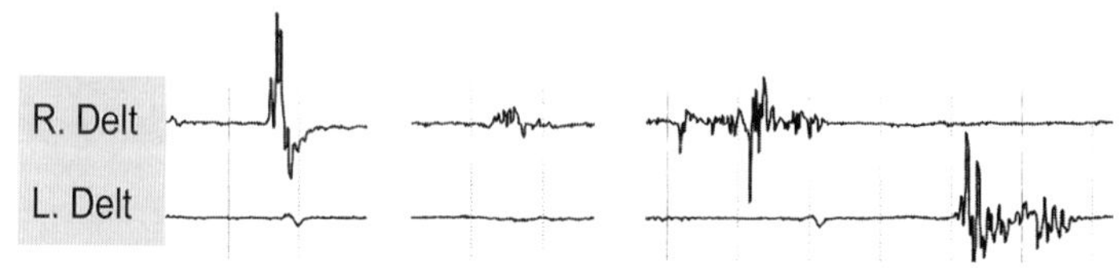

Figure b / Independent right and left myoclonic jerks recorded on the deltoid muscles.

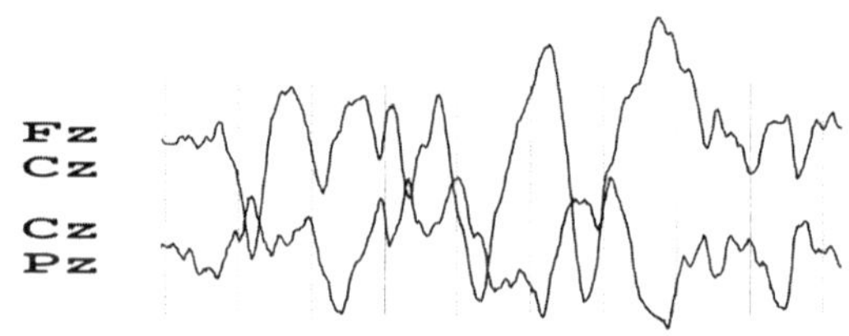

Figure c / V waves in phase reversal on Cz.

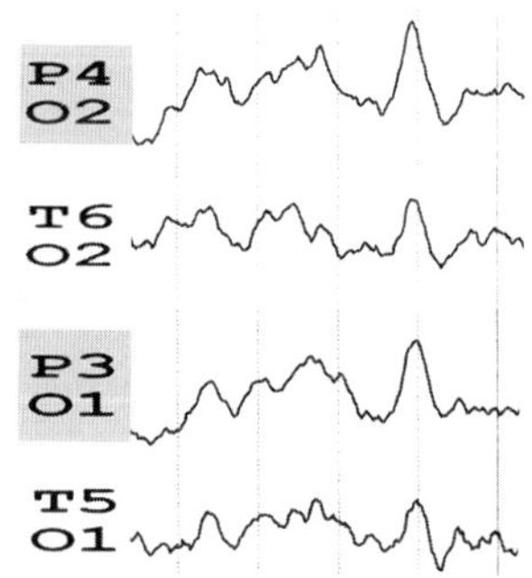

Figure d / A positive occipital sharp transient of sleep.

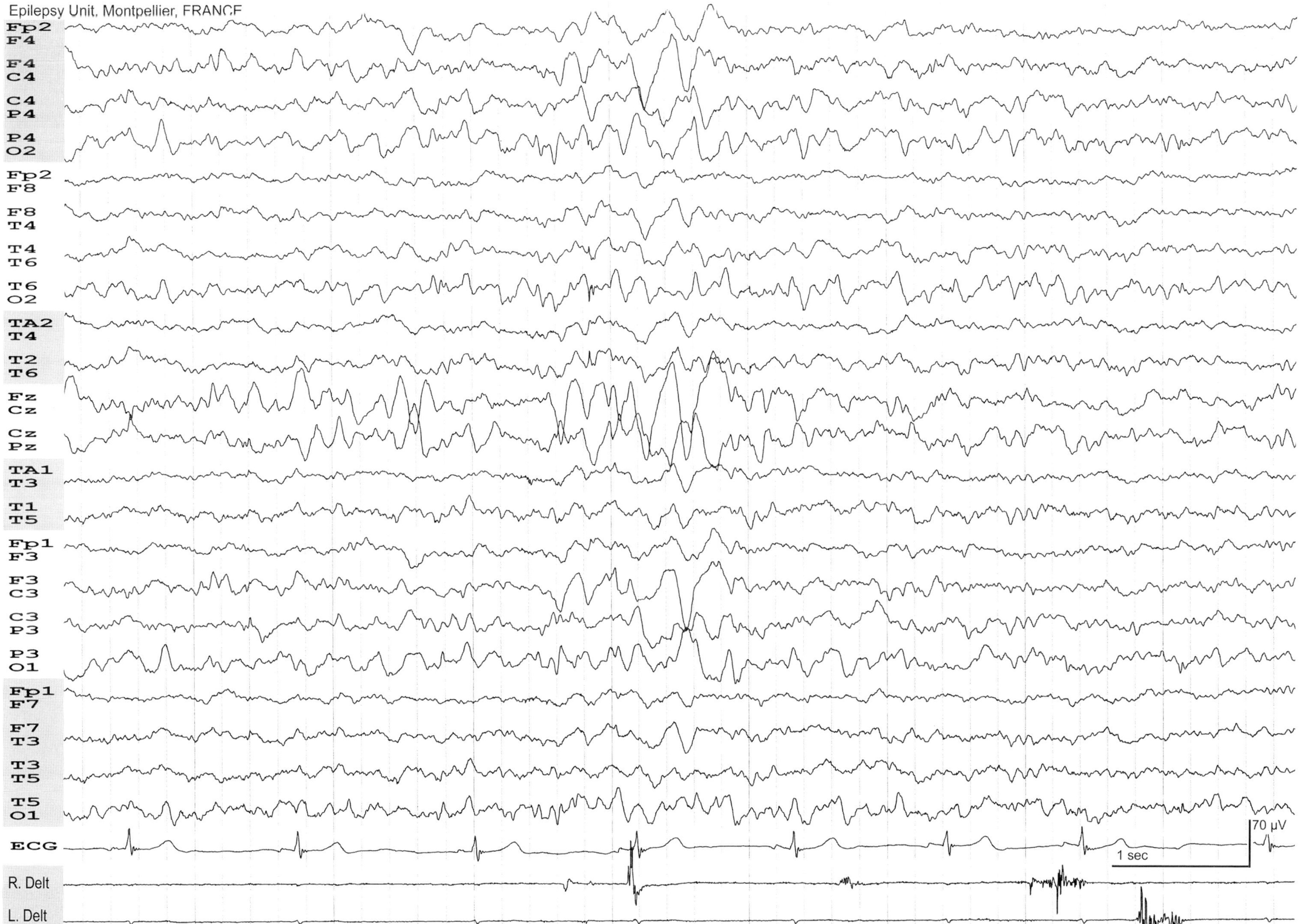
Epilepsy Unit, Montpellier, FRANCE
Fp2 F4
F4 C4
C4 P4
P4 O2
Fp2 F8
F8 T4
T4 T6
T6 O2
TA2 T4
T2 T6
Fz Cz
Cz Pz
TA1 T3
T1 T5
Fp1 F3
F3 C3
C3 P3
P3 O1
Fp1 F7
F7 T3
T3 T5
T5 O1
ECG
R. Delt
L. Delt
70 µV
1 sec

III • 19 NREM 2: Physiological elements in an adult (1)

Context

20-year-old man referred for a health certificate (airplane pilot).

What to note

Stage N2 sleep at sleep onset. V waves on the vertex. At the end of the plate, a K complex preceded and immediately followed by a sleep spindle can be observed. Note two physiological hypnic jerks on the deltoid muscles.

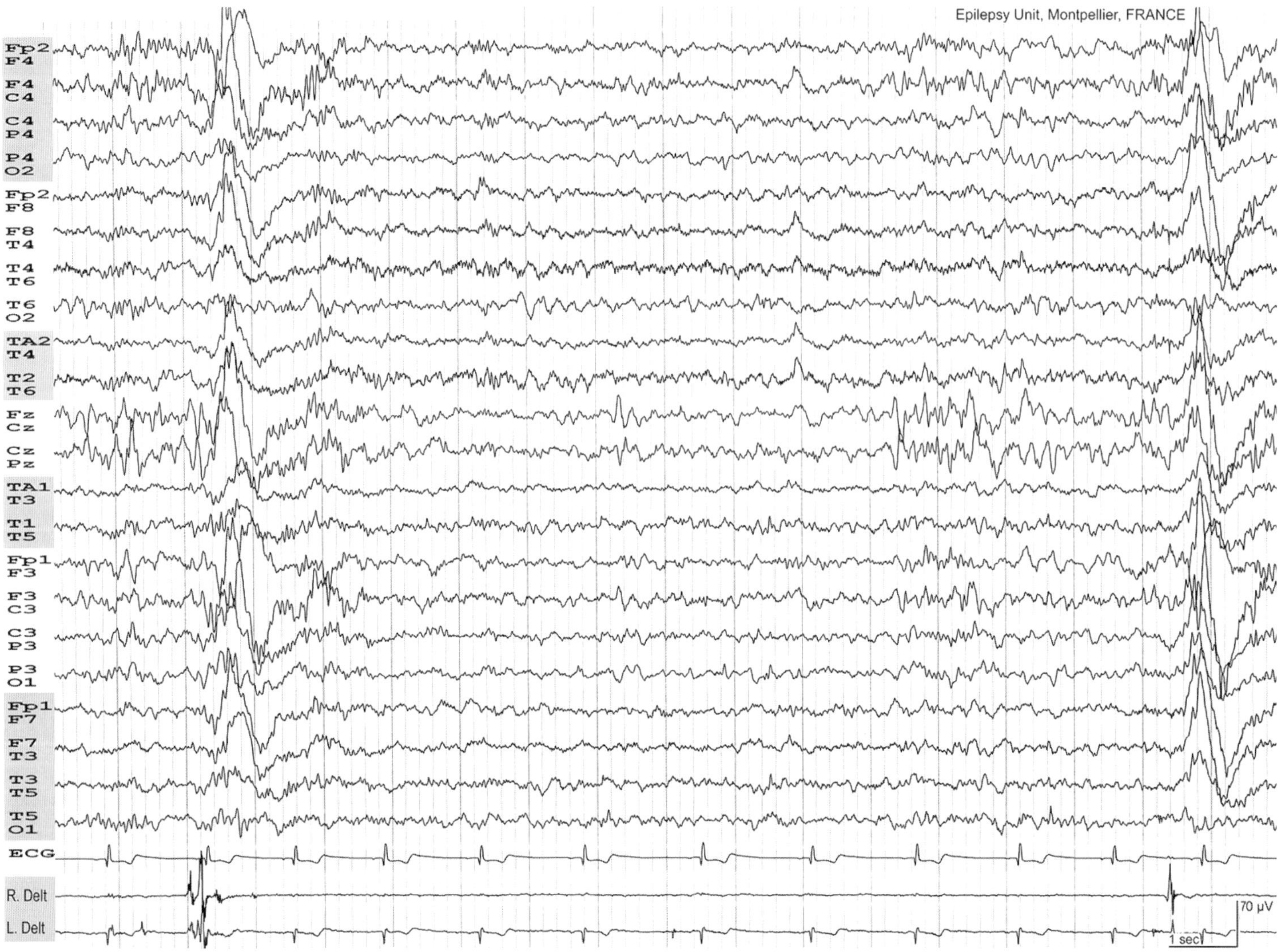

Figure a / Recording at 15 mm/s. At the end of the plate, a K complex and a physiological myoclonic jerk can be observed.

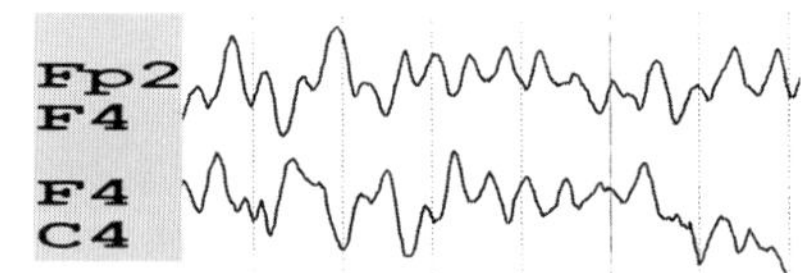

Figure b / Sleep spindle.

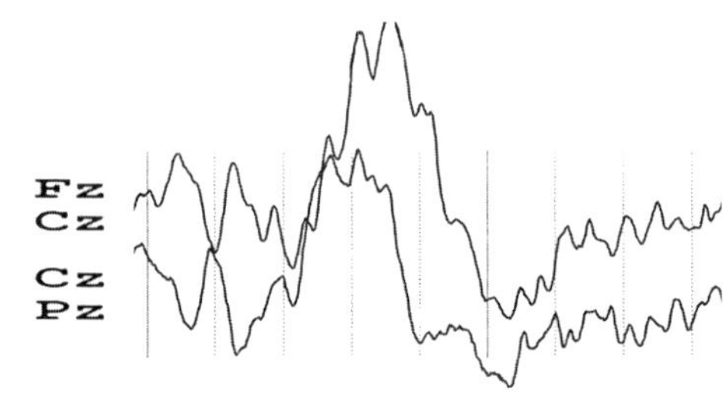

Figure c / K complex followed by a spindle.

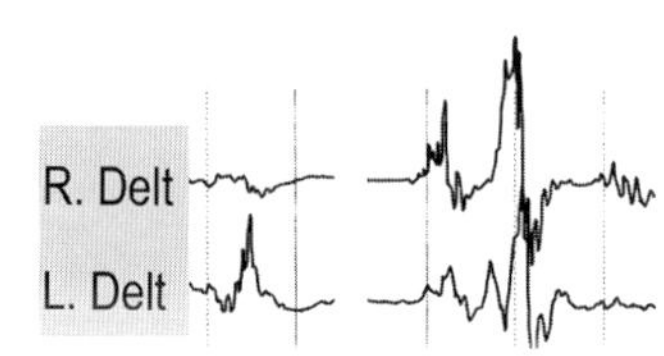

Figure d / Hypnic jerks.

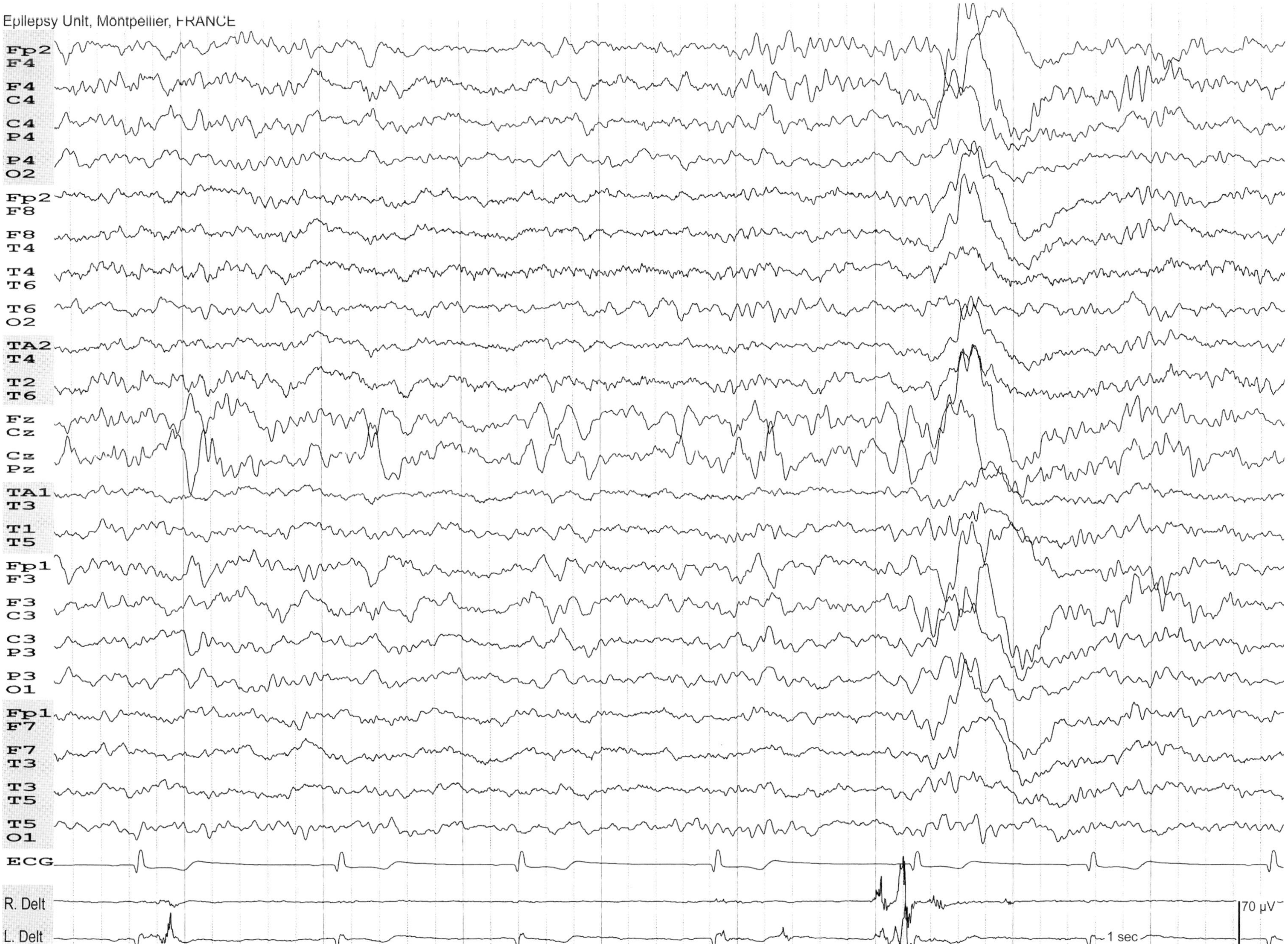
Epilepsy Unit, Montpellier, FRANCE
Fp2 F4
F4 C4
C4 P4
P4 O2
Fp2 F8
F8 T4
T4 T6
T6 O2
TA2 T4
T2 T6
Fz Cz
Cz Pz
TA1 T3
T1 T5
Fp1 F3
F3 C3
C3 P3
P3 O1
Fp1 F7
F7 T3
T3 T5
T5 O1
ECG
R. Delt
L. Delt
70 µV
1 sec

III • 20 NREM 2: Physiological elements in an adult (2)

Context

20-year-old woman with cryptogenic left occipital lobe epilepsy and migraine.

What to note

Stage N2 sleep during the third cycle of nocturnal sleep. At the beginning of the plate, a sleep spindle can be observed with higher amplitude on the right hemisphere. Then a first K complex (strong diphasic deflection) occurs followed two second later by a second K complex, immediately followed by a sleep spindle. In comparison with children, the amplitude of sleep spindles is lower in adolescents and young adults and of shorter duration (one second).

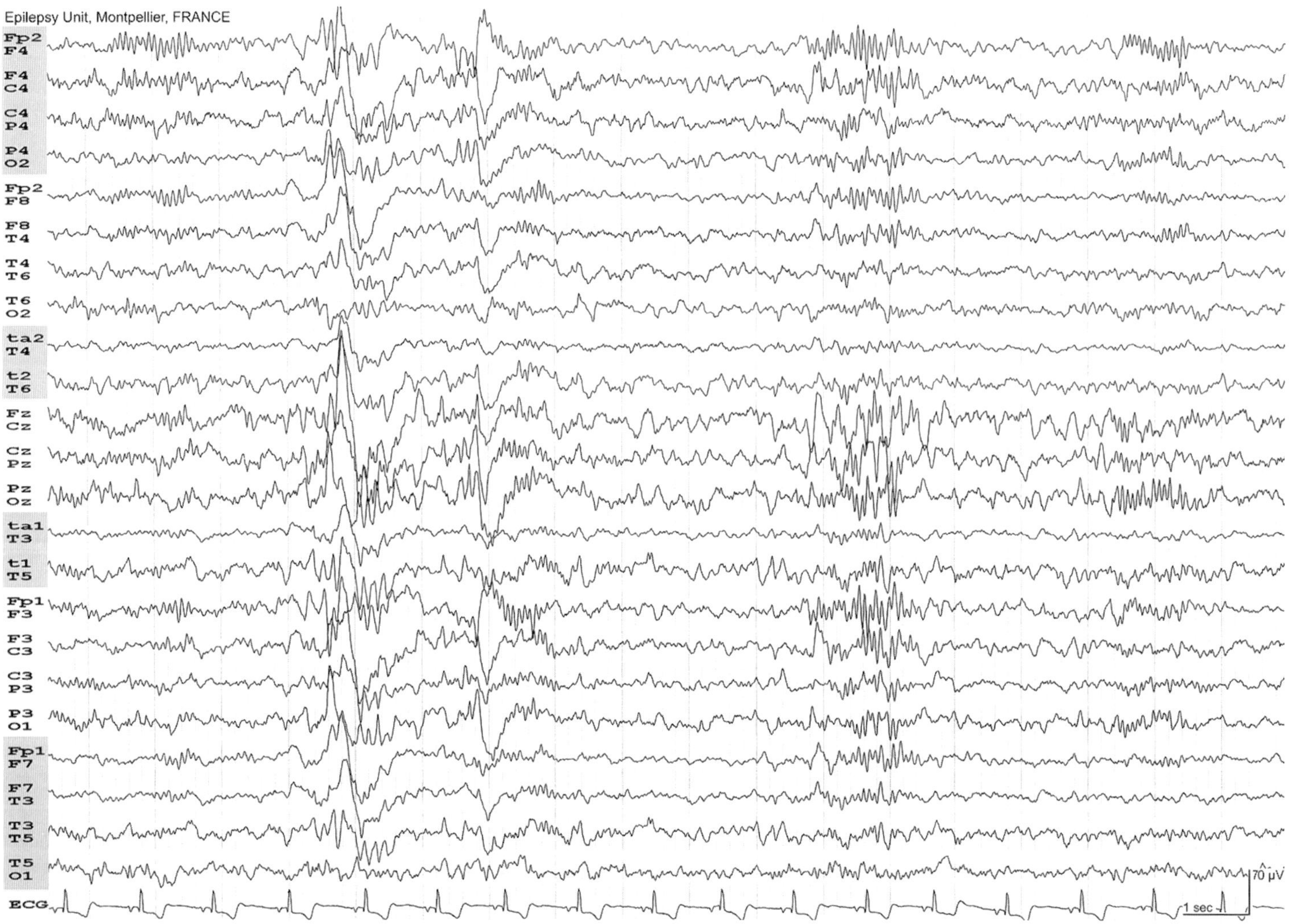

Figure a / Recording at 15 mm/s. Two sleep spindles occur after the second K complex. The spindle in the middle of the plate is intermixed with V waves conveying an impression of sharp waves.

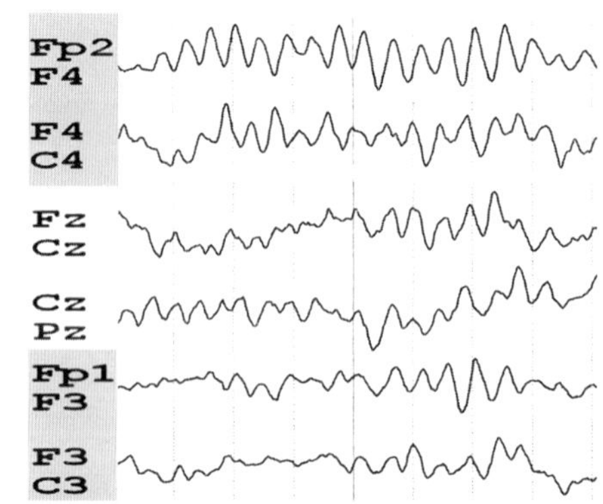

Figure b / Sleep spindle.

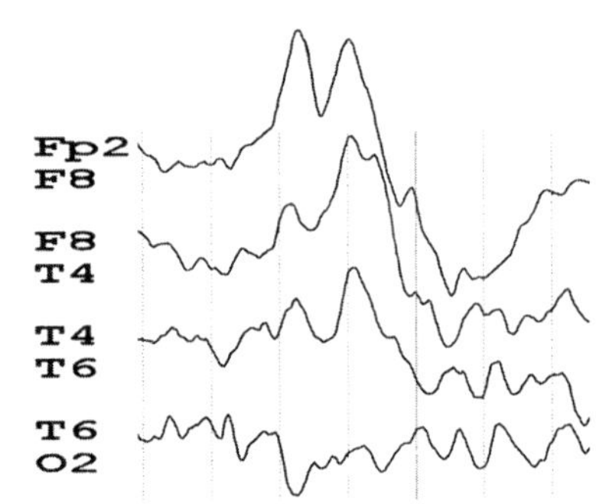

Figure c / First K complex.

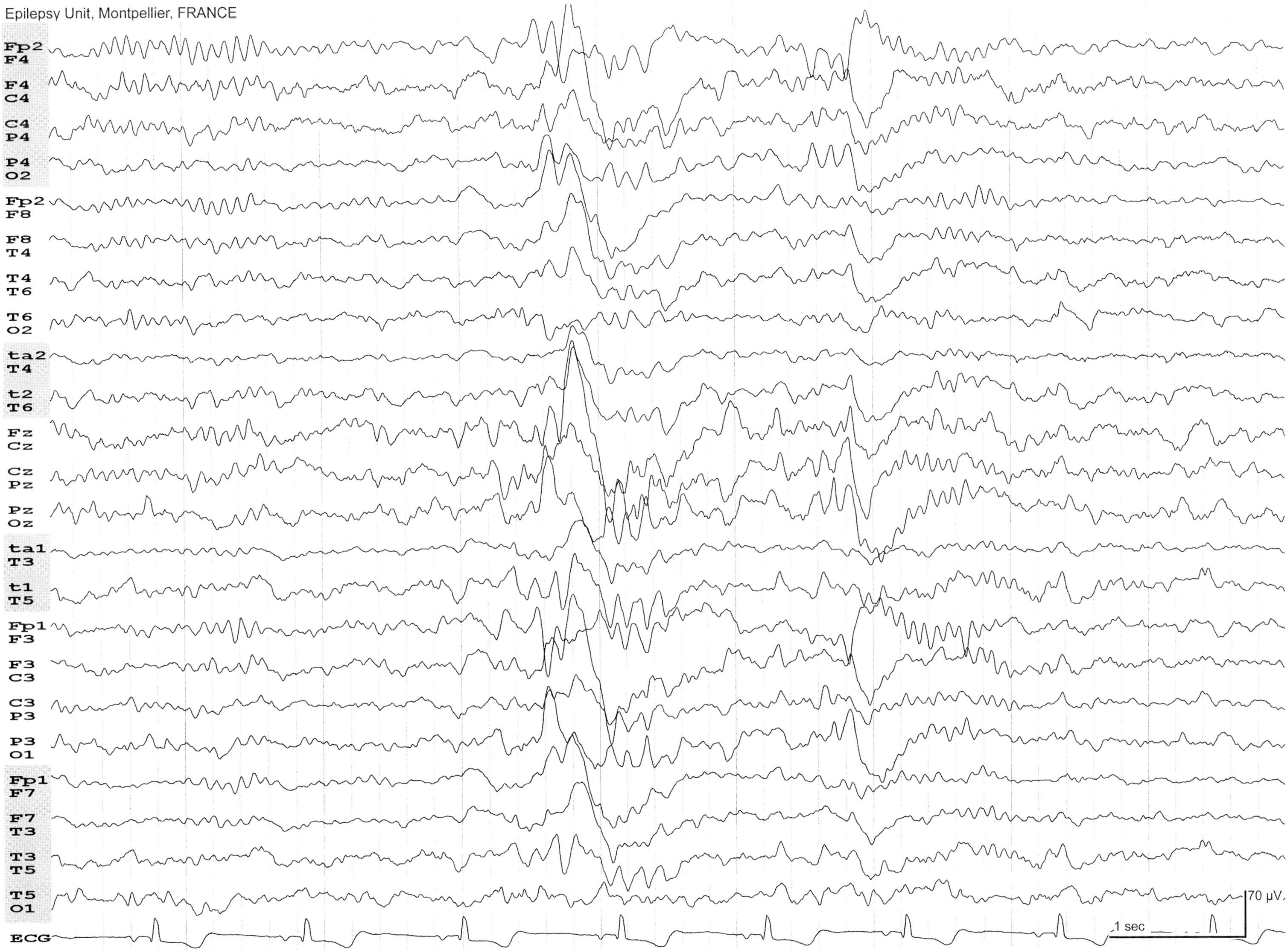

Epilepsy Unit, Montpellier, FRANCE
Fp2 F4
F4 C4
C4 P4
P4 O2
Fp2 F8
F8 T4
T4 T6
T6 O2
ta2 T4
t2 T6
Fz Cz
Cz Pz
Pz Oz
ta1 T3
t1 T5
Fp1 F3
F3 C3
C3 P3
P3 O1
Fp1 F7
F7 T3
T3 T5
T5 O1
ECG
70 µV
1 sec

• 21 NREM 2: Physiological elements in an adult (3)

Context

19-year-old man seen after episodes of loss of consciousness.

What to note

Two characteristic K complexes (strong diphasic deflection) immediately followed by spindles can be observed. These spindles are synchronous over the two hemispheres on this plate.

Comment

At this age, usually the sleep spindles occur bilaterally and simultaneously but sometimes independently with a shifting emphasis from side to side (see plate recorded at 15 mm/s). But a constant asymmetry of the spindles is abnormal. An EEG asymmetry depending to the epileptic focus side can be found in focal epilepsies (Crespel *et al.*, 1998; 2000). The spindles are better organized on the non-epileptic EEG side.

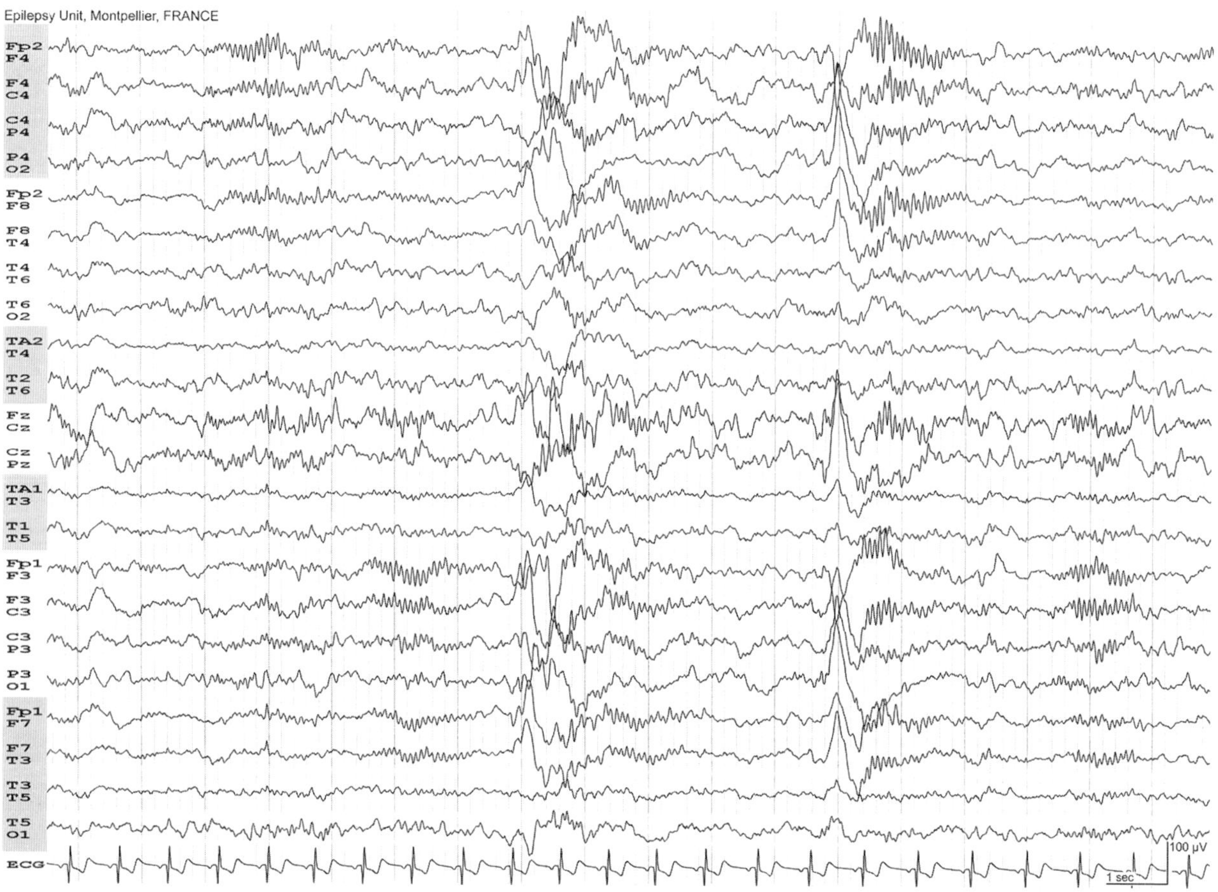

Figure a / Recording at 15 mm/s. Two asynchronous sleep spindles, first on the right then on the left hemisphere prior to the first K complex. At the end of the plate, spindle on the left fronto-central region.

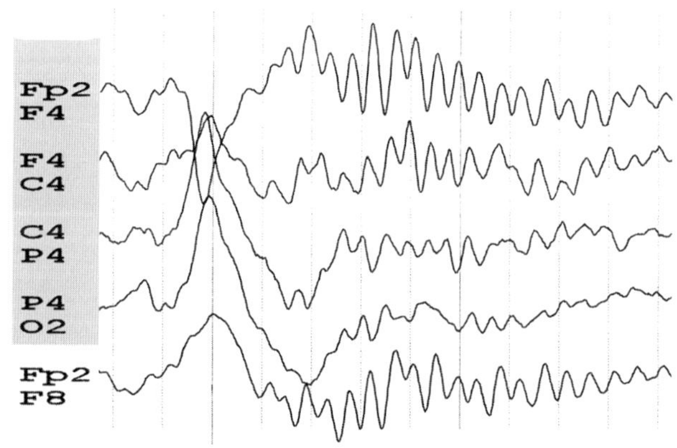

Figure b / K complex followed by a spindle.

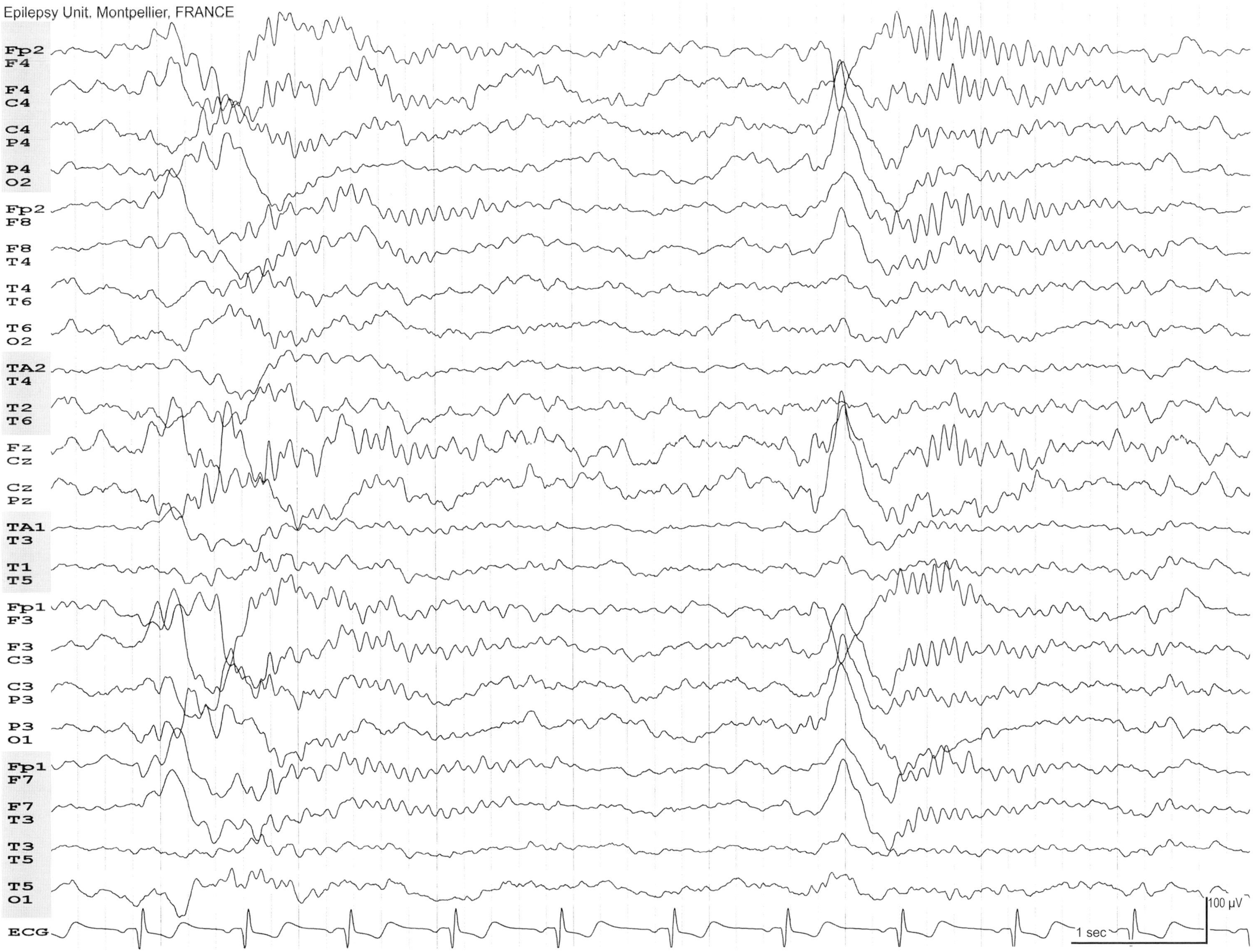
Epilepsy Unit, Montpellier, FRANCE
Fp2 F4
F4 C4
C4 P4
P4 O2
Fp2 F8
F8 T4
T4 T6
T6 O2
TA2 T4
T2 T6
Fz Cz
Cz Pz
TA1 T3
T1 T5
Fp1 F3
F3 C3
C3 P3
P3 O1
Fp1 F7
F7 T3
T3 T5
T5 O1
ECG
100 µV
1 sec

III • 22 NREM 3: Deep sleep in an infant

Context

14-month-old infant with benign myoclonic epilepsy of infancy. Same patient as plates III-15, III-28.

What to note

NREM sleep stage 3. Low sensitivity at 15 µV/mm. High amplitude slow wave activity. Occipital predominance of slow wave activity in deep sleep is usual in children under age 4 years. Note the difference with REM sleep (see plate III-28). REM sleep is monomorphous with a sinusoidal aspect at this age.

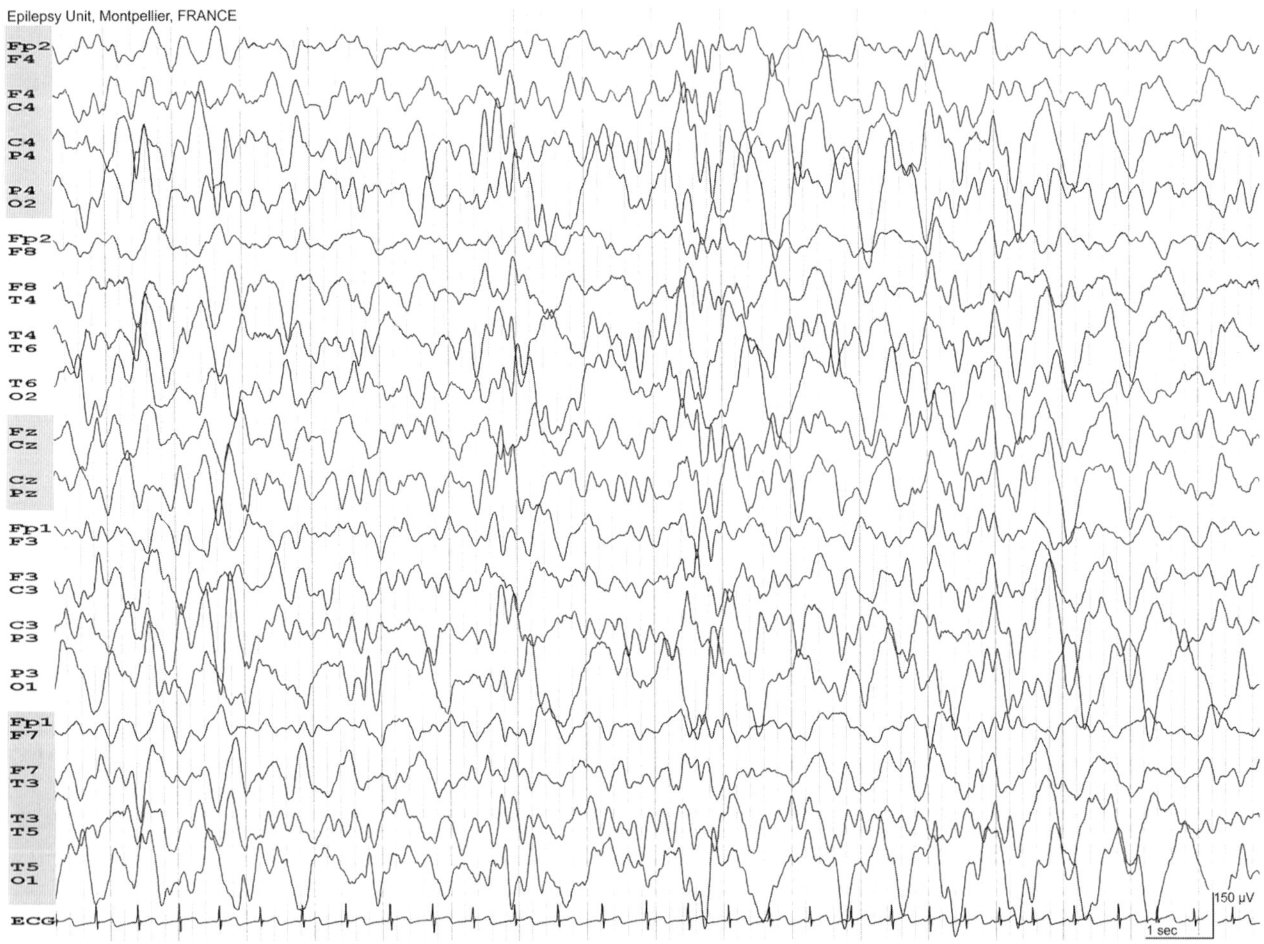

Figure a / Recording at 15 mm/s.

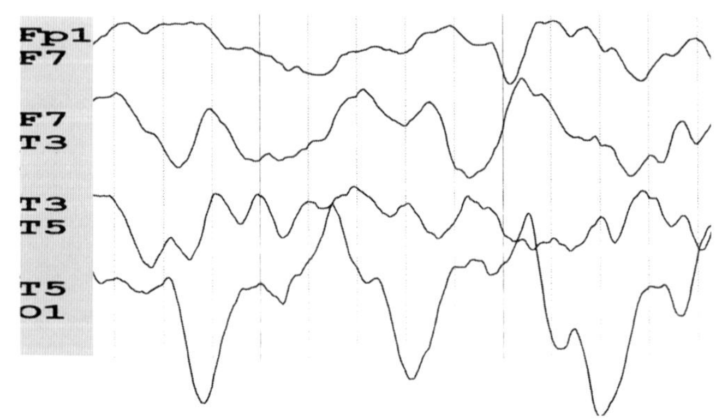

Figure b / High amplitude posteriorly predominant slow waves corresponding to deep sleep.

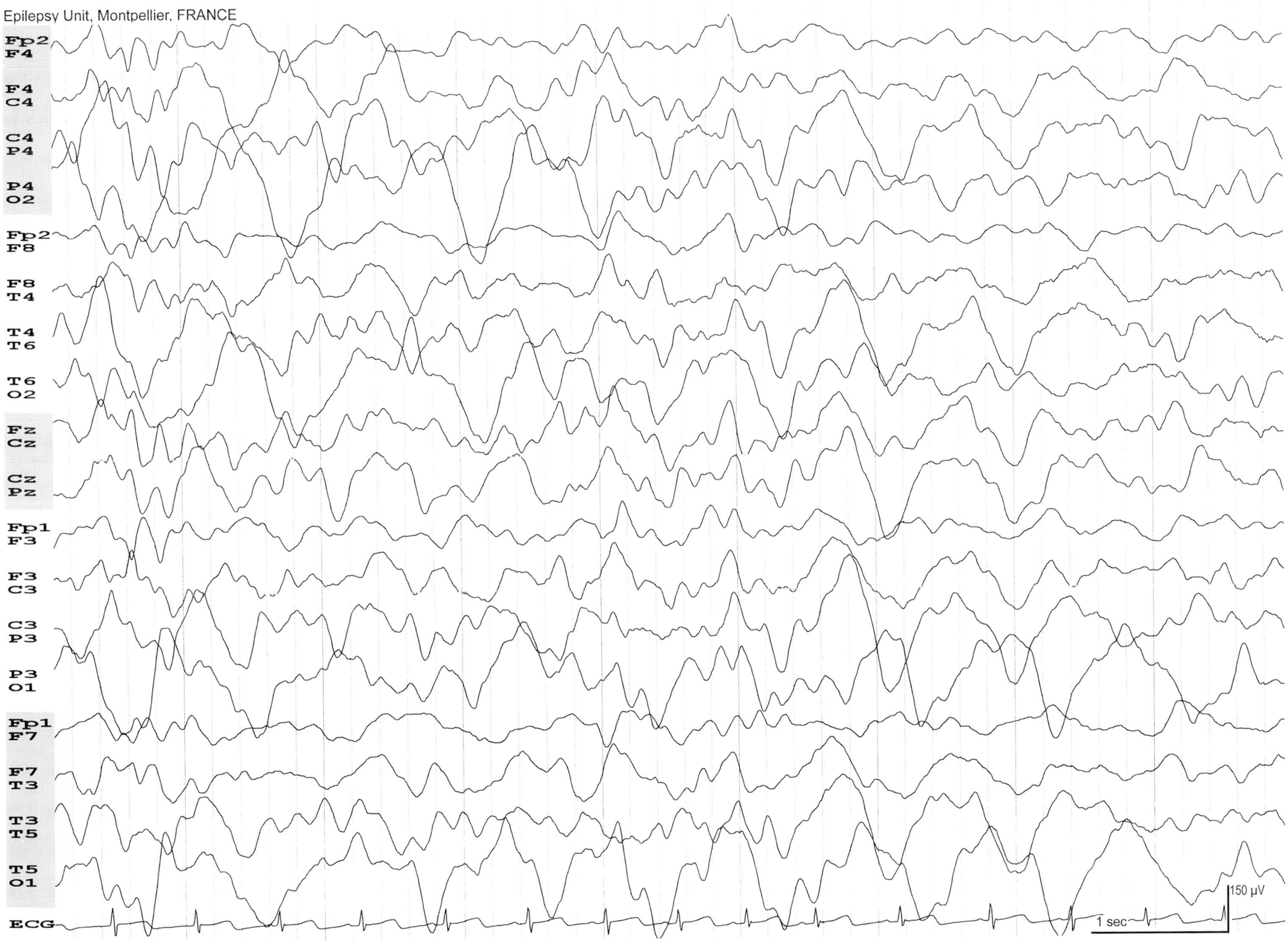
Epilepsy Unit, Montpellier, FRANCE
Fp2
F4
F4
C4
C4
P4
P4
O2
Fp2
F8
F8
T4
T4
T6
T6
O2
Fz
Cz
Cz
Pz
Fp1
F3
F3
C3
C3
P3
P3
O1
Fp1
F7
F7
T3
T3
T5
T5
O1
ECG
150 µV
1 sec

III • 23 NREM 3: Deep sleep in an adult

Context

19-year-old man seen after episodes of loss of consciousness. Same patient as plate III-21.

What to note

Stage N3 sleep. Residual sleep spindles and positive occipital sharp transients of sleep (POSTs) can be observed. In adults, the amplitude of slow wave activity in deep sleep tends to decrease with age. These waveforms are more prominent anteriorly.

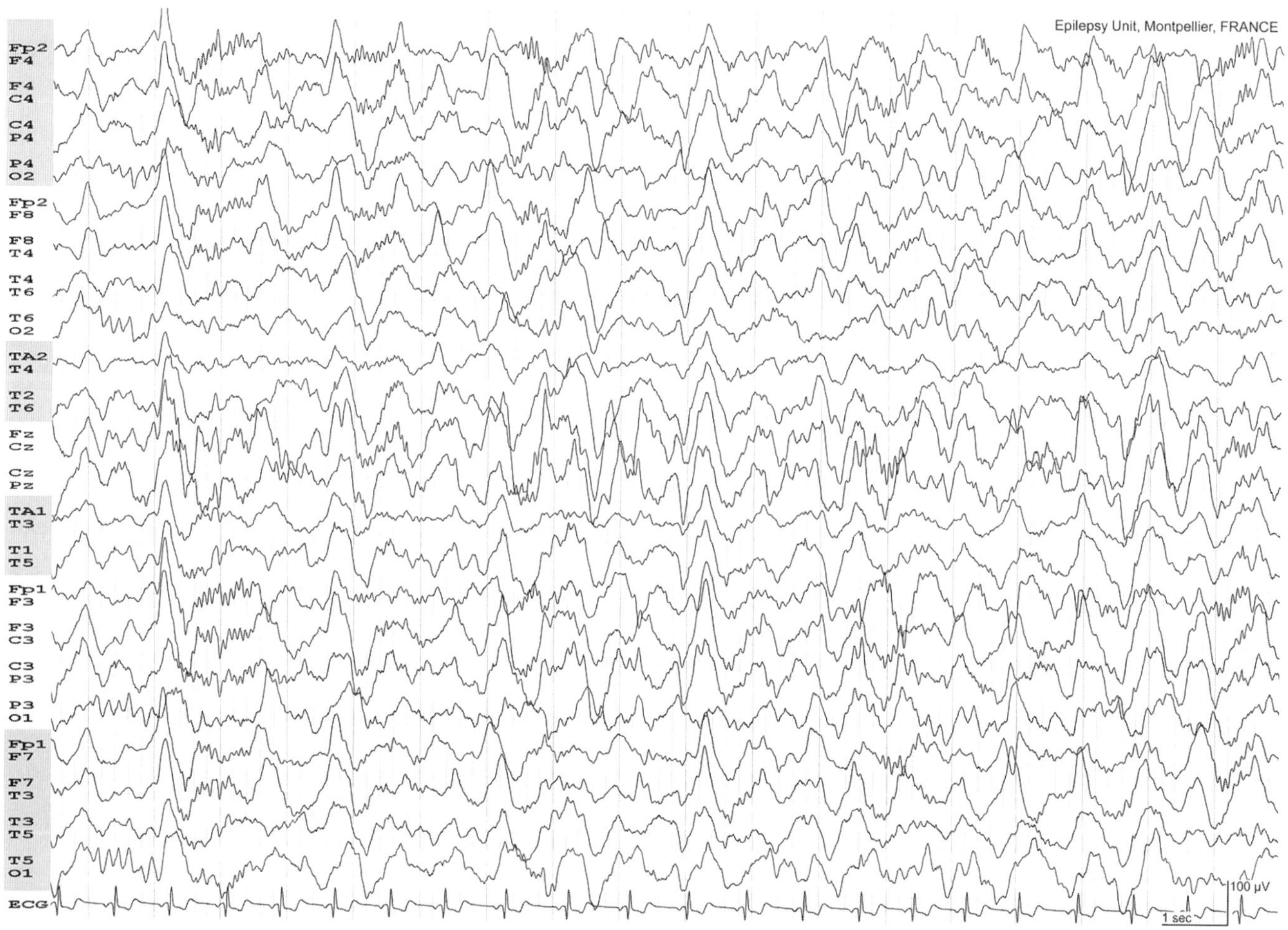

Figure a / Recording at 15 mm/s.

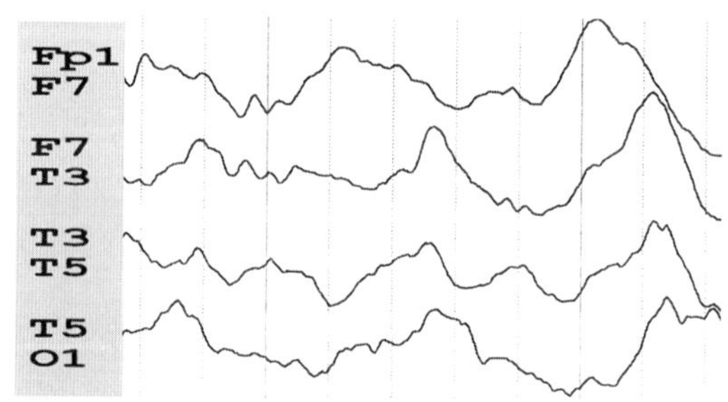

Figure b / Slow wave activity.

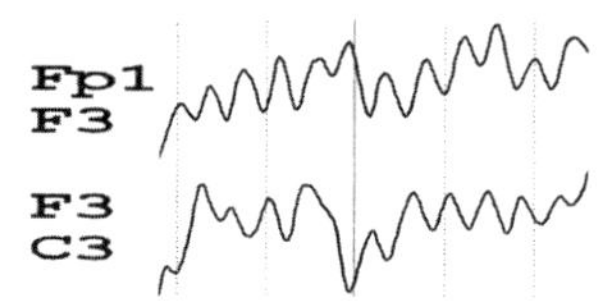

Figure c / Residual sleep spindle.

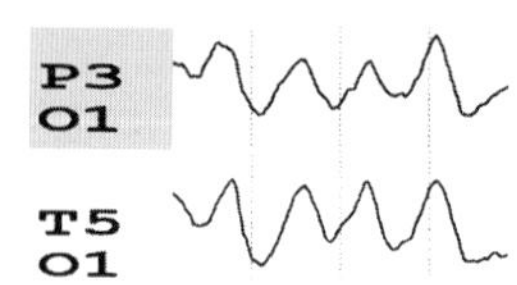

Figure d / Residual POSTs.

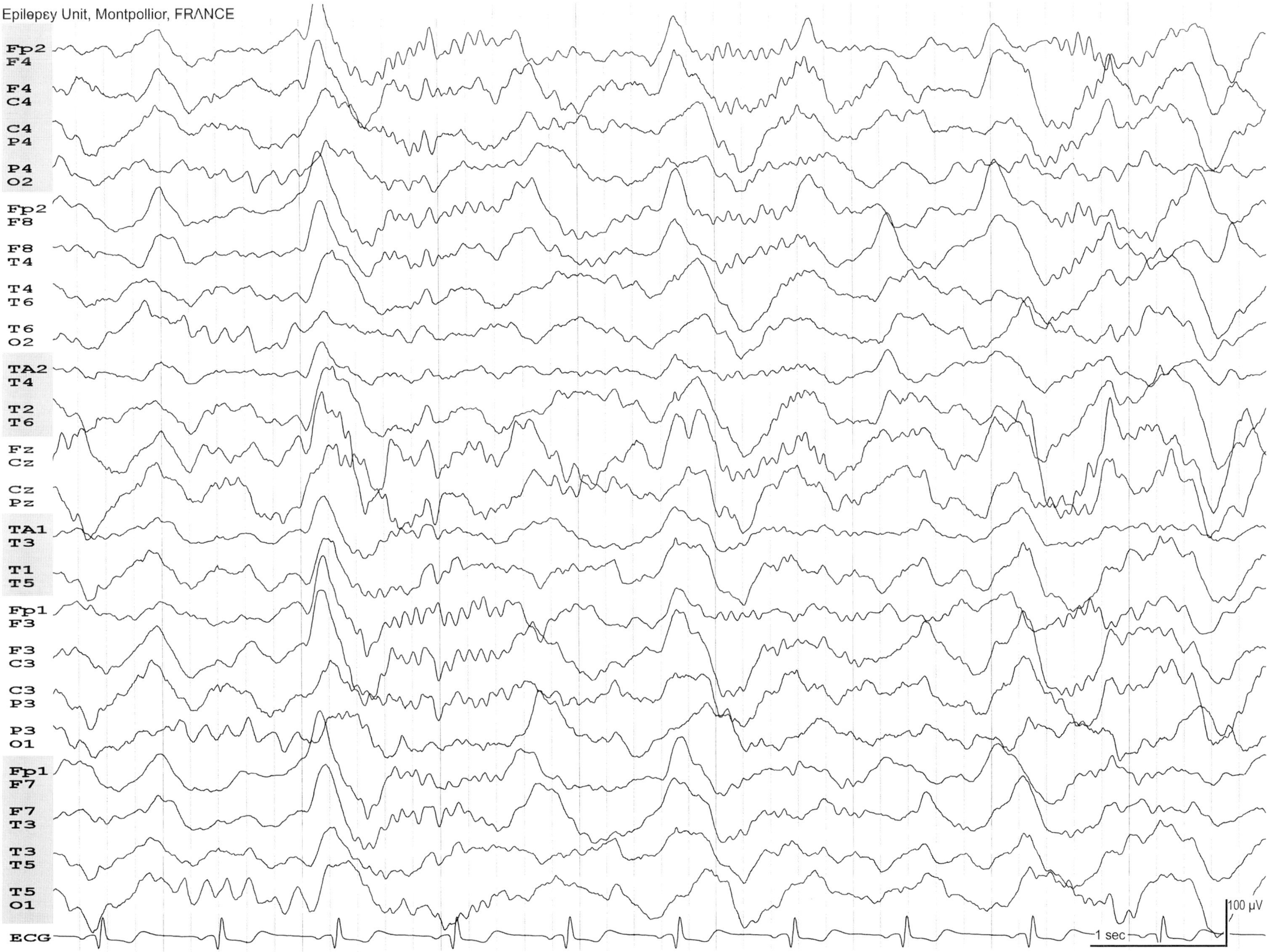
Epilepsy Unit, Montpellier, FRANCE
Fp2 F4
F4 C4
C4 P4
P4 O2
Fp2 F8
F8 T4
T4 T6
T6 O2
TA2 T4
T2 T6
Fz Cz
Cz Pz
TA1 T3
T1 T5
Fp1 F3
F3 C3
C3 P3
P3 O1
Fp1 F7
F7 T3
T3 T5
T5 O1
ECG
100 µV
1 sec

III • 24 Deep sleep in a child with superimposed theta rhythms

Context

6-year-old girl with type I neurofibromatosis.

What to note

Low sensitivity at 15 µV/mm. Stage N3 sleep. Theta rhythms close to the alpha frequency (7 to 8 Hz) are prominent over the anterior regions and admixed with slow wave activity. They were not present during lighter stages of sleep.

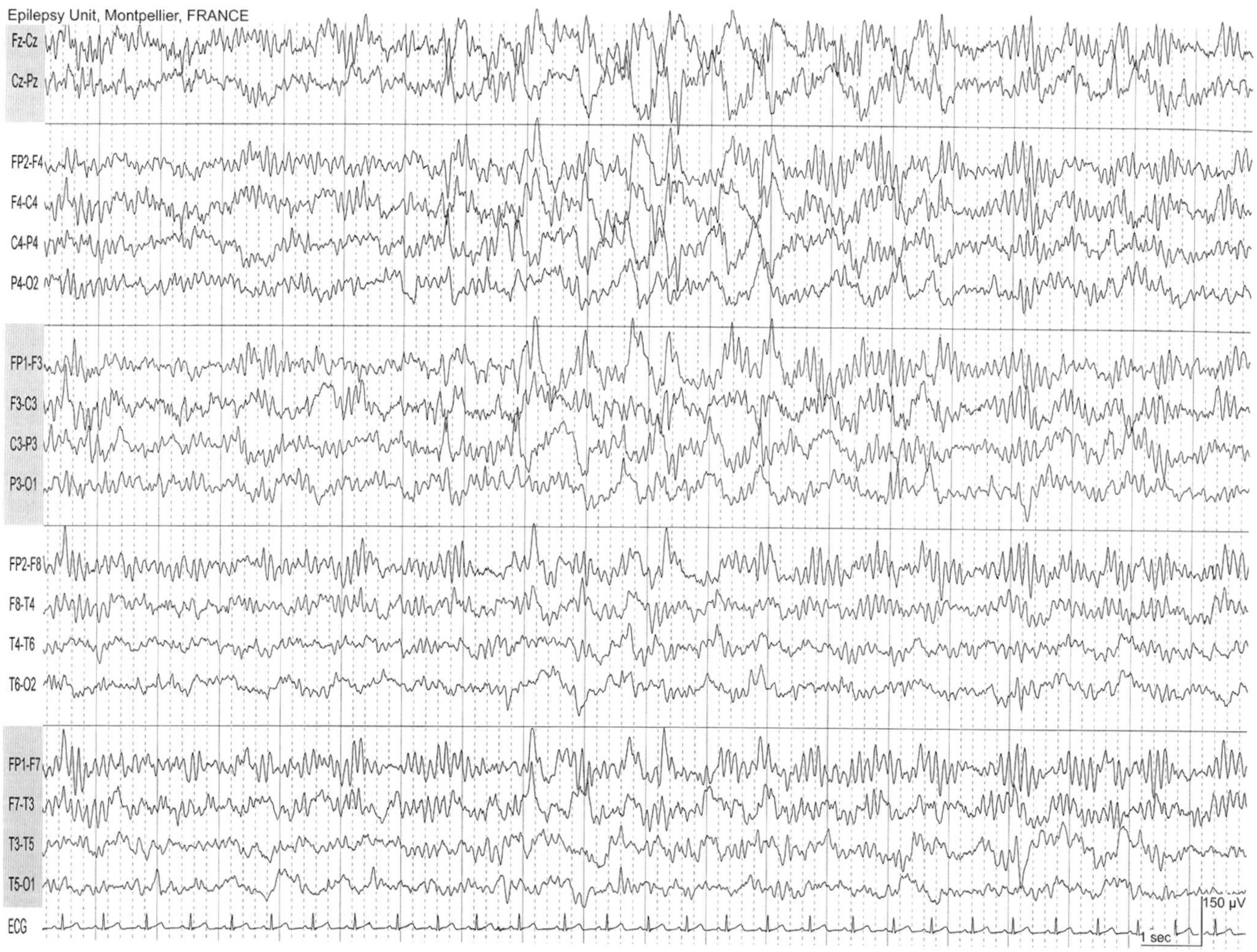

Figure a / Recording at 15 mm/s.

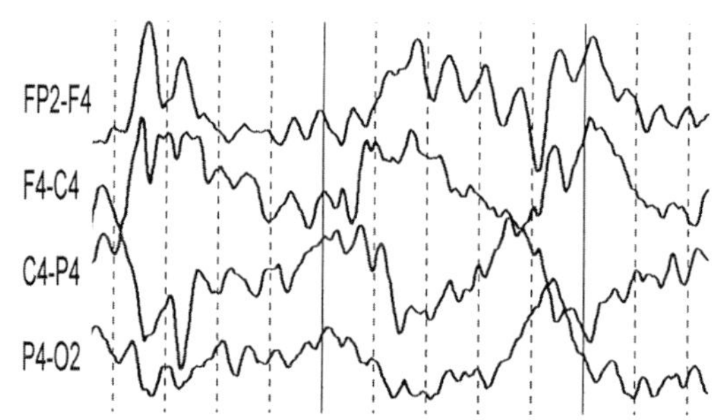

Figure b / Slow wave activity mixed with theta rhythms close to the alpha frequency (7 to 8 Hz) with anterior predominance.

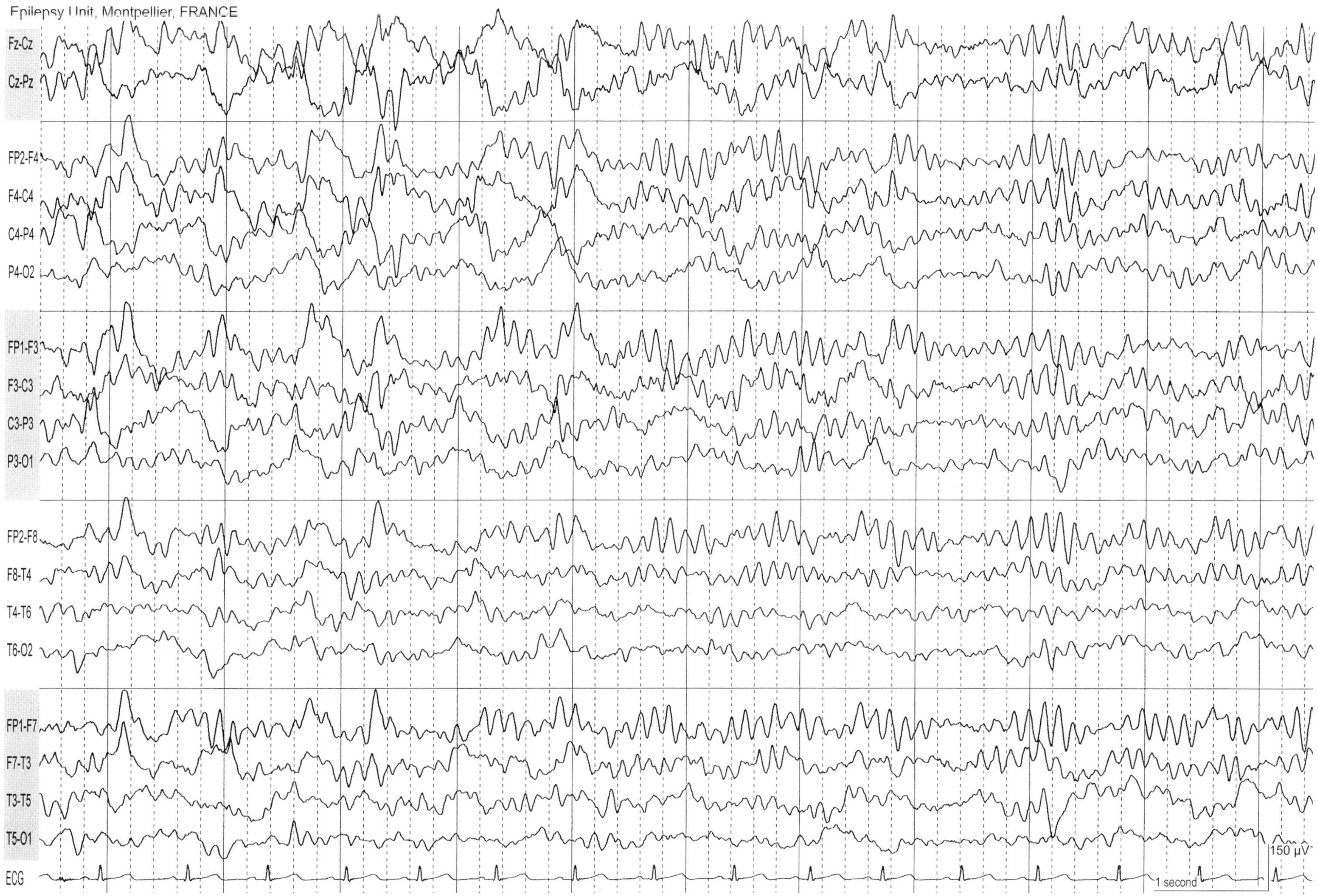
Epilepsy Unit, Montpellier, FRANCE
Fz-Cz
Cz-Pz
FP2-F4
F4-C4
C4-P4
P4-O2
FP1-F3
F3-C3
C3-P3
P3-O1
FP2-F8
F8-T4
T4-T6
T6-O2
FP1-F7
F7-T3
T3-T5
T5-O1
ECG
150 µV
1 second

III • 25 Deep sleep in an adult with superimposed alpha rhythms

Context

31-year-old woman with cryptogenic left temporal lobe epilepsy.

What to note

Stage N3 sleep. Note that the slow delta waves are superimposed with an alpha frequency (10 Hz). This alpha rhythm can be distinguished from the wakefulness alpha rhythm by the diffuse anterior spread over the two hemispheres. This pattern is unusual in sleep but not pathological. This pattern is referred to as alpha-delta sleep. When present, it generally persists in the same patient throughout deep sleep.

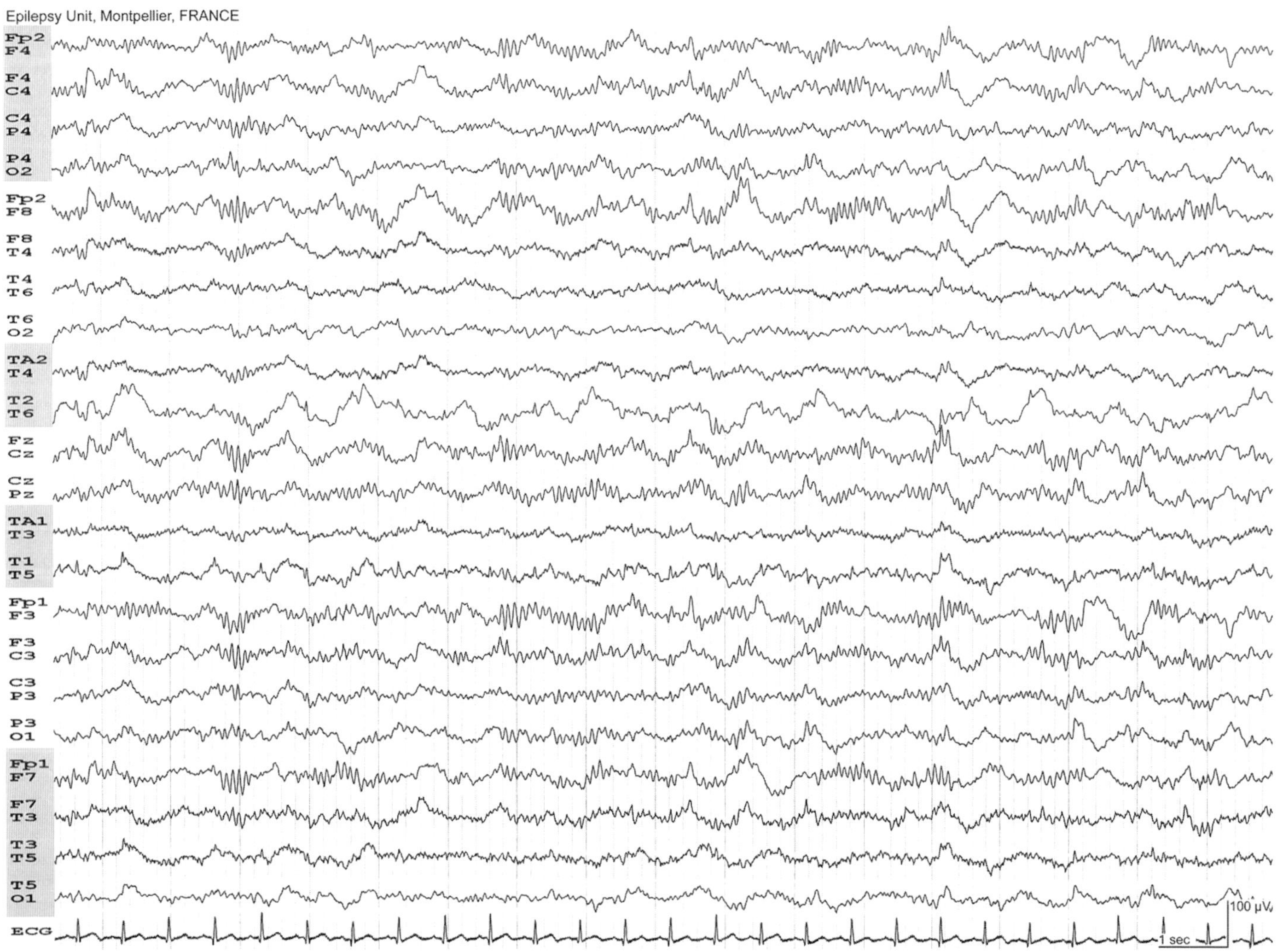

Figure a / Recording at 15 mm/s.

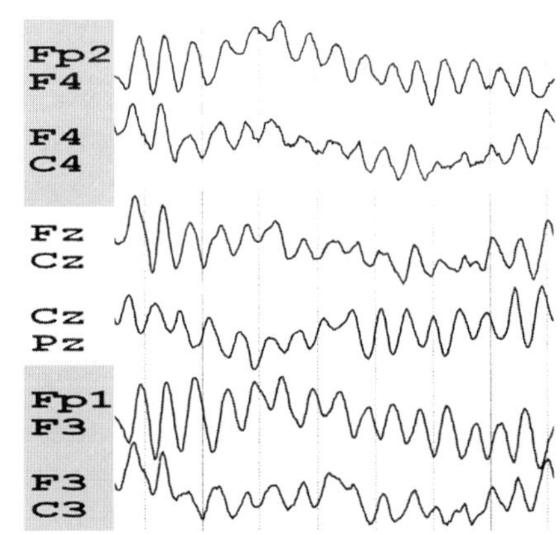

Figure b / Slow wave activity mixed with anterior dominant alpha rhythm.

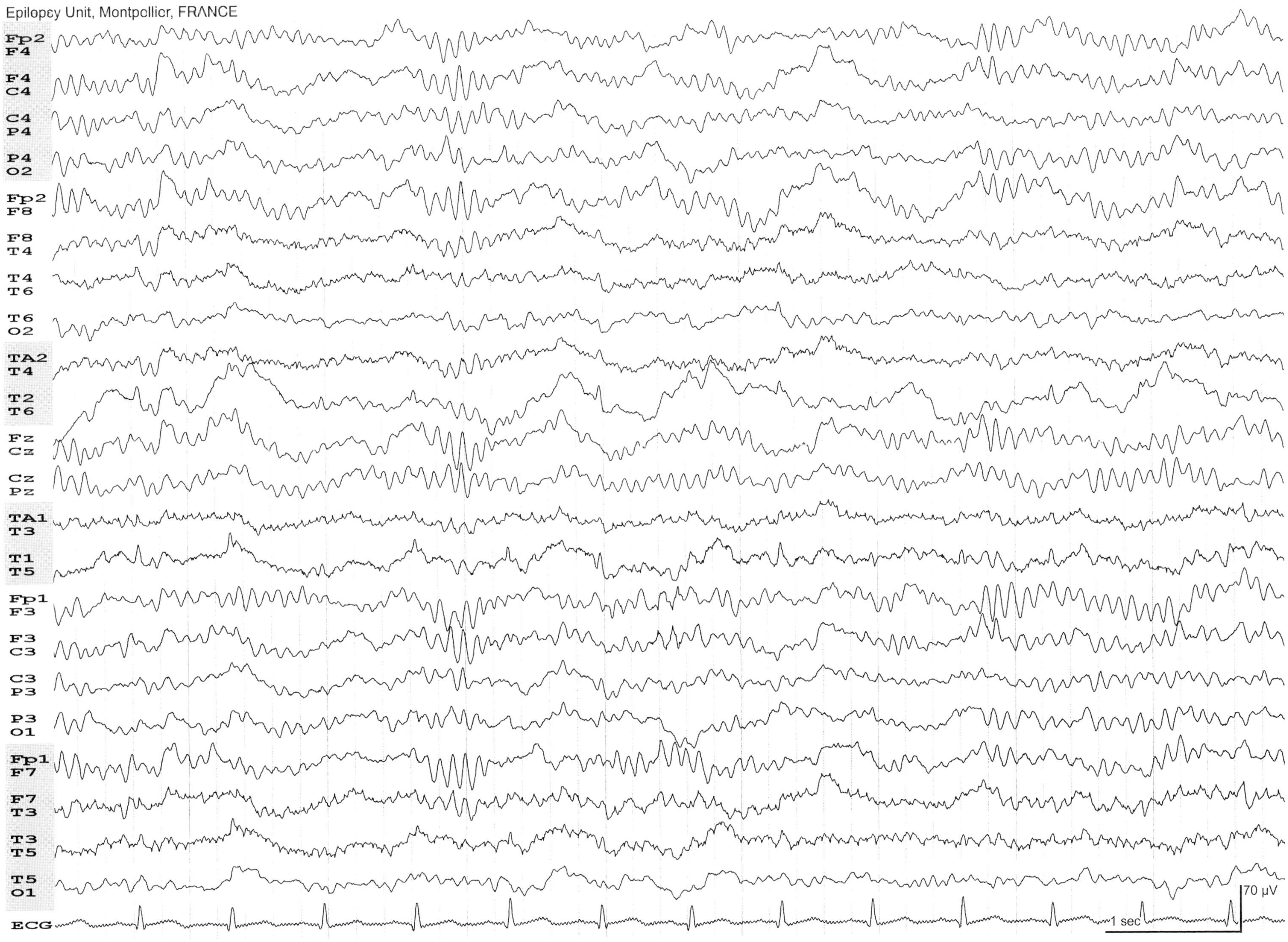
Epilepsy Unit, Montpellier, FRANCE
Fp2 F4
F4 C4
C4 P4
P4 O2
Fp2 F8
F8 T4
T4 T6
T6 O2
TA2 T4
T2 T6
Fz Cz
Cz Pz
TA1 T3
T1 T5
Fp1 F3
F3 C3
C3 P3
P3 O1
Fp1 F7
F7 T3
T3 T5
T5 O1
ECG
70 µV
1 sec

• 26 REM sleep: Transition from stage N2 sleep

Context

43-year-old man with cryptogenic right temporal lobe epilepsy, presurgical assessment.

What to note

Stage N2 sleep. A sleep spindle can be seen on the left fronto-central region, and muscle activity is observed on the chin EMG. Onset of REM sleep. Theta-like sawtooth waves can be seen over the vertex (see plate recorded at 15 mm/s). Reduced muscle activity (atonia) can be observed on the EMG. Lastly, respiration is not as deep as before (nasal (NAS) and thoracic (THO) respirations) (see plate recorded at 15 mm/s). This page corresponds to a transition from NREM stage 2 sleep to REM sleep.

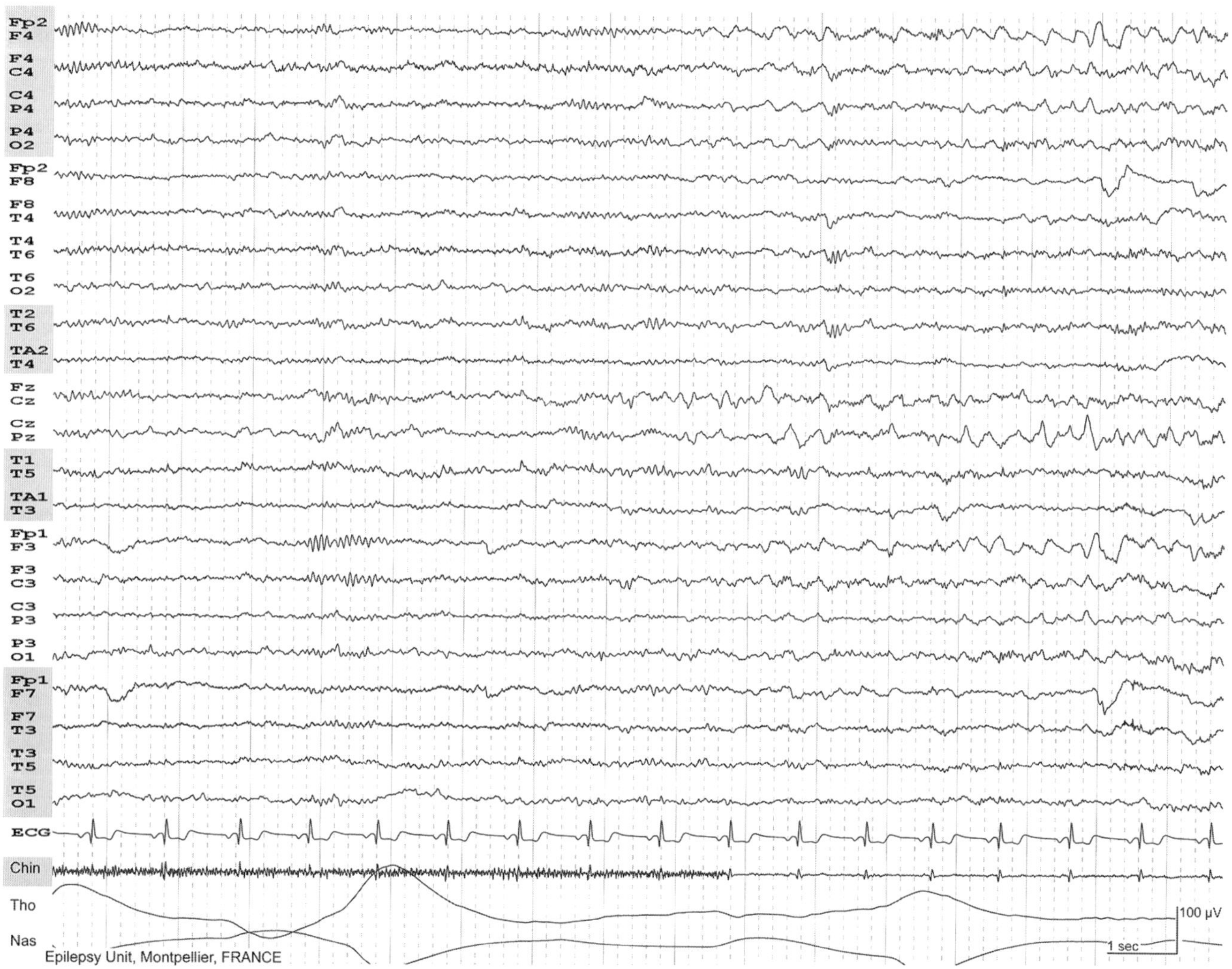

Figure a / Onset of REM sleep at the 11th second. Sawtooth waves can be seen over the vertex and the adjacent suprasylvian regions. Onset of rapid eye movements over the frontal polar regions at the end of the plate.

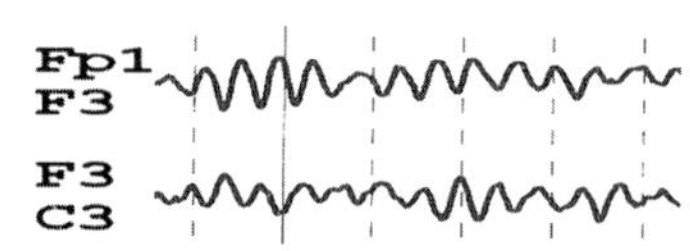

Figure b / Sleep spindle.

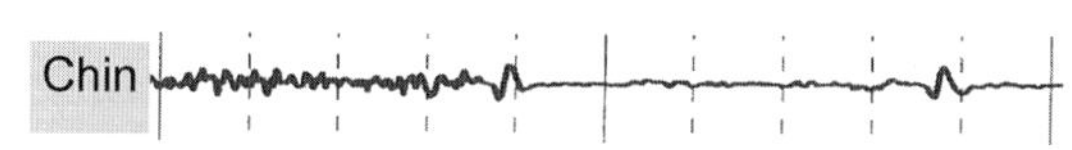

Figure c / Passage in muscle atonia.
EKG artifact.

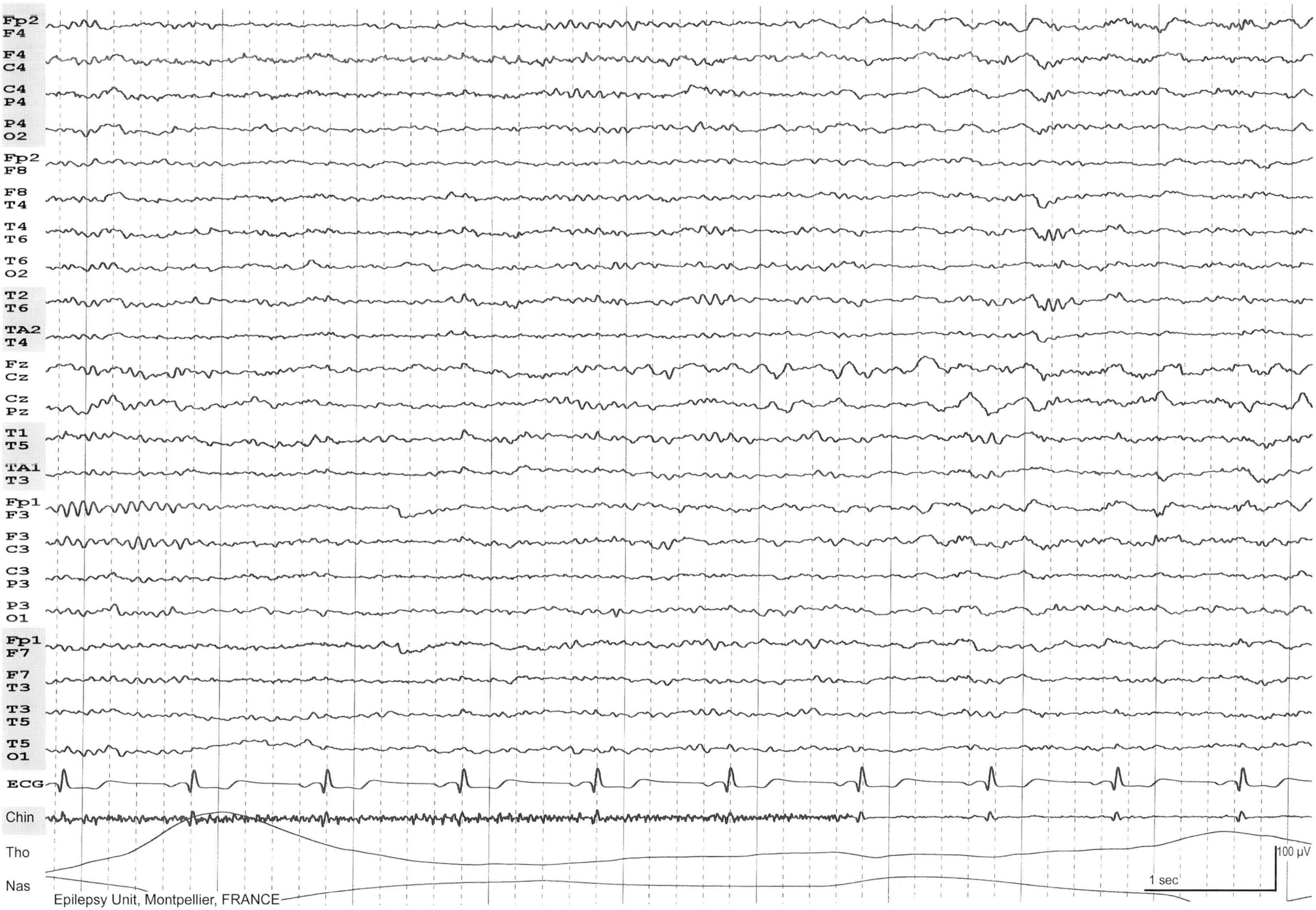
Fp2 F4
F4 C4
C4 P4
P4 O2
Fp2 F8
F8 T4
T4 T6
T6 O2
T2 T6
TA2 T4
Fz Cz
Cz Pz
T1 T5
TA1 T3
Fp1 F3
F3 C3
C3 P3
P3 O1
Fp1 F7
F7 T3
T3 T5
T5 O1
ECG
Chin
Tho
Nas
100 µV
1 sec
Epilepsy Unit, Montpellier, FRANCE

III • 27 REM sleep: Transition from stage N2 sleep

Context

43-year-old man with right temporal lobe epilepsy, referred for presurgical assessment.

What to note

Low amplitude K complex followed by a sleep spindle followed by sawtooth waves over the vertex region with higher amplitude on Fpz-Fz. Note on the plate recorded at 15 mm/s, the occurrence of rapid eye movements at the end of the plate.

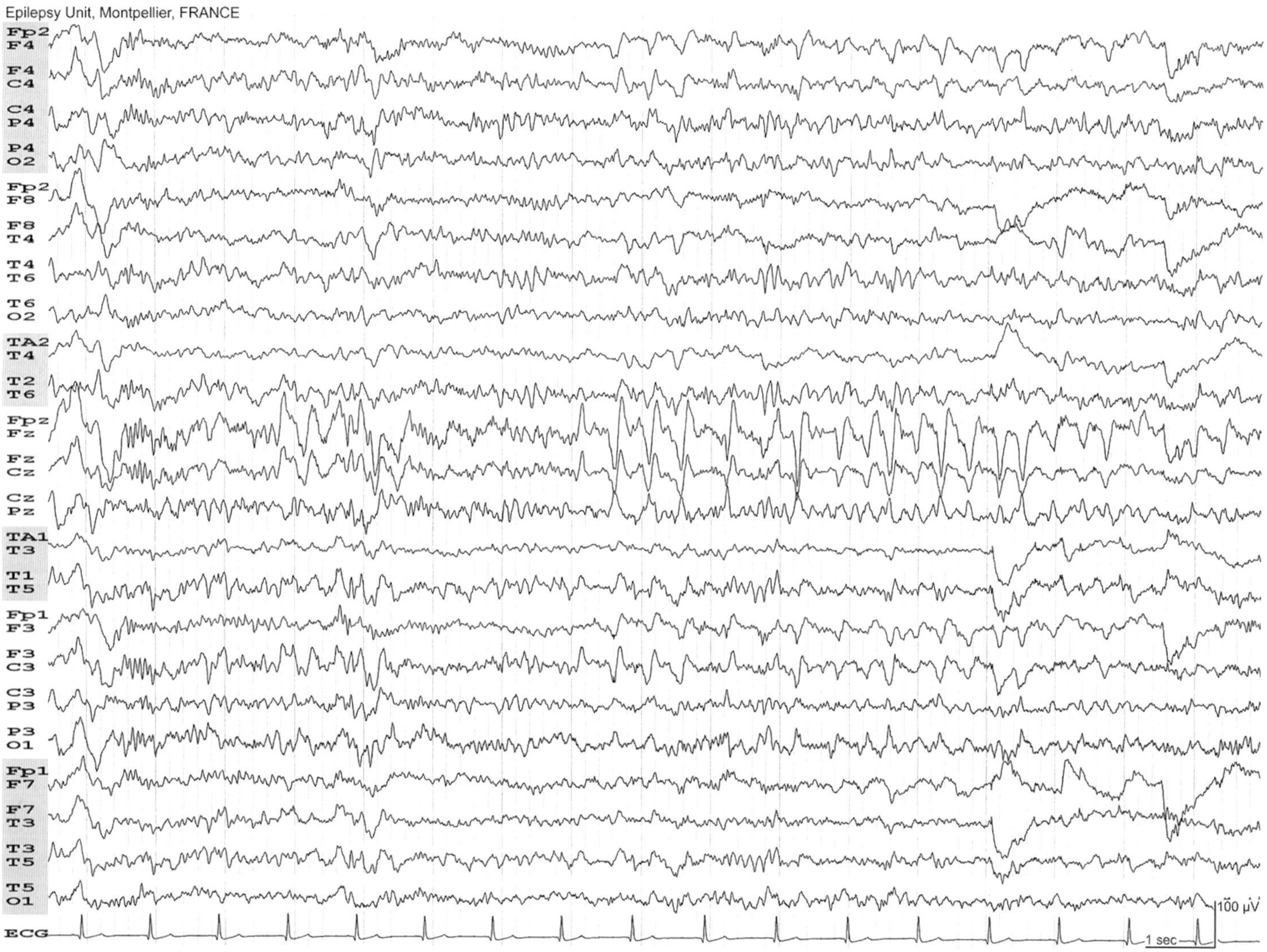

Figure a / Recording at 15 mm/s. Note at the beginning of the plate, a first K complex followed by a sleep spindle and the occurrence of rapid eye movements at the end of the plate.

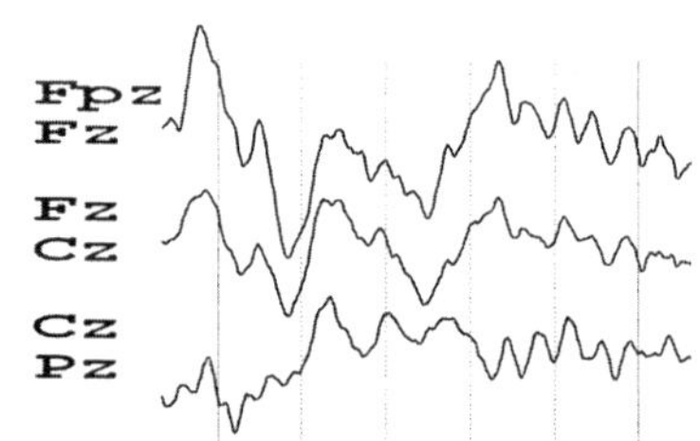

Figure b / K complex followed by a sleep spindle.

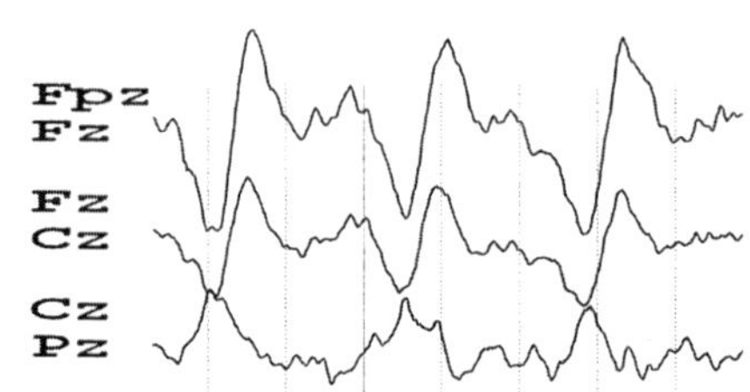

Figure c / Sawtooth waves over the vertex region.

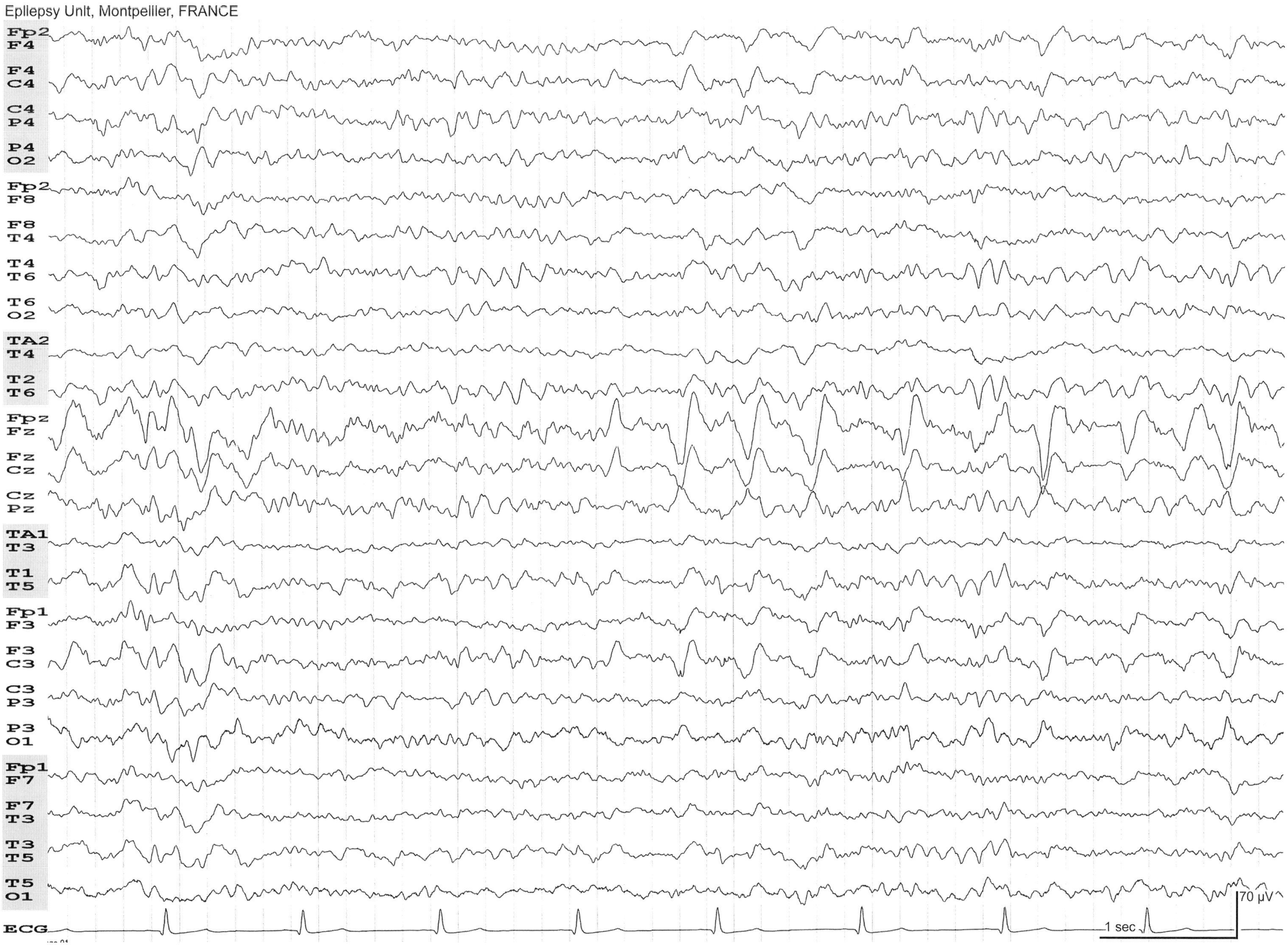
Epilepsy Unit, Montpellier, FRANCE
Fp2 F4
F4 C4
C4 P4
P4 O2
Fp2 F8
F8 T4
T4 T6
T6 O2
TA2 T4
T2 T6
Fpz Fz
Fz Cz
Cz Pz
TA1 T3
T1 T5
Fp1 F3
F3 C3
C3 P3
P3 O1
Fp1 F7
F7 T3
T3 T5
T5 O1
ECG
70 µV
1 sec

III • 28 REM sleep in an infant

Context

14-month-old infant with benign myoclonic epilepsy of infancy. Same patient as plates III-15 and 22.

What to note

Low sensitivity at 15 μV/mm. The infant is in REM sleep. Indeed, there is no sleep spindle. Note some very ample delta waves at 3.5 Hz with a sinusoidal form, which predominate occipitally. There are no sawtooth waves at this age.

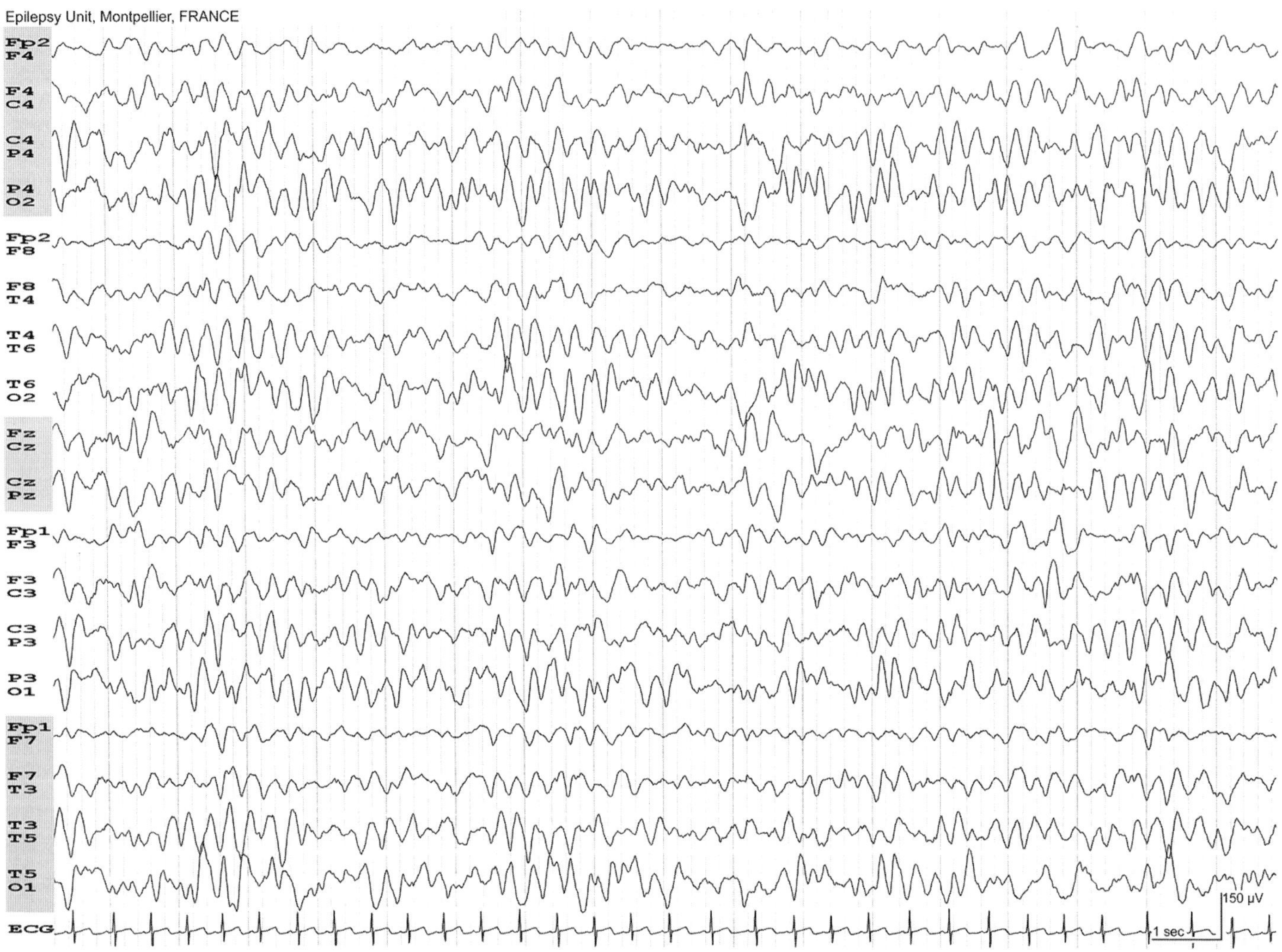

Figure a / Recording at 15 mm/s.

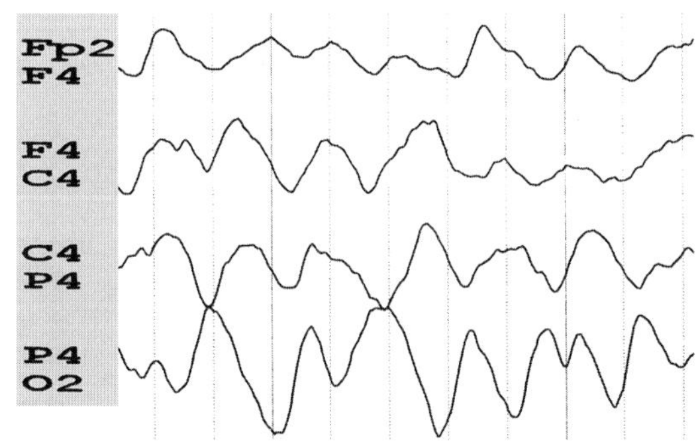

Figure b / Delta waves, which are occipital dominant.

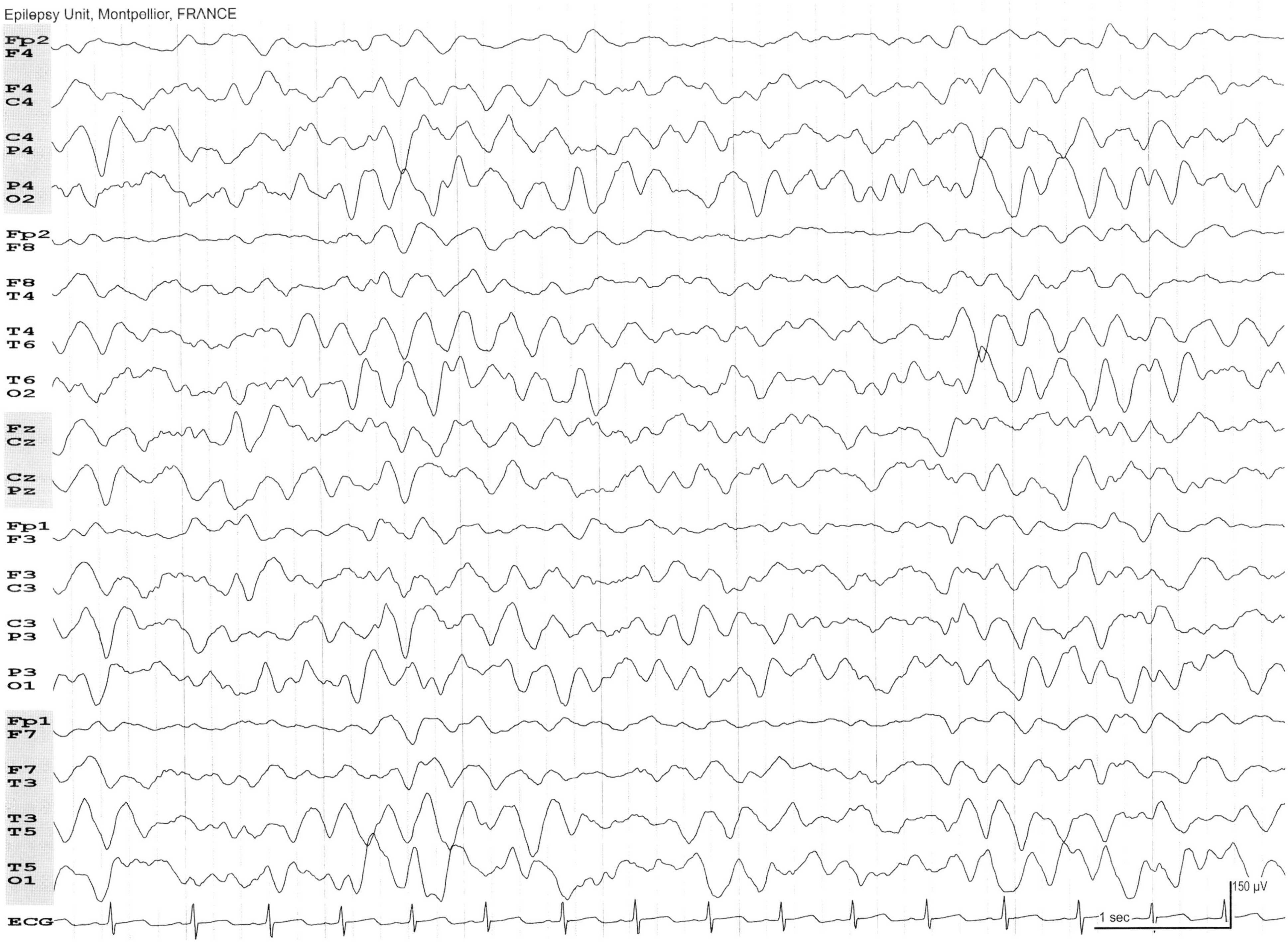
Epilepsy Unit, Montpellior, FRANCE
Fp2 F4
F4 C4
C4 P4
P4 O2
Fp2 F8
F8 T4
T4 T6
T6 O2
Fz Cz
Cz Pz
Fp1 F3
F3 C3
C3 P3
P3 O1
Fp1 F7
F7 T3
T3 T5
T5 O1
ECG
150 µV
1 sec

III • 29 REM sleep in a young child

Context

3.5 year-old child seen after a febrile seizure. Same patient as plate III-16.

What to note

Low sensitivity at 15 μV/mm. The child is in REM sleep. At this age, high amplitude sawtooth waves that spread to the right and left frontocentral regions.

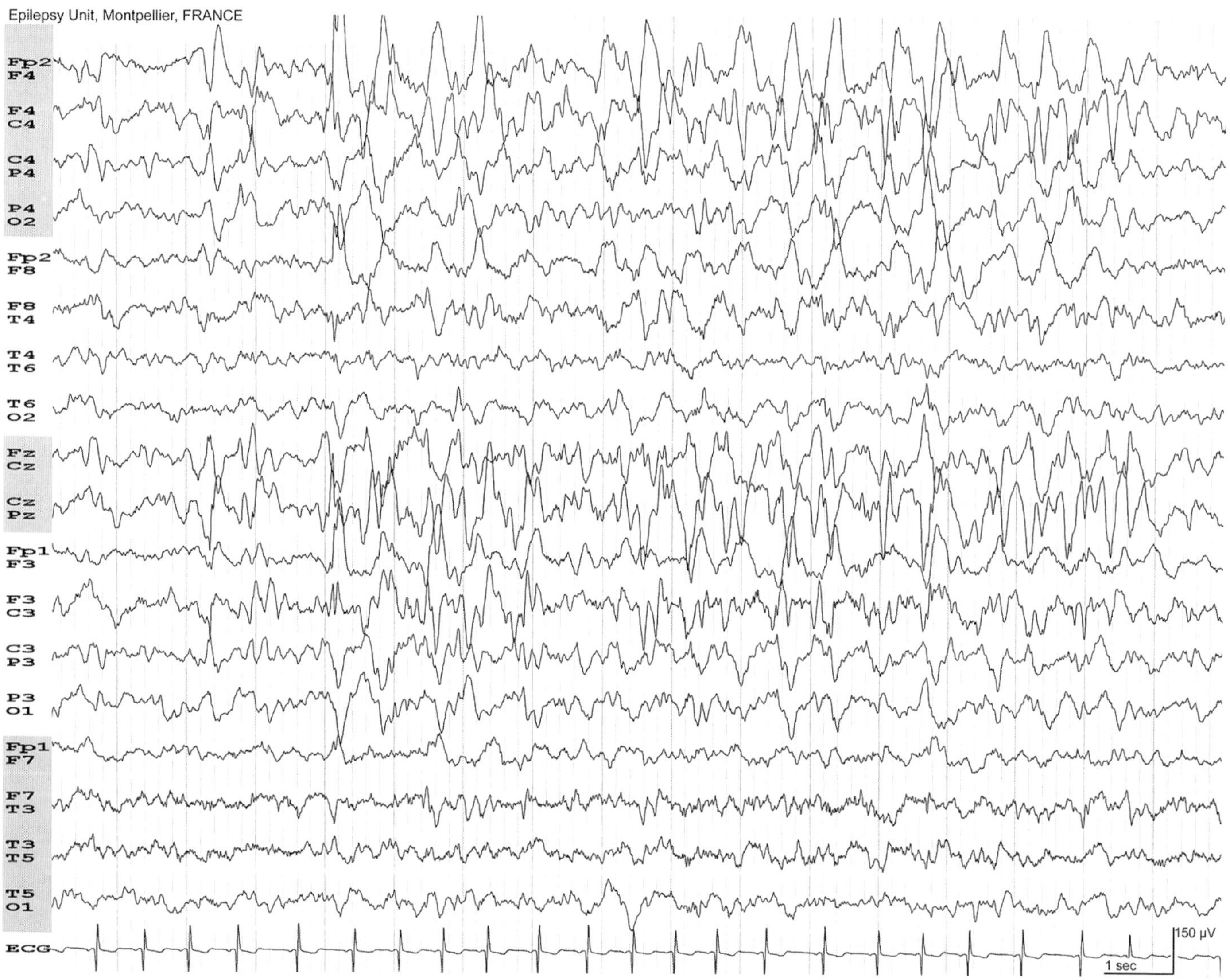

Figure a / Recording at 15 mm/s.

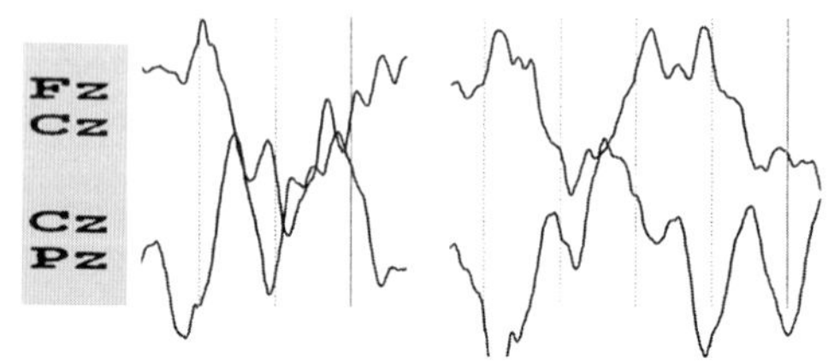

Figure b / Sawtooth waves on the vertex.

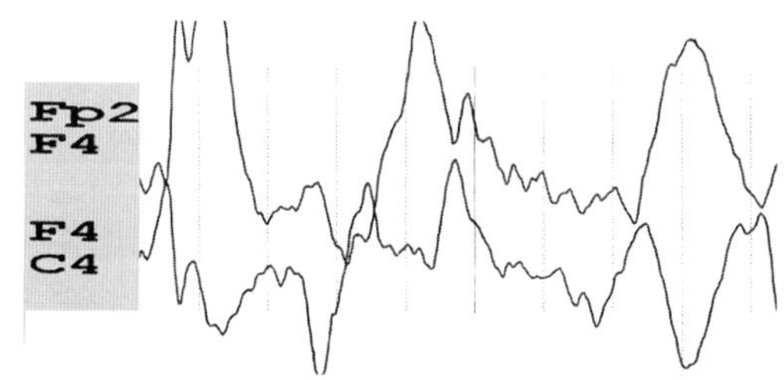

Figure c / Sawthooth waves that spread to the right fronto-central regions.

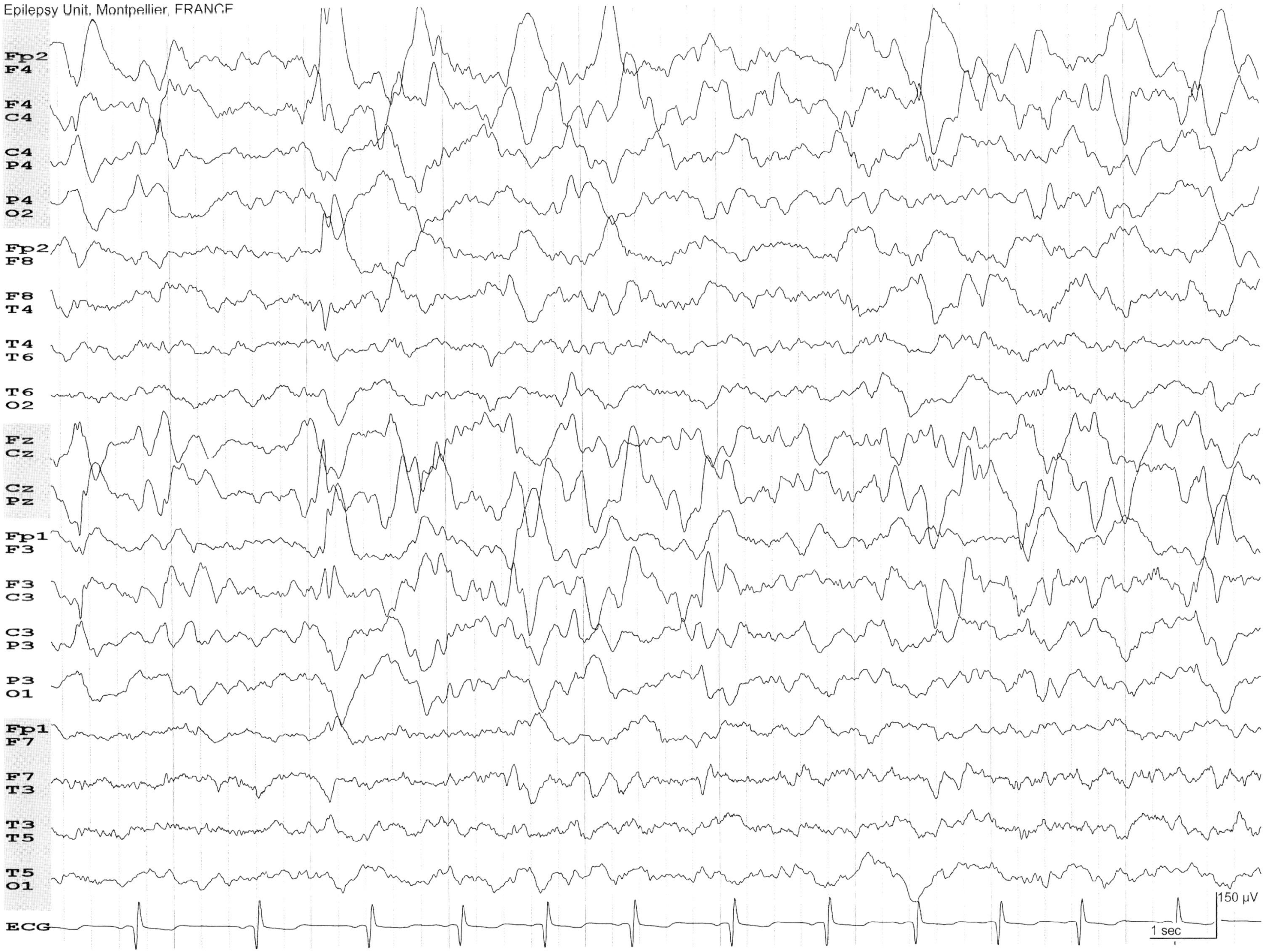
Epilepsy Unit, Montpellier, FRANCE
Fp2 F4
F4 C4
C4 P4
P4 O2
Fp2 F8
F8 T4
T4 T6
T6 O2
Fz Cz
Cz Pz
Fp1 F3
F3 C3
C3 P3
P3 O1
Fp1 F7
F7 T3
T3 T5
T5 O1
ECG
150 µV
1 sec

• 30 REM sleep in a child

Context

11-year-old girl with cryptogenic temporal lobe epilepsy.

What to note

REM sleep. Eye movements are detectable at Fp2-F8 and Fp1-F7. Reduced muscle activity (atonia) on the EMG and fast polyphasic potentials (facial twitch artifacts). Runs of 3-4 Hz waves over the vertex region (Fz-Cz-Pz) corresponding to sawtooth waves. Note that these sawtooth waves have not their typical aspect at this age. The amplitude of these waves is higher in children compared to adults.

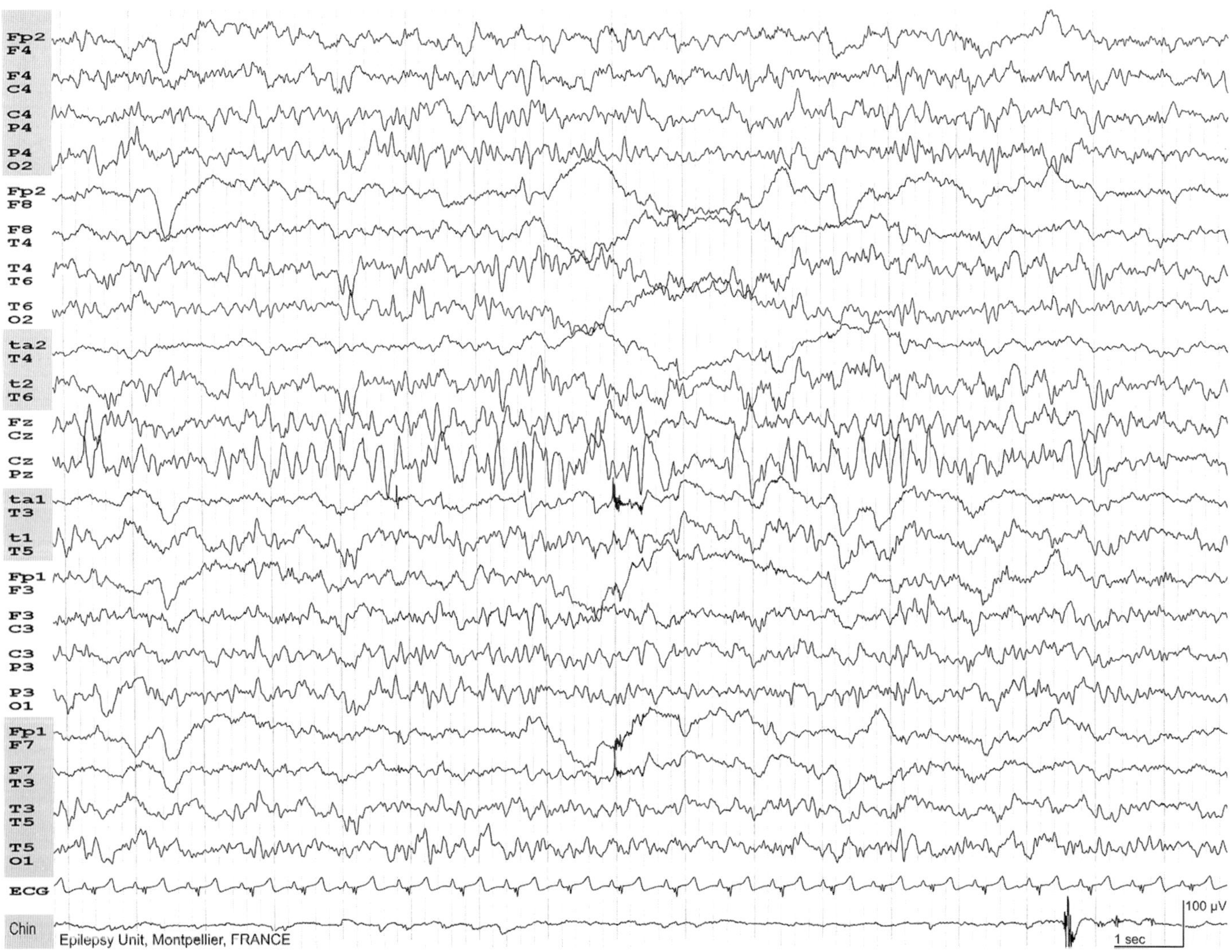

Figure a / Recording at 15 mm/s. Note at the end of the plate, the muscle twitches on the chin derivation.

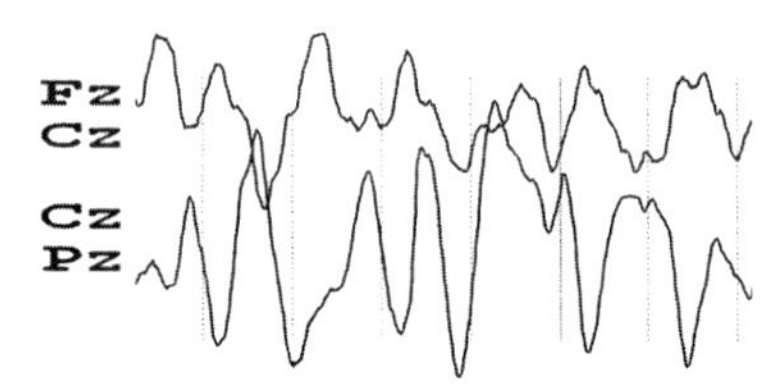

Figure b / Run of 3-4 Hz waves corresponding to sawtooth waves.

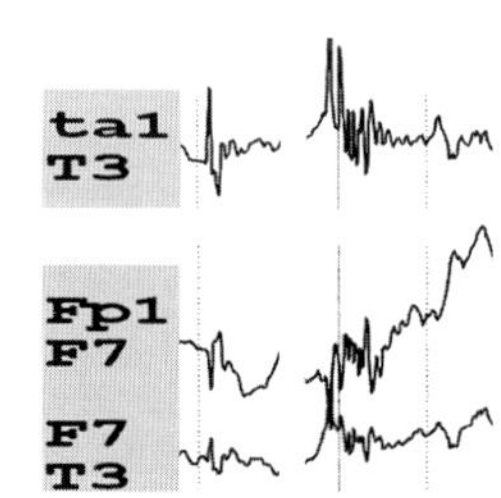

Figure c / Muscle twitches.

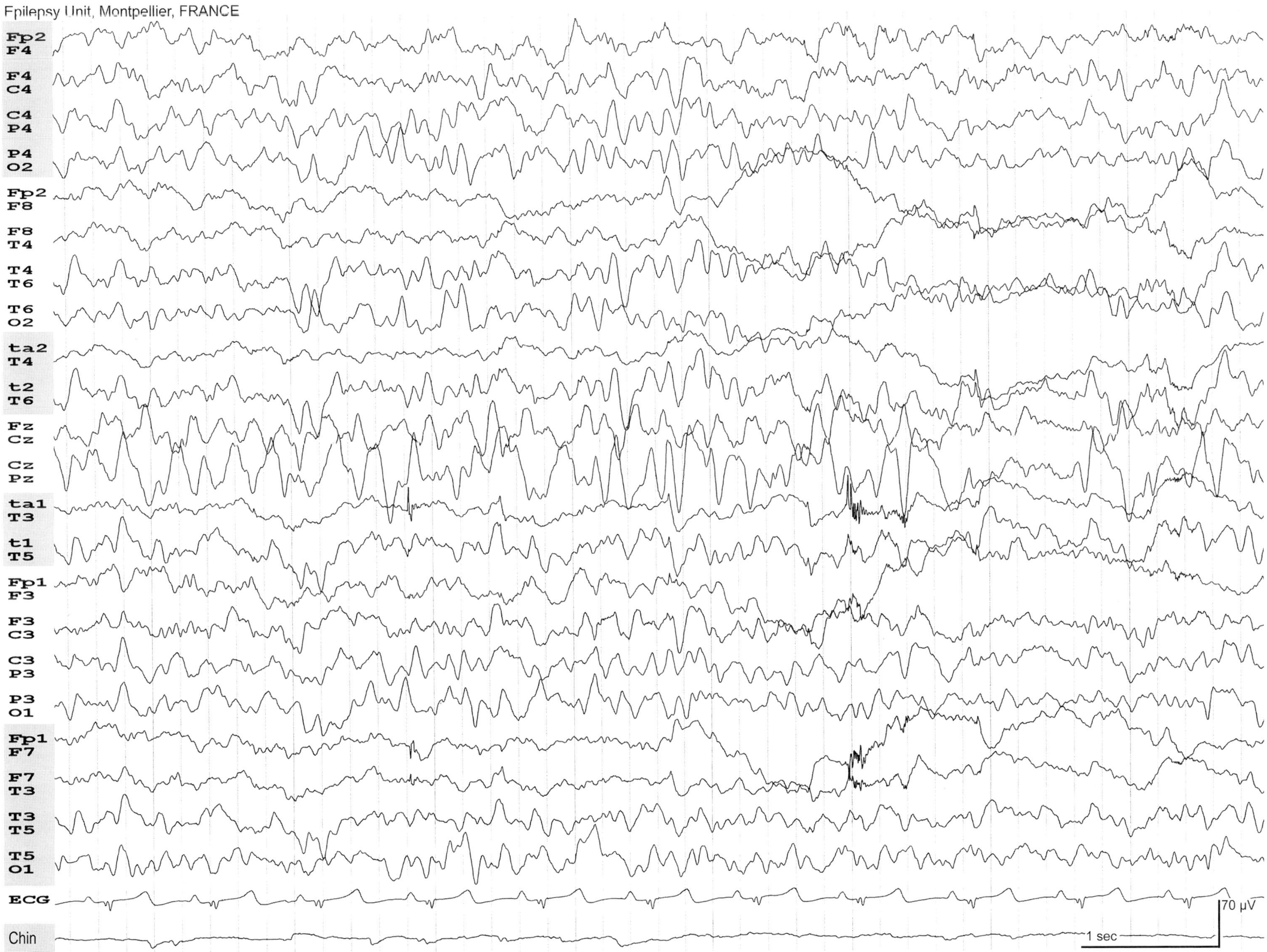
Epilepsy Unit, Montpellier, FRANCE
Fp2 F4
F4 C4
C4 P4
P4 O2
Fp2 F8
F8 T4
T4 T6
T6 O2
ta2 T4
t2 T6
Fz Cz
Cz Pz
ta1 T3
t1 T5
Fp1 F3
F3 C3
C3 P3
P3 O1
Fp1 F7
F7 T3
T3 T5
T5 O1
ECG
Chin
70 µV
1 sec

III • 31 REM sleep: alpha activity, sawtooth waves

Context

41-year-old woman seen after two confusional states.

What to note

REM sleep. Alpha background activity at 9.5 Hz. Compared to wakefulness, this rhythm is more monomorphic without sinusoidal aspect. The tracing also includes rapid eye movements and sawtooth waves on the vertex. The sawtooth waves mimic spikes.

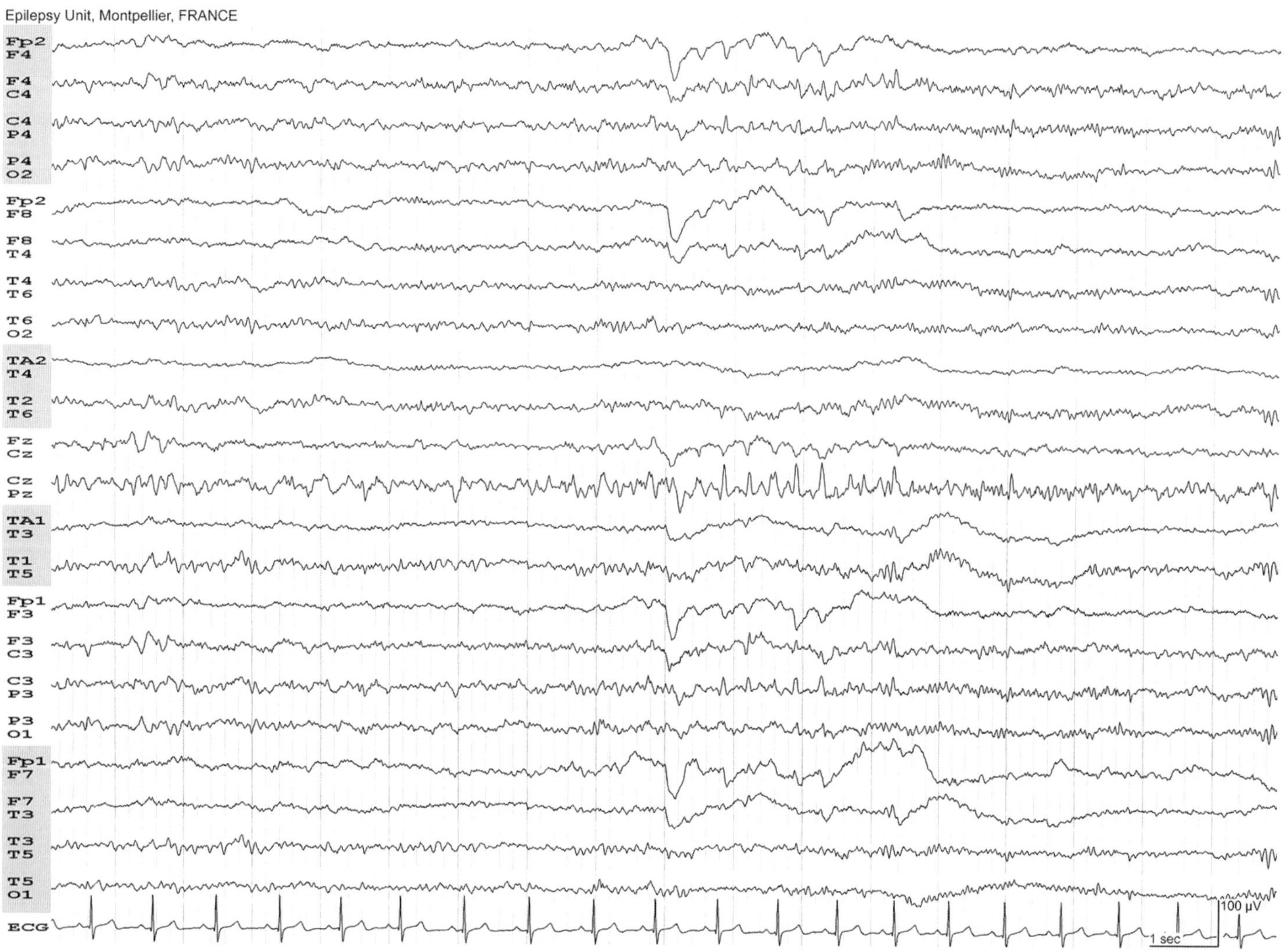

Figure a / Recording at 15 mm/s.

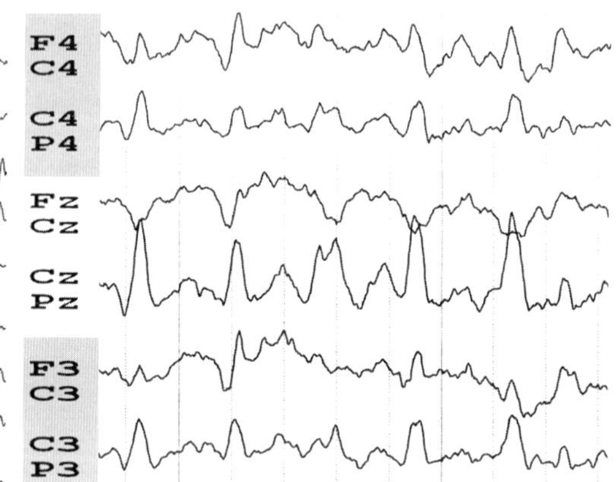

Figure b / Sawtooth waves resembling spikes.

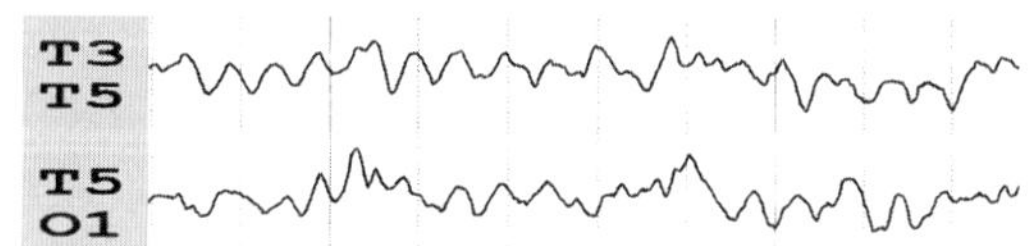

Figure c / Alpha background activity.

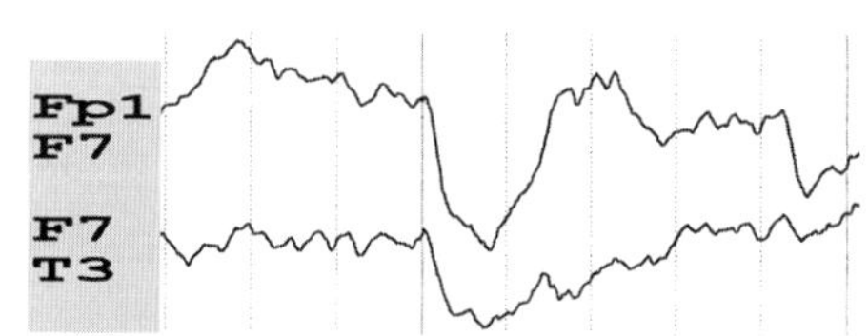

Figure d / Rapid eye movements.

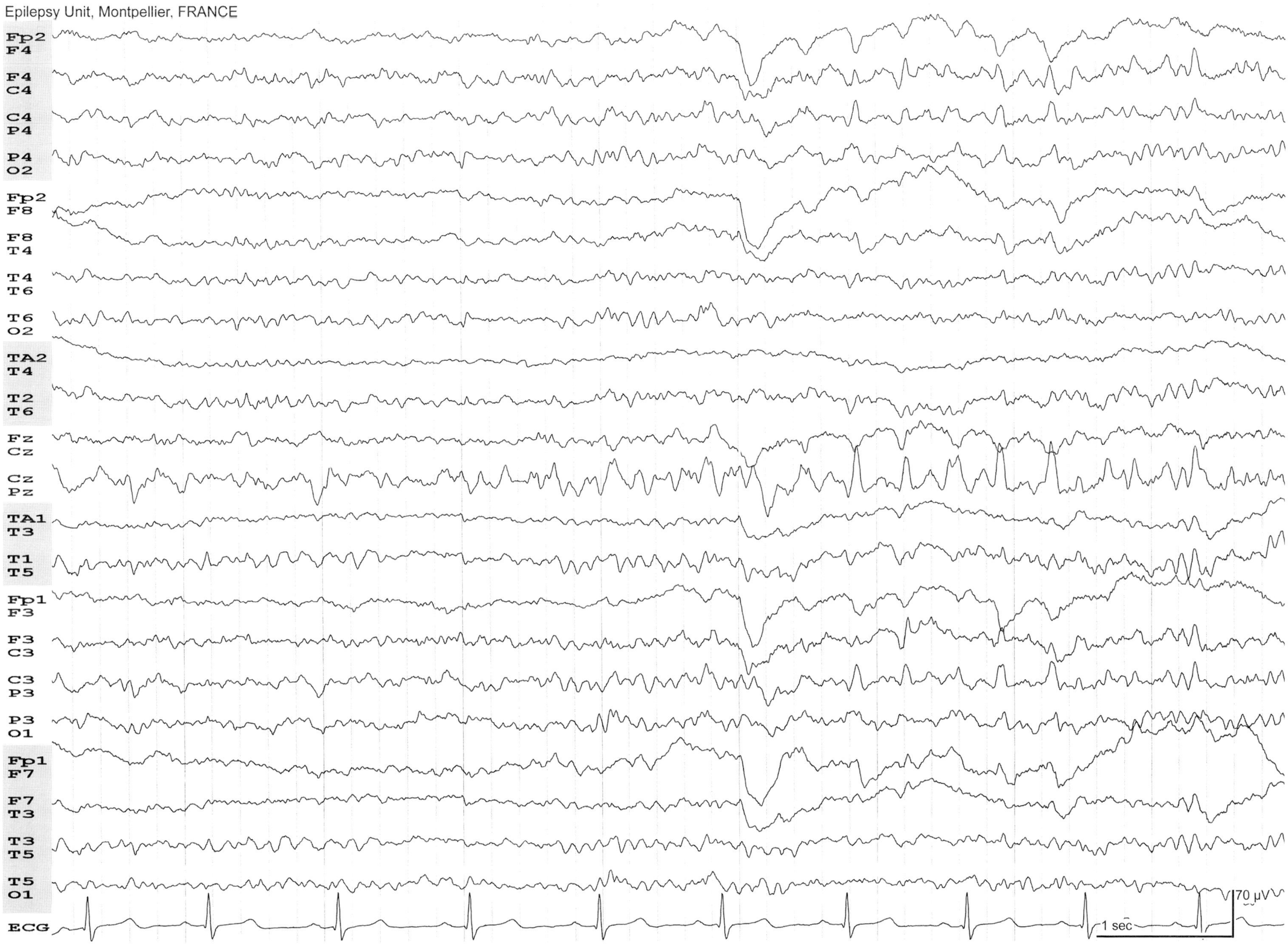
Epilepsy Unit, Montpellier, FRANCE
Fp2 F4
F4 C4
C4 P4
P4 O2
Fp2 F8
F8 T4
T4 T6
T6 O2
TA2 T4
T2 T6
Fz Cz
Cz Pz
TA1 T3
T1 T5
Fp1 F3
F3 C3
C3 P3
P3 O1
Fp1 F7
F7 T3
T3 T5
T5 O1
ECG
70 µV
1 sec

III • 32 REM sleep: alpha activity, sawtooth waves and mu rhythm

Context

42-year-old woman with temporal lobe epilepsy.

What to note

REM sleep. Low-voltage alpha background activity can be seen at the end of the plate. Runs of diphasic waves over the vertex region (Fz-Cz-Pz) corresponding to sawtooth waves. These are also visible at the right and left fronto-central derivations. Over the vertex, the sawtooth waves occur with an unusual morphology of sharply contoured theta waveforms. At the beginning of the plate, a mu rhythm can be observed on the right central region and the vertex.

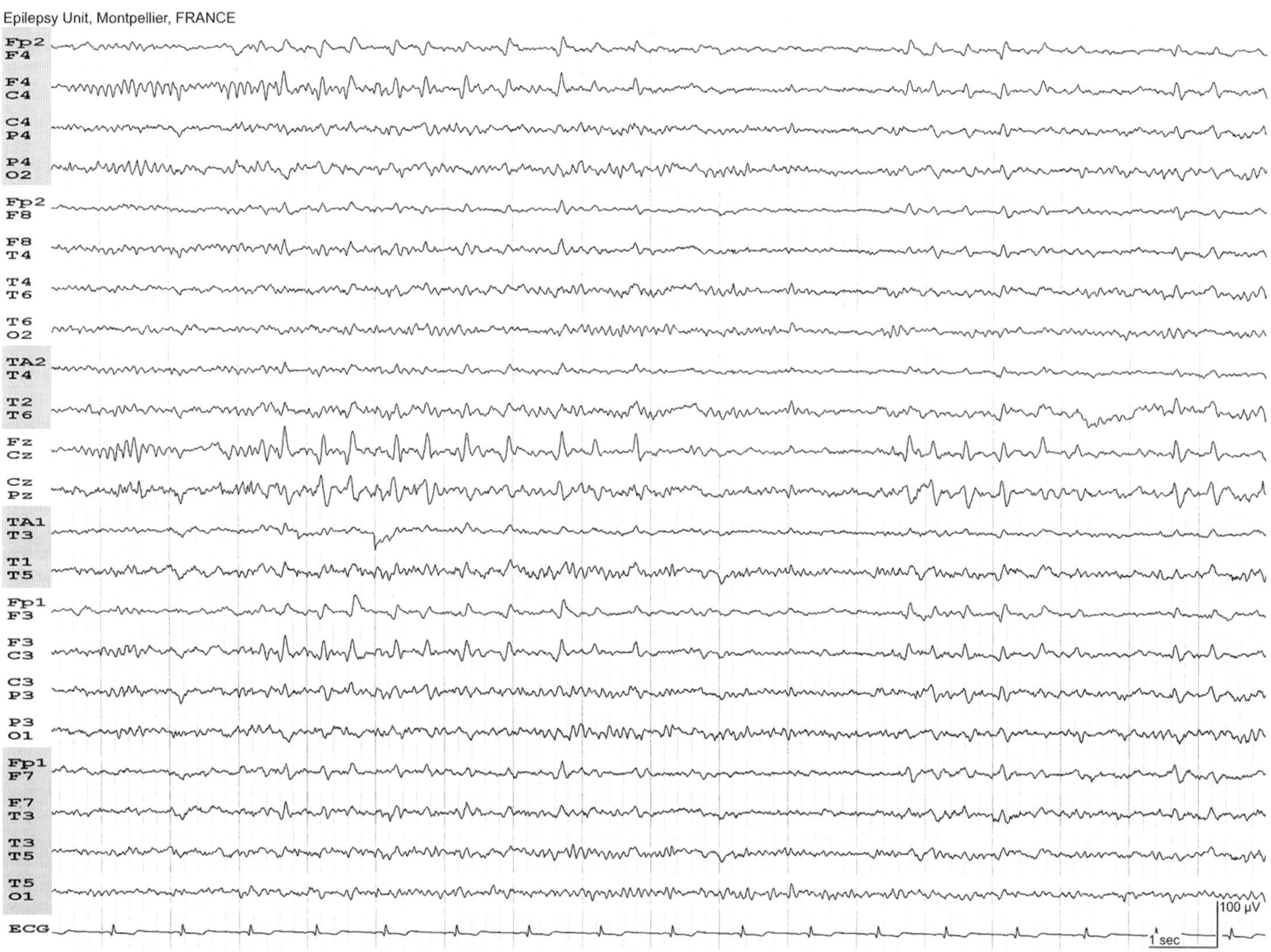

Figure a / Recording at 15 mm/s. Mu rhythm, swatooth waves and alpha activity.

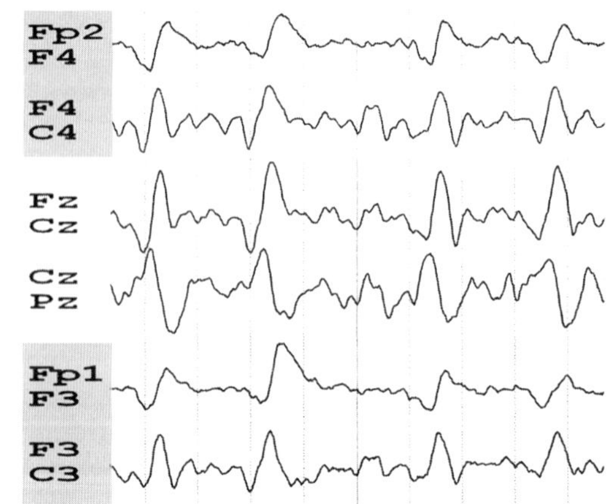

Figure b / Sawtooth waves.

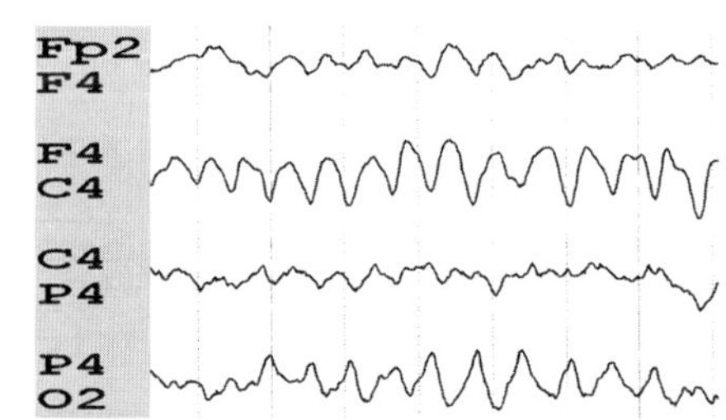

Figure c / Mu rhythm.

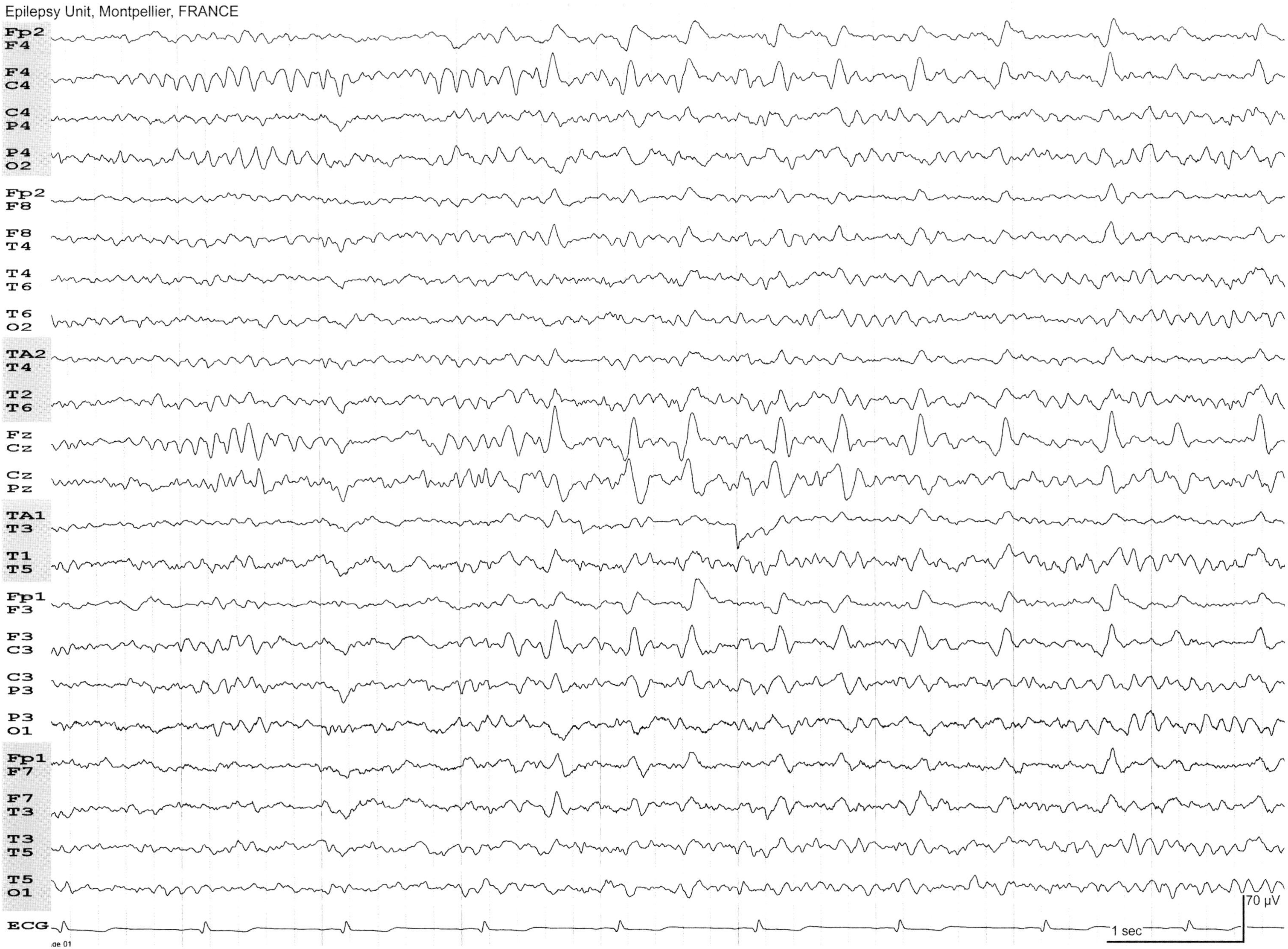
Epilepsy Unit, Montpellier, FRANCE
Fp2 F4
F4 C4
C4 P4
P4 O2
Fp2 F8
F8 T4
T4 T6
T6 O2
TA2 T4
T2 T6
Fz Cz
Cz Pz
TA1 T3
T1 T5
Fp1 F3
F3 C3
C3 P3
P3 O1
Fp1 F7
F7 T3
T3 T5
T5 O1
ECG
70 µV
1 sec

III • 33 REM sleep: sawtooth waves and muscle twitches

Context

42-year-old woman with cryptogenic left temporal lobe epilepsy, presurgical assessment.

What to note

REM sleep. Low-voltage background activity and sawtooth waves on the vertex. Note the muscle artifacts over the right and left hemispheres corresponding to muscle twitches.

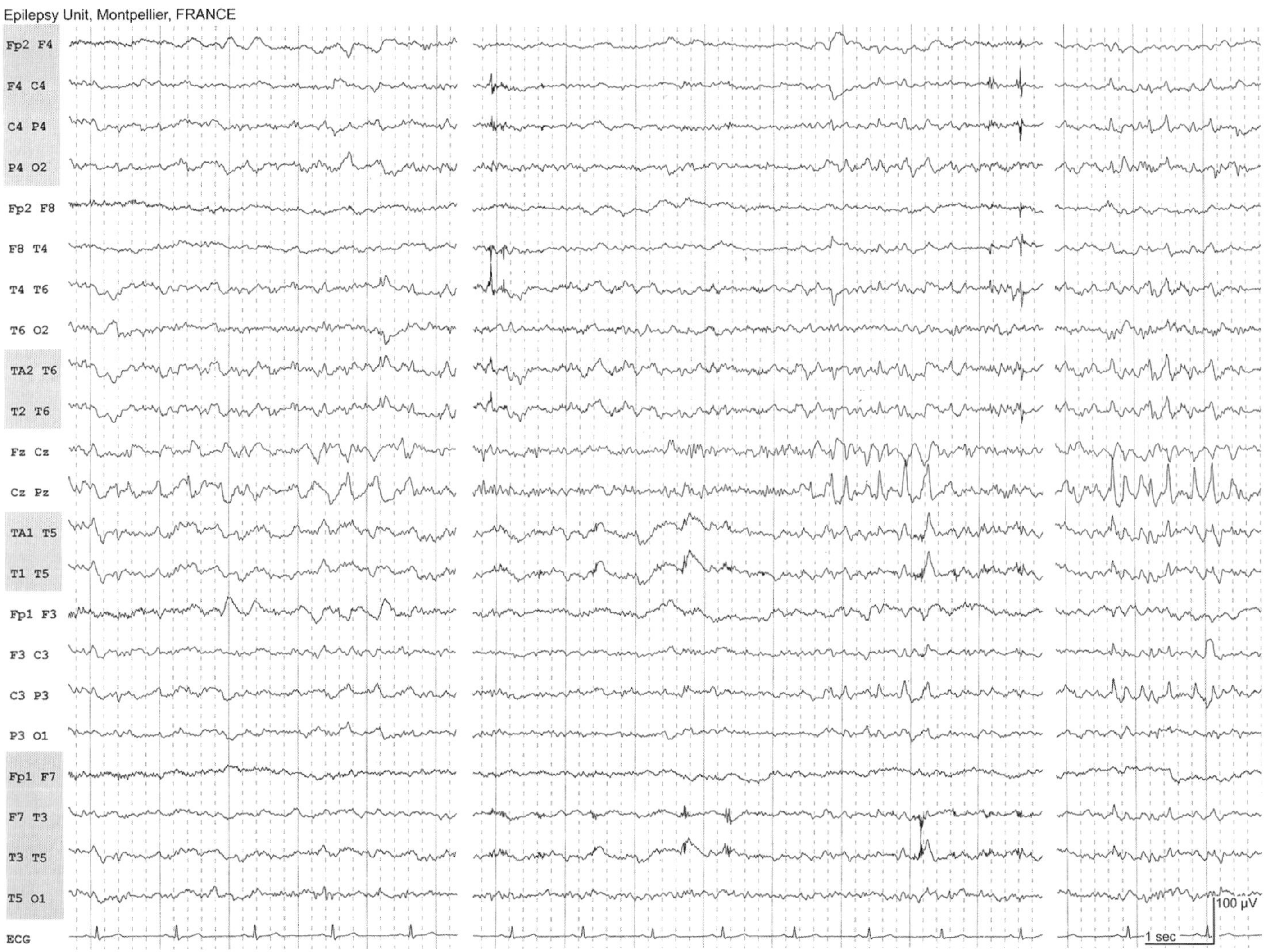

Figure a / Recording at 15 mm/s. Note that several presentations of sawtooth waves can occur in the same patient. At center and on right, the sawtooth waves mimic spikes.

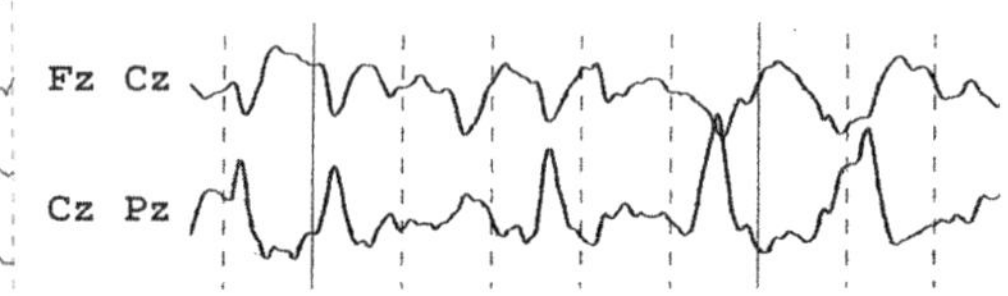

Figure b / Sawtooth waves.

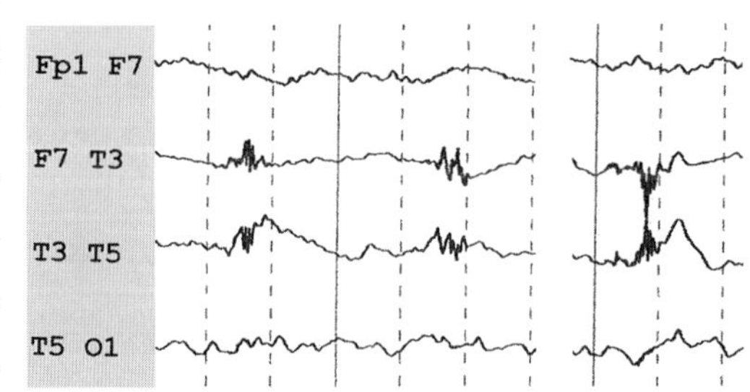

Figure c / Muscle twitches.

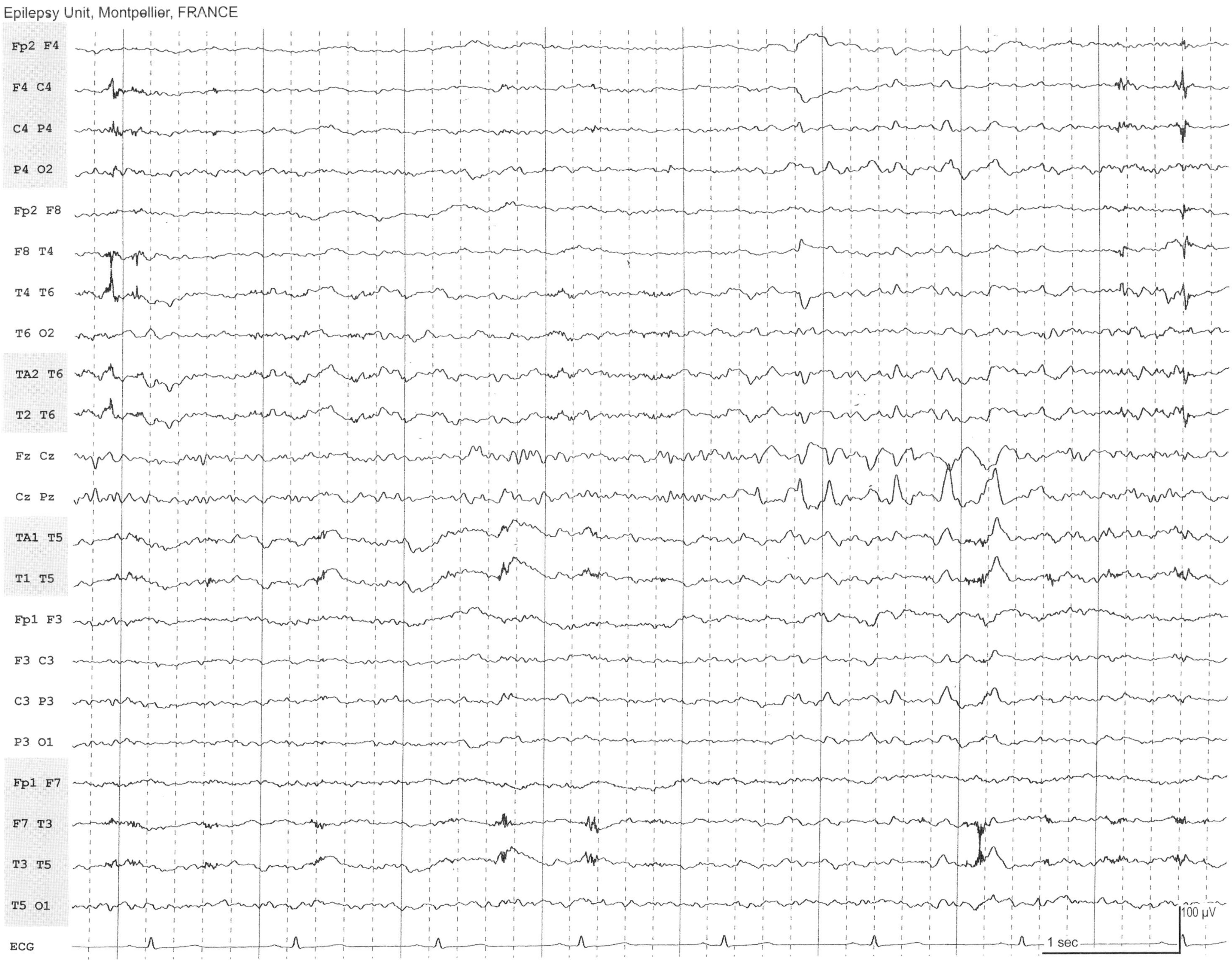
Epilepsy Unit, Montpellier, FRANCE
Fp2 F4
F4 C4
C4 P4
P4 O2
Fp2 F8
F8 T4
T4 T6
T6 O2
TA2 T6
T2 T6
Fz Cz
Cz Pz
TA1 T5
T1 T5
Fp1 F3
F3 C3
C3 P3
P3 O1
Fp1 F7
F7 T3
T3 T5
T5 O1
ECG
100 µV
1 sec

III • 34 REM sleep: posterior theta rhythm

Context

64-year-old woman with drug resistant epilepsy, later diagnosed as psychogenic seizures.

What to note

REM sleep with rapid eye movements at the end of the plate. Background theta activity at 4.5 Hz. Some waves are forked. Note the electrode artifact at Cz due to poor impedance.

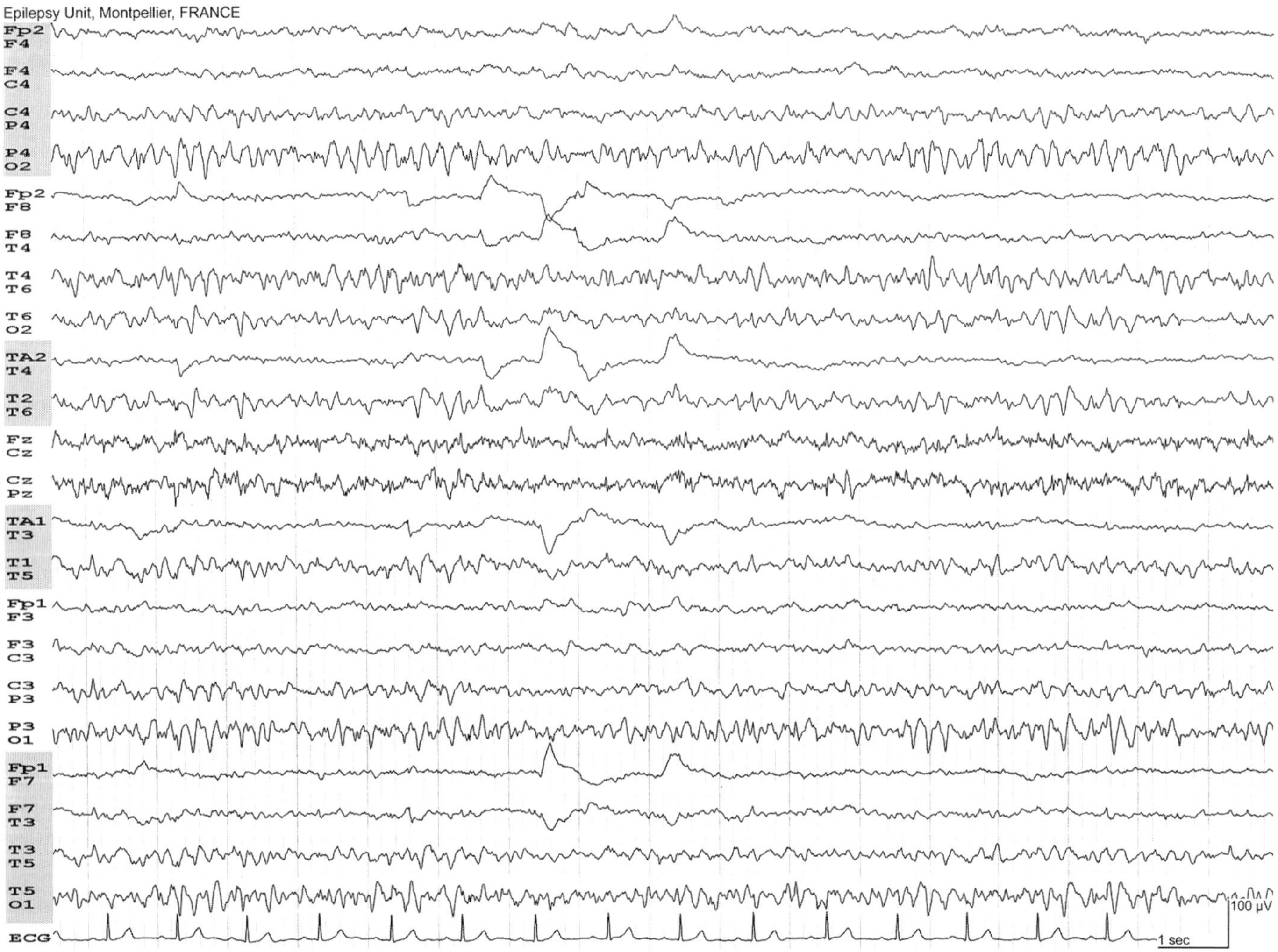

Figure a / Recording at 15 mm/s.

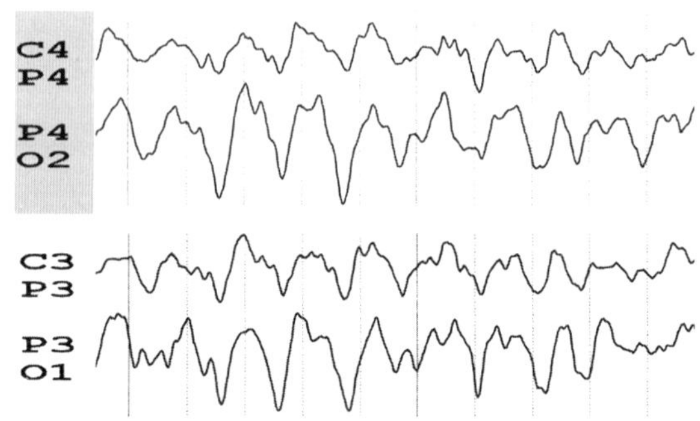

Figure b / Theta activity.

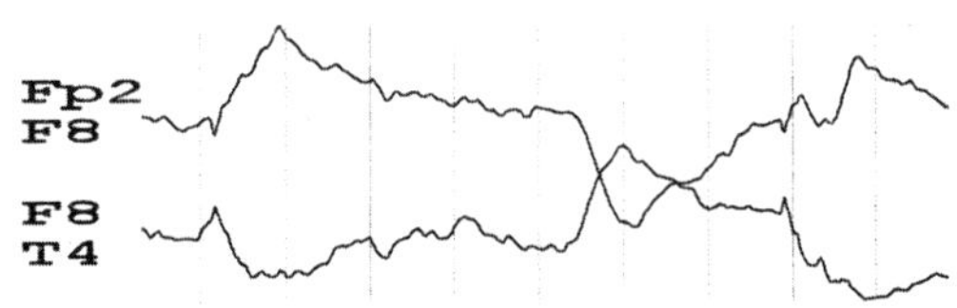

Figure c / Rapid eye movements over the right frontal polar region.

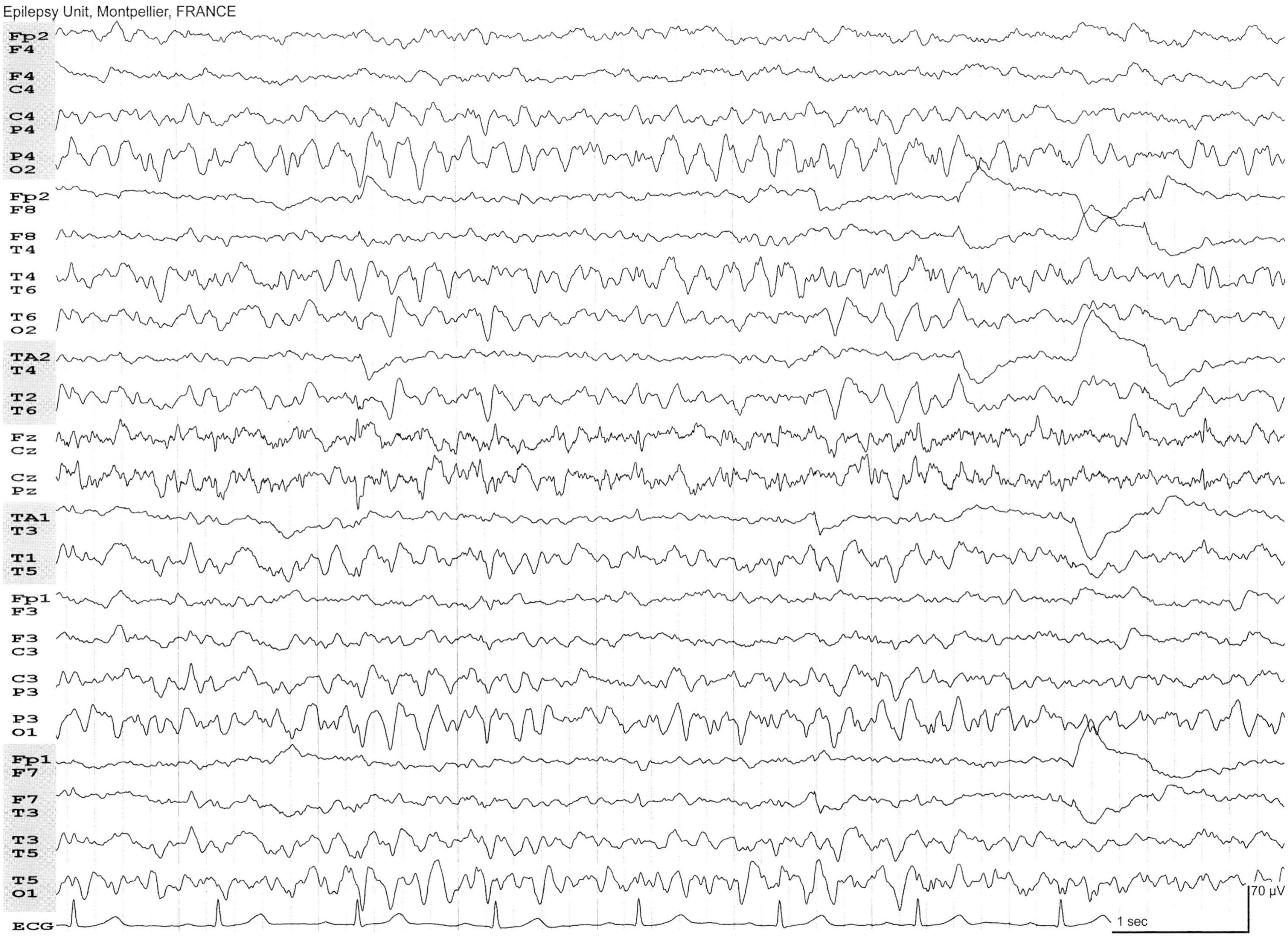

Epilepsy Unit, Montpellier, FRANCE
Fp2 F4
F4 C4
C4 P4
P4 O2
Fp2 F8
F8 T4
T4 T6
T6 O2
TA2 T4
T2 T6
Fz Cz
Cz Pz
TA1 T3
T1 T5
Fp1 F3
F3 C3
C3 P3
P3 O1
Fp1 F7
F7 T3
T3 T5
T5 O1
ECG
70 µV
1 sec

III • 35 REM sleep: Slow alpha variant

Context

49-year-old woman referred for epilepsy follow-up. Same patient as plate I-8.

What to note

REM sleep with atonia on the chin EMG derivation and rapid eye movement artifacts on the right segment. On the occipital regions, burst of notched theta waves at 5 Hz corresponding to a slow alpha variant. See plate I-8 for the same patient during wakefulness. The morphology and the topography of the theta waves are identical.

Comment

REM sleep is a stage of sleep that contains rhythms similar to those seen during wakefulness and drowsiness. Slow alpha variant has been reported in REM sleep especially during the tonic phases (Gelisse & Crespel; 2008; Crespel *et al.*, 2009). This observation confirms that the slow alpha-variant rhythm shares the same characteristics of the alpha rhythm.

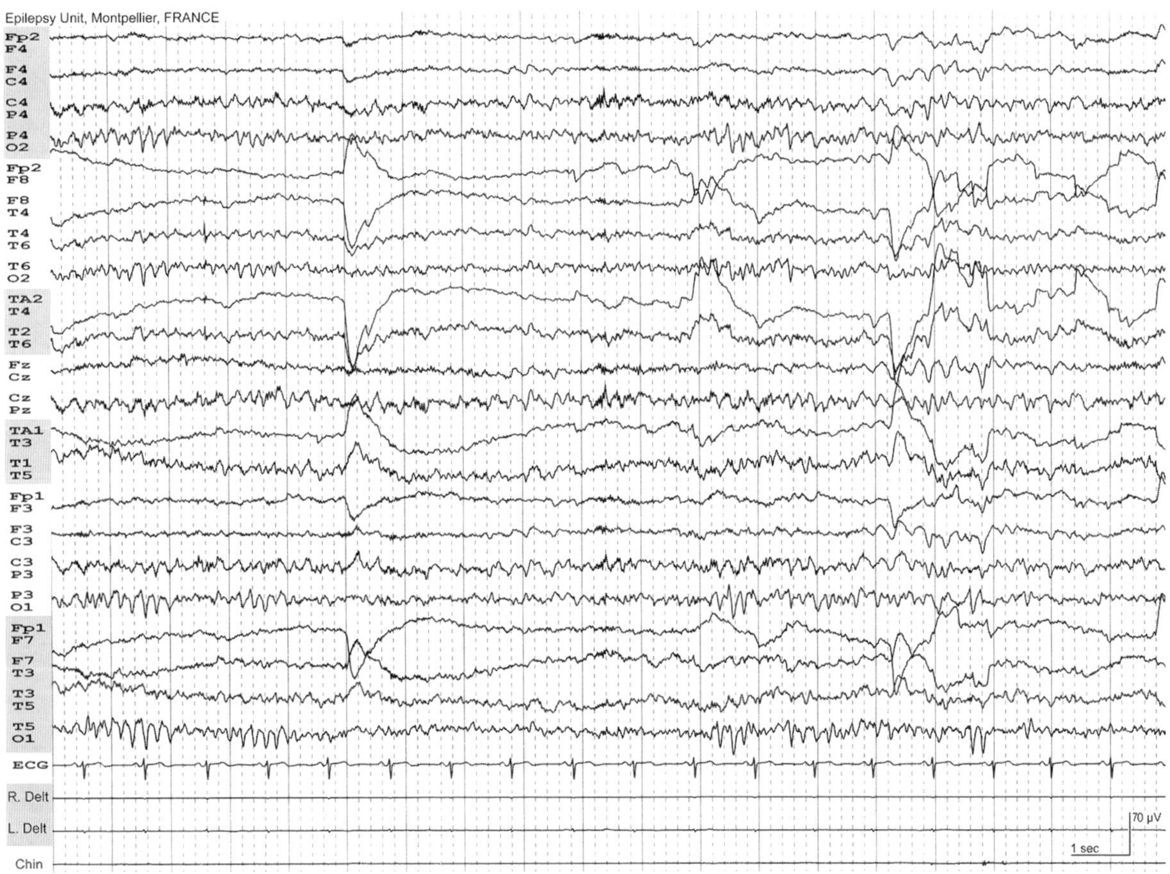

Figure a / Recording at 15 mm/s. Another example of slow alpha variant during REM sleep during the same recording.

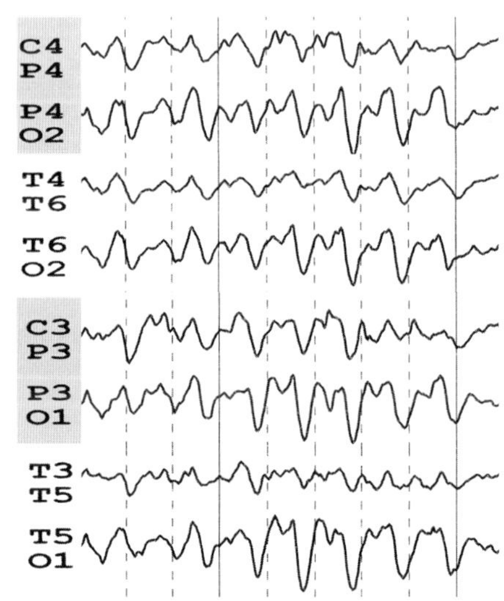

Figure b / Slow alpha variant during REM sleep.

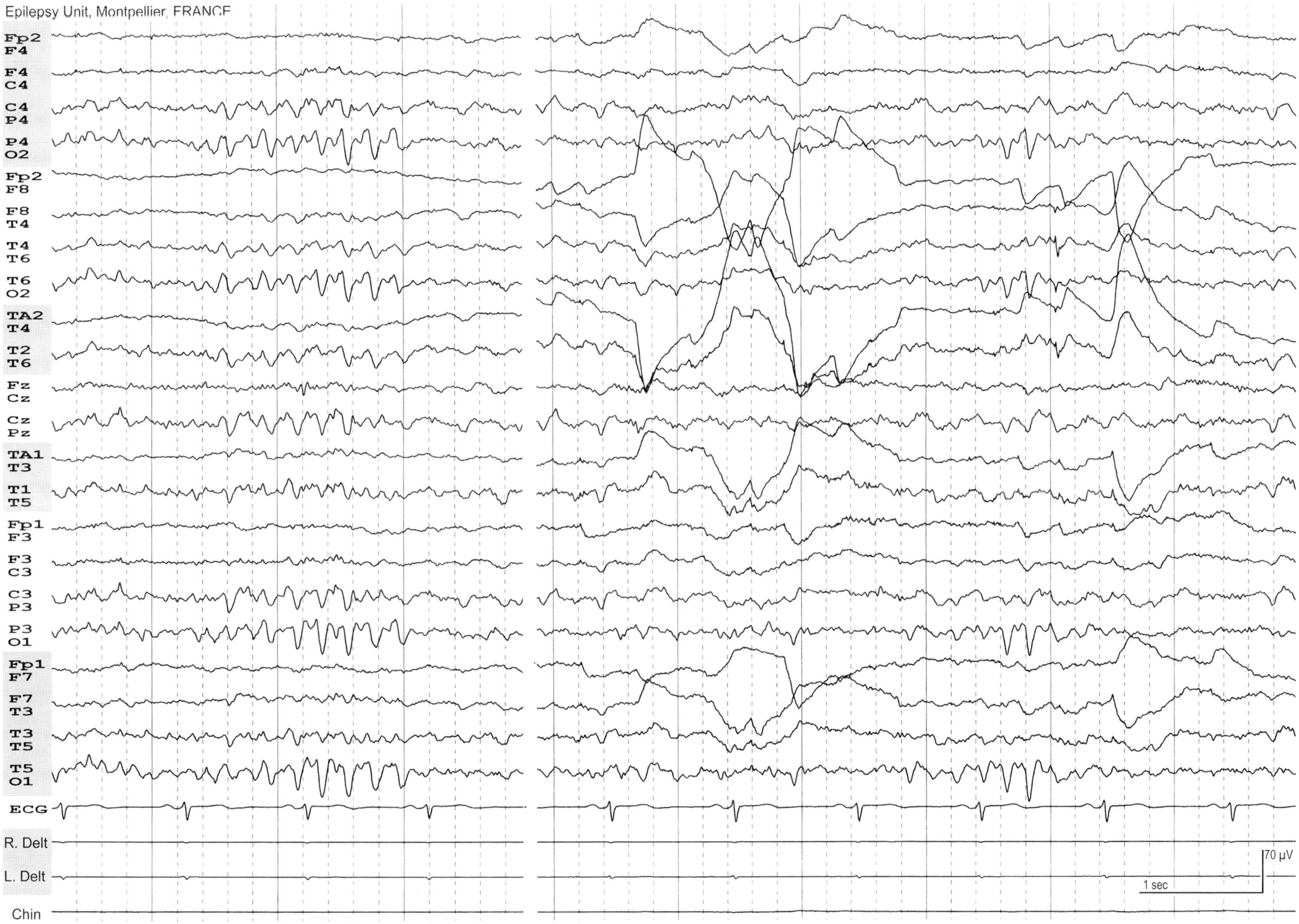
Epilepsy Unit, Montpellier, FRANCE
Fp2 F4
F4 C4
C4 P4
P4 O2
Fp2 F8
F8 T4
T4 T6
T6 O2
TA2 T4
T2 T6
Fz Cz
Cz Pz
TA1 T3
T1 T5
Fp1 F3
F3 C3
C3 P3
P3 O1
Fp1 F7
F7 T3
T3 T5
T5 O1
ECG
R. Delt
L. Delt
Chin
70 µV
1 sec

III • 36 REM sleep: beta rhythms

Context

59-year-old man with focal epilepsy symptomatic of right insular cavernoma.

What to note

REM sleep. Rapid eye movements and muscle atonia (chin) can be observed. Low-voltage background. Note the occurrence of beta rhythms over the anterior regions on this plate.

Comment

Beta rhythms are usually enhanced during drowsiness, disappear in NREM sleep and reappear in REM sleep.

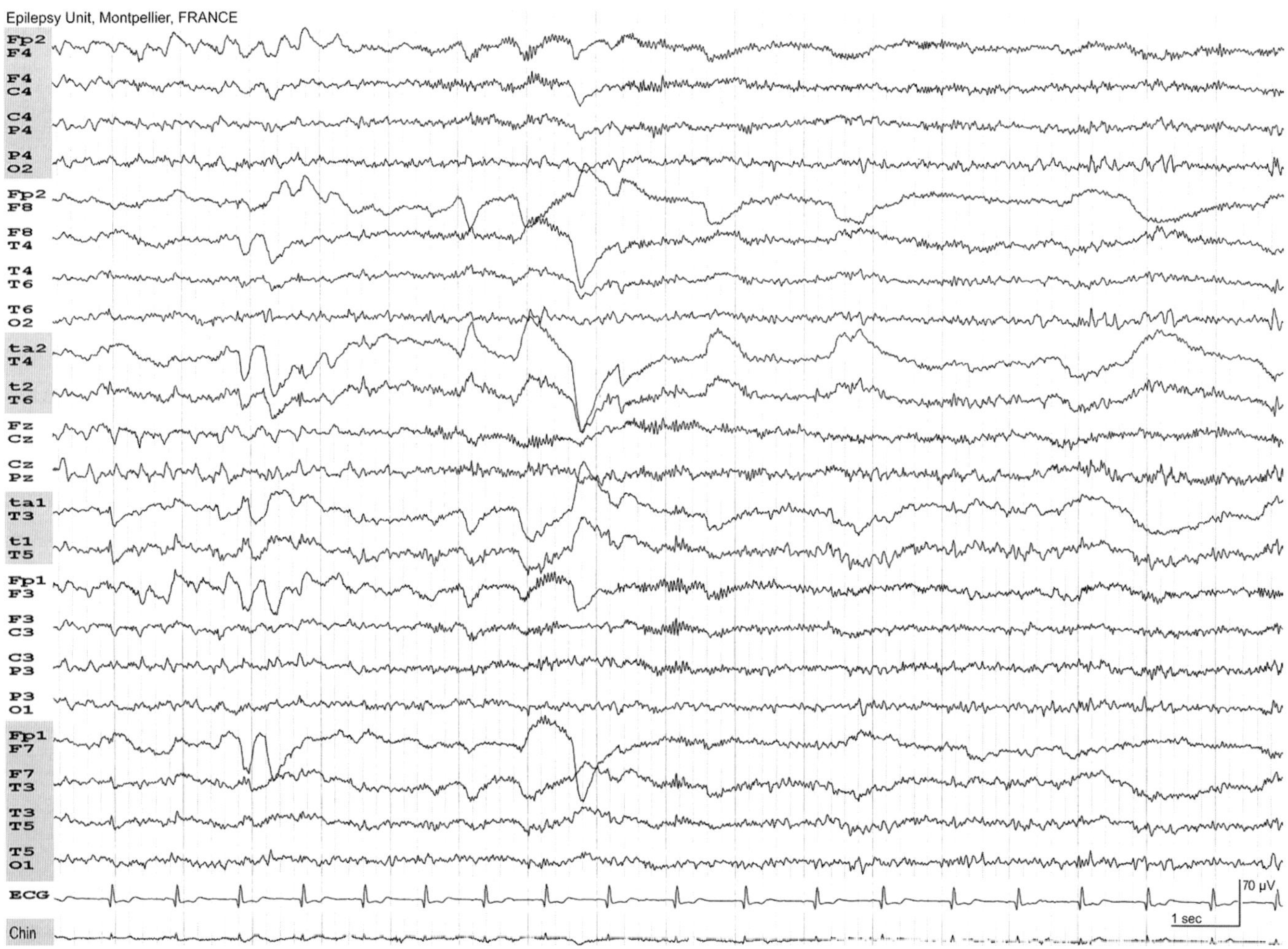

Figure a / Recording at 15 mm/s. Note at the beginning of the plate, the presence of sawtooth waves on the vertex.

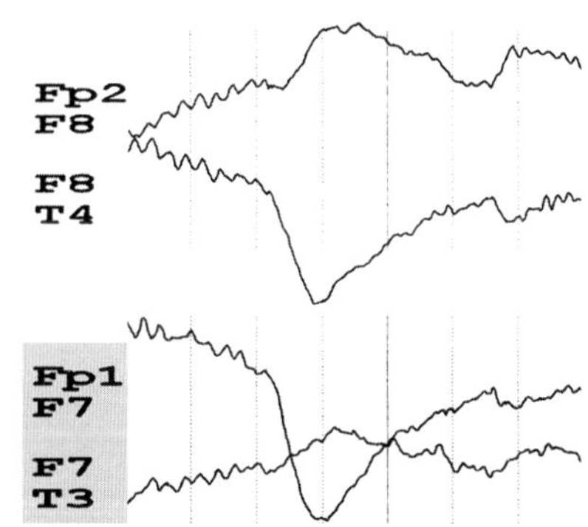

Figure b / Rapid eye movements over the frontal polar regions.

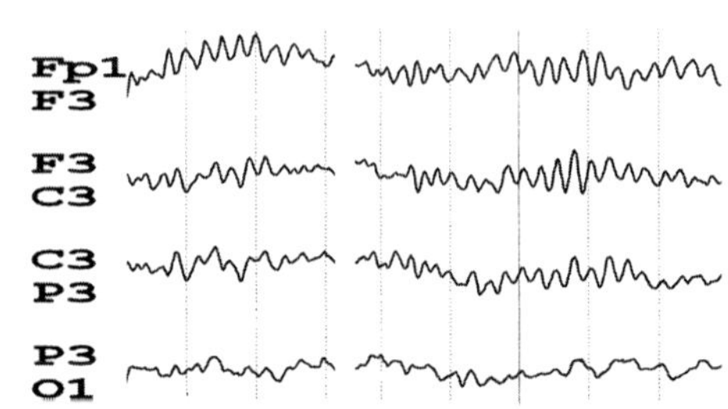

Figure c / Beta rhythms.

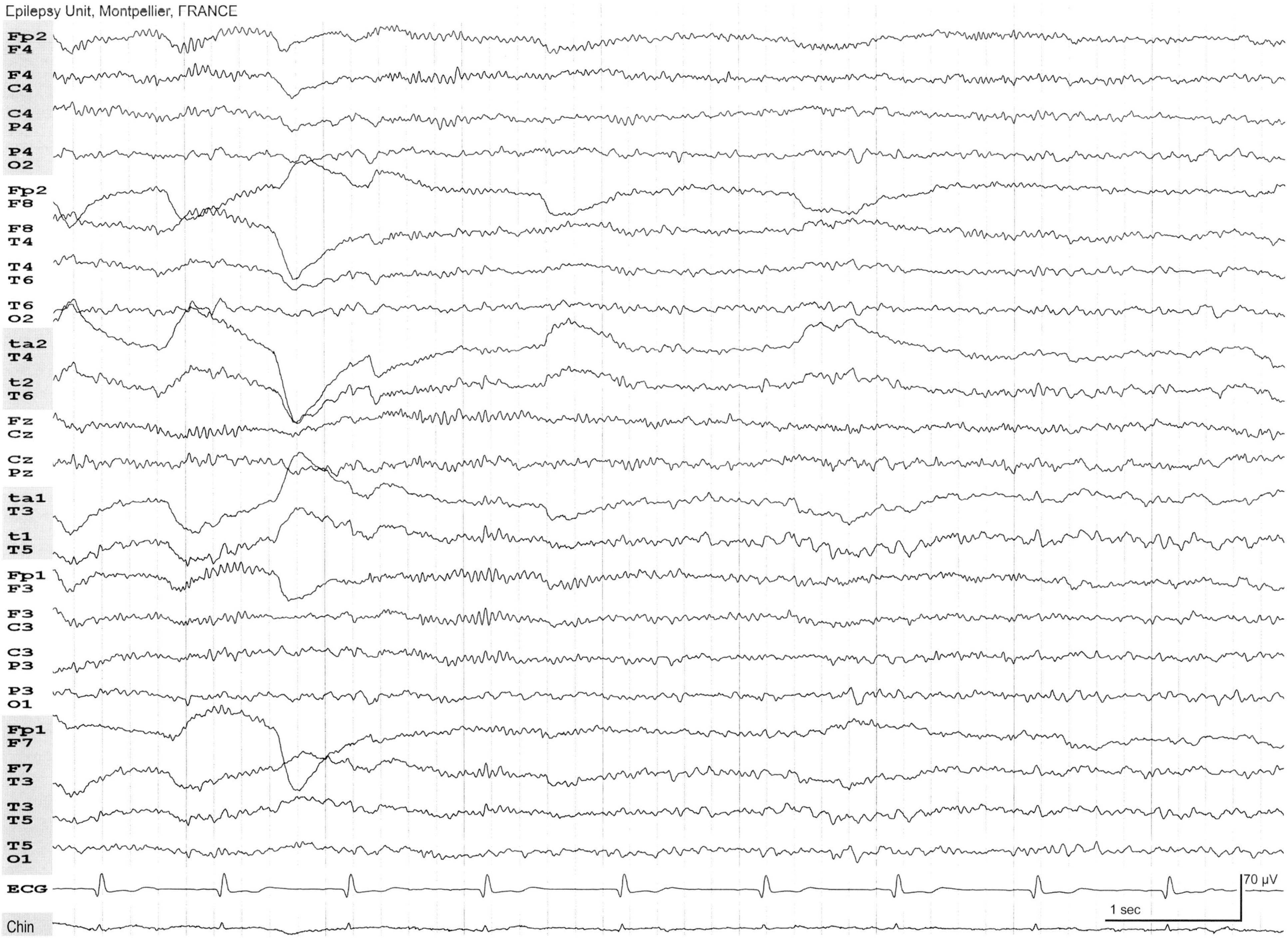
Epilepsy Unit, Montpellier, FRANCE
Fp2 F4
F4 C4
C4 P4
P4 O2
Fp2 F8
F8 T4
T4 T6
T6 O2
ta2 T4
t2 T6
Fz Cz
Cz Pz
ta1 T3
t1 T5
Fp1 F3
F3 C3
C3 P3
P3 O1
Fp1 F7
F7 T3
T3 T5
T5 O1
ECG
Chin
70 µV
1 sec

• 37 REM sleep: beta rhythms, muscle atonia and muscle twitches

Context

43-year-old man with cryptogenic right medial temporal lobe epilepsy, presurgical assessment.

What to note

REM sleep. Left, theta-like sawtooth waves on the vertex, rapid eye movements over the frontal polar regions, physiological fast beta rhythms and muscle atonia. Right, rapid eye movements, theta-like sawtooth waves, and muscle atonia can be observed alternating with twitches recorded only at the EMG chin derivation.

Comment

Pharmacological substances such as benzodiazepines, barbiturates induce reactivation of beta rhythms in REM sleep.

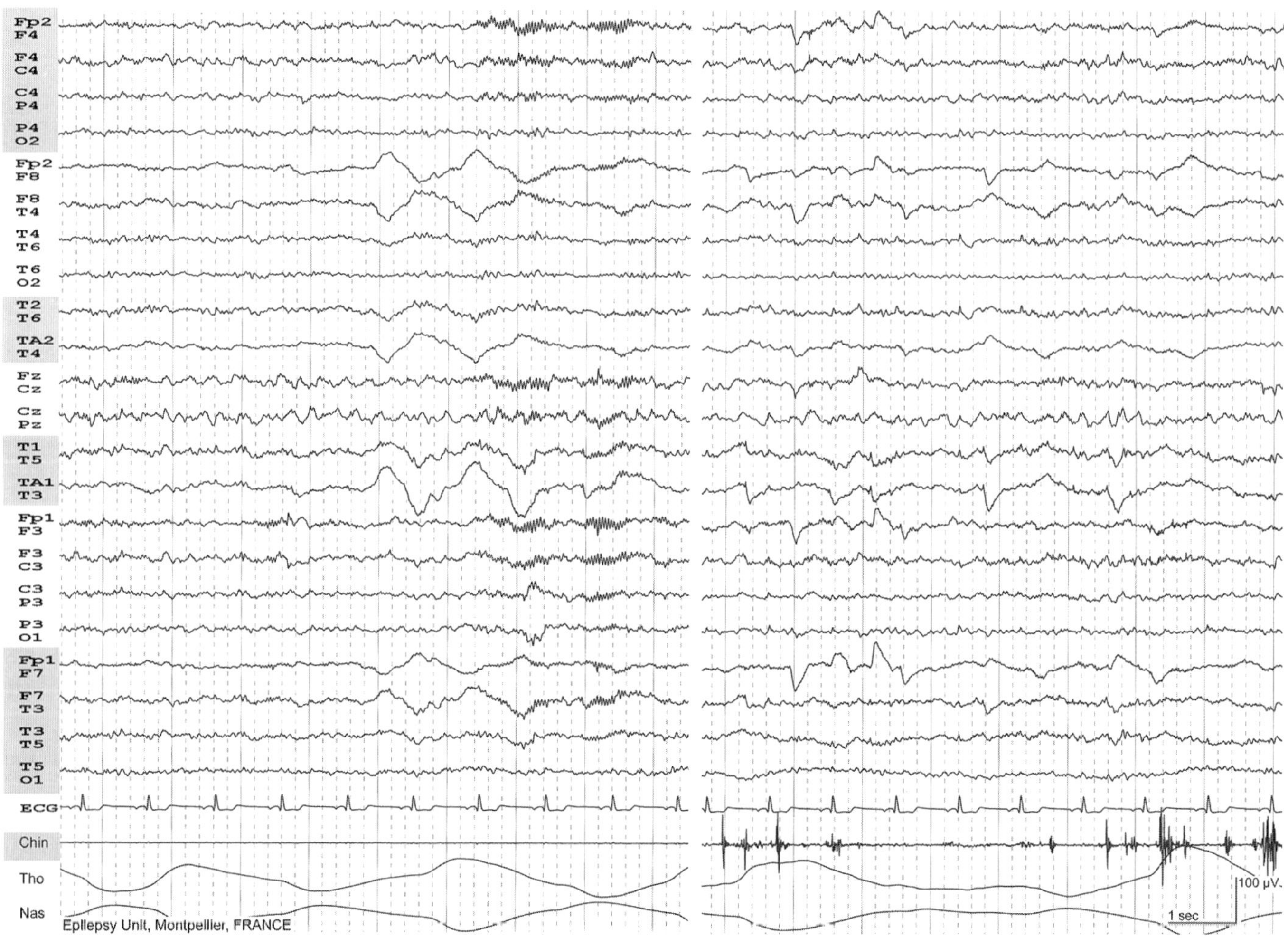

Figure a / Recording at 15 mm/s.

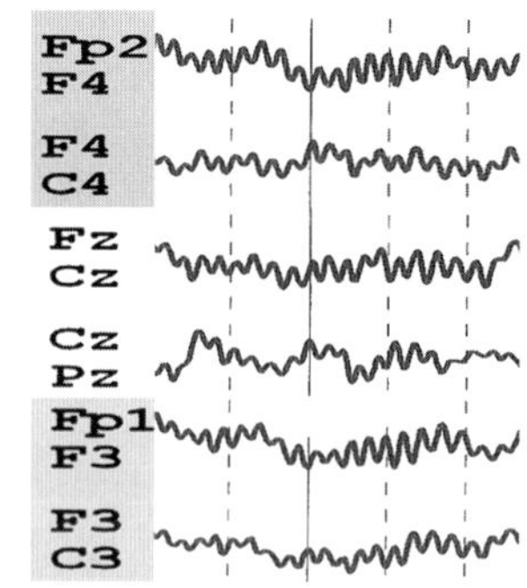

Figure b / Beta rhythms.

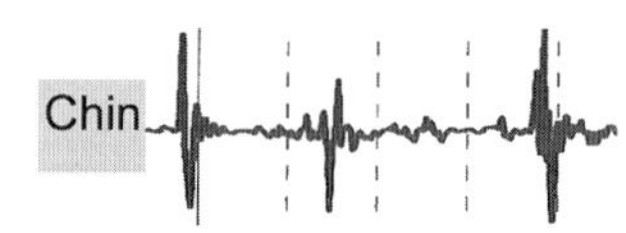

Figure c / Muscle twitches on the chin EMG alternating with muscle atonia.

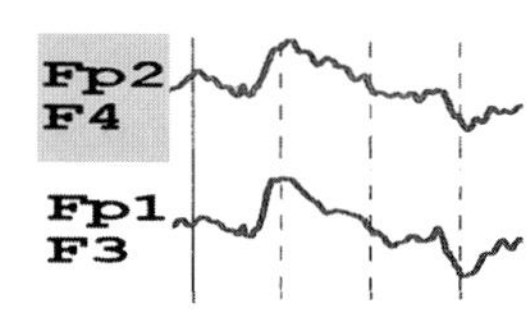

Figure d / Rapid eye movements.

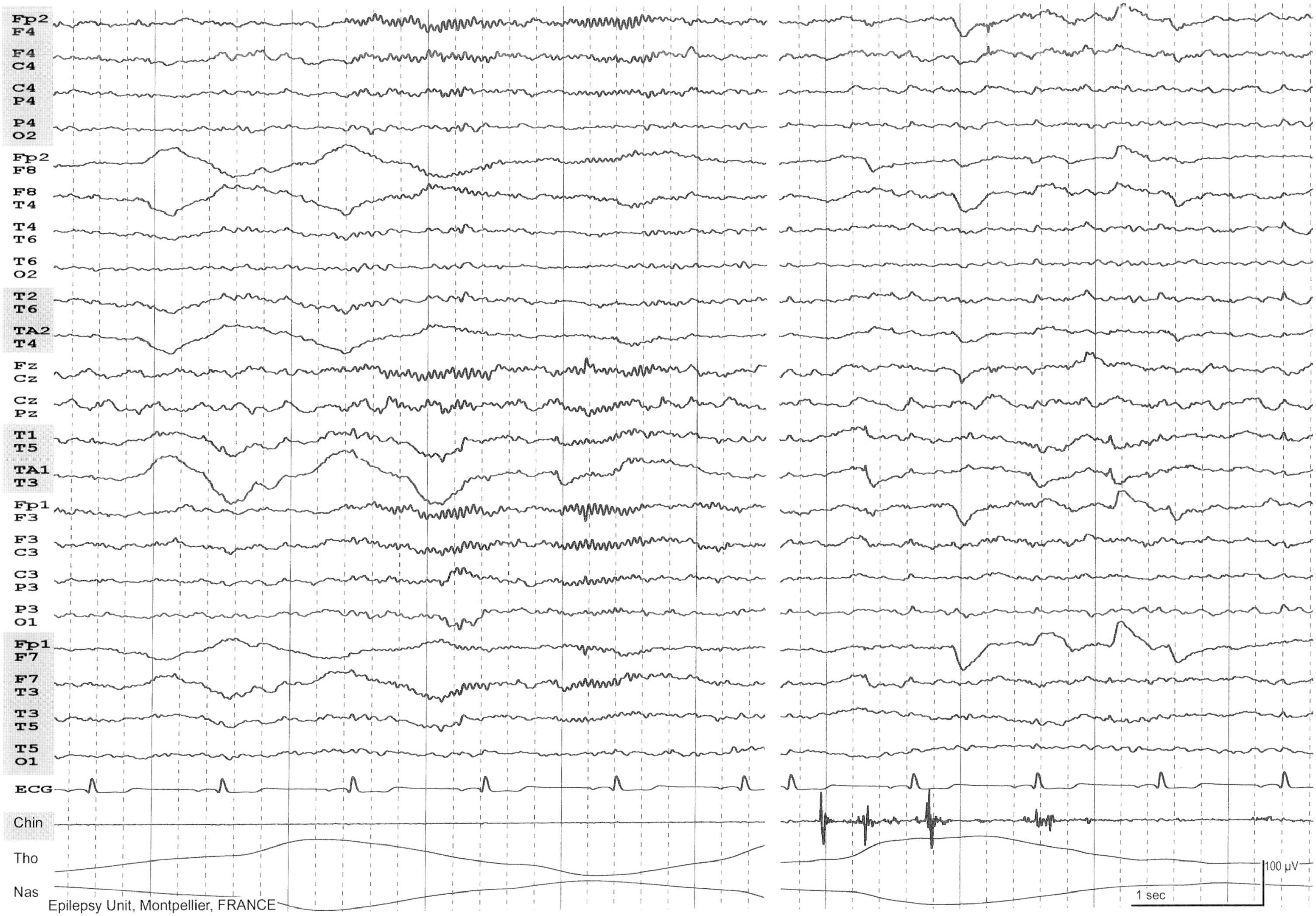

Fp2 F4
F4 C4
C4 P4
P4 O2
Fp2 F8
F8 T4
T4 T6
T6 O2
T2 T6
TA2 T4
Fz Cz
Cz Pz
T1 T5
TA1 T3
Fp1 F3
F3 C3
C3 P3
P3 O1
Fp1 F7
F7 T3
T3 T5
T5 O1
ECG
Chin
Tho
Nas
Epilepsy Unit, Montpellier, FRANCE
100 µV
1 sec

III • 38 Transient arousal

Context

48-year-old woman, operated 3 years earlier for right mesial temporal lobe epilepsy.

What to note

The patient is asleep. Fast activities (20 Hz) with predominance over the right fronto-temporal regions intermixed with theta and alpha waves. This corresponds to a transient arousal reaction from NREM sleep stage 1.

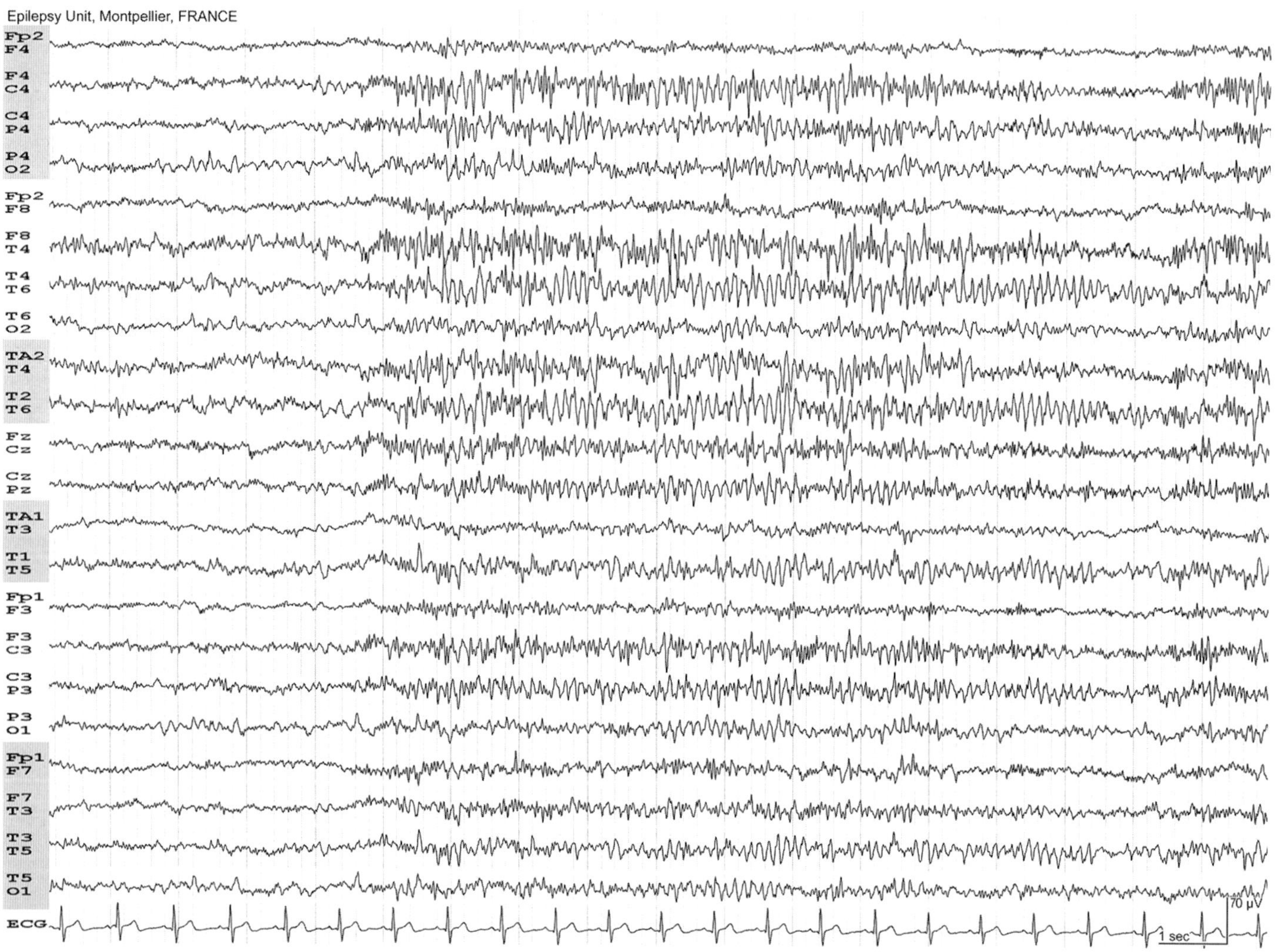

Figure a / Recording at 15 mm/s.

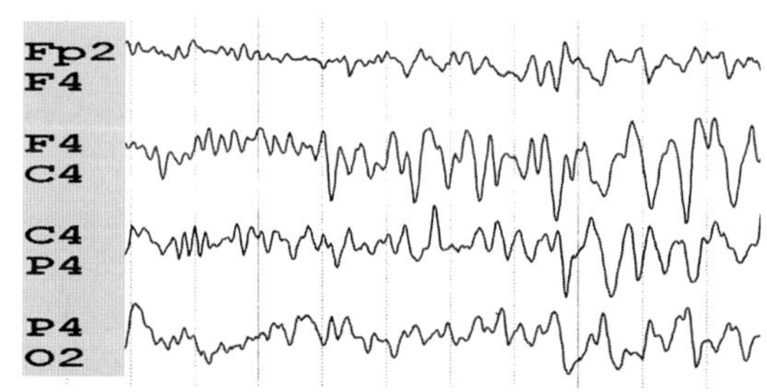

Figure b / Fast activities over the right fronto-central region intermixed with theta waves.

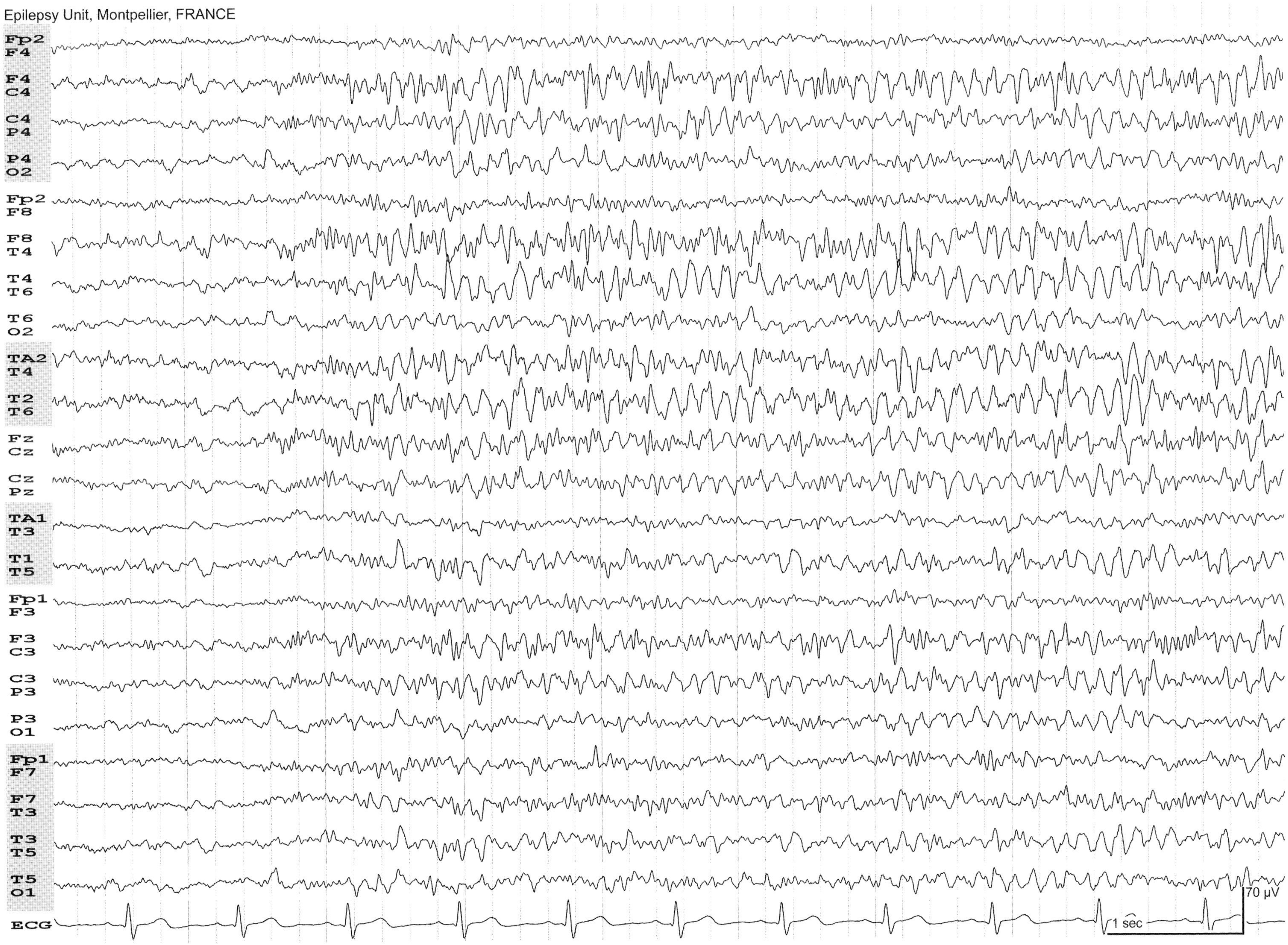
Epilepsy Unit, Montpellier, FRANCE
Fp2 F4
F4 C4
C4 P4
P4 O2
Fp2 F8
F8 T4
T4 T6
T6 O2
TA2 T4
T2 T6
Fz Cz
Cz Pz
TA1 T3
T1 T5
Fp1 F3
F3 C3
C3 P3
P3 O1
Fp1 F7
F7 T3
T3 T5
T5 O1
ECG
70 µV
1 sec

III • 39 Arousal: K alpha

Context

27-year-old man with faints later diagnosed as vasovagal syncopes.

What to note

Stage N2 sleep. K complex preceded by a clearly detectable sleep spindle at Fp2-F4. The morphology of this K complex is characteristic with a strong diphasic deflection over the anterior regions. The K complex is immediately followed by a sleep spindle then a rhythm at 8 Hz lasting 10 seconds corresponding to a "K alpha".

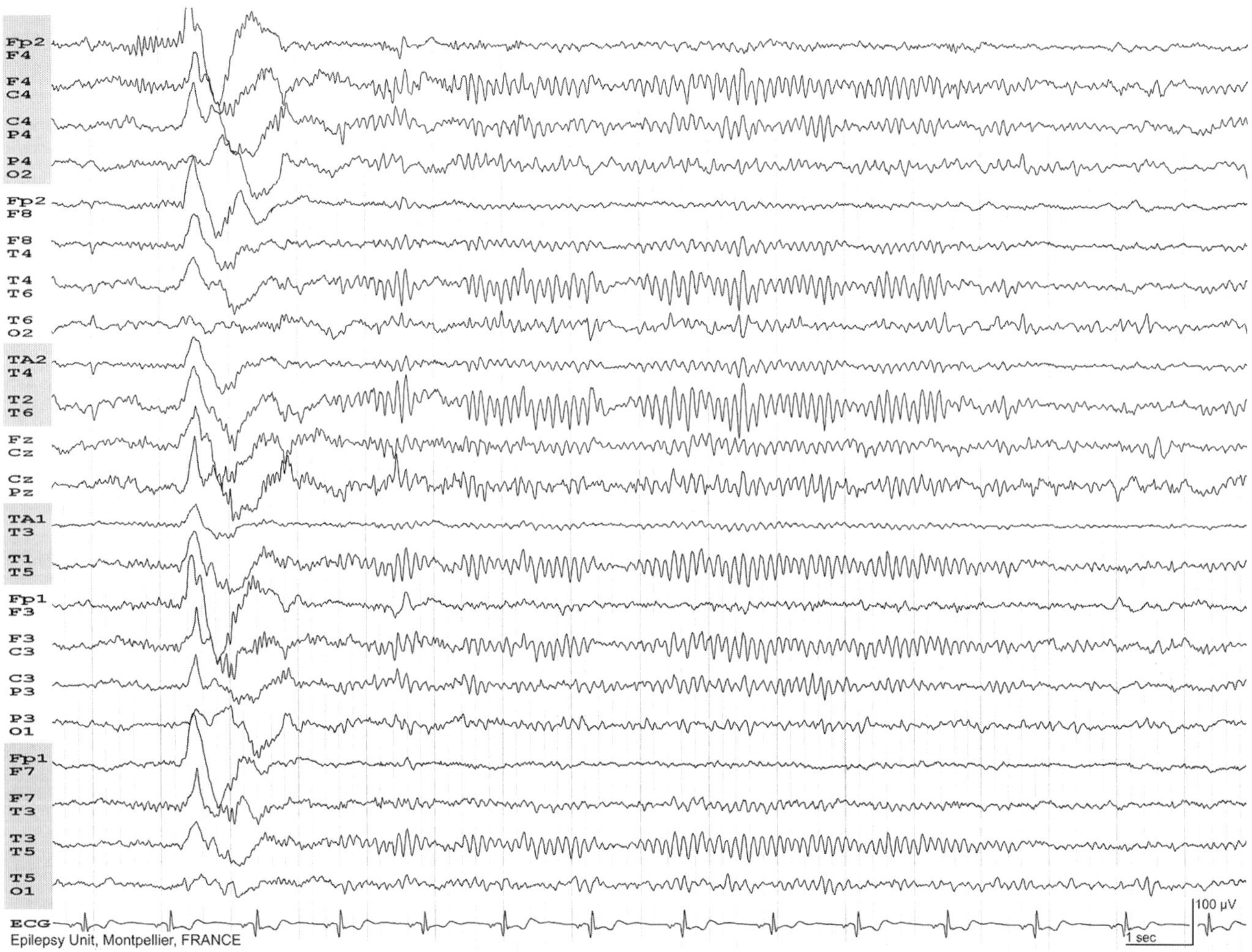

Figure a / Recording at 15 mm/s.

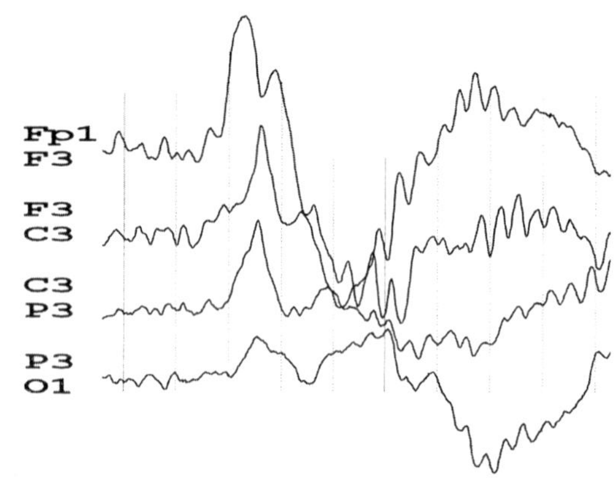

Figure b / K complex immediately followed by a sleep spindle.

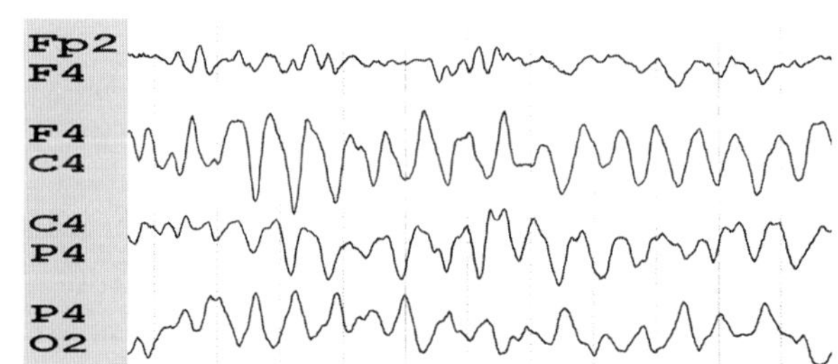

Figure c / Activity at 8 Hz.

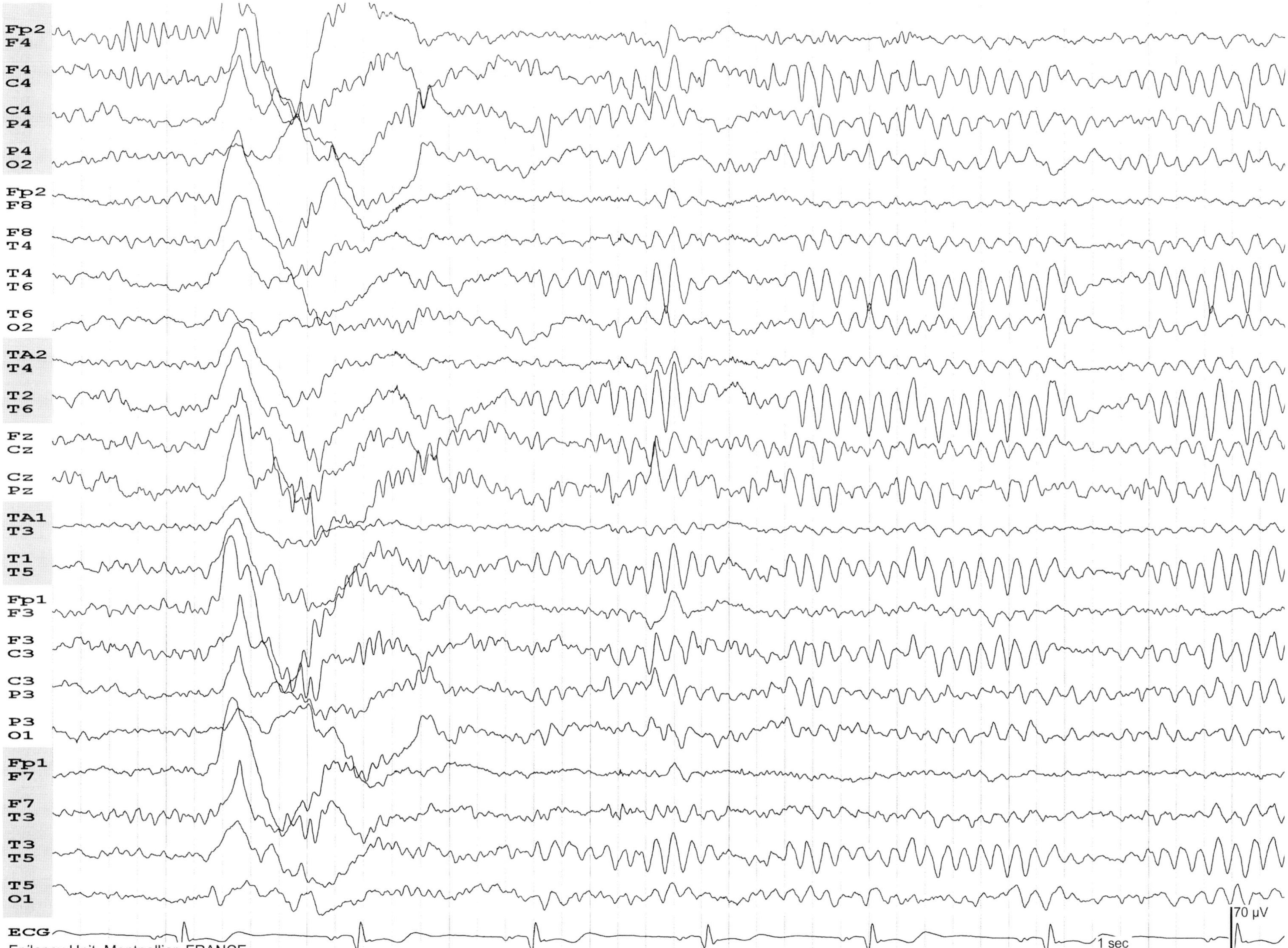

Epilepsy Unit, Montpellier, FRANCE

III • 40 Arousal: Postarousal hypersynchrony in an infant

Context

26-month-old infant referred for assessment after an episode of loss of consciousness.

What to note

Low sensitivity at 20 µV/mm. The infant was woken up from deep sleep at the end of the EEG recording. Note some very ample delta waves with a sinusoidal form which are fronto-central dominant. These delta waves correspond to a postarousal hypersychrony, which is physiological and commonly seen in children under age 5 years. Also note the presence of fast EMG activity at the temporal derivations due to jaw clenching upon arousal.

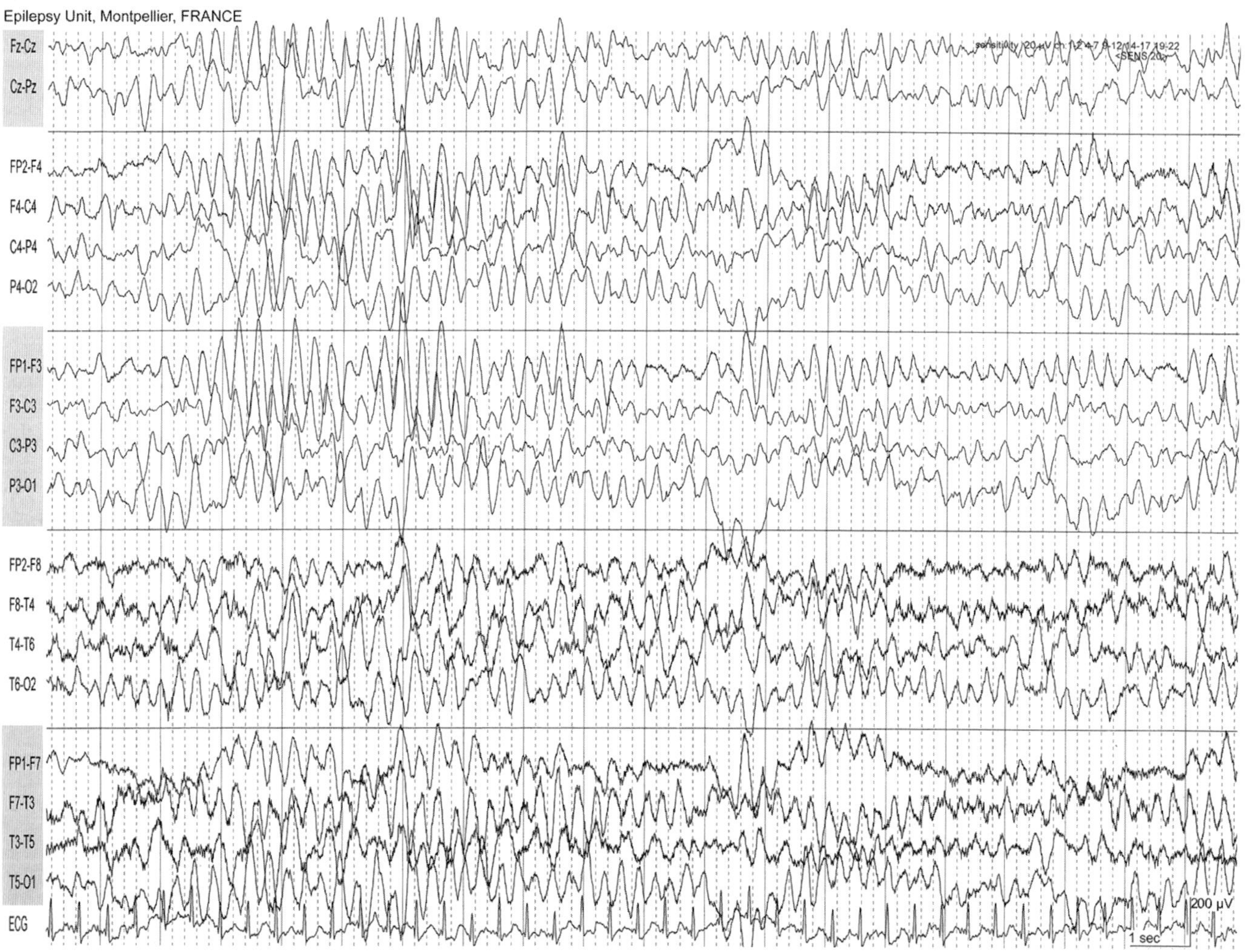

Figure a / Recording at 15 mm/s.

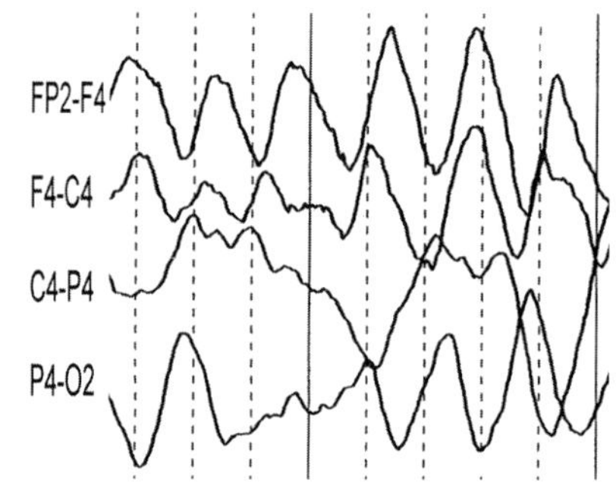

Figure b / During arousal, very ample sinusoidal delta waves occurring with fronto-central predominance (postarousal hypersychrony).

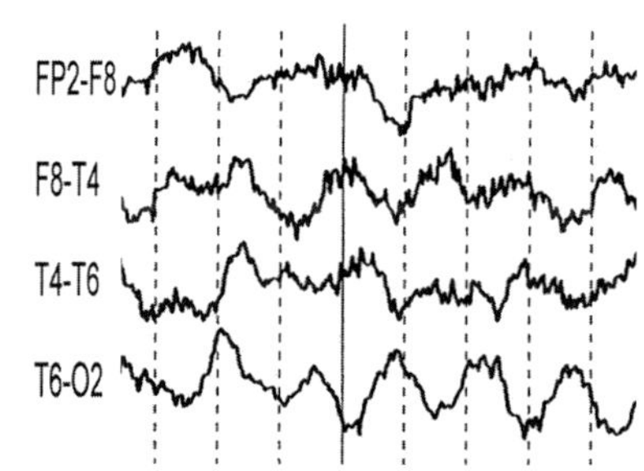

Figure c / Fast EMG activity at the temporal derivations, jaw clenching upon arousal.

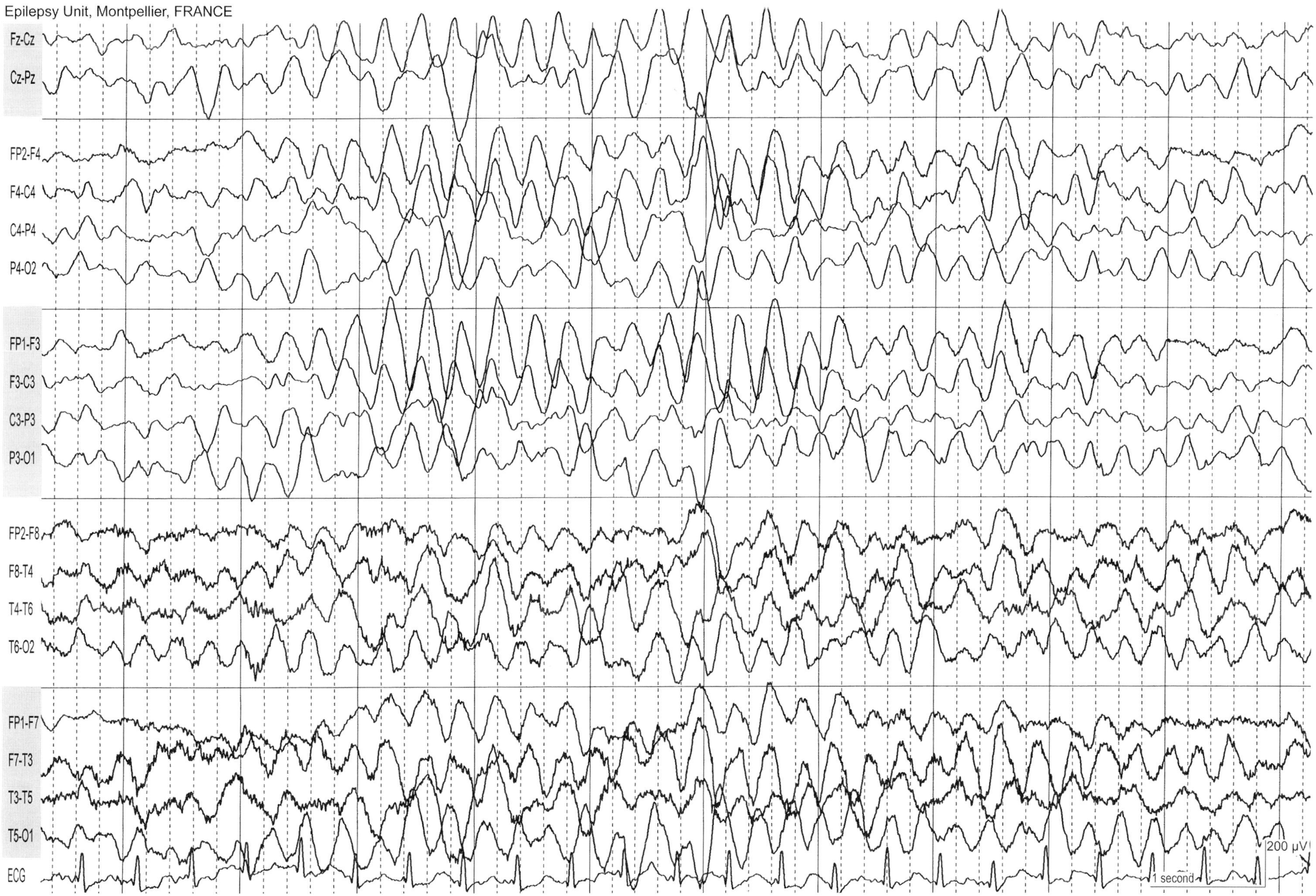
Epilepsy Unit, Montpellier, FRANCE
Fz-Cz
Cz-Pz
FP2-F4
F4-C4
C4-P4
P4-O2
FP1-F3
F3-C3
C3-P3
P3-O1
FP2-F8
F8-T4
T4-T6
T6-O2
FP1-F7
F7-T3
T3-T5
T5-O1
ECG
200 µV
1 second

III • 41 Arousal reaction: Hypersynchronous delta activity (1)

Context

19-year-old woman with photogenic epilepsy (Jeavons syndrome).

What to note

Stage N3 sleep. Arousal reaction with ample delta waves at 1 Hz, predominating frontally. Fast EMG activity at the temporal derivations due to jaw clenching upon arousal.

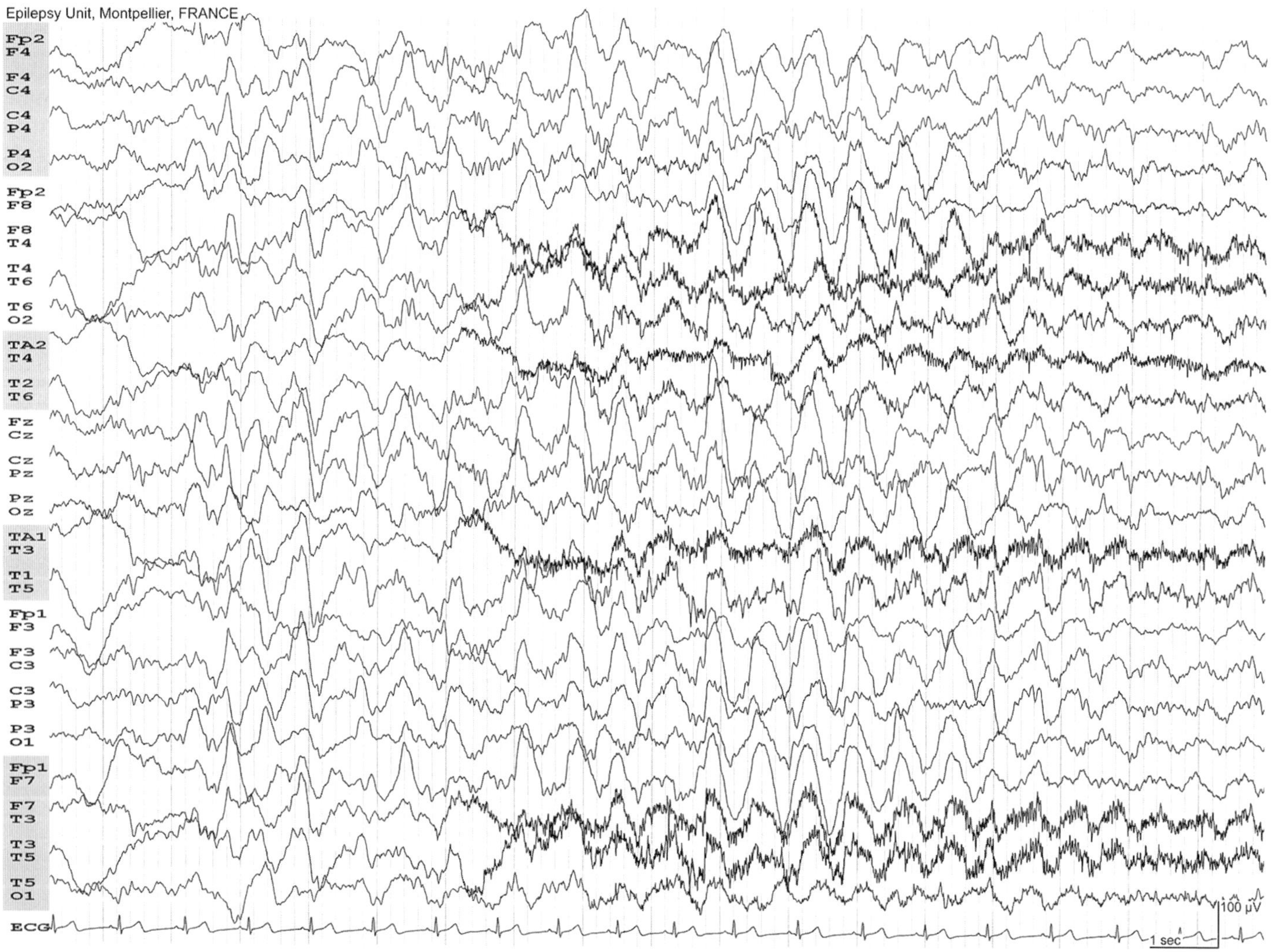

Figure a / Recording at 15 mm/s.

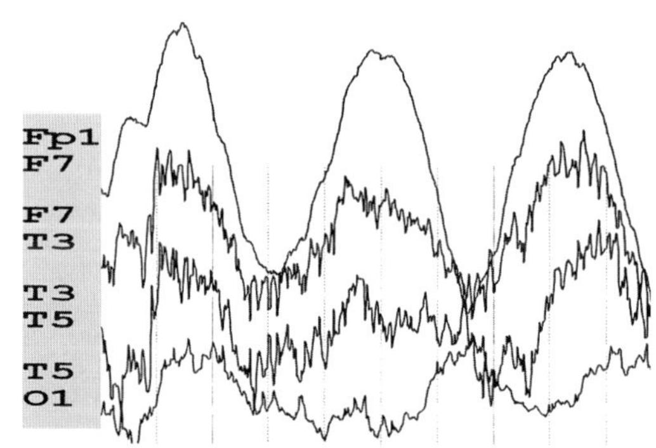

Figure b / Delta waves at 1 Hz.

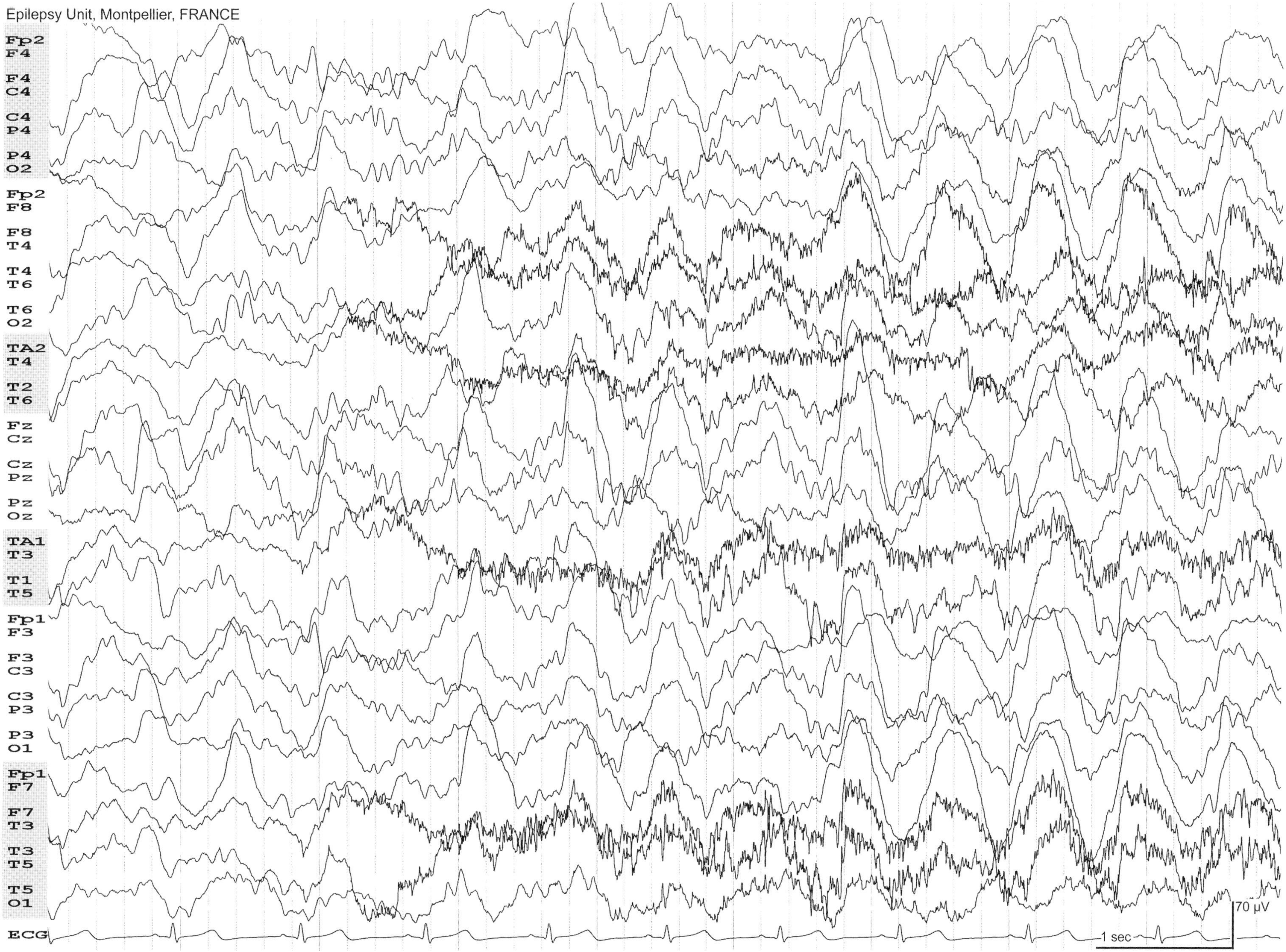
Epilepsy Unit, Montpellier, FRANCE
Fp2 F4
F4 C4
C4 P4
P4 O2
Fp2 F8
F8 T4
T4 T6
T6 O2
TA2 T4
T2 T6
Fz Cz
Cz Pz
Pz Oz
TA1 T3
T1 T5
Fp1 F3
F3 C3
C3 P3
P3 O1
Fp1 F7
F7 T3
T3 T5
T5 O1
ECG
70 µV
1 sec

III • 42 Arousal reaction: Hypersynchronous delta activity (2)

Context

20-year-old man with left temporal lobe epilepsy, presurgical assessment.

What to note

The man is in NREM stage 3 with high-amplitude slow wave activity. Arousal reaction with very-high-amplitude monomorphous, hypersynchronic slow waves, lasting approximately 20 seconds and occurring several times during deep sleep without any clinical signs. Accelerated heart rate and increased muscle activity on the chin and on the temporal derivations indicate lighter sleep.

Comment

These hypersynchronic slow waves correspond to arousal reactions, which occur during stage N3 sleep. These waves, which express a change of deep sleep organization, occur mostly in patients with parasomnias in deep sleep (arousal disorders).

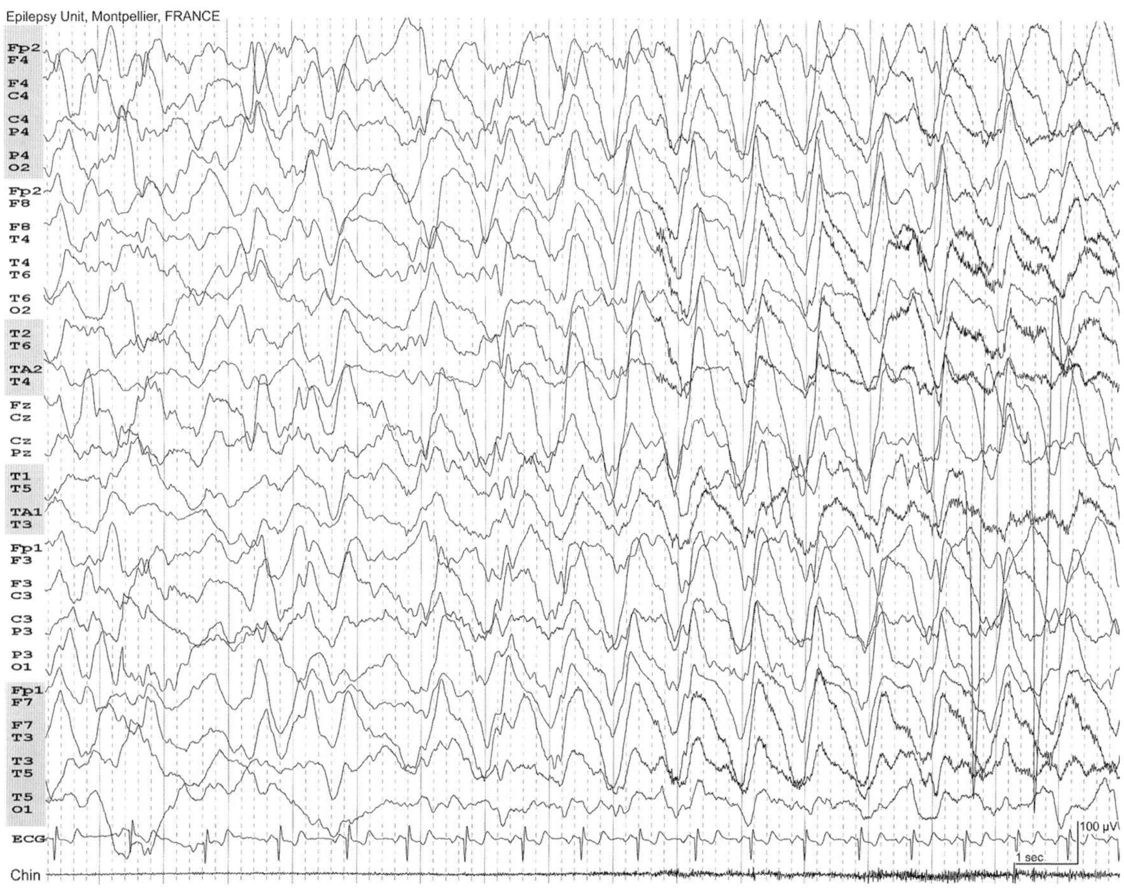

Figure a / Recording at 15 mm/s. Note the accelerated cardiac rhythm.

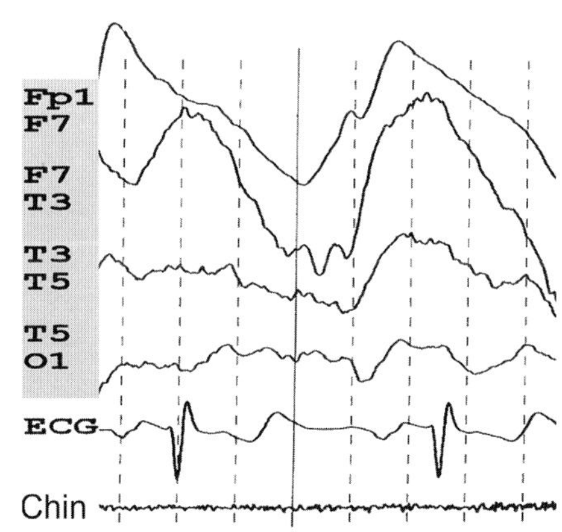

Figure b / Monomorphic hypersynchronic slow waves on the anterior derivations.

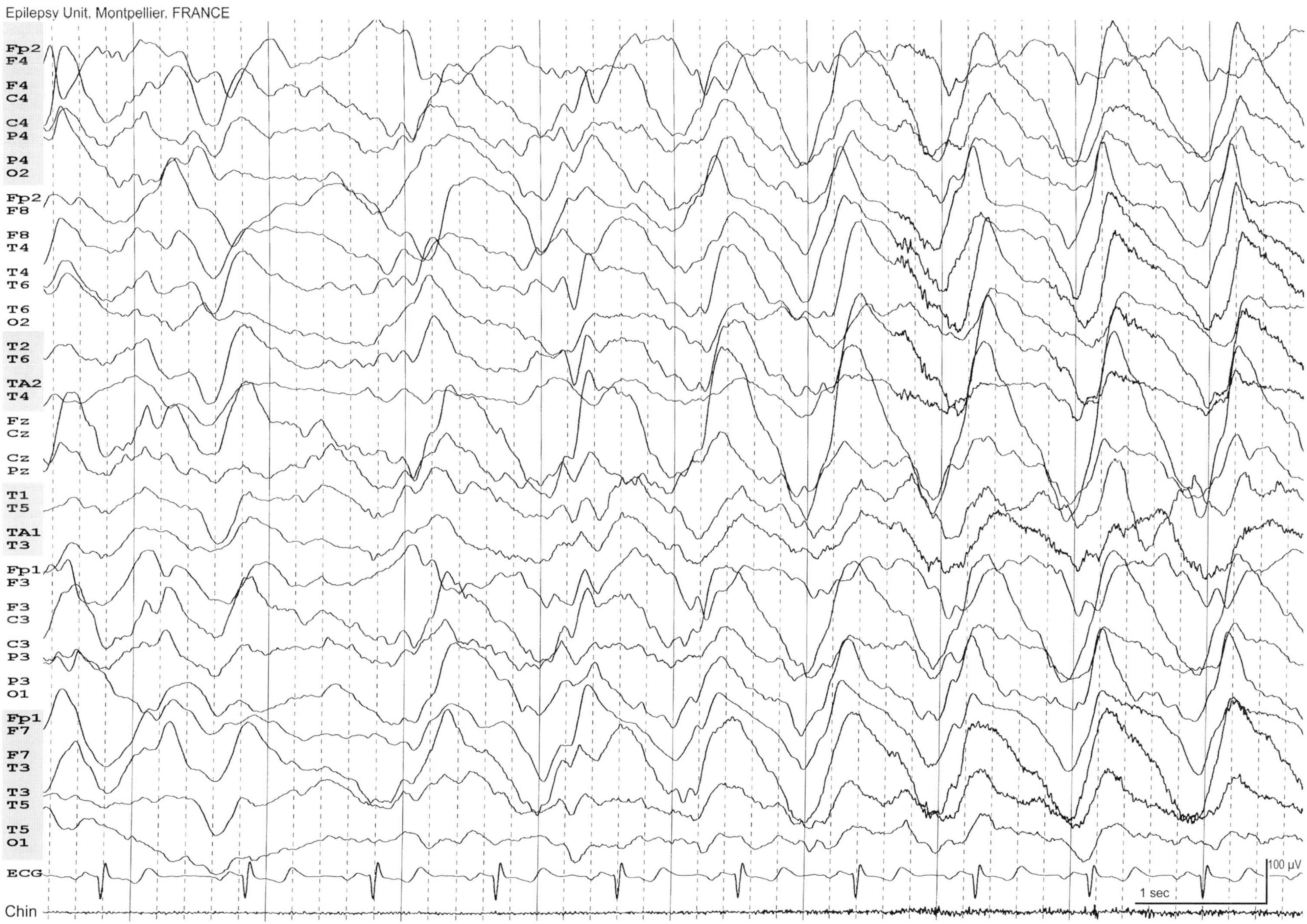
Epilepsy Unit, Montpellier, FRANCE
Fp2 F4
F4 C4
C4 P4
P4 O2
Fp2 F8
F8 T4
T4 T6
T6 O2
T2 T6
TA2 T4
Fz Cz
Cz Pz
T1 T5
TA1 T3
Fp1 F3
F3 C3
C3 P3
P3 O1
Fp1 F7
F7 T3
T3 T5
T5 O1
ECG
Chin
100 µV
1 sec

• 43 Arousal reaction: Frontal arousal rhythms in a young child

Context

5-year-old boy with occiptal lobe epilepsy.

What to note

Low sensitivity at 15 µV/mm. Stage N3 sleep. Theta waves at 6 Hz over the frontal regions. They are intermixed with the slow waves of sleep conveying an impression of polyspike-waves. This pattern corresponds to a frontal arousal rhythm in a young child. Note the presence of fast EMG activity at the temporal derivations due to jaw clenching upon arousal.

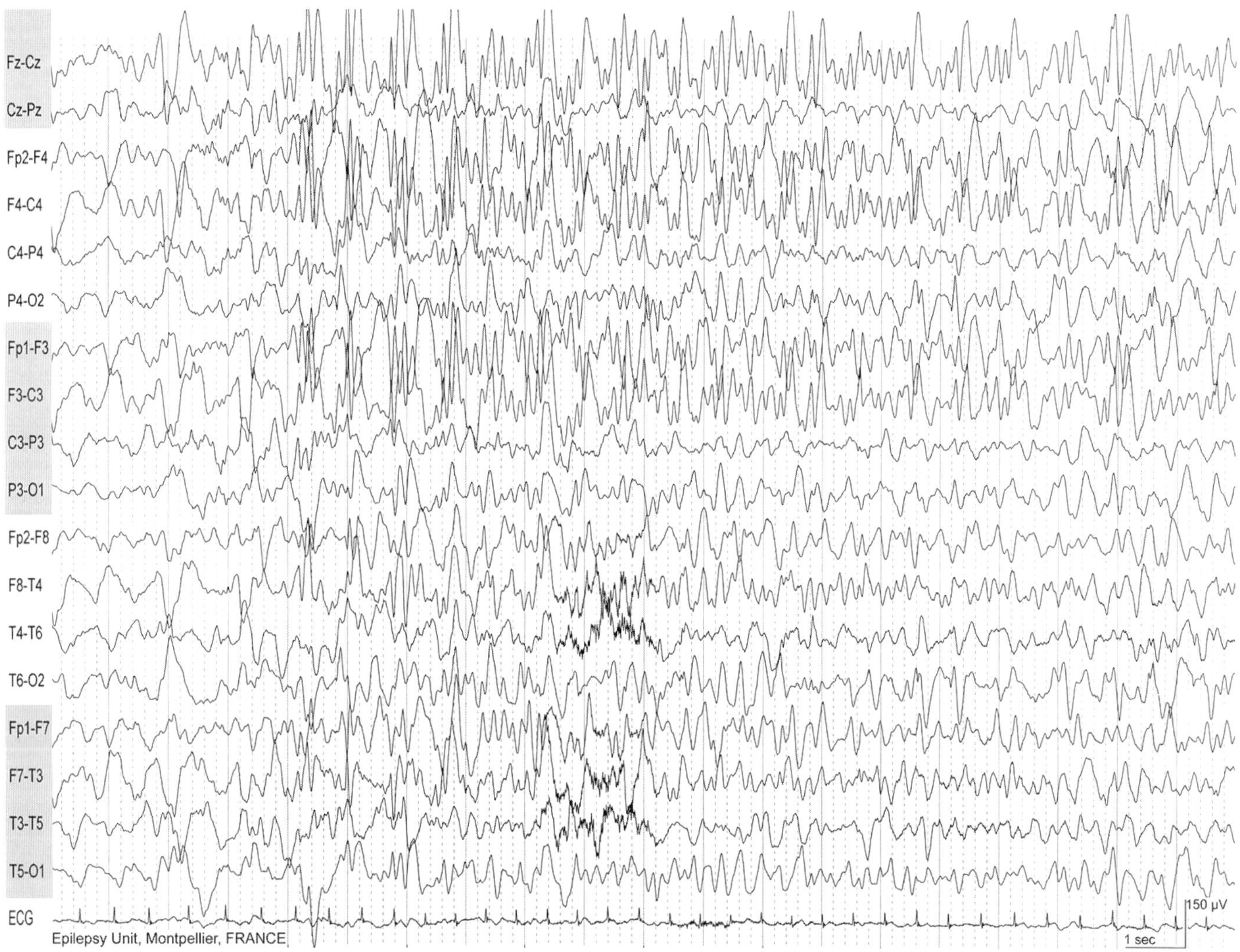

Figure a / Recording at 15 mm/s.

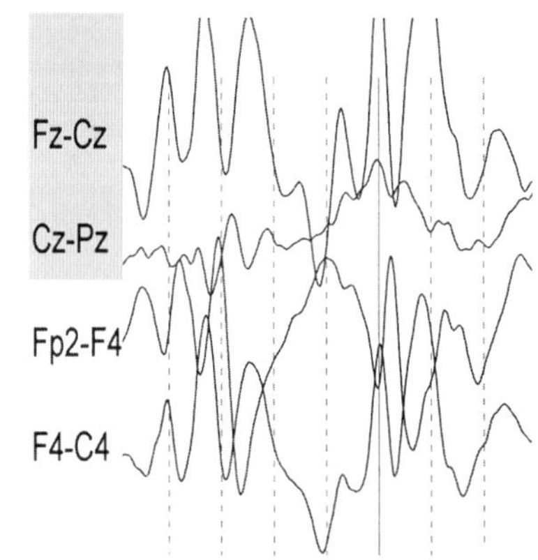

Figure b / Theta waves at 6 Hz intermixed with slow delta waves of sleep.

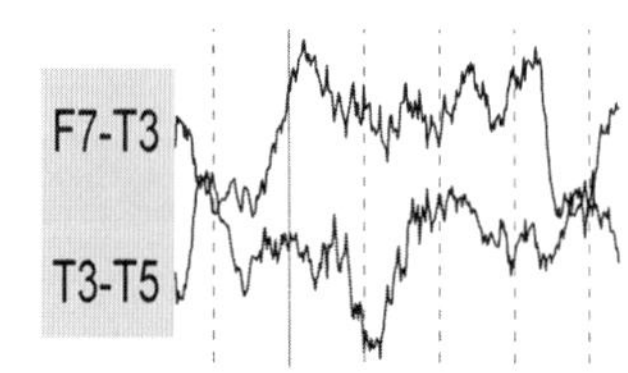

Figure c / Fast EMG activity at T3.

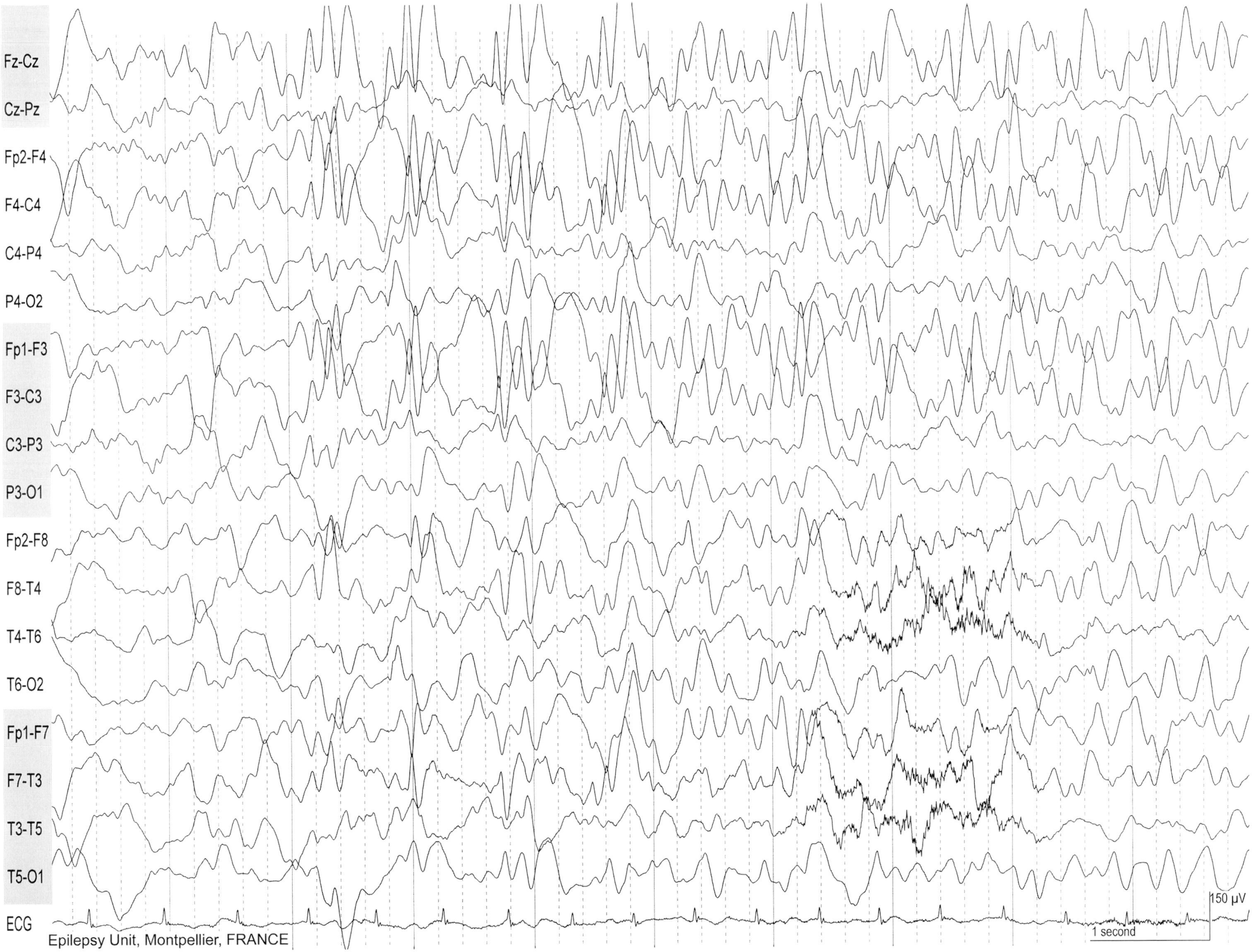
Fz-Cz
Cz-Pz
Fp2-F4
F4-C4
C4-P4
P4-O2
Fp1-F3
F3-C3
C3-P3
P3-O1
Fp2-F8
F8-T4
T4-T6
T6-O2
Fp1-F7
F7-T3
T3-T5
T5-O1
ECG
150 µV
1 second
Epilepsy Unit, Montpellier, FRANCE

• 44 Arousal reaction: Frontal arousal rhythms in a child

Context

9-year-old girl with poor school performance.

What to note

Low sensitivity at 15 µV/mm. Stage N2 sleep. First a cluster of three V waves, then activities at 13 Hz over the frontal regions. This pattern is typical and corresponds to a frontal arousal rhythm. The sharply contoured waveforms are physiological and must not be confused with epileptiform elements or even a seizure. The heart rate slightly increases upon arousal. Also note the presence of fast EMG activity upon arousal.

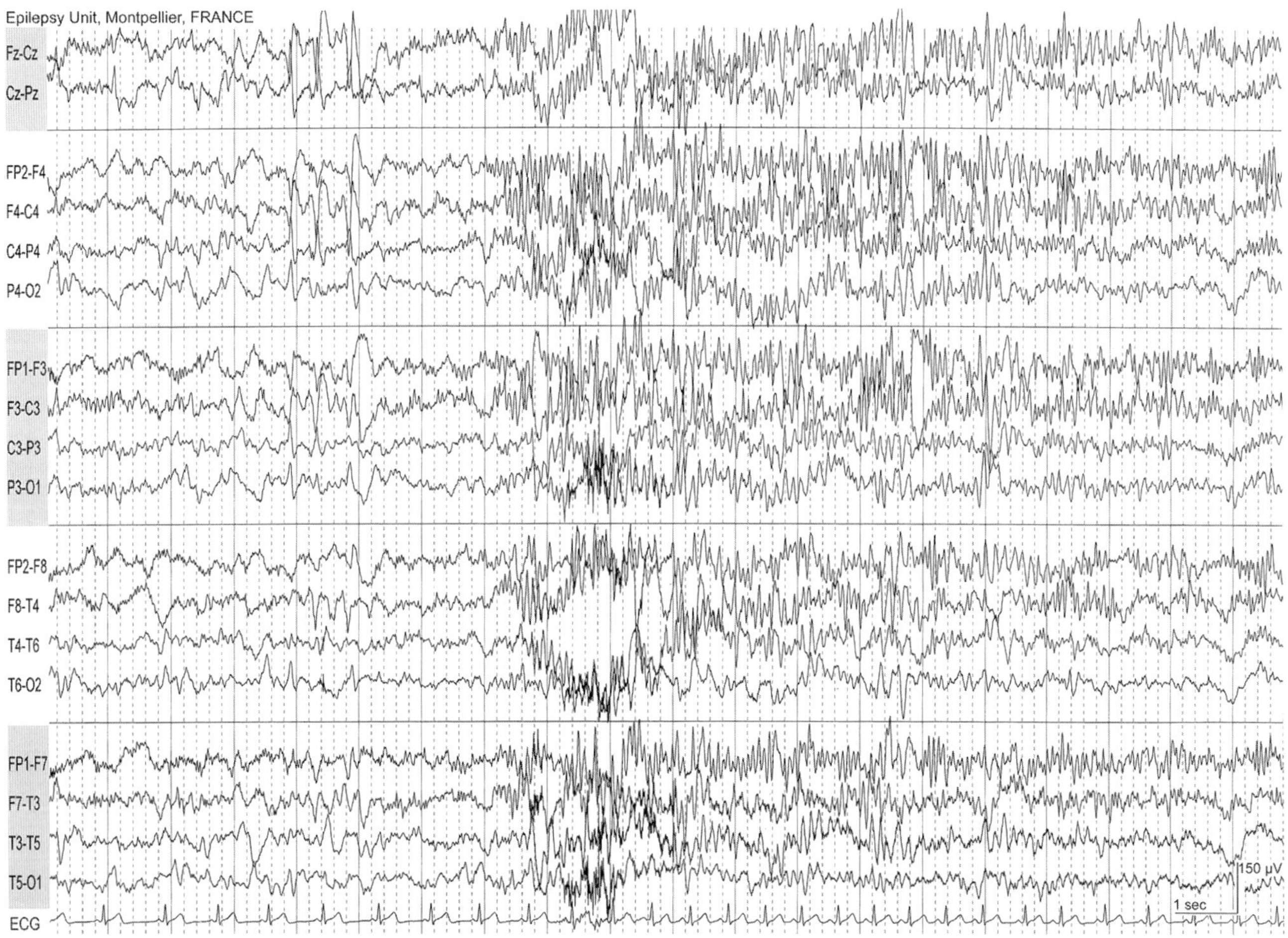

Figure a / Recording at 15 mm/s. First a sleep spindle can be seen at F3-C3 followed by a cluster of three V waves, then activities at 13 Hz.

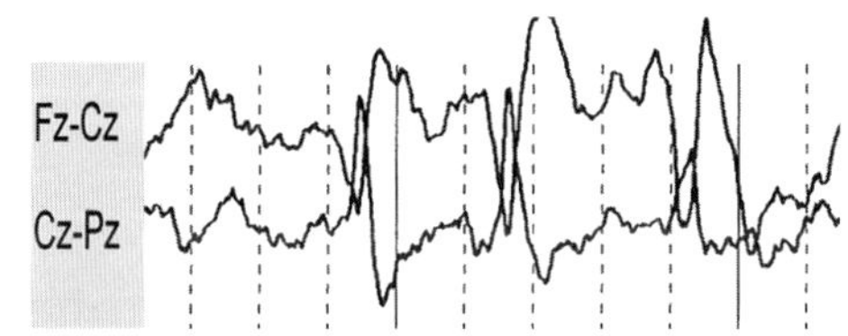

Figure b / Burst of three V waves.

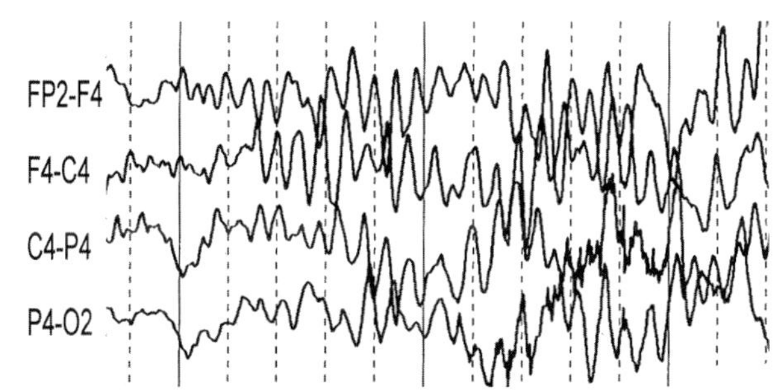

Figure c / Rhythm at 13 Hz over the right frontal region with sharply contoured waveforms corresponding to a physiological frontal arousal rhythm of children.

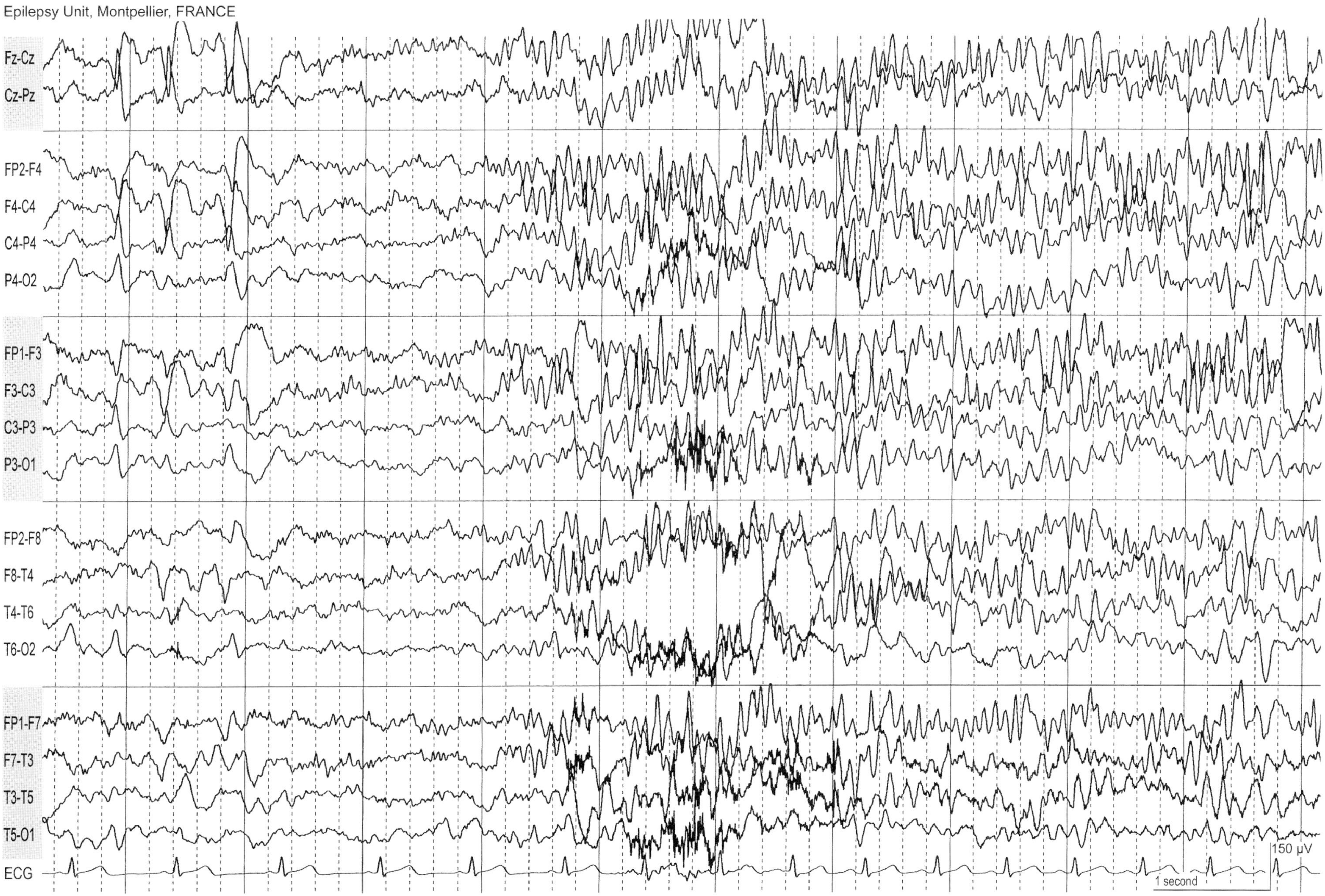
Epilepsy Unit, Montpellier, FRANCE
Fz-Cz
Cz-Pz
FP2-F4
F4-C4
C4-P4
P4-O2
FP1-F3
F3-C3
C3-P3
P3-O1
FP2-F8
F8-T4
T4-T6
T6-O2
FP1-F7
F7-T3
T3-T5
T5-O1
ECG
150 µV
1 second

III • 45 Arousal reaction: Frontal arousal rhythms in an adolescent

Context

16-year-old man seen after a loss of consciousness.

What to note

Stage N3 sleep. Arousal with 10 Hz activities over the frontal regions. Note the presence of fast EMG activity at the temporal derivations due to jaw clenching upon arousal. Frontal arousal rhythms are physiological and must not be confused with frontal seizure. The heart rate slightly increases upon arousal.

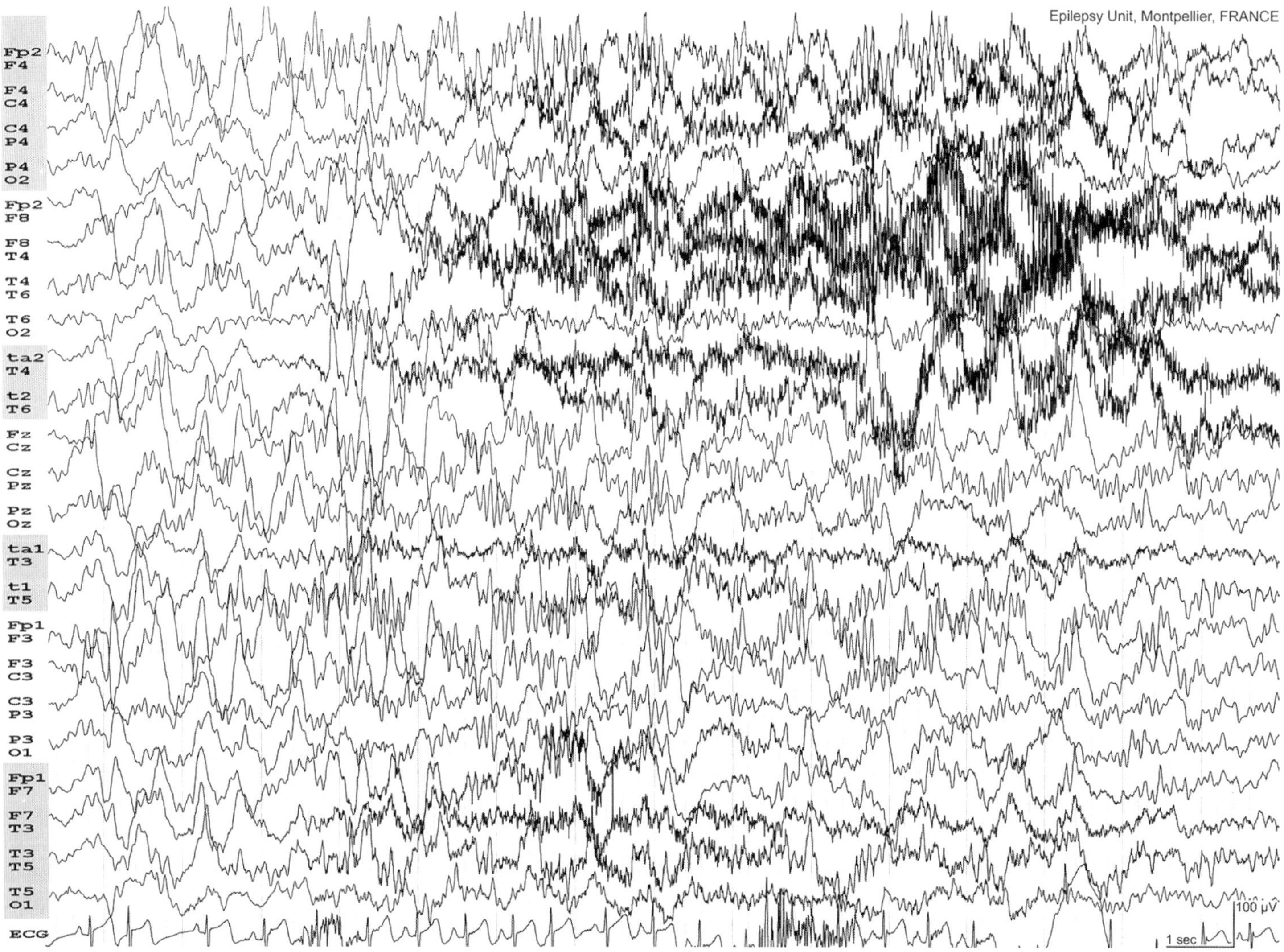

Figure a / Recording at 15 mm/s.

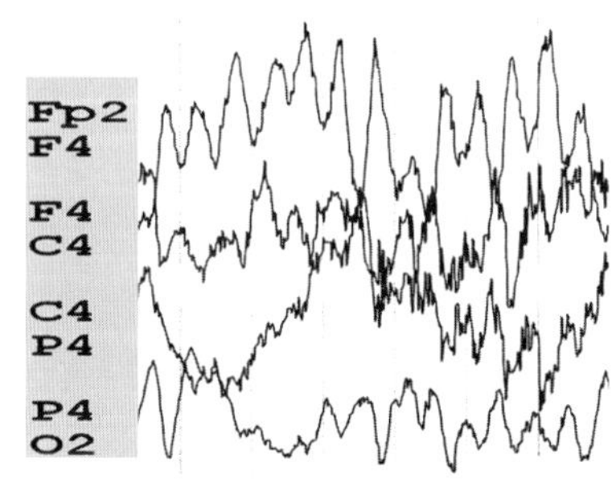

Figure b / Activity at 10 Hz on the right frontal region.

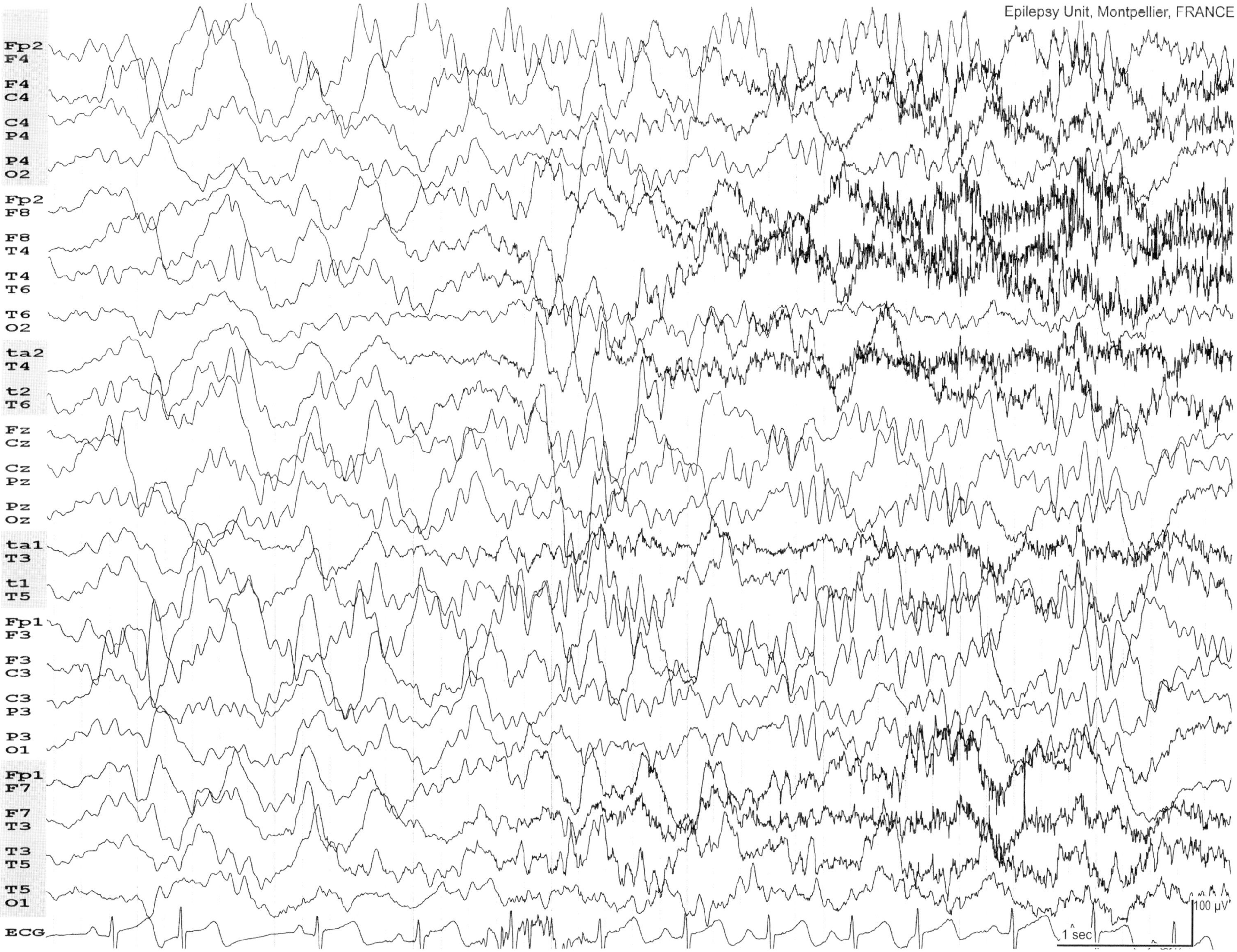
Epilepsy Unit, Montpellier, FRANCE
Fp2 F4
F4 C4
C4 P4
P4 O2
Fp2 F8
F8 T4
T4 T6
T6 O2
ta2 T4
t2 T6
Fz Cz
Cz Pz
Pz Oz
ta1 T3
t1 T5
Fp1 F3
F3 C3
C3 P3
P3 O1
Fp1 F7
F7 T3
T3 T5
T5 O1
ECG
100 µV
1 sec

III

• 46 Positive occipital sharp transients of sleep (POSTs) in NREM sleep stage 2 (1)

Context

37-year-old woman with left temporal lobe epilepsy.

What to note

Stage N2 sleep. Typical positive occipital sharp transients of sleep (POSTs) are present over the occipital regions. Occurrence of a typical K complex at the end of the plate.

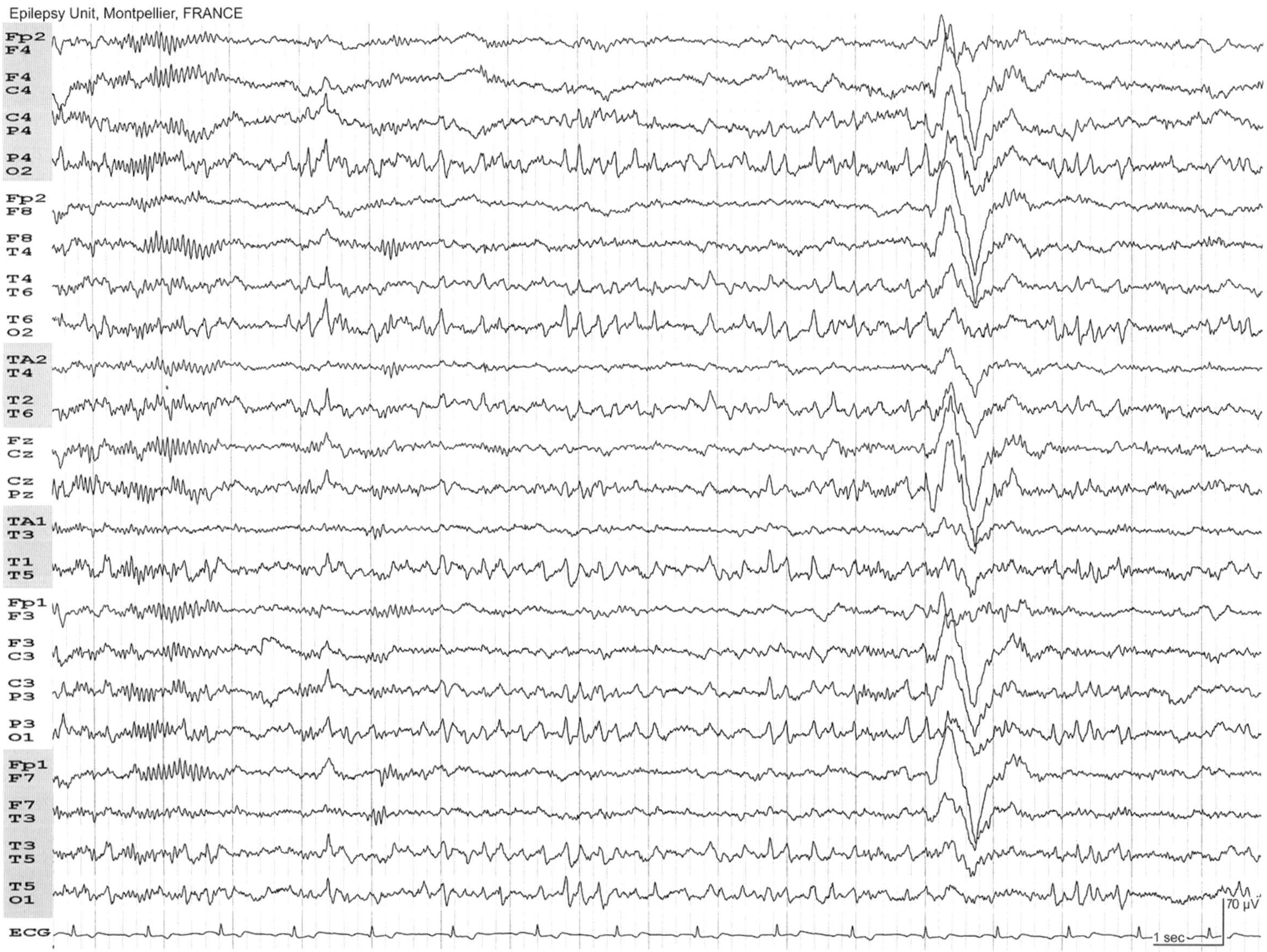

Figure a / Recording at 15 mm/s. A bilateral sleep spindle at the beginning of the plate.

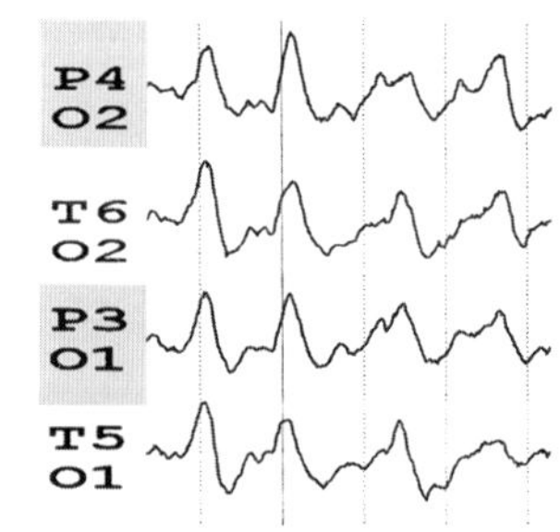

Figure b / POSTs.

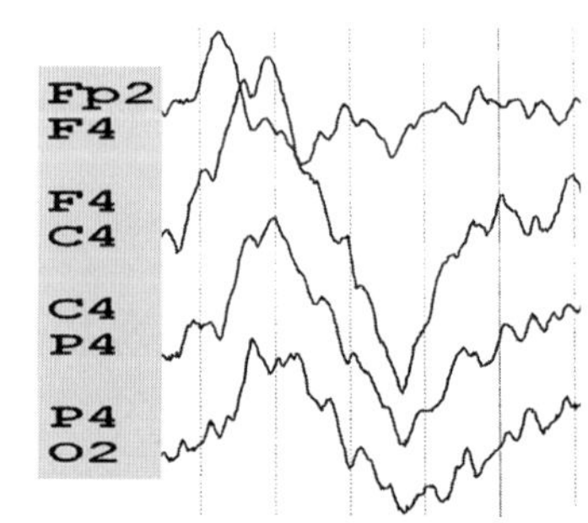

Figure c / K complex.

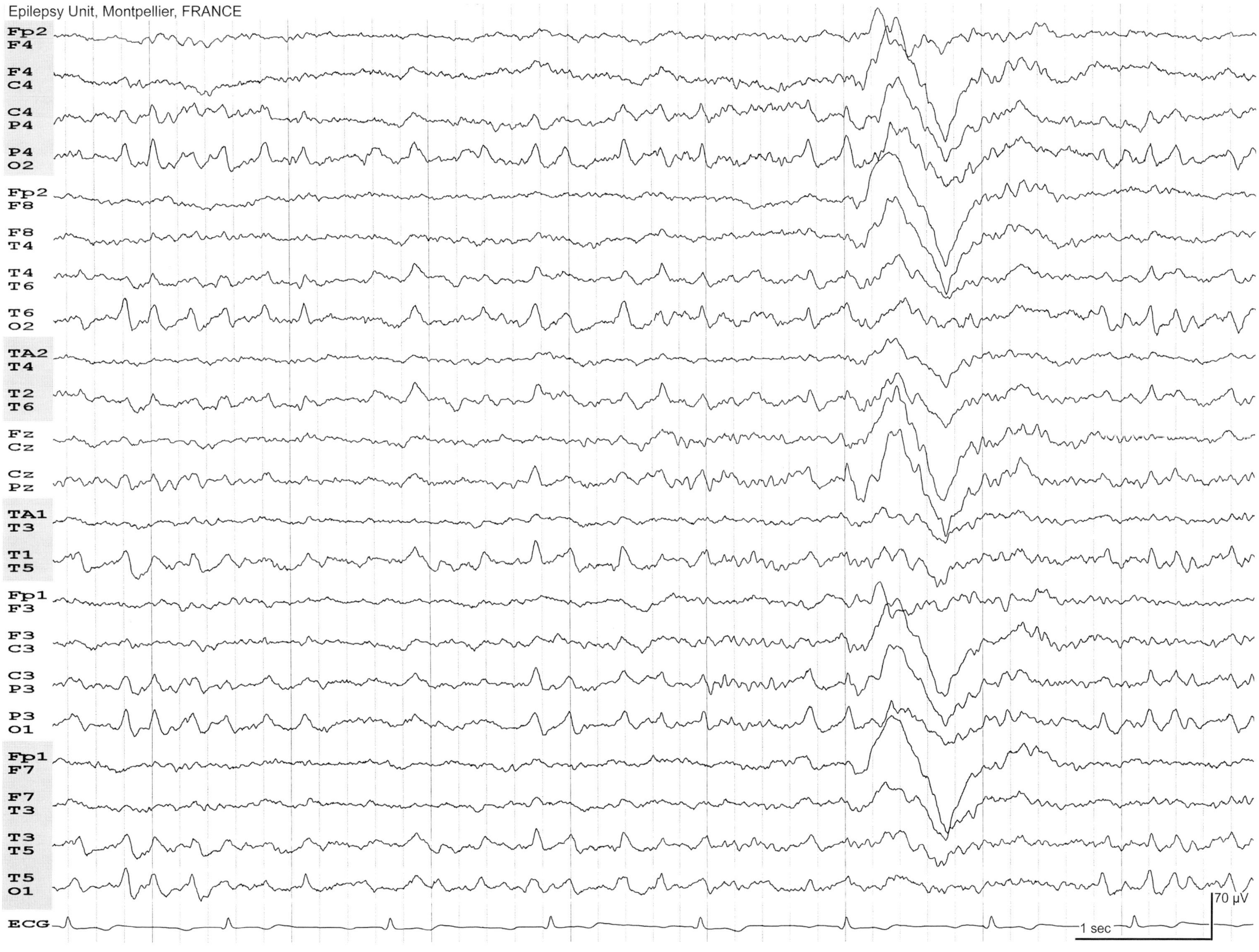
Epilepsy Unit, Montpellier, FRANCE
Fp2 F4
F4 C4
C4 P4
P4 O2
Fp2 F8
F8 T4
T4 T6
T6 O2
TA2 T4
T2 T6
Fz Cz
Cz Pz
TA1 T3
T1 T5
Fp1 F3
F3 C3
C3 P3
P3 O1
Fp1 F7
F7 T3
T3 T5
T5 O1
ECG
70 µV
1 sec

III • 47 Positive occipital sharp transients of sleep (POSTs) in NREM sleep stage 2 (2)

Context

27-year-old woman with cryptogenic left temporo-parieto-occipital juction epilepsy. Same patient as plate I-19 and III-50.

What to note

The woman is in stage N2 sleep with at the beginning the plate, a K complex with its characteristic strong deflection. Ample, mono or diphasic sharp waves over the occipital regions. Theses waves correspond to positive occipital sharp transients of sleep (POSTs). They are particularly abundant in this patient. POSTs are physiological.

Comment

When lambda waves are of high amplitude, POSTs are usually of high amplitude.

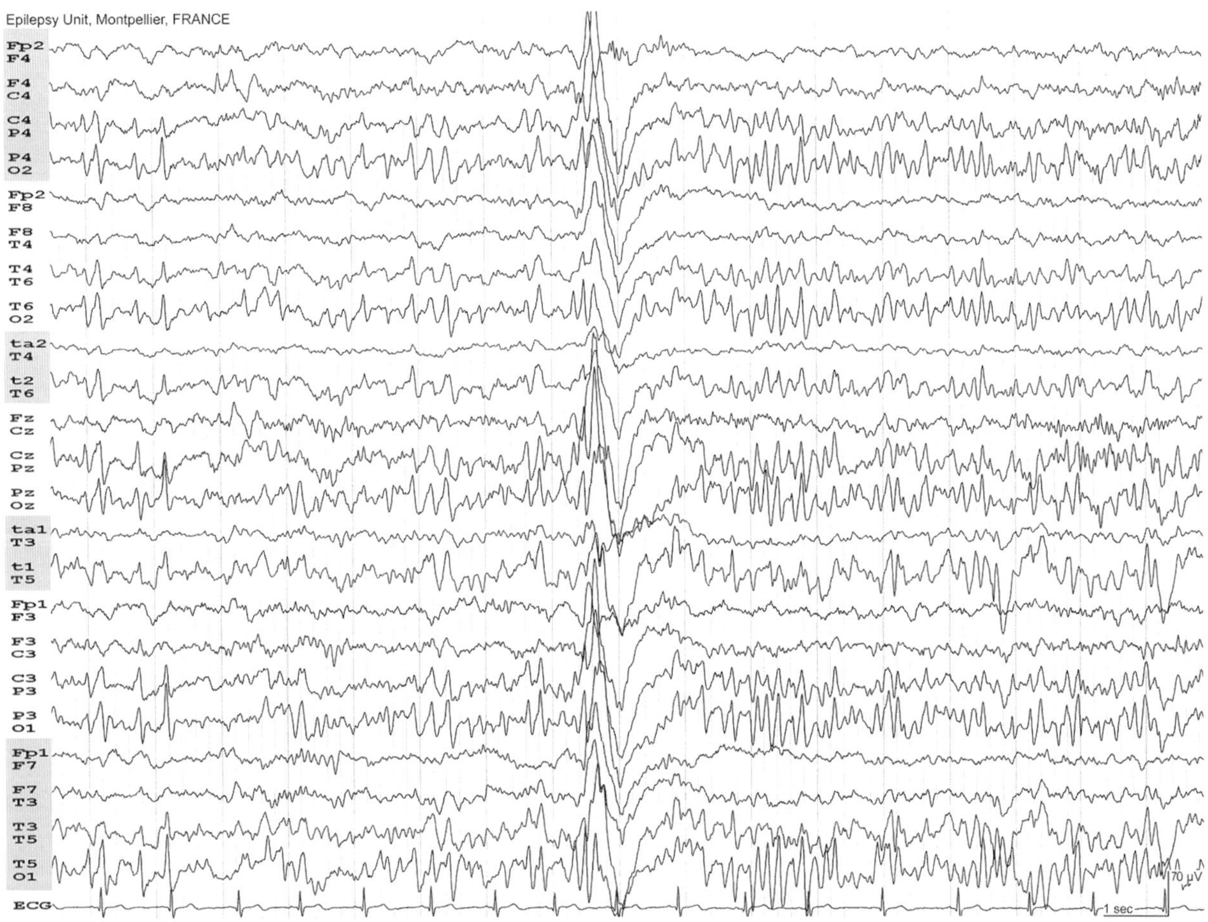

Figure a / Recording at 15 mm/s. On this plate, the POSTs occur either in bursts or isolated mono or diphasic.

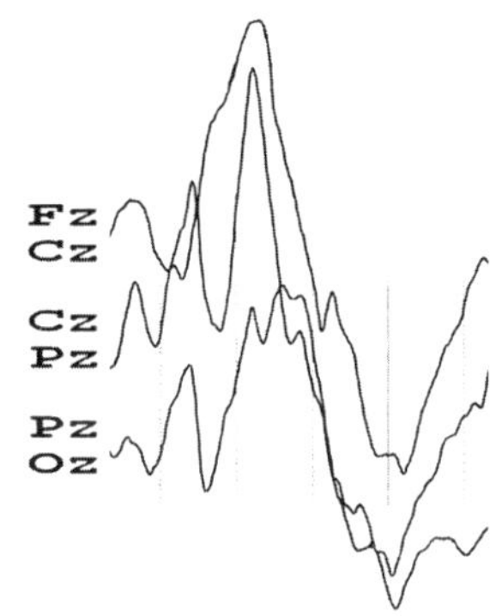

Figure b / K complex.

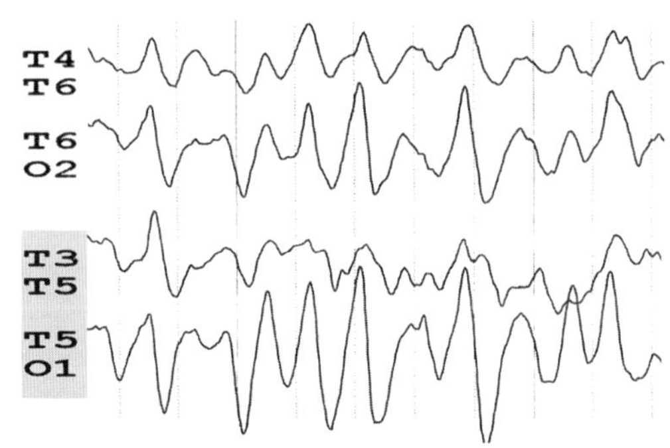

Figure c / Ample, sharp, diphasic waves over the occipital regions corresponding to POSTs.

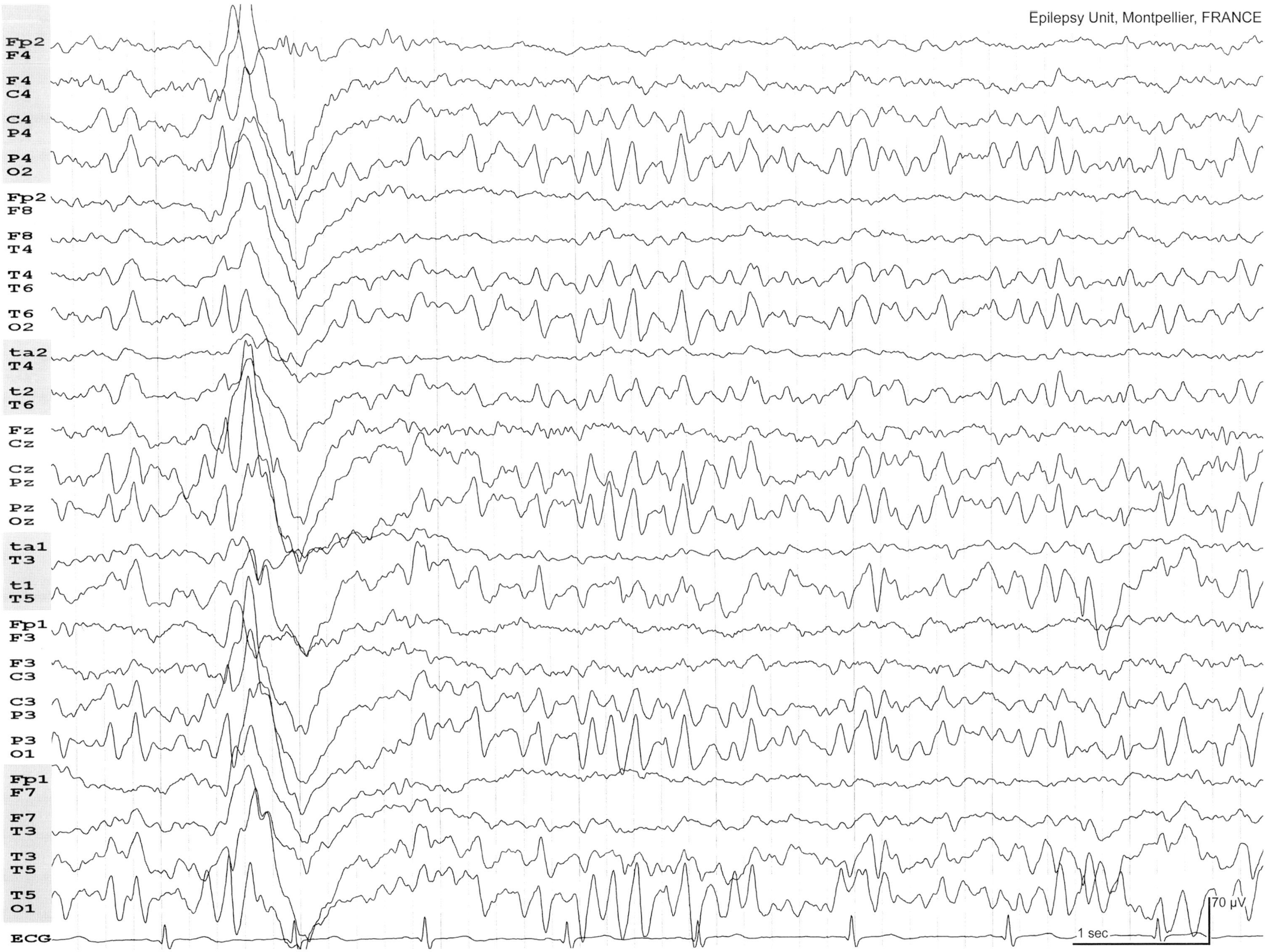
Epilepsy Unit, Montpellier, FRANCE
Fp2 F4
F4 C4
C4 P4
P4 O2
Fp2 F8
F8 T4
T4 T6
T6 O2
ta2 T4
t2 T6
Fz Cz
Cz Pz
Pz Oz
ta1 T3
t1 T5
Fp1 F3
F3 C3
C3 P3
P3 O1
Fp1 F7
F7 T3
T3 T5
T5 O1
ECG
70 µV
1 sec

III • 48 Positive occipital sharp transients of sleep (POSTs) in NREM sleep stage 2 (3)

Context

19-year-old woman with juvenile myoclonic epilepsy. Same patient as plate II-29.

What to note

Stage N2 sleep. An asymmetrical sleep spindle with higher amplitude on the right hemisphere can be observed prior to a K complex with its characteristic strong deflection. Mostly symmetrical diphasic sharp waves occur over the occipital regions. These correspond to positive occipital sharp transients of sleep (POSTs).

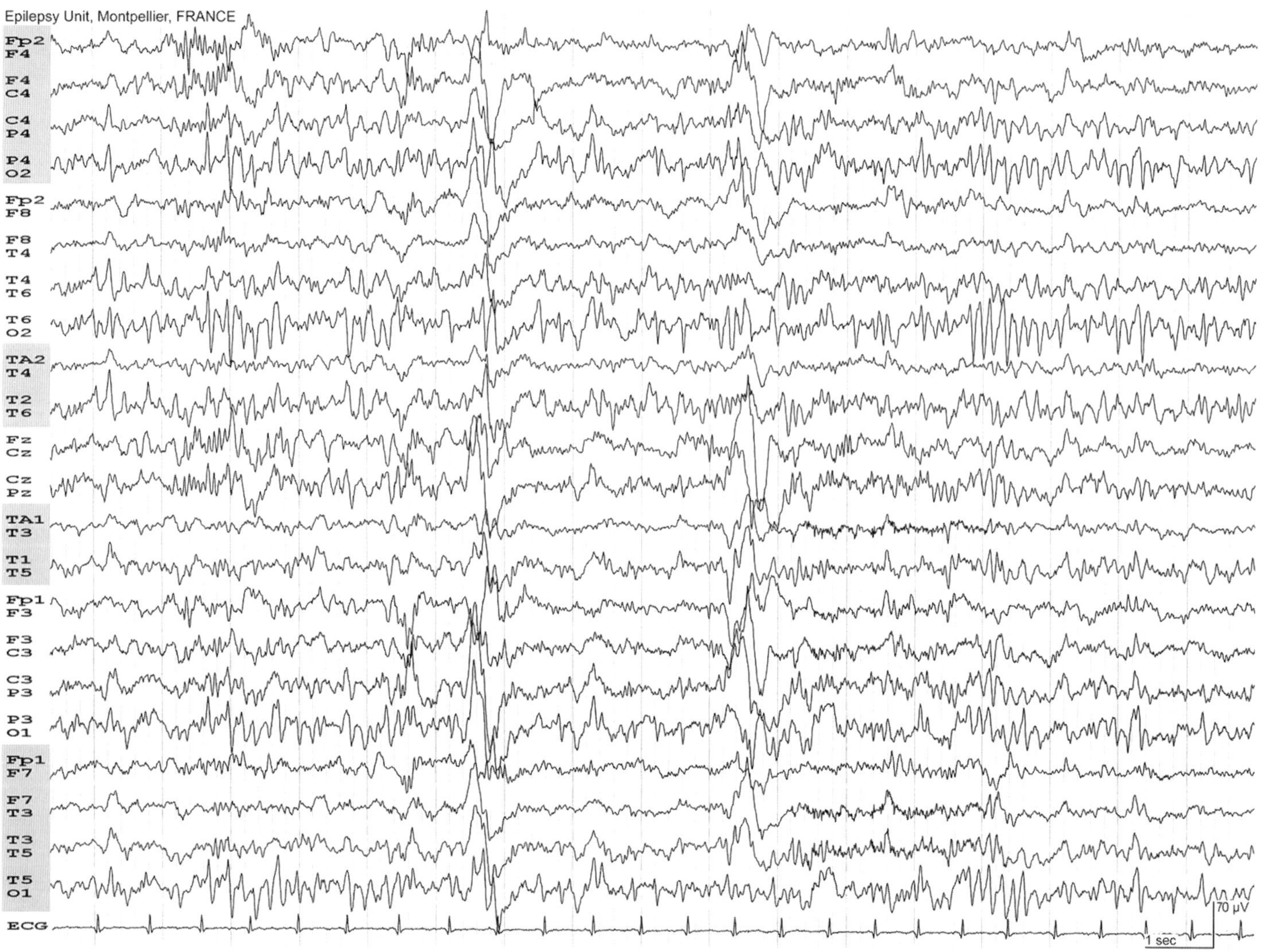

Figure a / Recording at 15 mm/s. POSTs occur either isolated or in bursts after the second K complex.

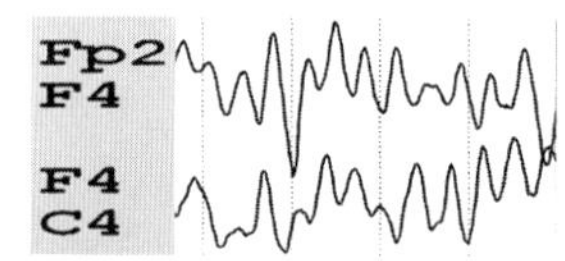

Figure b / Sleep spindle.

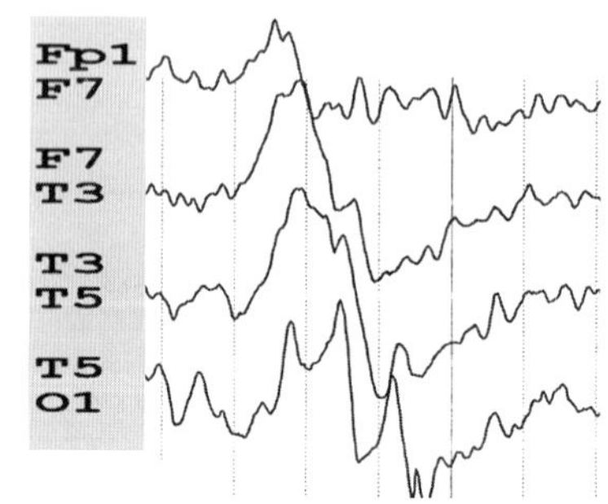

Figure c / K complex.

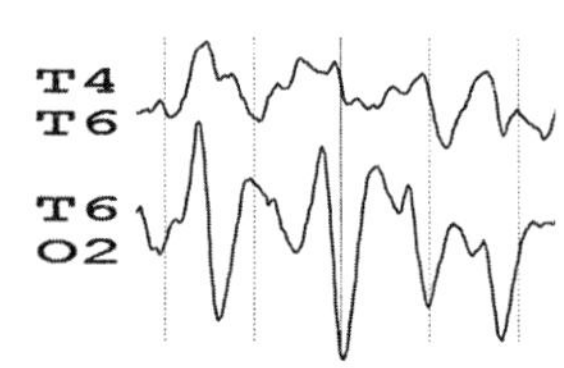

Figure d / Diphasic POSTs.

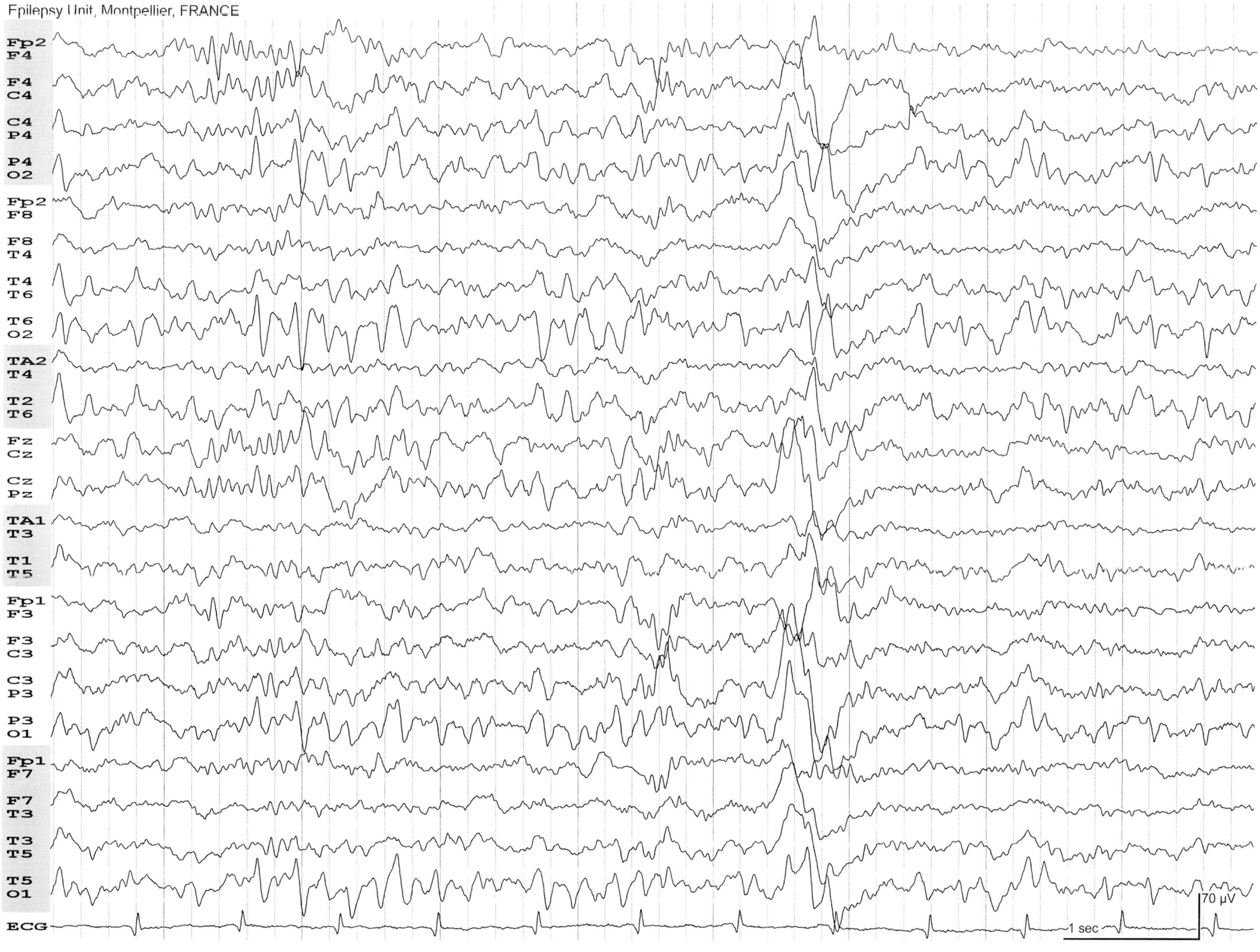
Epilepsy Unit, Montpellier, FRANCE
Fp2 F4
F4 C4
C4 P4
P4 O2
Fp2 F8
F8 T4
T4 T6
T6 O2
TA2 T4
T2 T6
Fz Cz
Cz Pz
TA1 T3
T1 T5
Fp1 F3
F3 C3
C3 P3
P3 O1
Fp1 F7
F7 T3
T3 T5
T5 O1
ECG
70 µV
1 sec

III • 49 A train of positive occipital sharp transients of sleep (POSTs) in NREM sleep stage 2

Context

24-year-old woman with idiopathic generalized epilepsy.

What to note

Stage N2 sleep with sleep spindles. Repetitive POSTs evolving into a sharp theta activity at 6 Hz over the occipital regions. The sharply contoured aspect and the bursts should not be misinterpreted as epileptiform abnormalities.

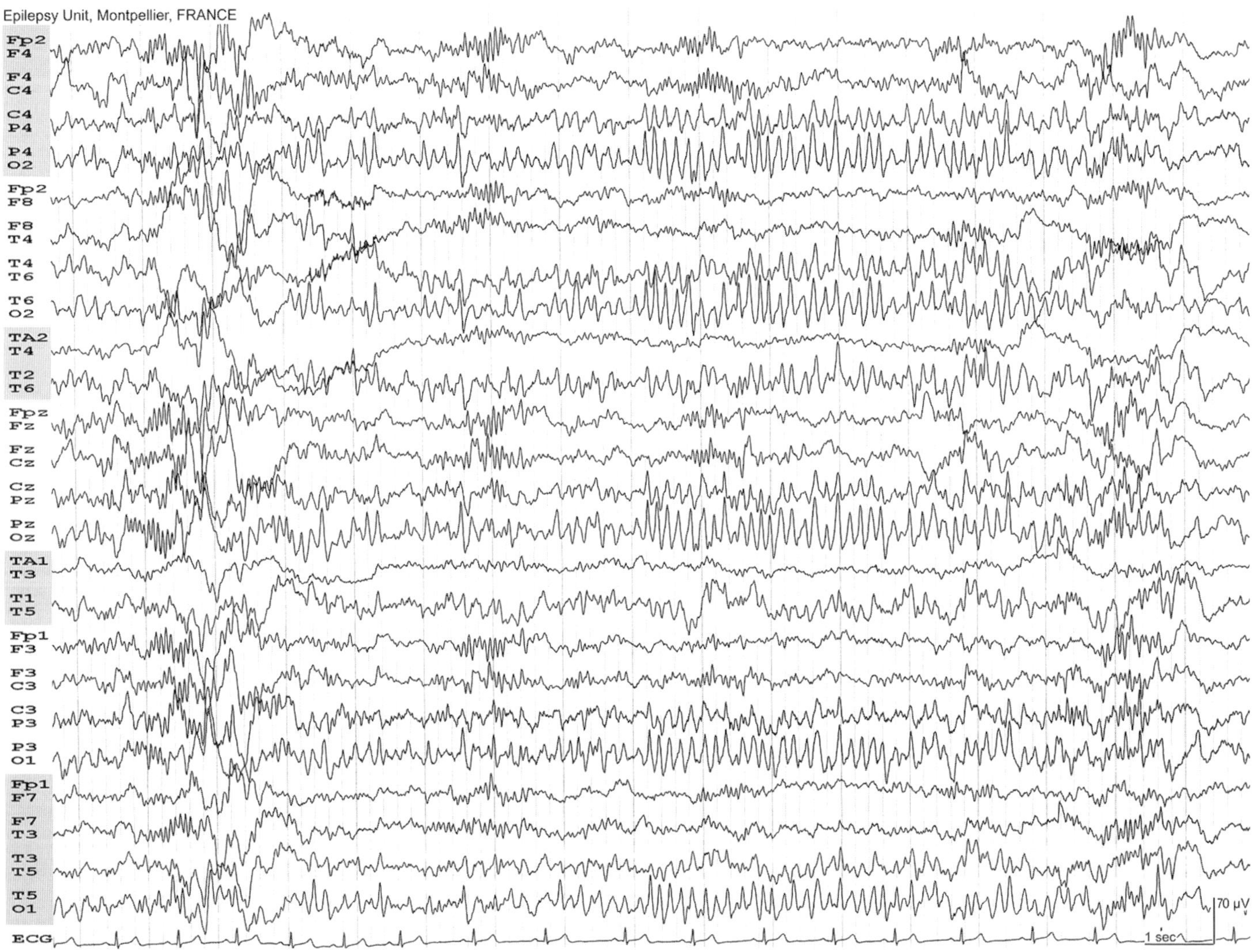

Figure a / Recording at 15 mm/s. At the beginning of the plate, a sleep spindle that spread to the occipital regions followed by a K complex can be observed.

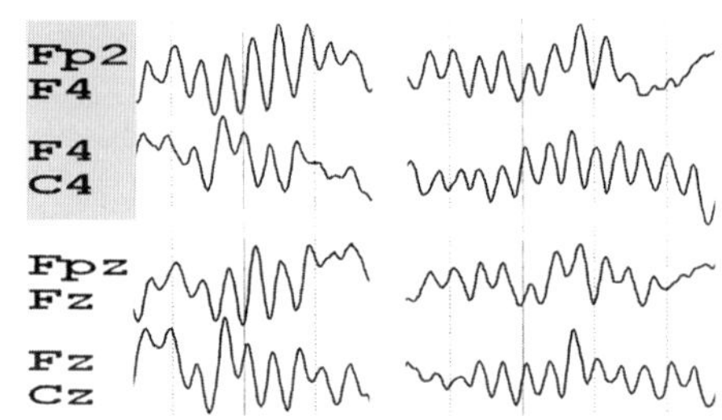

Figure b / Sleep spindles.

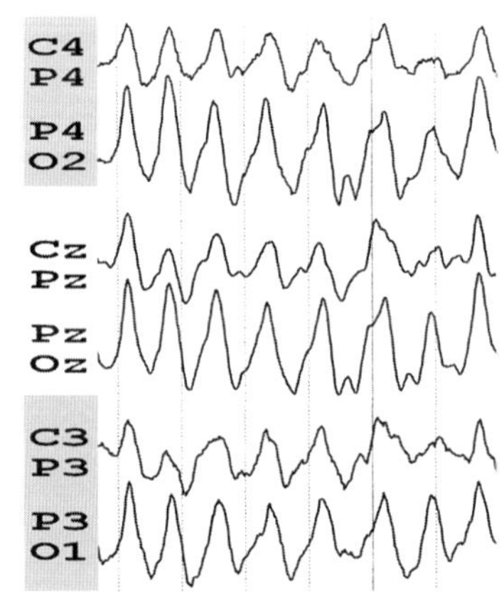

Figure c / Repetitive POSTs at a frequency of 6 Hz.

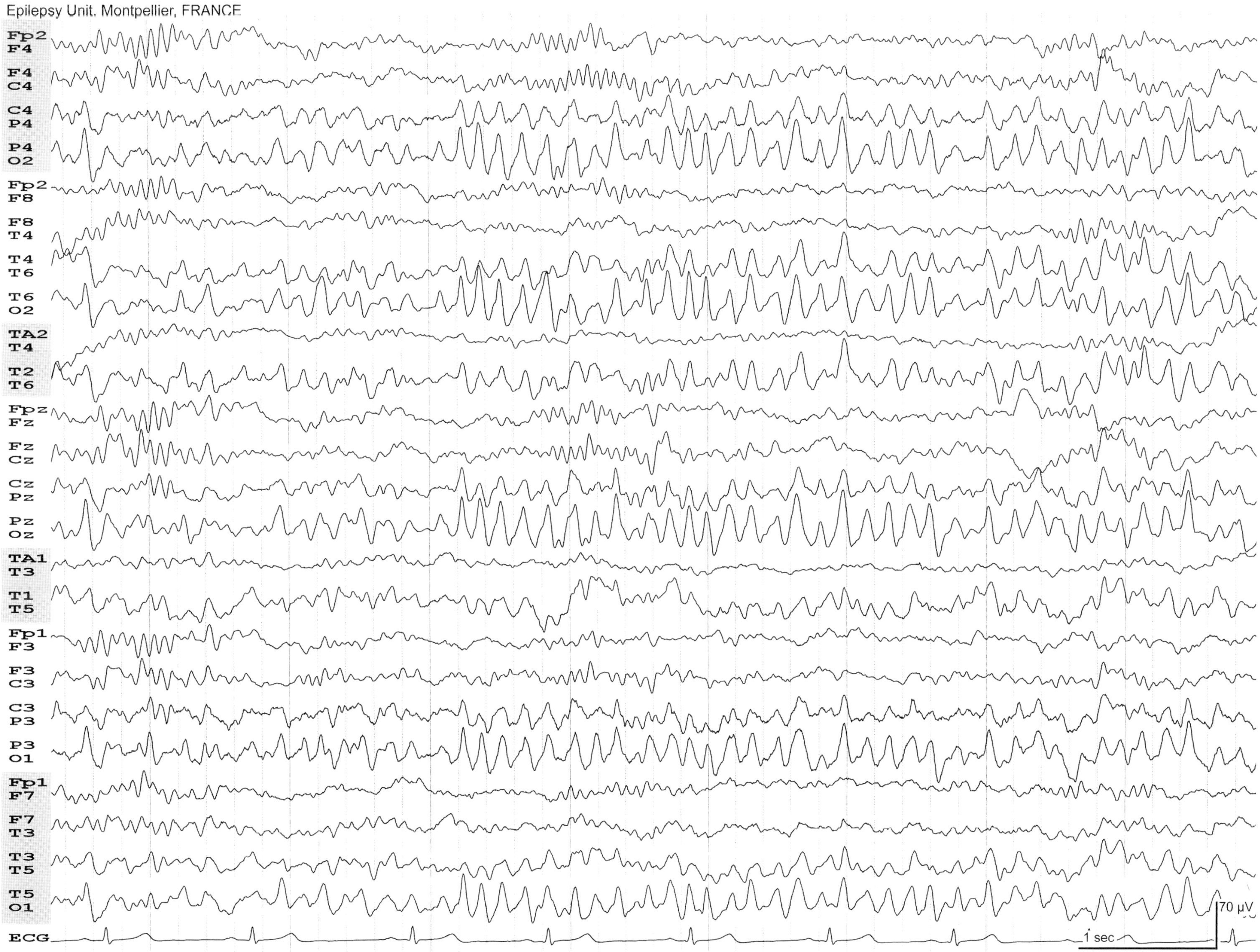
Epilepsy Unit, Montpellier, FRANCE
Fp2 F4
F4 C4
C4 P4
P4 O2
Fp2 F8
F8 T4
T4 T6
T6 O2
TA2 T4
T2 T6
Fpz Fz
Fz Cz
Cz Pz
Pz Oz
TA1 T3
T1 T5
Fp1 F3
F3 C3
C3 P3
P3 O1
Fp1 F7
F7 T3
T3 T5
T5 O1
ECG
70 µV
1 sec

III • 50 Positive occipital sharp transients of sleep (POSTs) in NREM sleep stage 3

Context

27-year-old woman with cryptogenic left temporo-parieto-occipital junction epilepsy. Same patient as plates I-19 and III-47.

What to note

The woman is in deep sleep. Slow delta waves are intermixed with POSTs. POSTs generally occur in NREM sleep stage 2 and they may persist in NREM sleep stage 3 but usually not so frequent.

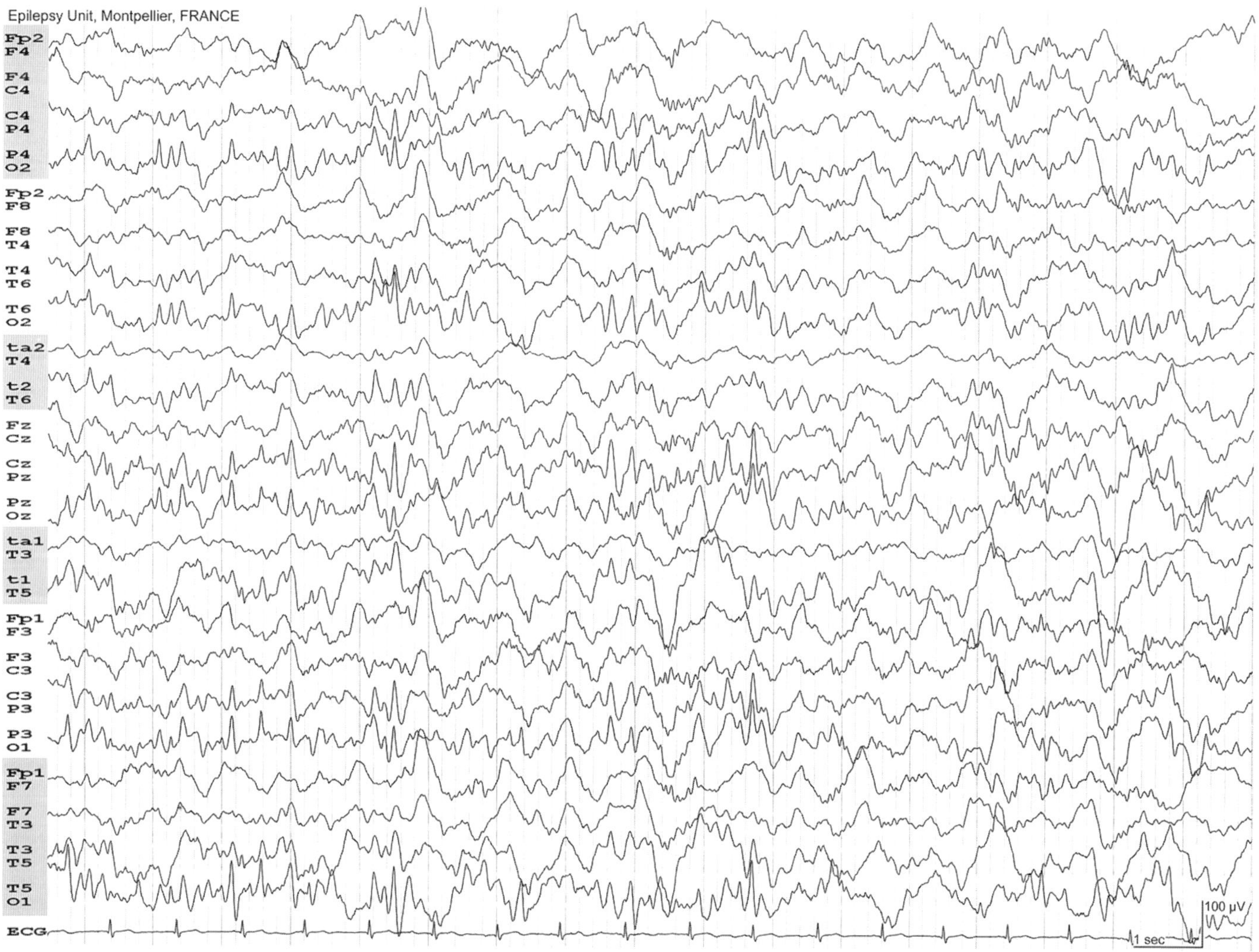

Figure a / Recording at 15 mm/s.

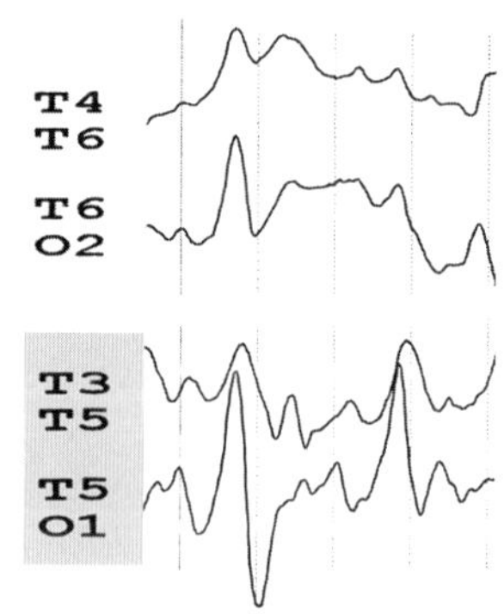

Figure b / POSTs.

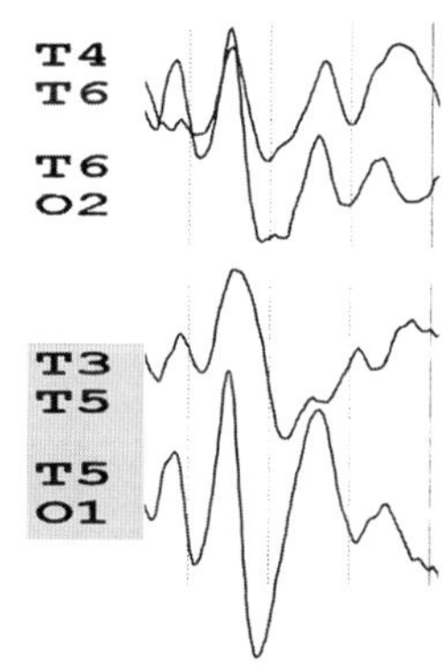

Figure c / Superimposition of the two rhythms conveying an impression of sharp waves.

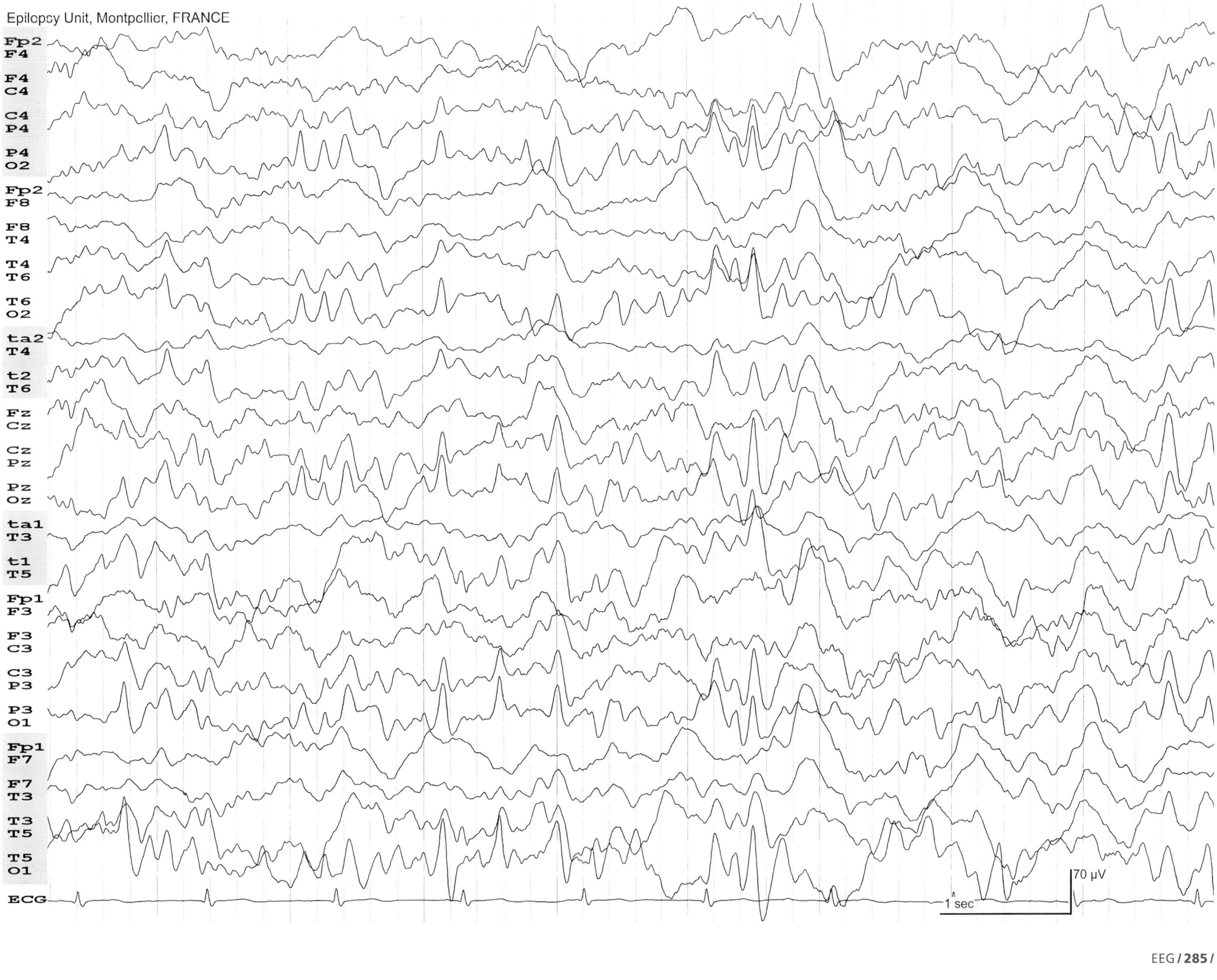
Epilepsy Unit, Montpellier, FRANCE
Fp2 F4
F4 C4
C4 P4
P4 O2
Fp2 F8
F8 T4
T4 T6
T6 O2
ta2 T4
t2 T6
Fz Cz
Cz Pz
Pz Oz
ta1 T3
t1 T5
Fp1 F3
F3 C3
C3 P3
P3 O1
Fp1 F7
F7 T3
T3 T5
T5 O1
ECG
1 sec
70 µV

III • 51 Alpha-like activity in NREM Sleep

Context

22-year-old woman with cryptogenic left centro-parietal lobe epilepsy, presurgical assessment.

What to note

Stage N2 sleep. Left segment, before a typical K complex, bilateral rhythm at 8 Hz without arousal (no muscular activity, no change in breathing) over the parietal and the posterior temporal regions. This pattern corresponds to alpha-like activity of NREM sleep. Right segment, short burst of alpha activity. If taken alone, it can be mistaken for "epileptic" spikes. But the same elements, when seen in longer runs, are clearly alpha activity of NREM sleep.

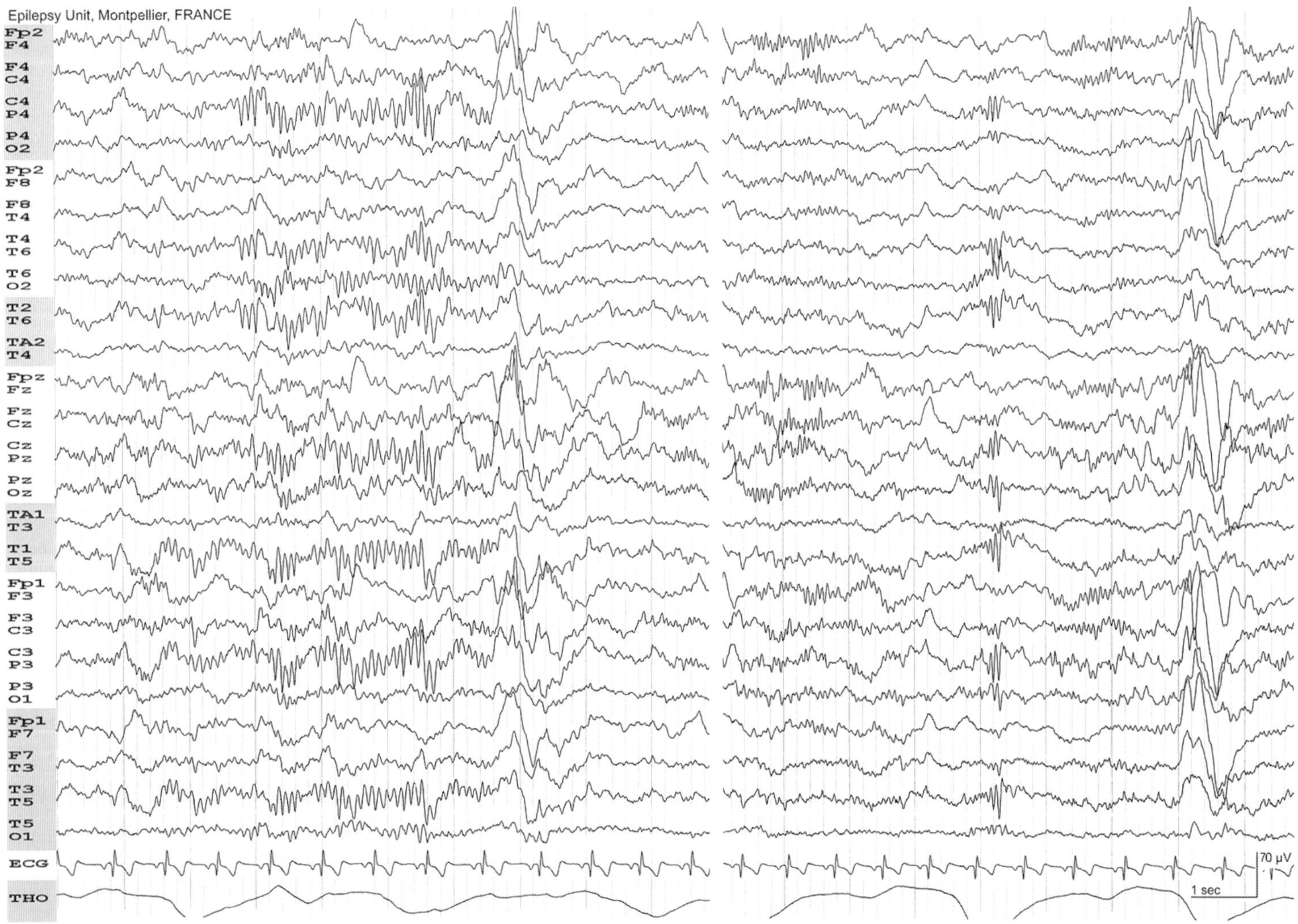

Figure a / Recording at 15 mm/s. Right segment, sleep spindles at the beginning of the plate, in the middle and just after a typical K complex.

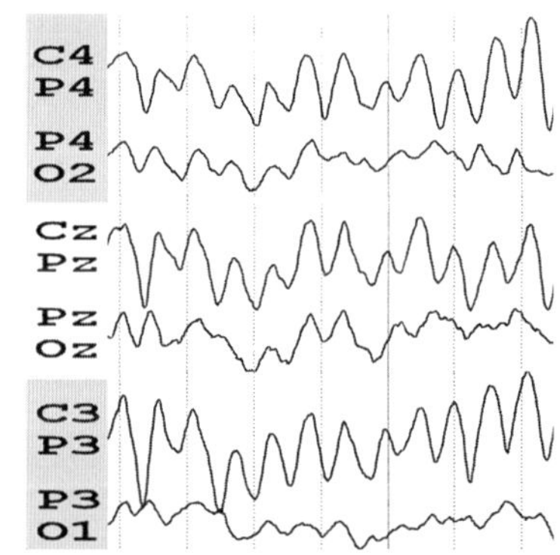

Figure b / Alpha-like activity.

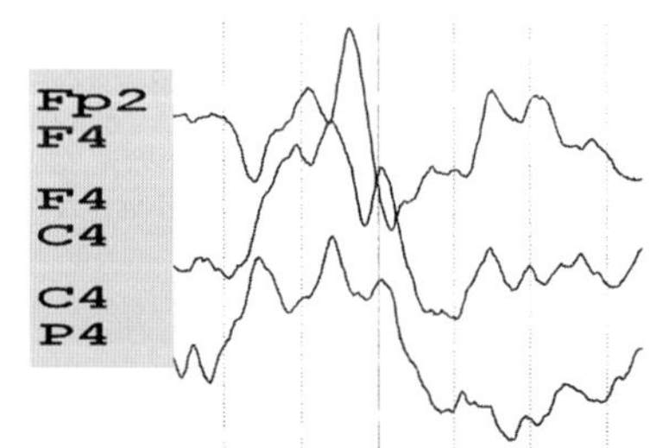

Figure c / K complex.

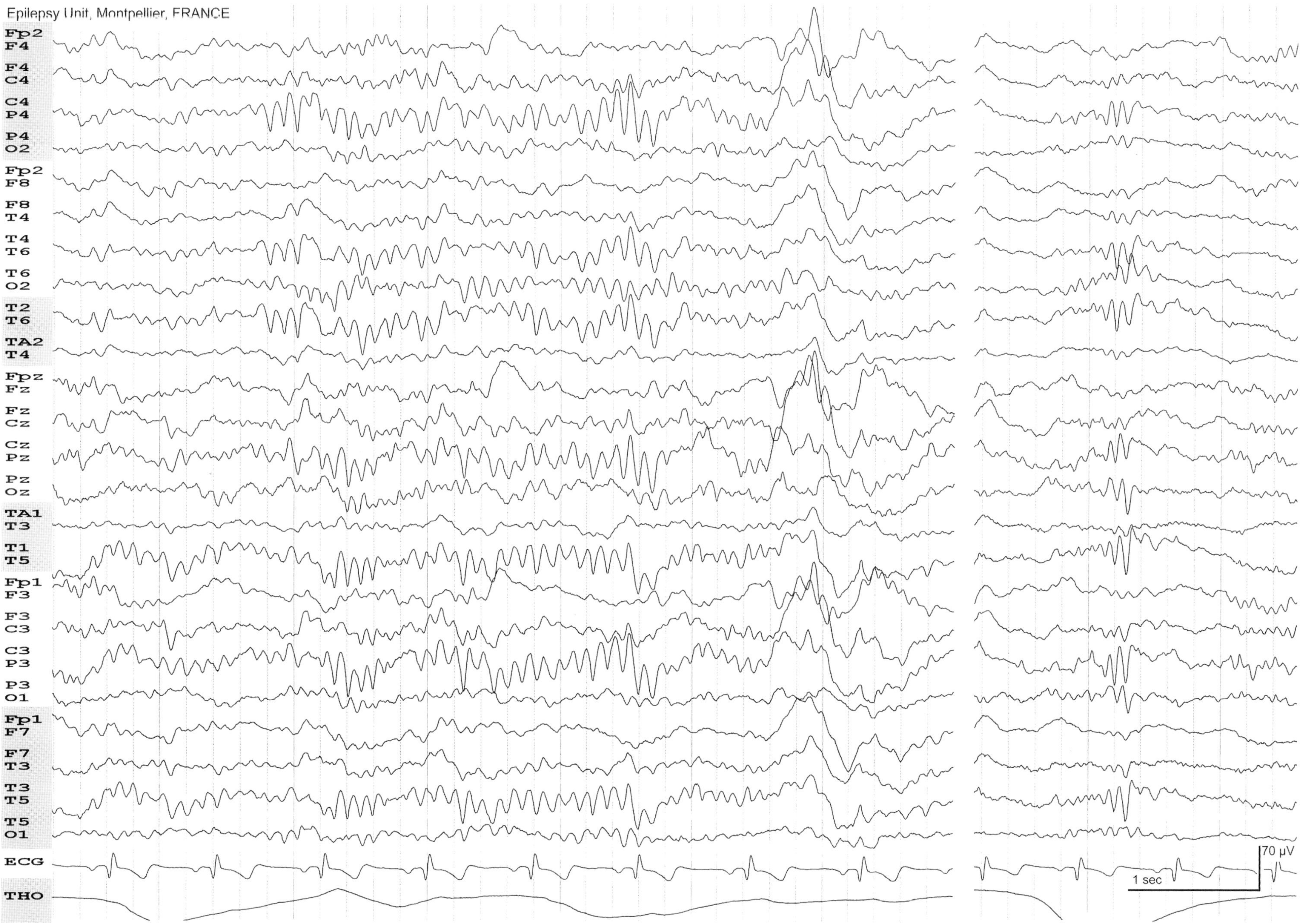
Epilepsy Unit, Montpellier, FRANCE
Fp2 F4
F4 C4
C4 P4
P4 O2
Fp2 F8
F8 T4
T4 T6
T6 O2
T2 T6
TA2 T4
Fpz Fz
Fz Cz
Cz Pz
Pz Oz
TA1 T3
T1 T5
Fp1 F3
F3 C3
C3 P3
P3 O1
Fp1 F7
F7 T3
T3 T5
T5 O1
ECG
THO
70 µV
1 sec

III • 52 Wicket spikes (1)

Context

70-year-old woman, full night sleep EEG, finally diagnosed with REM sleep behavioral disorder.

What to note

In the left segment, stage N1 sleep. Arciform waves can be seen at 8 Hz over the left temporal region with phase reversal at F7-T3. In the right segment, stage N1 sleep, two discharges of wicket spikes occur over the right temporal regions. The first one spreads to the left temporal region. Note the last element of the run of the last one and compare with the wicket spikes on the following plate.

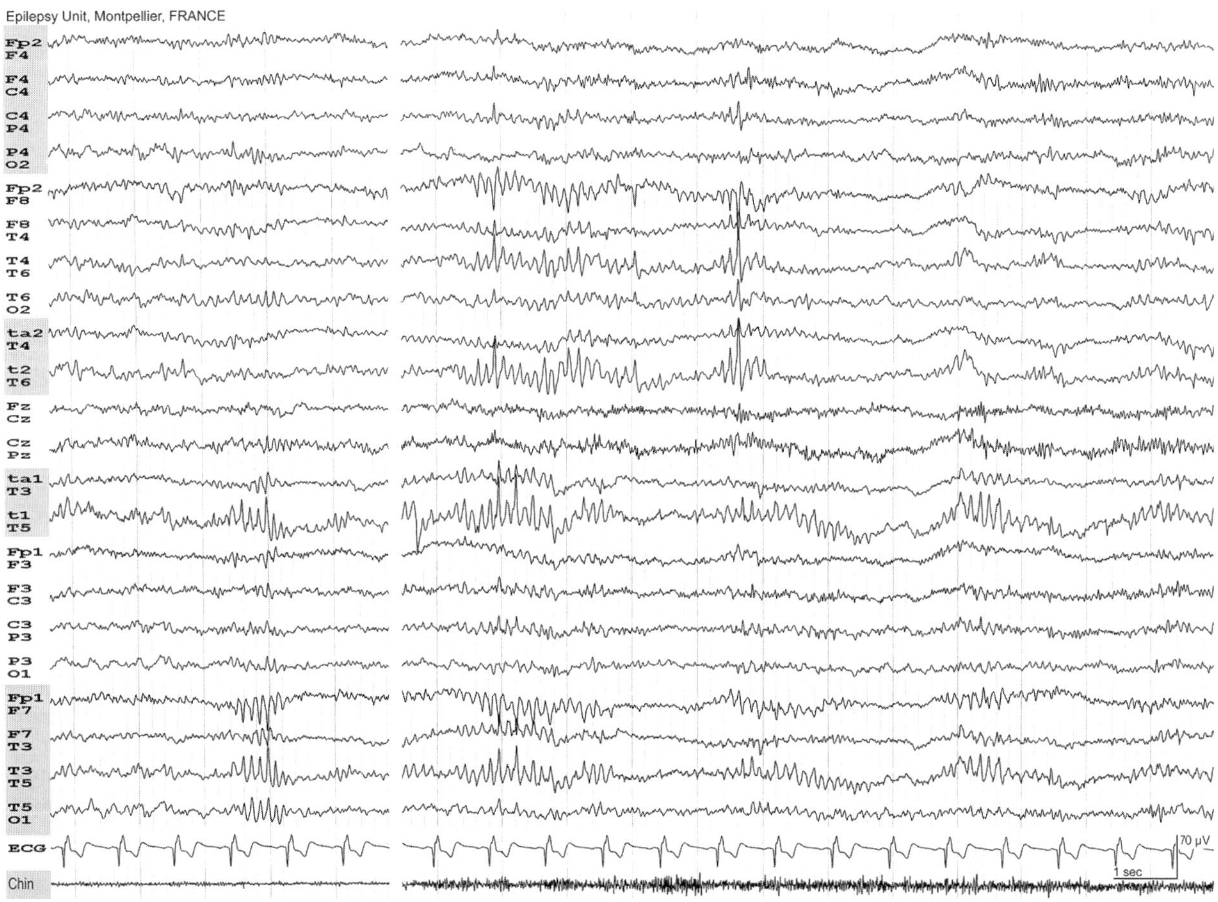

Figure a / Recording at 15 mm/s.

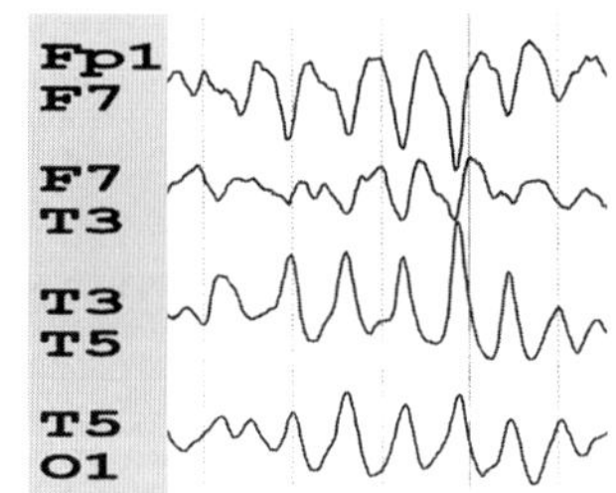

Figure b / Arciform waves at 8 Hz over the left temporal region (wicket spikes), phase reversal at F7-T3.

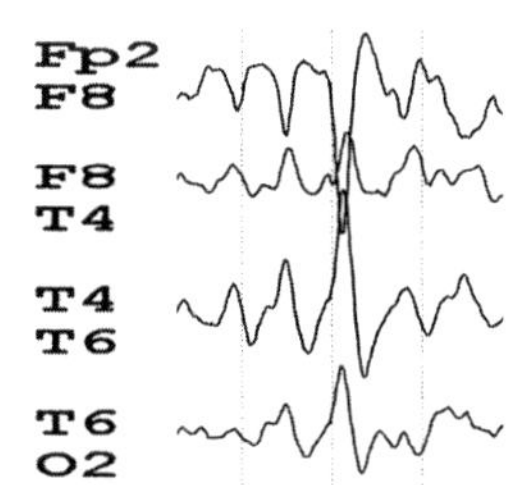

Figure c / Short run of wicket spikes over the right temporal region. Note the last element of the run which, if taken alone, resembles an "epileptic" spike.

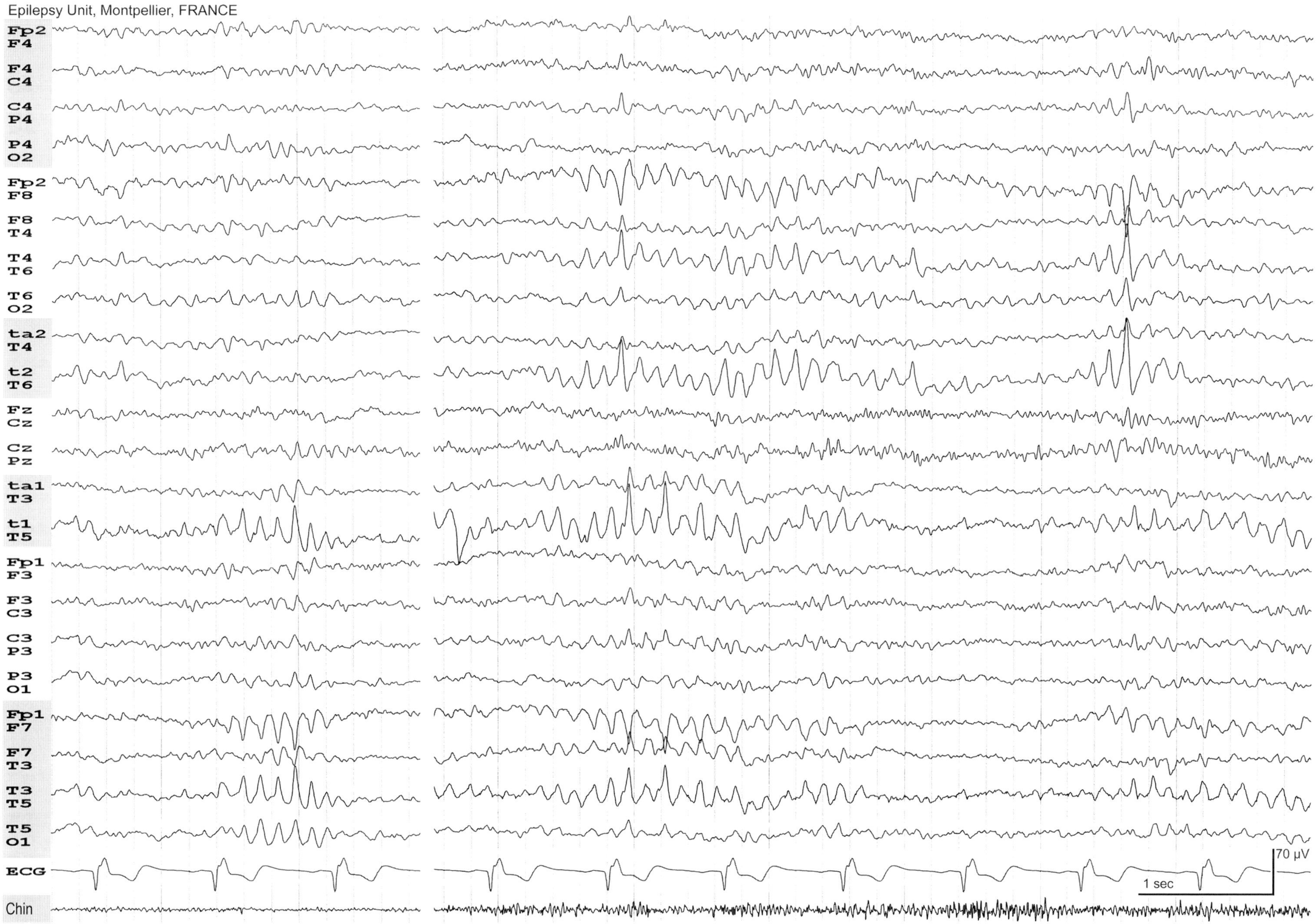
Epilepsy Unit, Montpellier, FRANCE
Fp2 F4
F4 C4
C4 P4
P4 O2
Fp2 F8
F8 T4
T4 T6
T6 O2
ta2 T4
t2 T6
Fz Cz
Cz Pz
ta1 T3
t1 T5
Fp1 F3
F3 C3
C3 P3
P3 O1
Fp1 F7
F7 T3
T3 T5
T5 O1
ECG
Chin
70 µV
1 sec

III • 53 Wicket spikes (2)

Context

70-year-old woman, same patient as on the previous plate.

What to note

In the left segment, stage N2 sleep. In the central segment, stage N3 sleep. In the right segment, REM sleep with atonia on the EMG. In the left and central segments, a very sharply contoured waveform can be observed which, if taken alone, can be mistaken for an "epileptic" spike. But the same element, when seen in longer runs, is clearly a wicket spike. Indeed, the morphology of this sharply contoured wave is identical to the morphology of the most sharply contoured waveforms in the runs of wicket spikes on the previous plate. In REM sleep, the wicket spikes are not quite as ample but their morphology and distribution remain unchanged. Note that several different presentations of wicket spikes can occur in the same patient.

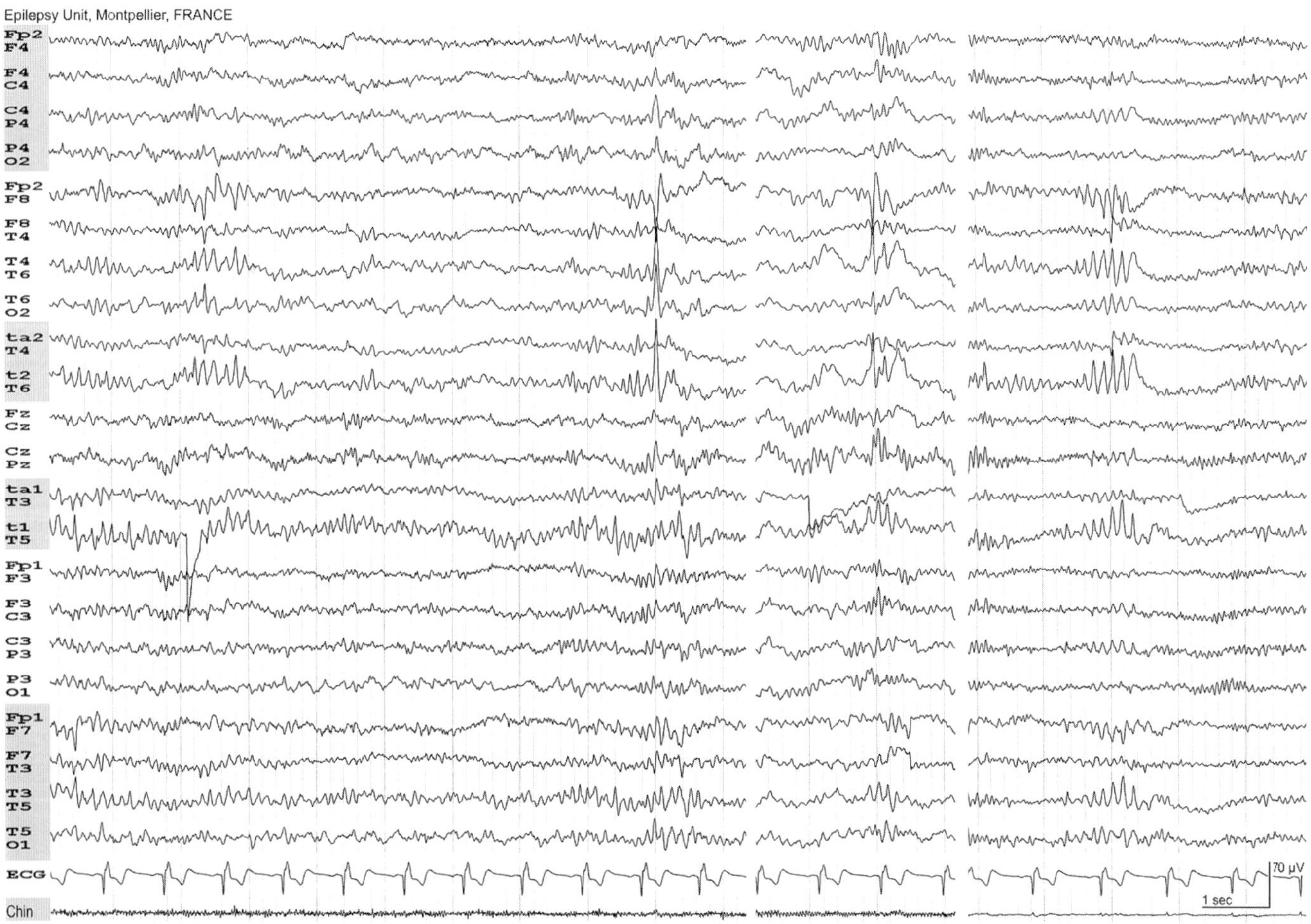

Figure a / Recording at 15 mm/s. In the left segment, wicket spikes occurs independently over the left then over the right temporal region.

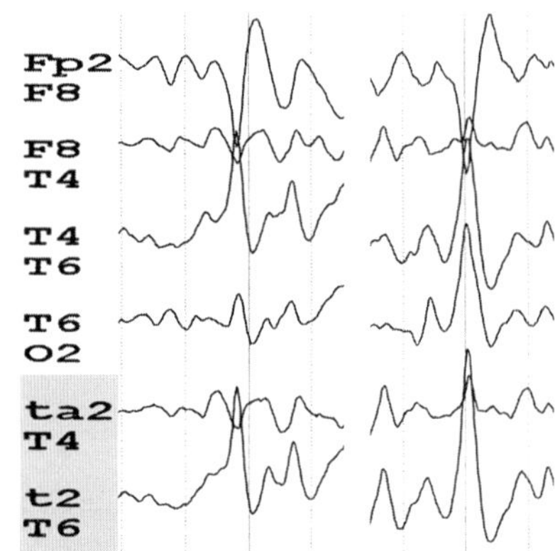

Figure b / NREM sleep. Isolated wicket spike which can be mistaken for an "epileptic" abnormality. Its morphology is identical to the most sharply contoured waveform in the run on the previous plate.

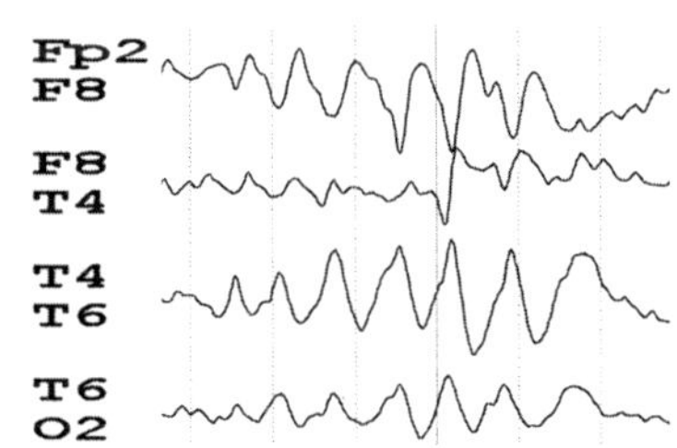

Figure c / REM sleep. Wicket spikes over the right temporal region.

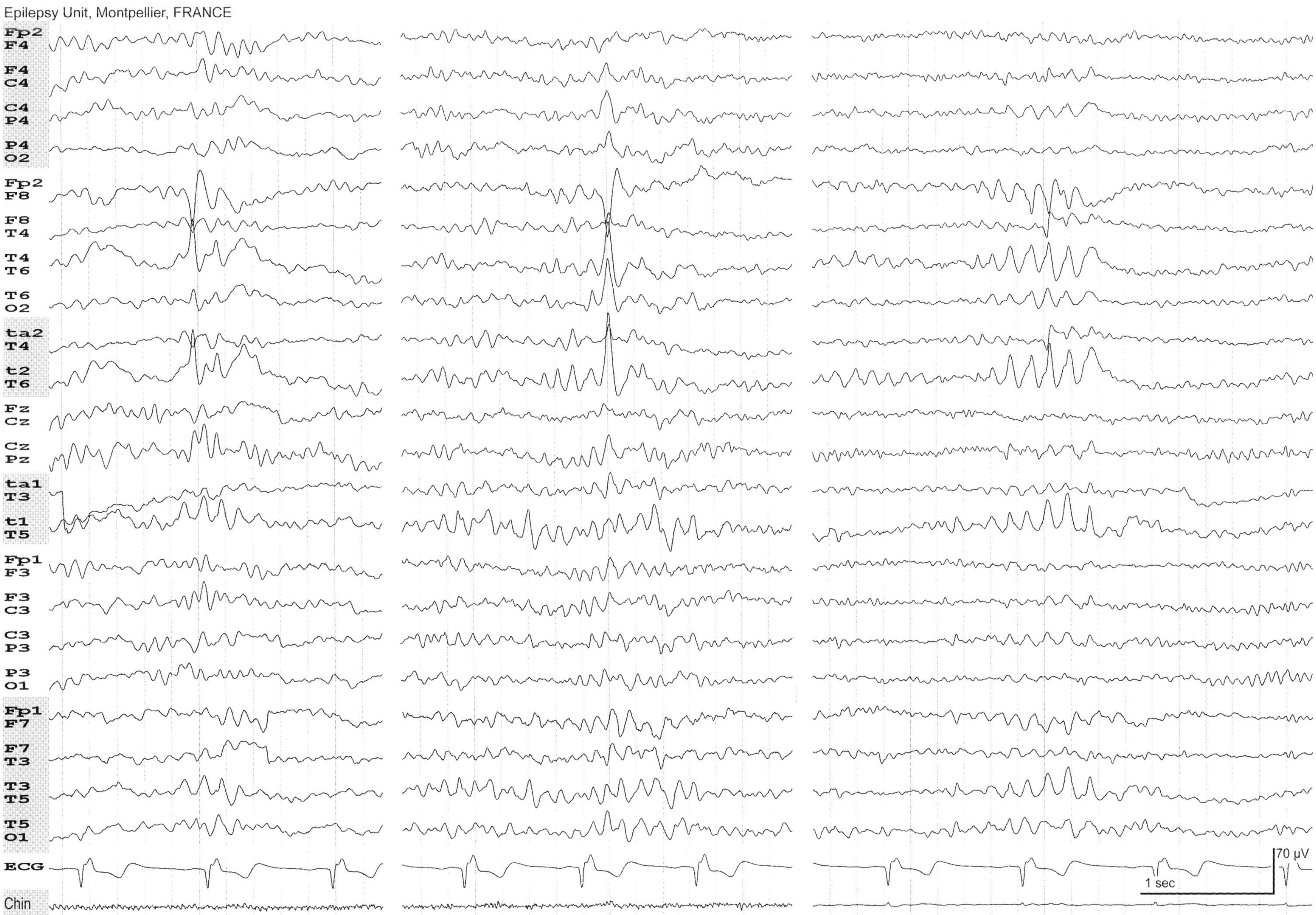
Epilepsy Unit, Montpellier, FRANCE
Fp2 F4
F4 C4
C4 P4
P4 O2
Fp2 F8
F8 T4
T4 T6
T6 O2
ta2 T4
t2 T6
Fz Cz
Cz Pz
ta1 T3
t1 T5
Fp1 F3
F3 C3
C3 P3
P3 O1
Fp1 F7
F7 T3
T3 T5
T5 O1
ECG
Chin
70 µV
1 sec

III • 54 Wicket spikes (3)

Context

70-year-old man with cryptogenic left lateral temporal lobe epilepsy.

What to note

Stage N2 sleep. The physiologic elements of sleep are poorly developed. A sleep spindle can be seen. At the beginning of the plate, a run of arciform waves at 7 Hz with phase reversal under T4-T6, corresponding to wicket spikes. In the middle of the plate, a burst of fast activities over the left temporal region. This pattern corresponds to interictal abnormalities in this man. In this man, the wicket spikes are controlateral to the left temporal epileptic focus.

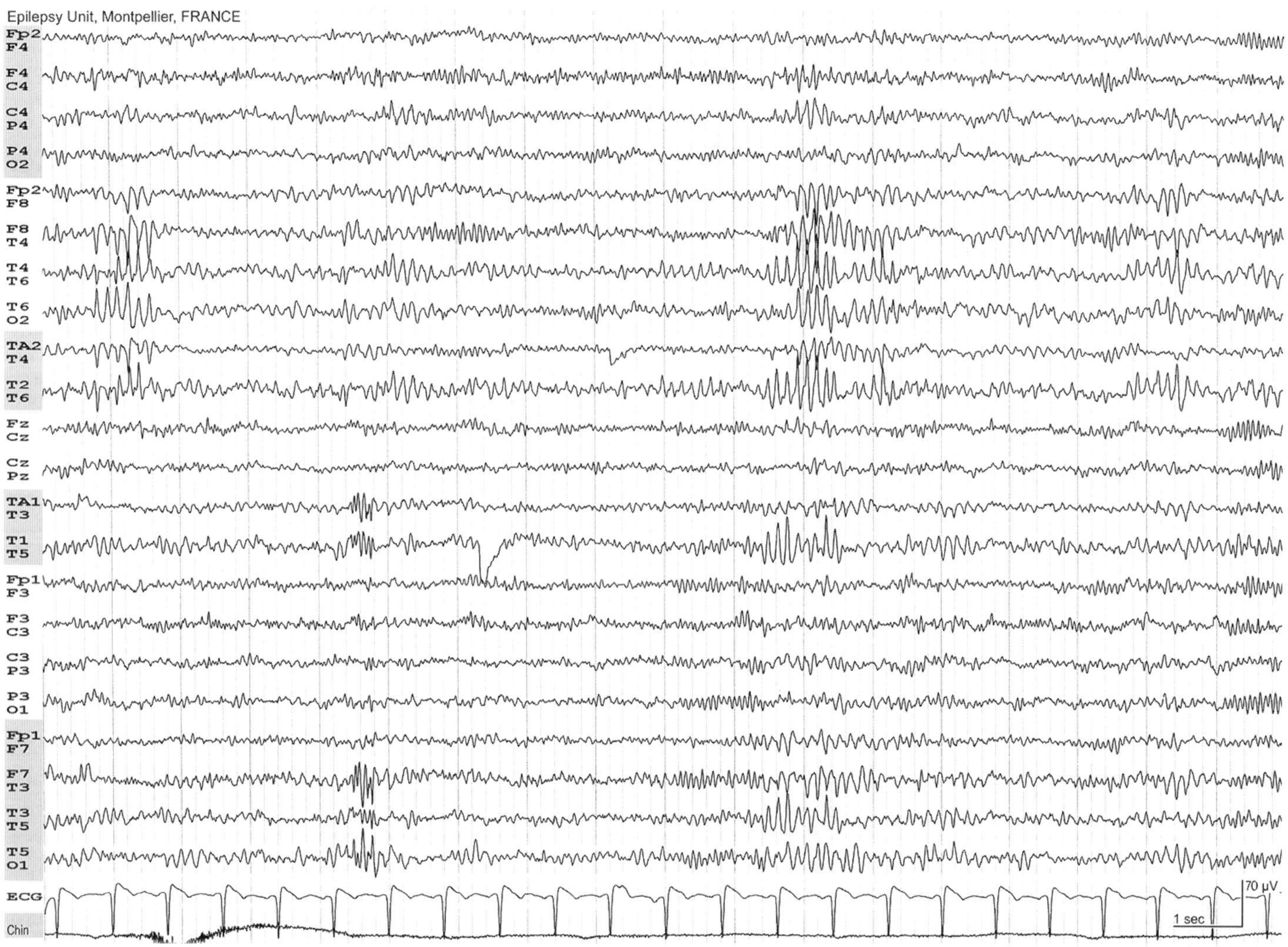

Figure a / Recording at 15 mm/s. Some wicket spikes spread to the left temporal region. Sleep spindle at the end of the plate.

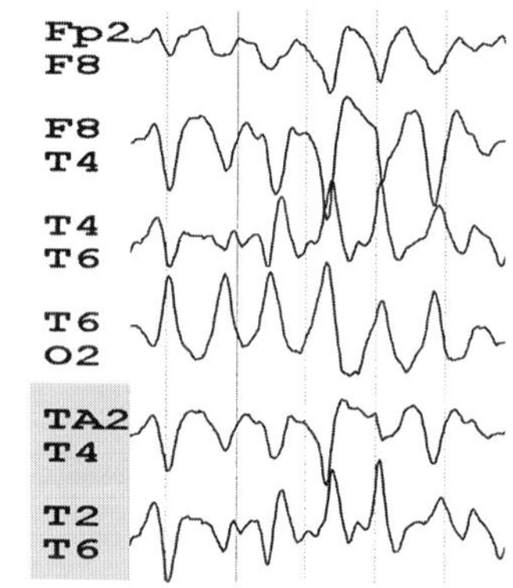

Figure b / Wicket spikes.

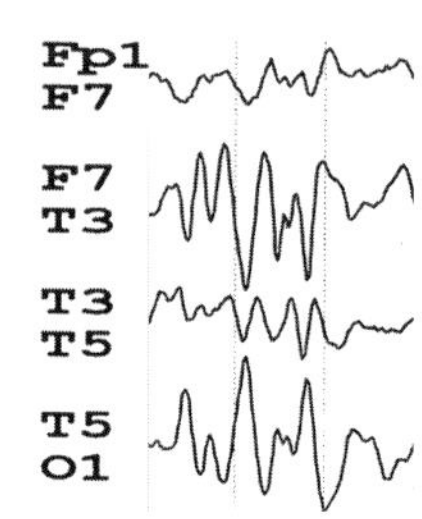

Figure c / Fast rhythms (interictal focus).

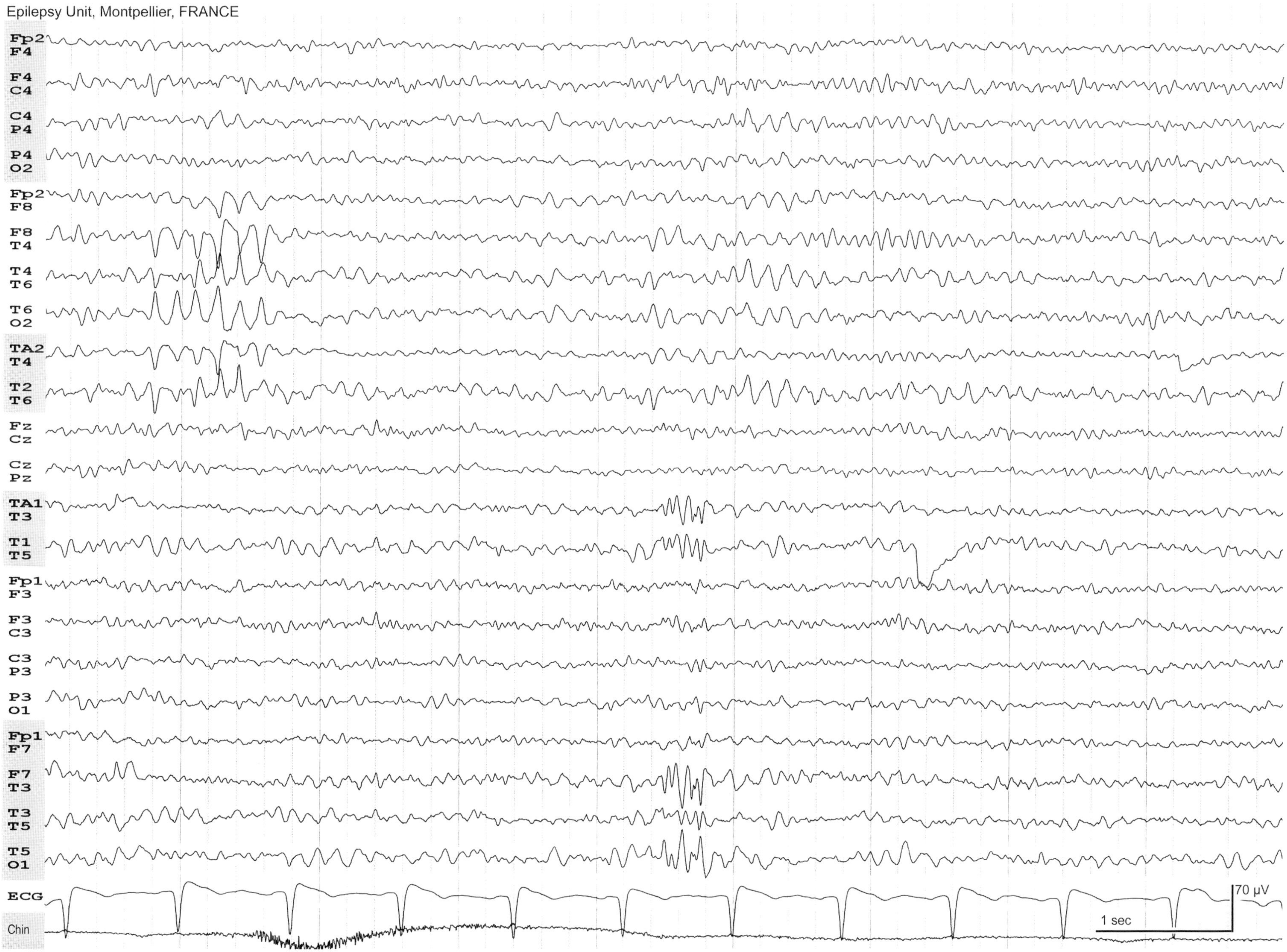
Epilepsy Unit, Montpellier, FRANCE
Fp2 F4
F4 C4
C4 P4
P4 O2
Fp2 F8
F8 T4
T4 T6
T6 O2
TA2 T4
T2 T6
Fz Cz
Cz Pz
TA1 T3
T1 T5
Fp1 F3
F3 C3
C3 P3
P3 O1
Fp1 F7
F7 T3
T3 T5
T5 O1
ECG
Chin
70 µV
1 sec

III • 55 Wicket spikes (4)

Context

42-year-old woman with right lateral temporal lobe epilepsy, presurgical assessment.

What to note

Stage N2 sleep. Poorly developed K complex and sleep spindles predominating on the left hemisphere. Run of 8 Hz arciform waves can be observed in phase reversal under F7-T3, particularly visible at the T1-T5 derivation. These waveforms correspond to wicket spikes. At the 4th second, a sharp wave can also be seen in this part of the plate over the right temporal region prior to slow waves. This pattern corresponds to interictal abnormalities in this woman. In this woman, the wicket spikes are controlateral to the right temporal epileptic focus.

Comment

In focal epilepsy, an EEG asymmetry depending to the epileptic focus side can be found especially for spindles (Crespel *et al.*, 1998; 2000). Spindles are better organized on the non-epileptic EEG side.

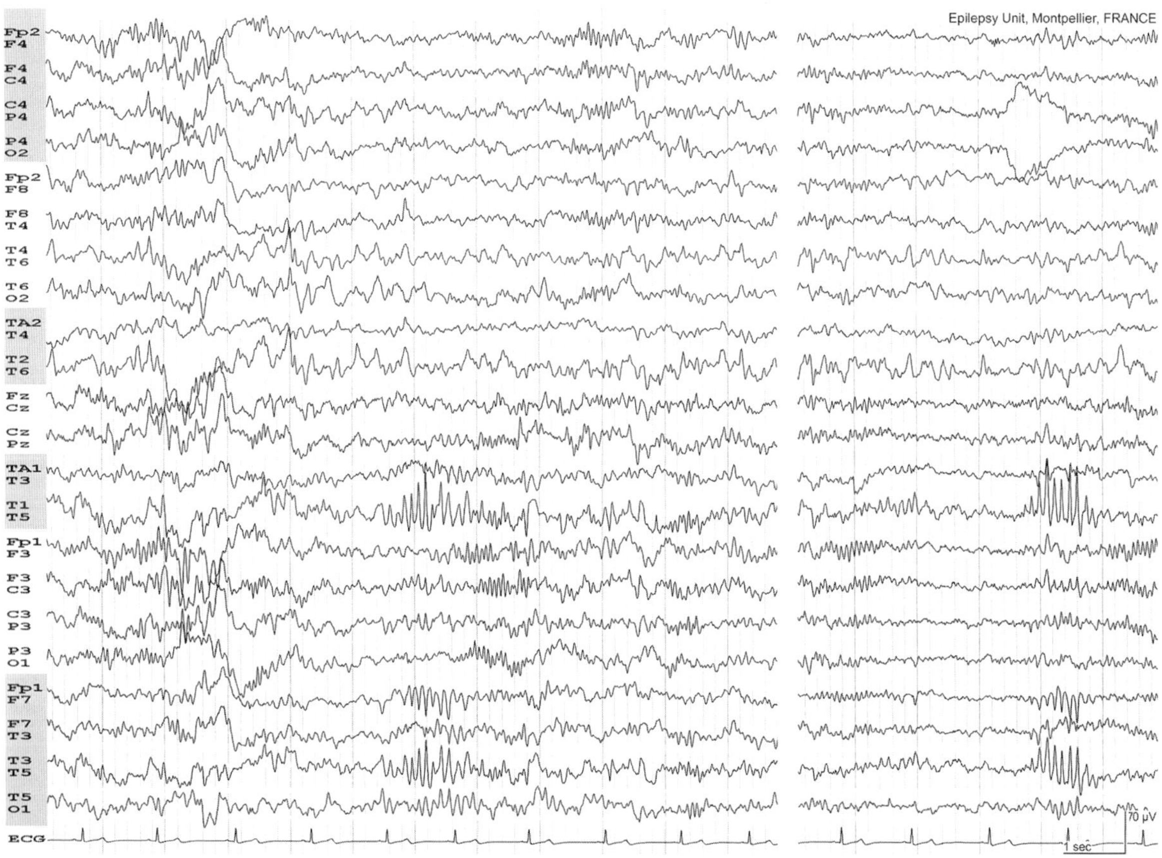

Figure a / Recording at 15 mm/s. Right segment: at the 1st second sleep spindle predominating on the left; at the 4th second, wicket spikes. The differences between spindles and wicket spikes are clear, the latter being slower, with more ample waveforms, and midtemporal distribution.

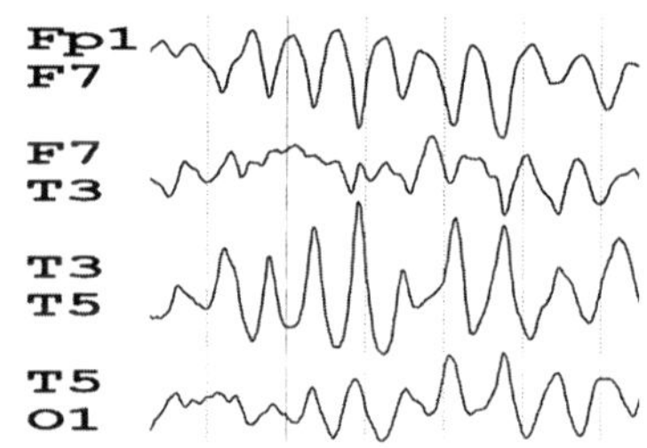

Figure b / Wicket spikes.

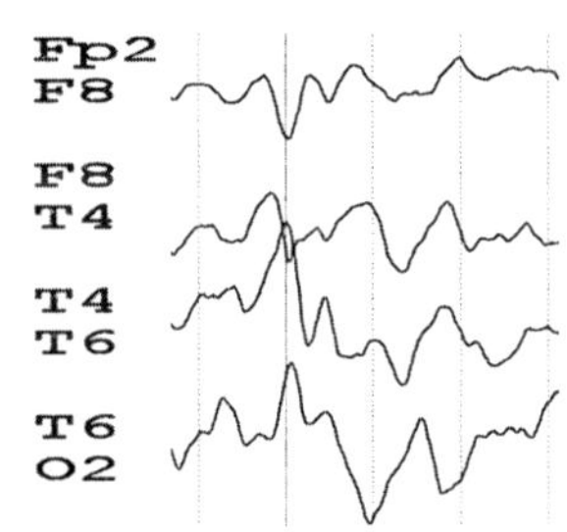

Figure c / Sharp wave followed by slow waves over the right temporal region (interictal focus).

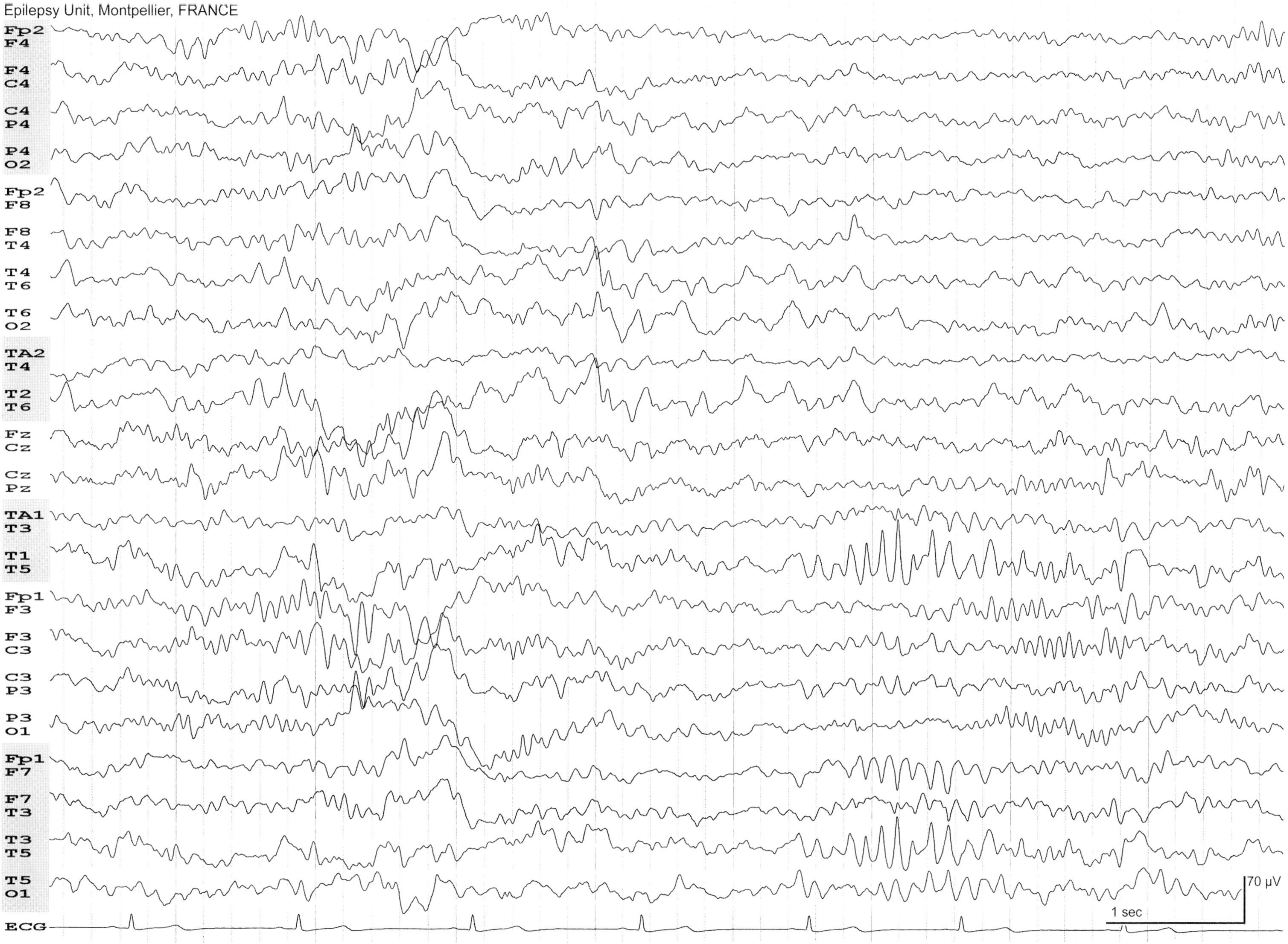

Epilepsy Unit, Montpellier, FRANCE
Fp2 F4
F4 C4
C4 P4
P4 O2
Fp2 F8
F8 T4
T4 T6
T6 O2
TA2 T4
T2 T6
Fz Cz
Cz Pz
TA1 T3
T1 T5
Fp1 F3
F3 C3
C3 P3
P3 O1
Fp1 F7
F7 T3
T3 T5
T5 O1
ECG
70 µV
1 sec

III • 56 Wicket spikes in REM sleep

Context

42-year-old woman, same patient as on the previous plate.

What to note

The woman is now in REM sleep, with sawtooth waves over the vertex that spread to the adjacent regions and rapid eye movements at the frontal polar derivations. Over the left temporal region, wicket spikes can still be observed in REM sleep. Compared to the previous plate, they are not quite as ample but their morphology and distribution remain unchanged. Moreover, right temporal lobe epileptiform abnormalities can be observed.

Comment

Wicket spikes appear in relaxation, drowsiness, and stages N1 and N2. They disappear in NREM deep sleep and reappear in REM sleep: in the latter stage, they have an identical morphology as in drowsiness or stage N2 sleep with only slightly lower amplitude. Their location remains identical (Gelisse *et al.*, 2003). Sérafini *et al.* (2014) reported an activation of wicket spikes by REM sleep in some patients.

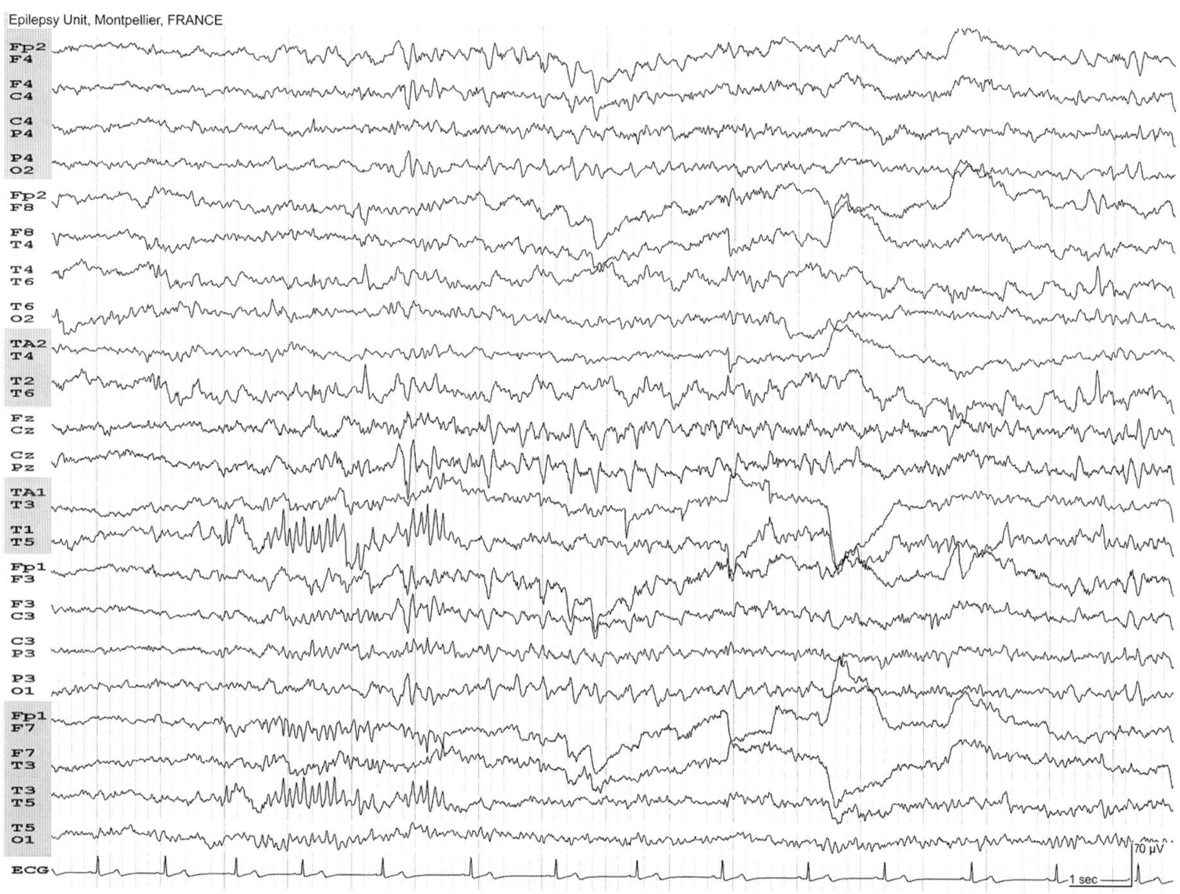

Figure a / Recording at 15 mm/s.

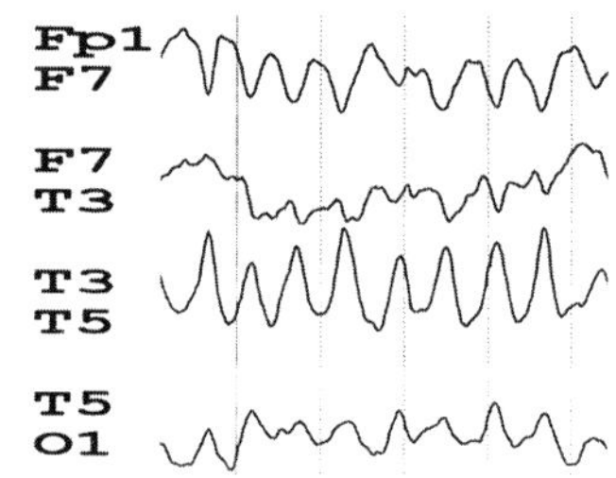

Figure b / Wicket spikes over the left temporal region.

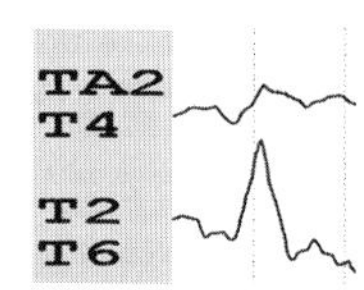

Figure c / Spike on the right temporal lobe (interictal focus).

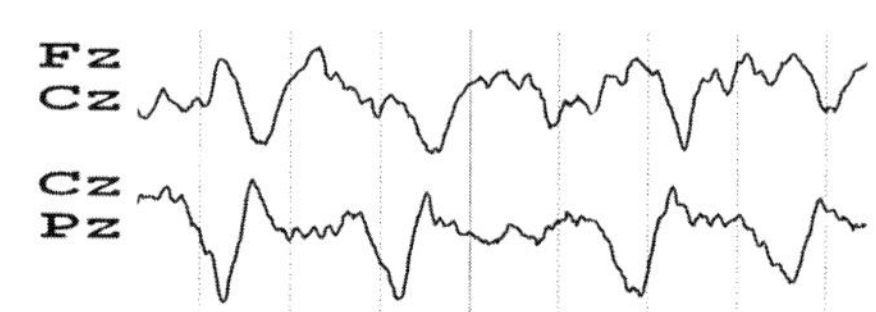

Figure d / Sawtooth waves.

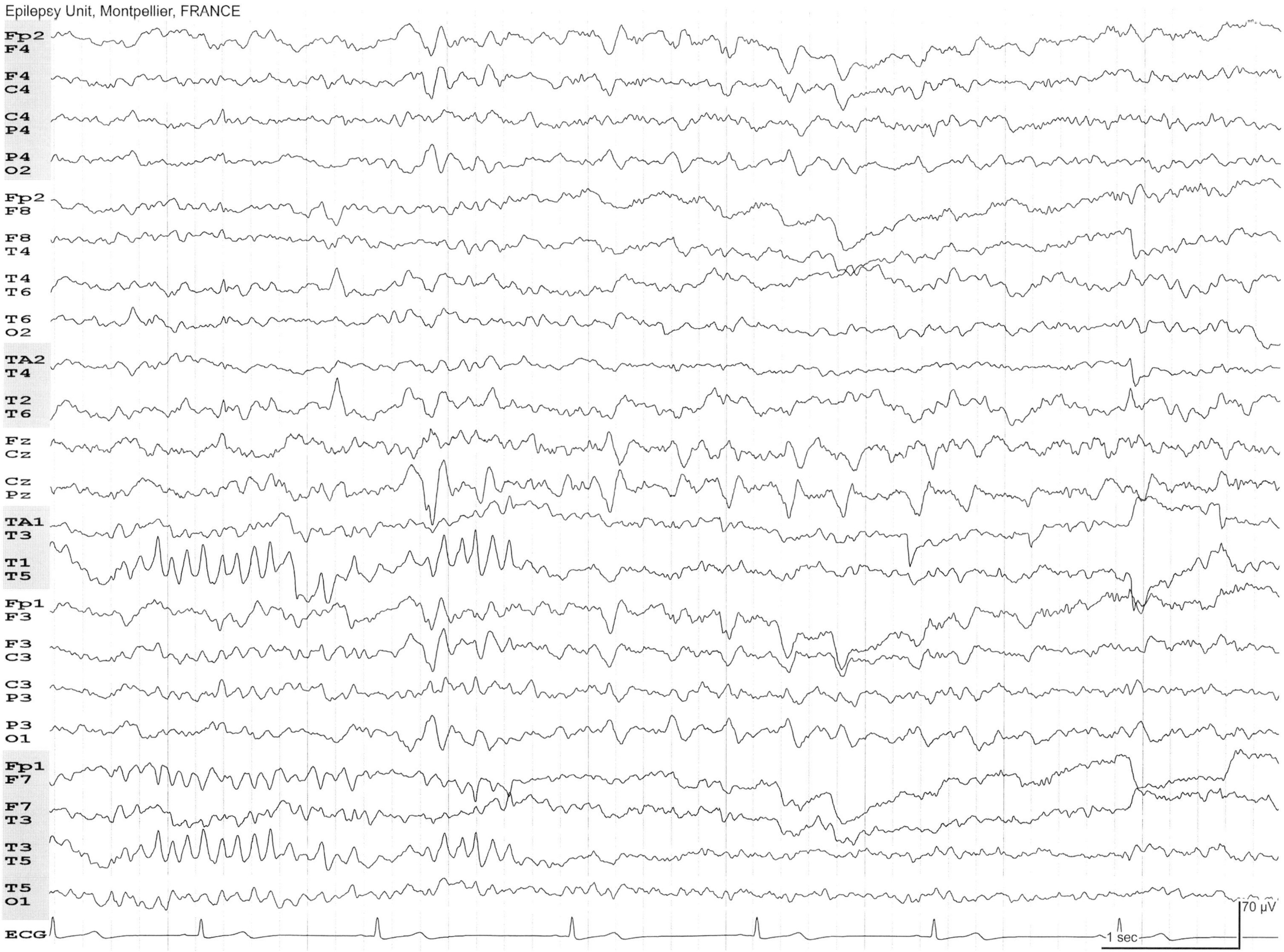
Epilepsy Unit, Montpellier, FRANCE
Fp2 F4
F4 C4
C4 P4
P4 O2
Fp2 F8
F8 T4
T4 T6
T6 O2
TA2 T4
T2 T6
Fz Cz
Cz Pz
TA1 T3
T1 T5
Fp1 F3
F3 C3
C3 P3
P3 O1
Fp1 F7
F7 T3
T3 T5
T5 O1
ECG
70 µV
1 sec

• 57 Small Sharp Spikes (SSS)/ Benign sporadic sleep spikes/ Benign epileptiform transients of sleep (1)

Context

72-year-old woman, nightly sleep EEG after two episodes of confusion.

What to note

Stage N2 sleep. On the left and right, low-voltage, short duration, spikes occur singly and predominantly over the temporal regions. They spread to the central regions. These small spikes correspond to small sharp spikes (SSS). They have no known pathological significance although several authors have indicated an increased occurrence in patients with a psychiatric, epileptic, or cardiovascular history.

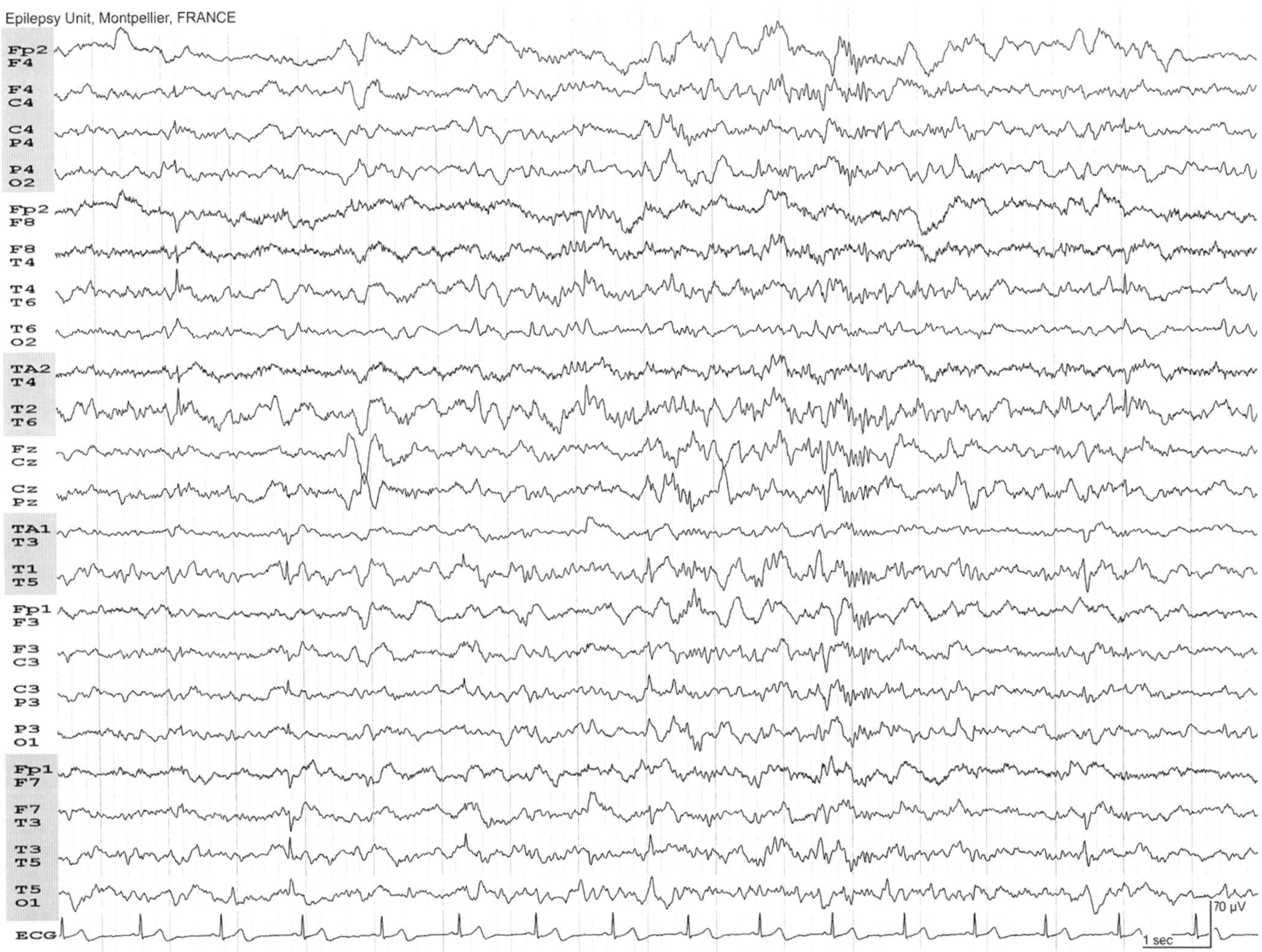

Figure a / Recording at 15 mm/s. Sleep spindle in the middle of the plate. Independent SSS on the left and right temporal region at the end of the plate.

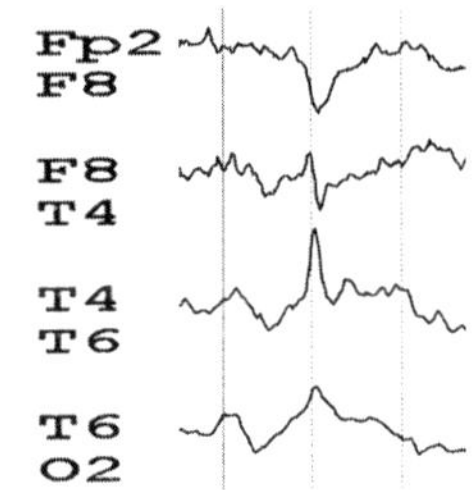

Figure b / SSS over the right temporal region.

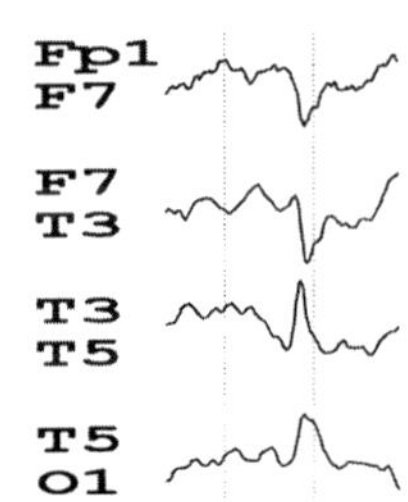

Figure c / Independent SSS over the left temporal lobe.

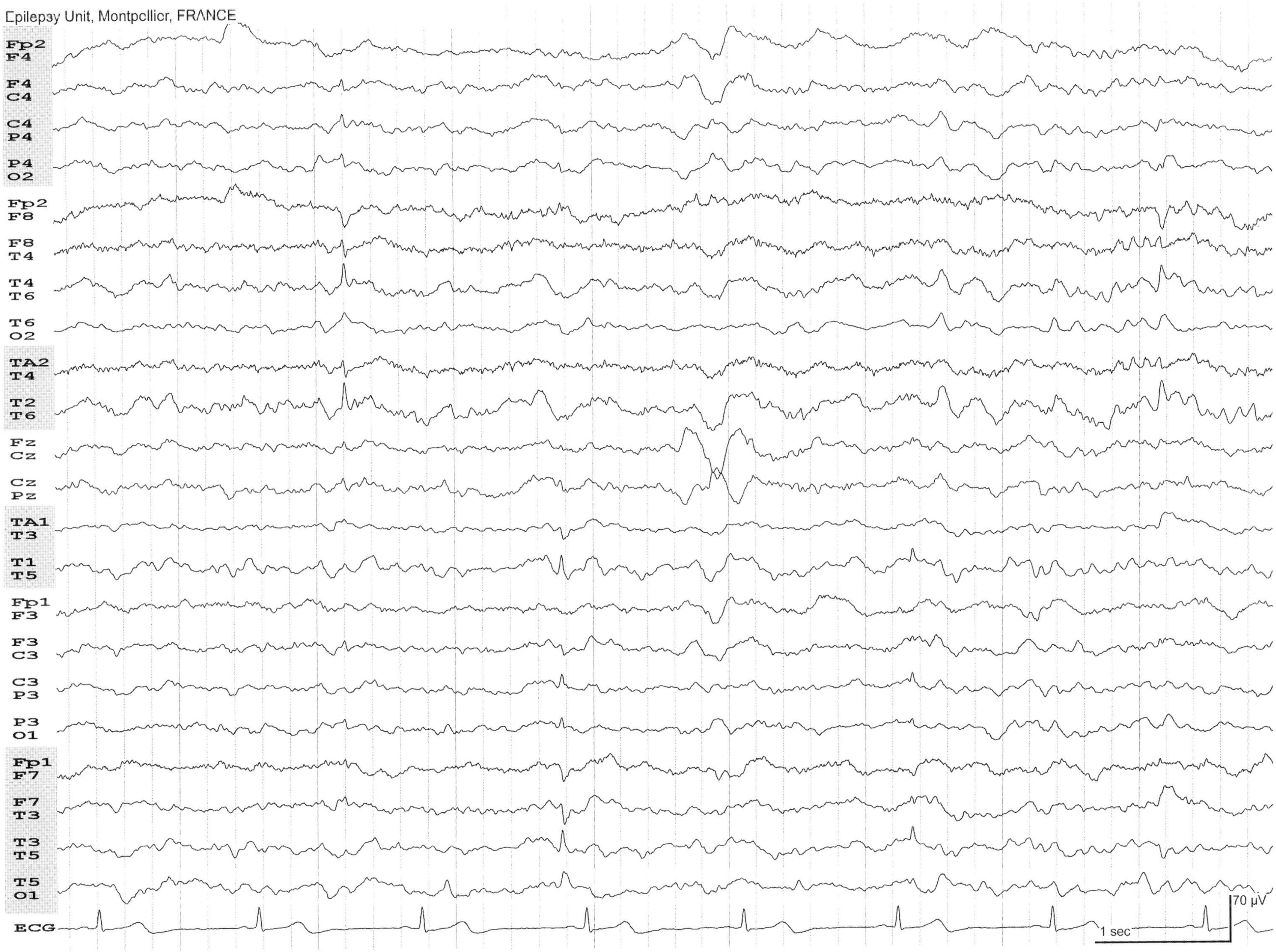
Epilepsy Unit, Montpellier, FRANCE
Fp2 F4
F4 C4
C4 P4
P4 O2
Fp2 F8
F8 T4
T4 T6
T6 O2
TA2 T4
T2 T6
Fz Cz
Cz Pz
TA1 T3
T1 T5
Fp1 F3
F3 C3
C3 P3
P3 O1
Fp1 F7
F7 T3
T3 T5
T5 O1
ECG
70 µV
1 sec

• 58 Small Sharp Spikes (SSS)/ Benign sporadic sleep spikes/ Benign epileptiform transients of sleep (2)

Context

61-year-old woman referred after a first generalized tonic-clonic seizure (acute symptomatic seizure).

What to note

On the left and right, low-voltage, short duration, mono or diphasic spikes or spike-waves occur singly and predominantly over the midtemporal regions (phase reversal at T3 and at T4). In this patient, they occur more frequently on the left. These small diphasic spikes correspond to small sharp spikes (SSS). SSS occur independently shifting from side to side.

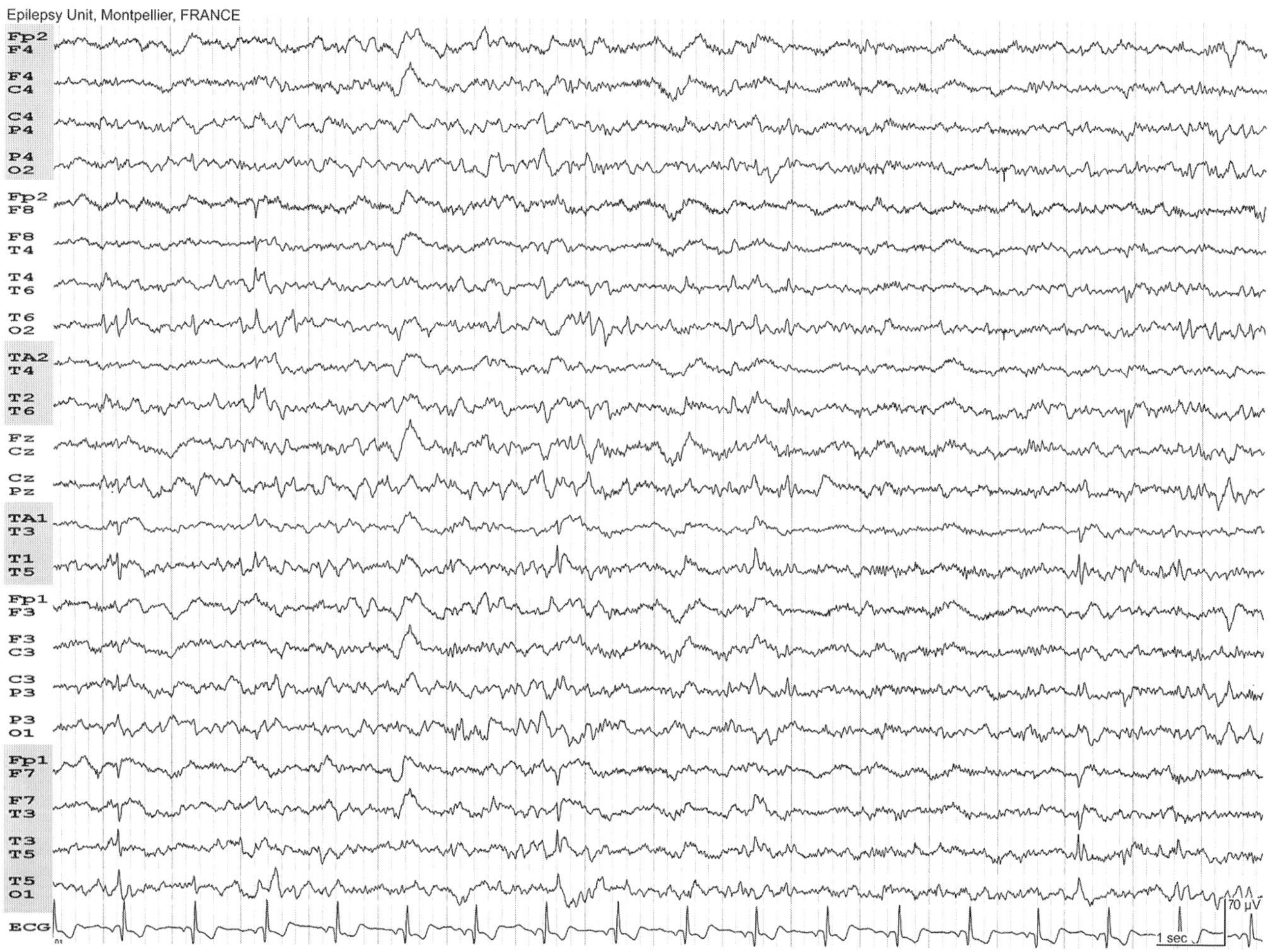

Figure a / Recording at 15 mm/s.

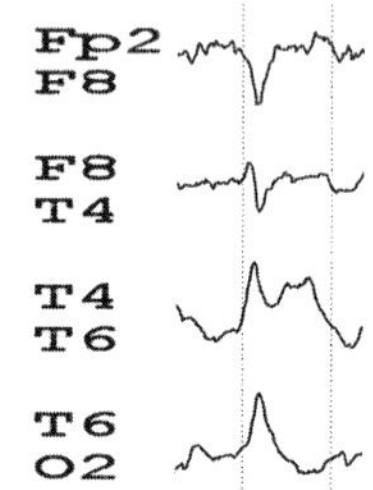

Figure b / SSS on the right midtemporal region.

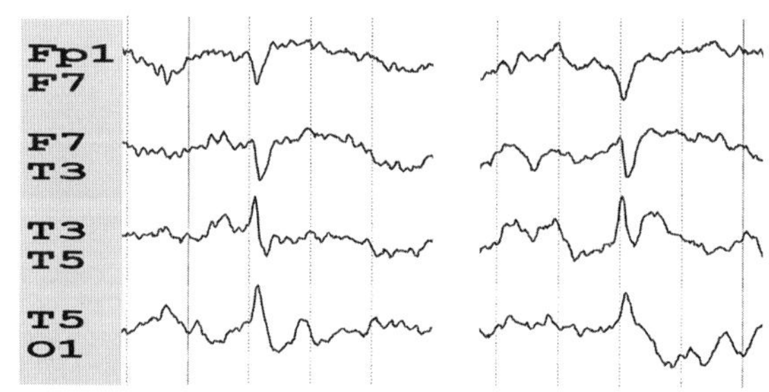

Figure c / SSS on the left midtemporal region.

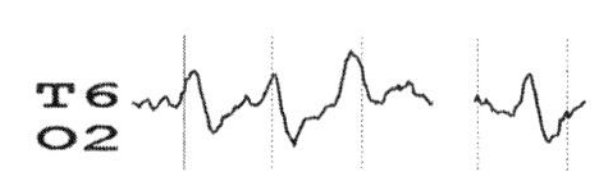

Figure d / Positive occipital transients of sleep.

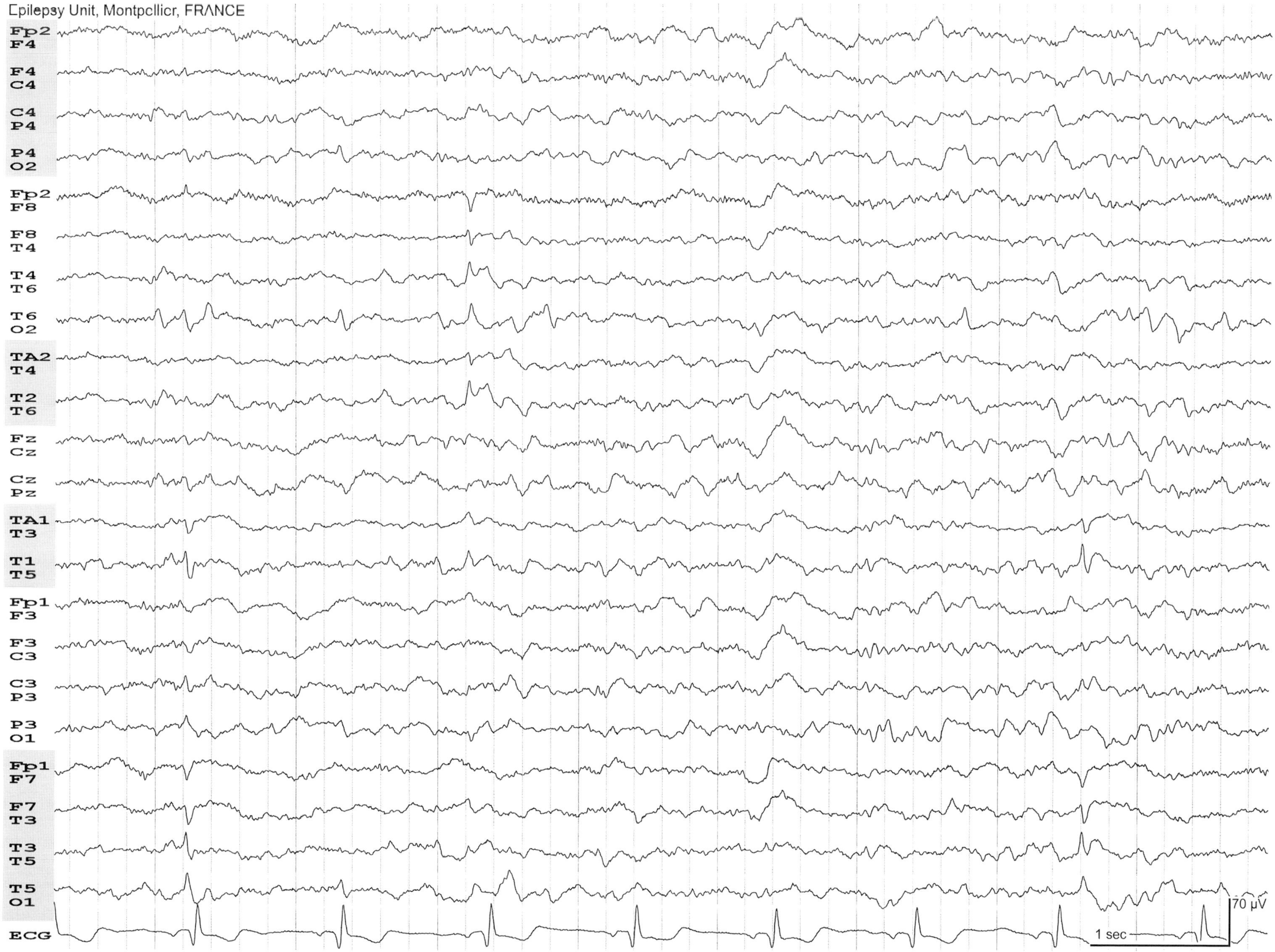
Epilepsy Unit, Montpellier, FRANCE
Fp2 F4
F4 C4
C4 P4
P4 O2
Fp2 F8
F8 T4
T4 T6
T6 O2
TA2 T4
T2 T6
Fz Cz
Cz Pz
TA1 T3
T1 T5
Fp1 F3
F3 C3
C3 P3
P3 O1
Fp1 F7
F7 T3
T3 T5
T5 O1
ECG
70 µV
1 sec

III • 59 Fourteen- and six-Hertz positive bursts during REM sleep in a child

Context

5-year-old boy with a history of febrile seizures.

What to note

The child is in REM sleep with sawtooth waves over the vertex. The amplitude of these waves is higher in children compared to adults. A14- and 6-Hertz positive burst can be observed on the left temporal region especially on T1-T5.

Comment

Based on our experience, 14- and 6-Hz positive bursts are mainly seen during REM sleep. The use of a lower temporal line that explores the inferior part of the temporal lobe significantly increases the visualization of the 14- and 6-Hertz positive bursts. They have the highest amplitude over the temporal leads, formed with the additional temporal electrodes (T1, TA1, T2, TA2) especially with the bipolar derivations T2-T6 and T1-T5 (Velizarova *et al.*, 2011).

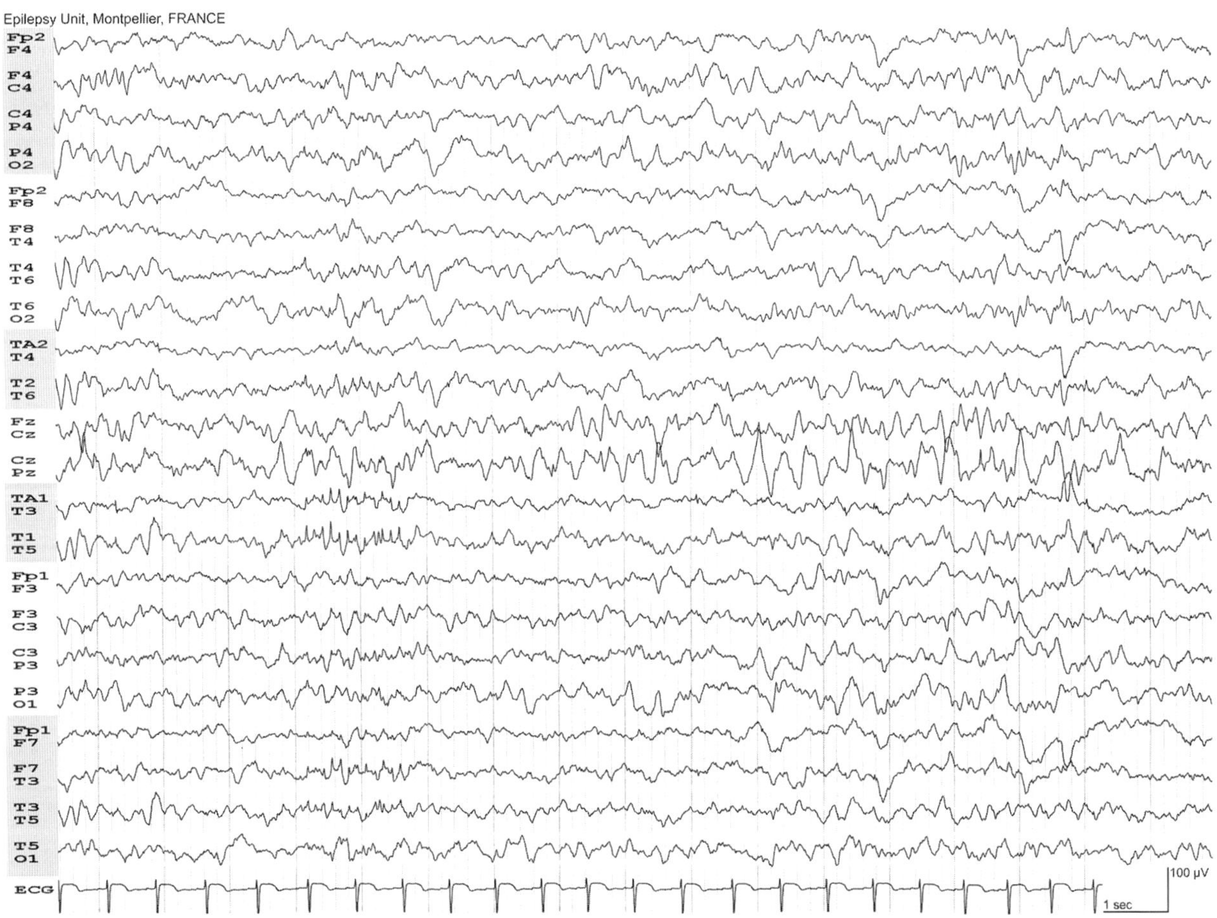

Figure a / Recording at 15 mm/s.

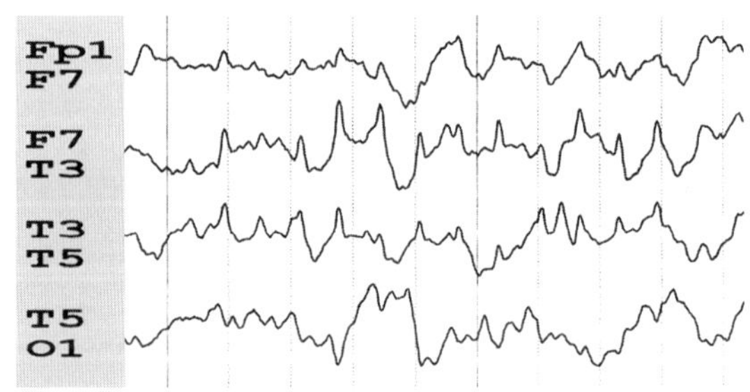

Figure b / 14- and 6-Hz positive burst during REM sleep.

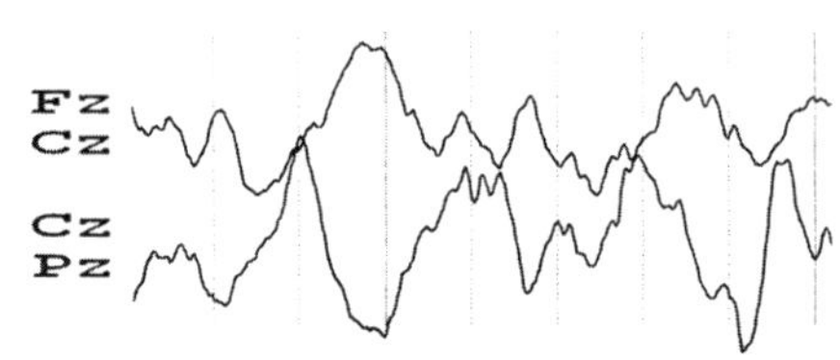

Figure c / Sawtooth waves.

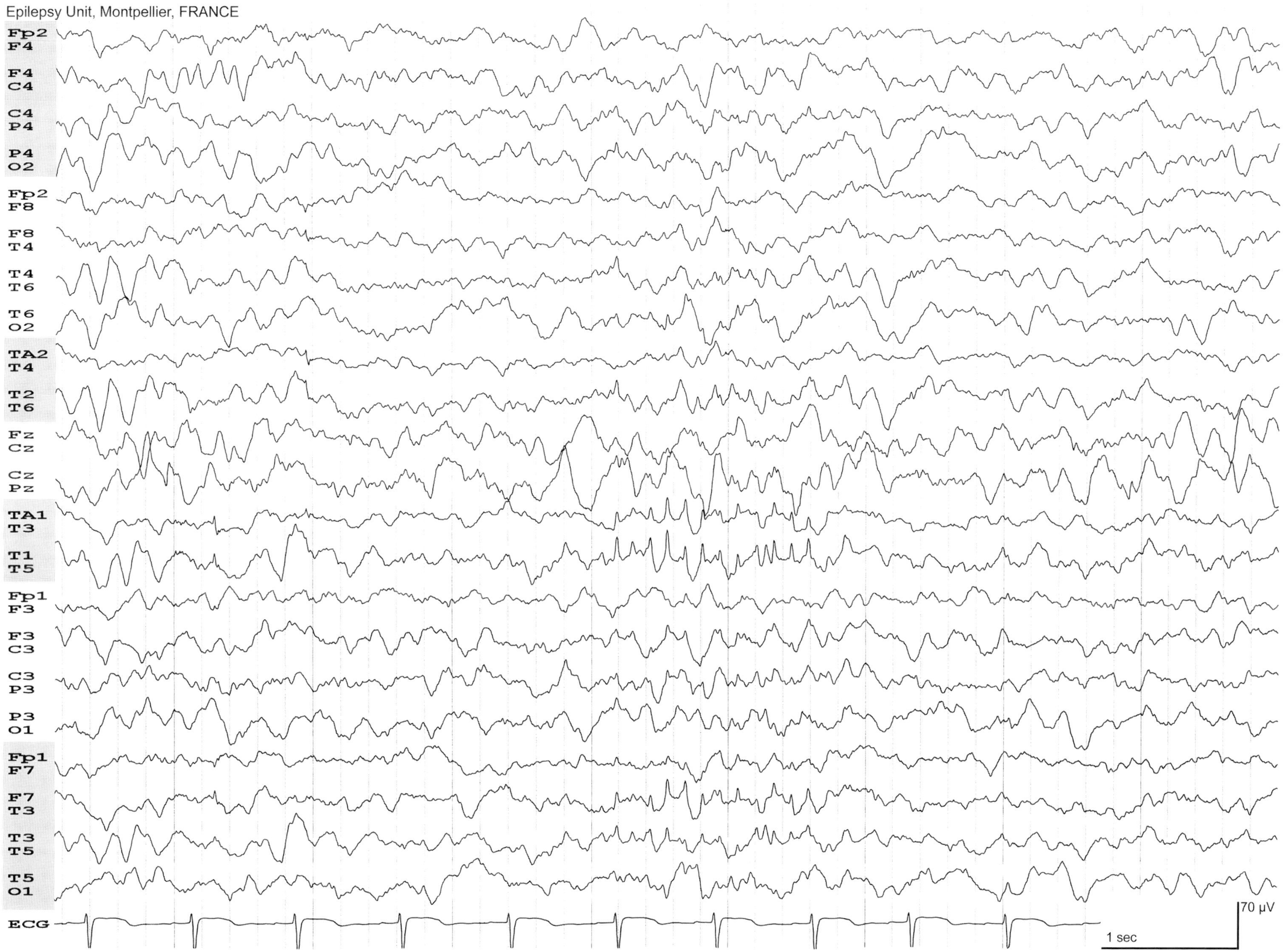
Epilepsy Unit, Montpellier, FRANCE
Fp2 F4
F4 C4
C4 P4
P4 O2
Fp2 F8
F8 T4
T4 T6
T6 O2
TA2 T4
T2 T6
Fz Cz
Cz Pz
TA1 T3
T1 T5
Fp1 F3
F3 C3
C3 P3
P3 O1
Fp1 F7
F7 T3
T3 T5
T5 O1
ECG
70 µV
1 sec

III • 60 Fourteen- and six-Hertz positive bursts during REM sleep in an adult (1)

Context

19-year-old man with psychogenic seizures.

What to note

REM sleep with rapid eye movements at the beginning of the plate and reduced muscle activity (atonia) on the EMG (Chin). Activity at 7 Hz localized over the right posterior temporal region, especially at T2-T6. This burst corresponds to the slow variant of 14- and 6-Hz positive bursts. In this patient, 14- and 6-Hertz positive bursts were also found in NREM sleep but there was a clear activation in REM sleep.

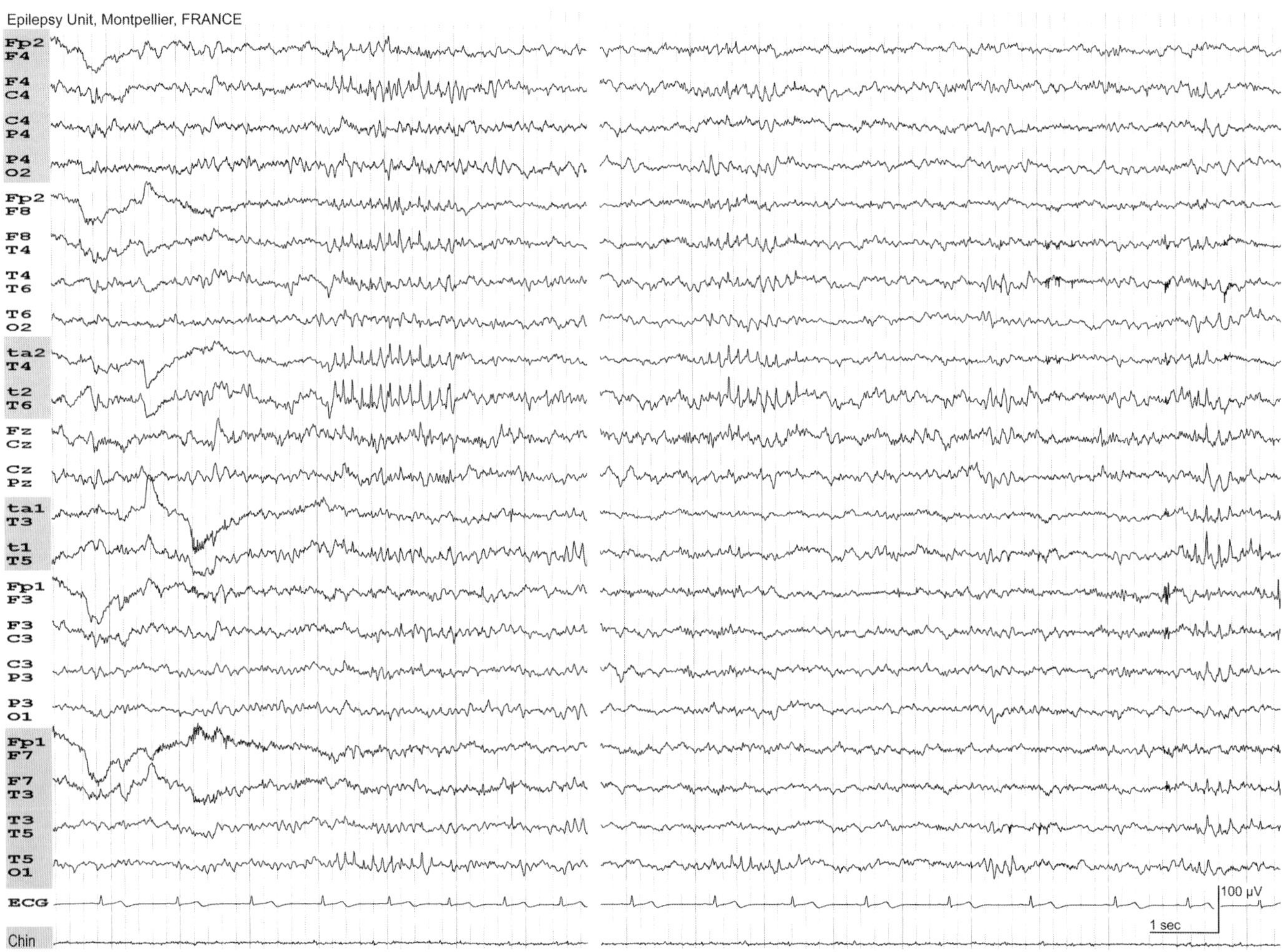

Figure a / Recording at 15 mm/s. Right segment. REM sleep. Occurrence of independant 14- and 6-Hertz positive bursts.

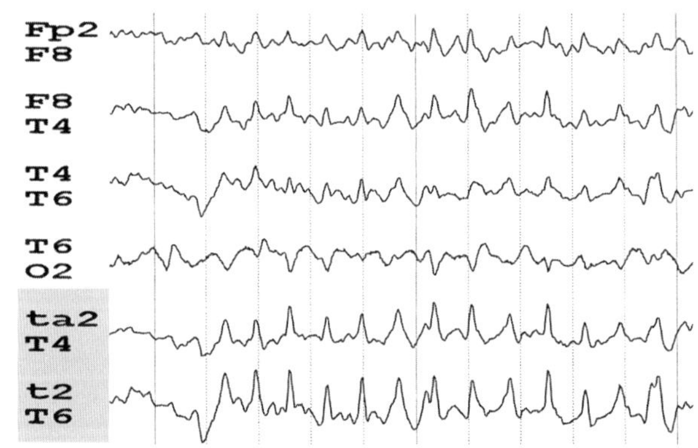

Figure b / 14- and 6-Hz positive burst (slow variant).

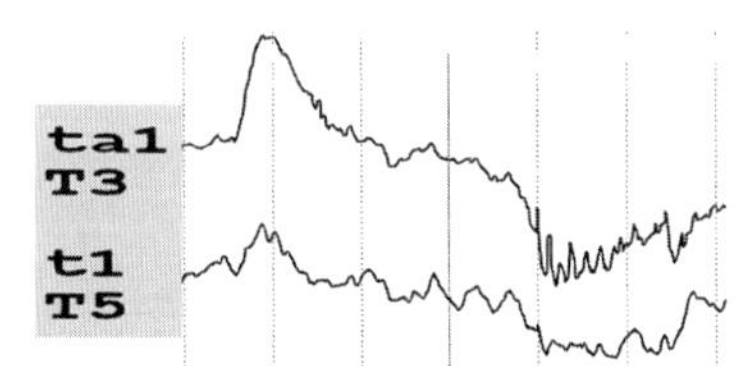

Figure c / Rapid eye movements.

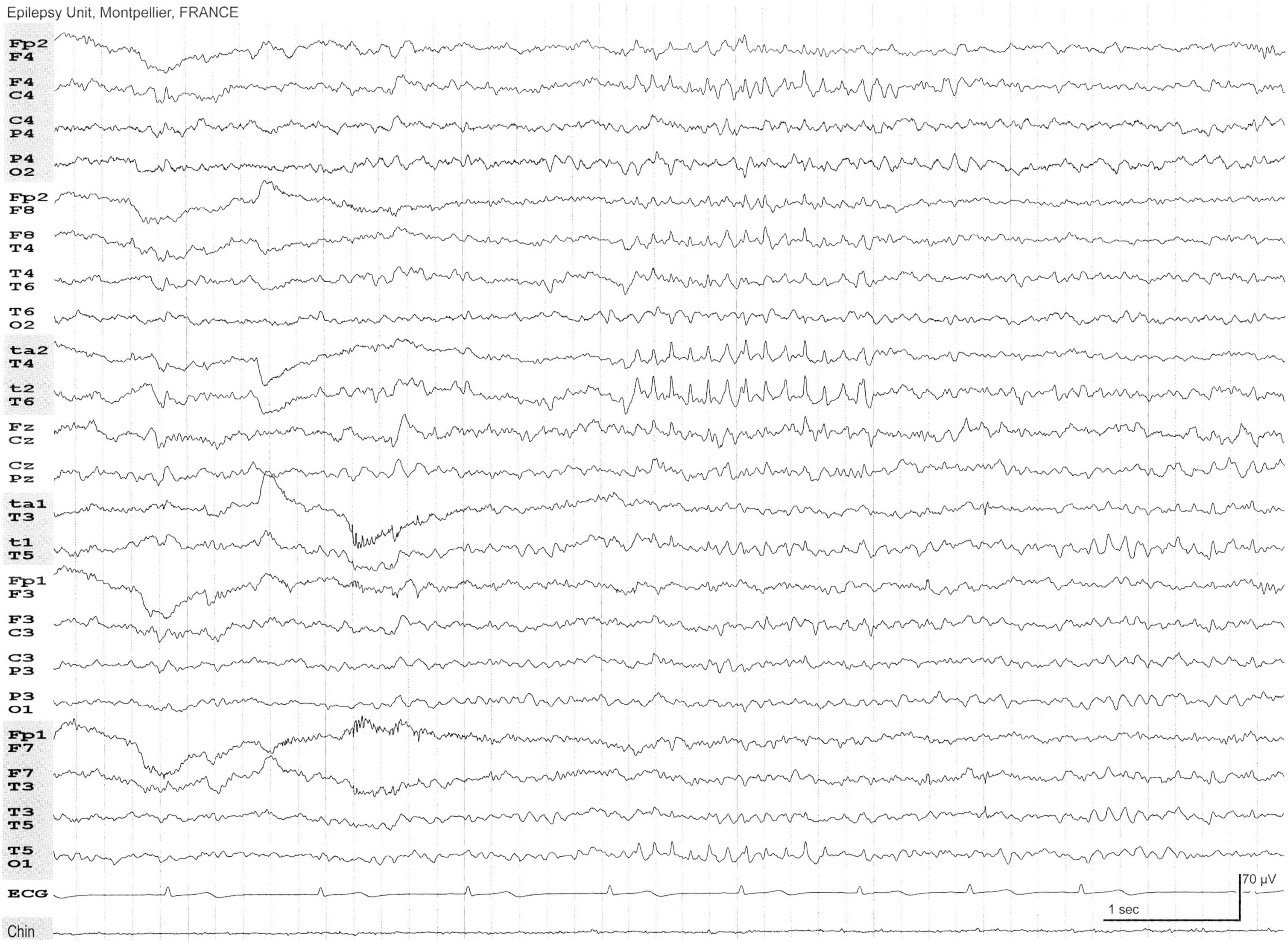
Epilepsy Unit, Montpellier, FRANCE
Fp2 F4
F4 C4
C4 P4
P4 O2
Fp2 F8
F8 T4
T4 T6
T6 O2
ta2 T4
t2 T6
Fz Cz
Cz Pz
ta1 T3
t1 T5
Fp1 F3
F3 C3
C3 P3
P3 O1
Fp1 F7
F7 T3
T3 T5
T5 O1
ECG
Chin
70 µV
1 sec

III • 61 Fourteen- and six-Hertz positive bursts during REM sleep in an adult (2)

Context

21-year-old woman with idiopathic generalized epilepsy.

What to note

REM sleep with reduced muscle activity (atonia) on the EMG (Chin). 14- and 6-Hertz positive bursts. The second burst is localized on the right posterior temporal region whereas the first one is more diffuse. These bursts correspond to the fast variant of 14- and 6-Hz positive bursts. In this patient, 14- and 6-Hertz positive bursts were also found in NREM sleep but there was a clear activation in REM sleep.

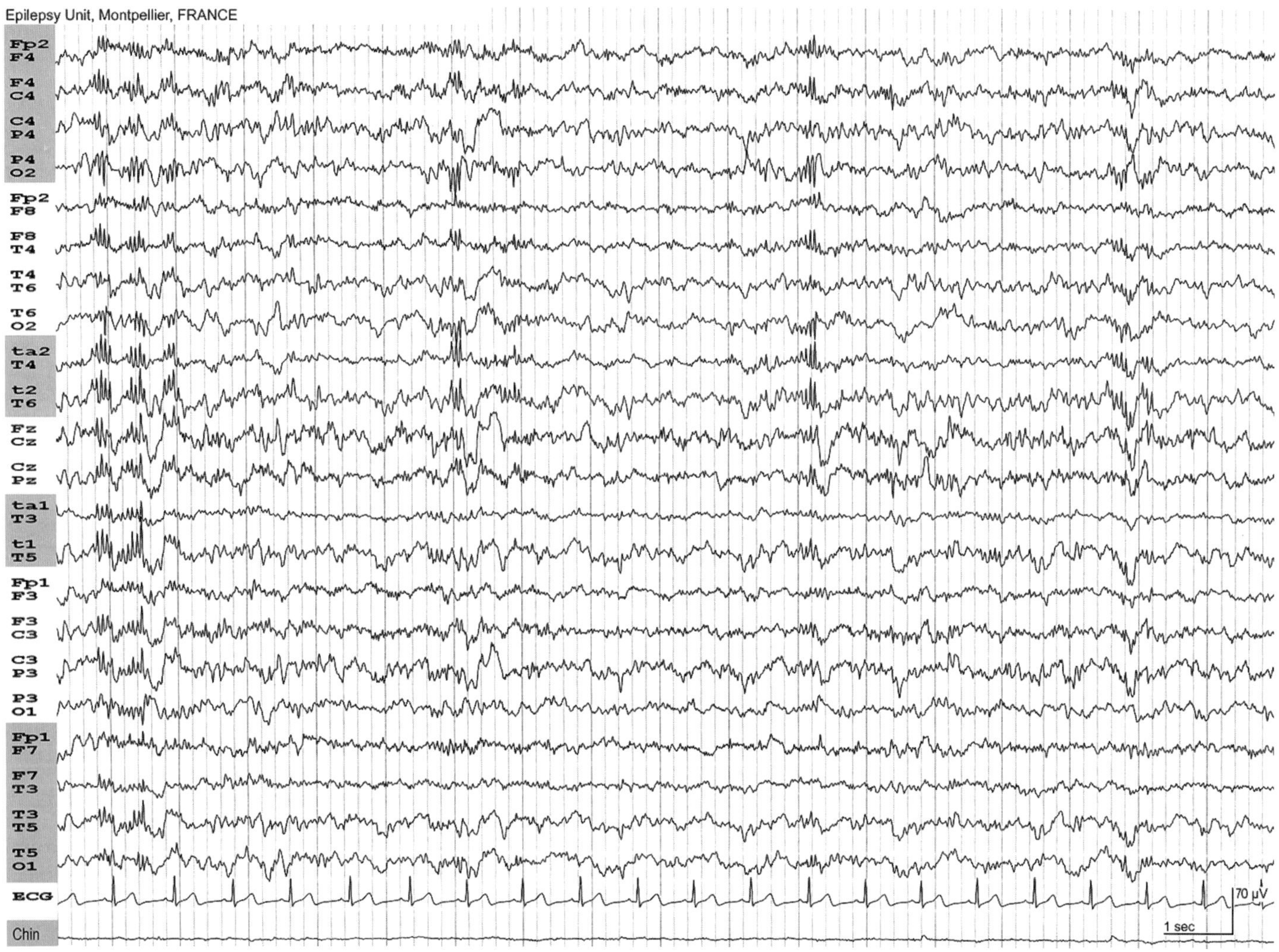

Figure a / Recording at 15 mm/s. Clear activation of 14- and 6-Hertz positive bursts in REM sleep.

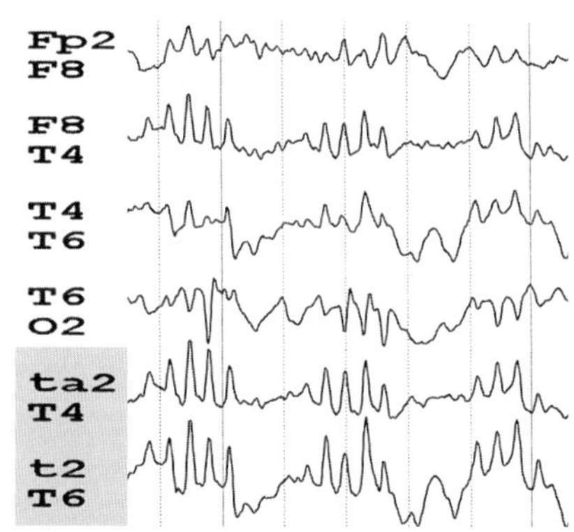

Figure b / 14- and 6-Hz positive burst (fast variant).

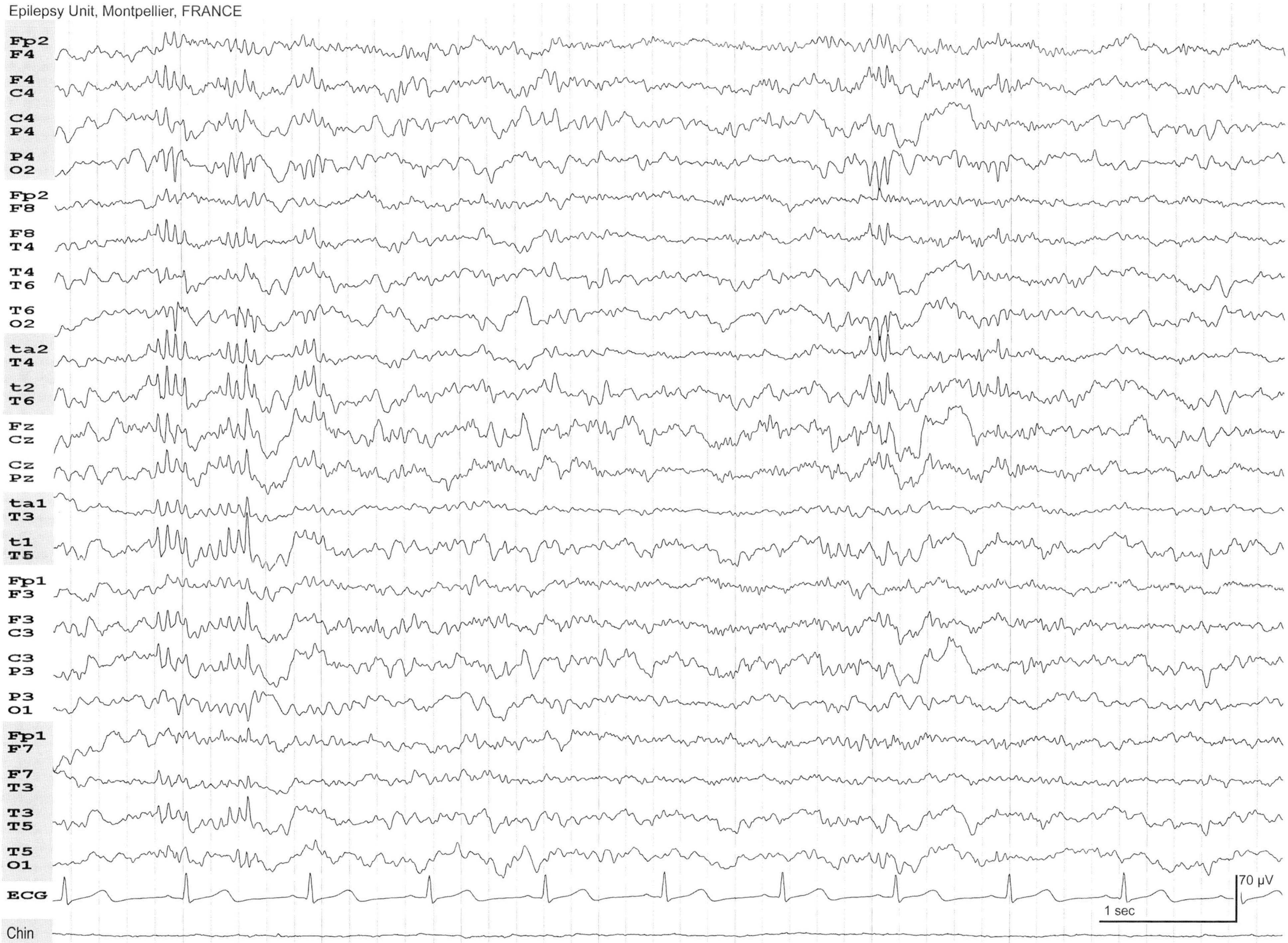
Epilepsy Unit, Montpellier, FRANCE
Fp2 F4
F4 C4
C4 P4
P4 O2
Fp2 F8
F8 T4
T4 T6
T6 O2
ta2 T4
t2 T6
Fz Cz
Cz Pz
ta1 T3
t1 T5
Fp1 F3
F3 C3
C3 P3
P3 O1
Fp1 F7
F7 T3
T3 T5
T5 O1
ECG
Chin
70 µV
1 sec

III • 62 Fourteen- and six-Hertz positive bursts during REM sleep in an adult (3)

Context

18-year-old woman with idiopathic generalized epilepsy.

What to note

REM sleep. Low-voltage background activity. A 14- and 6-Hertz can be observed over the right posterior temporal region especially on T2-T6. Note the presence of the fast variant at the beginning of the burst followed by slow variant (6 Hz).

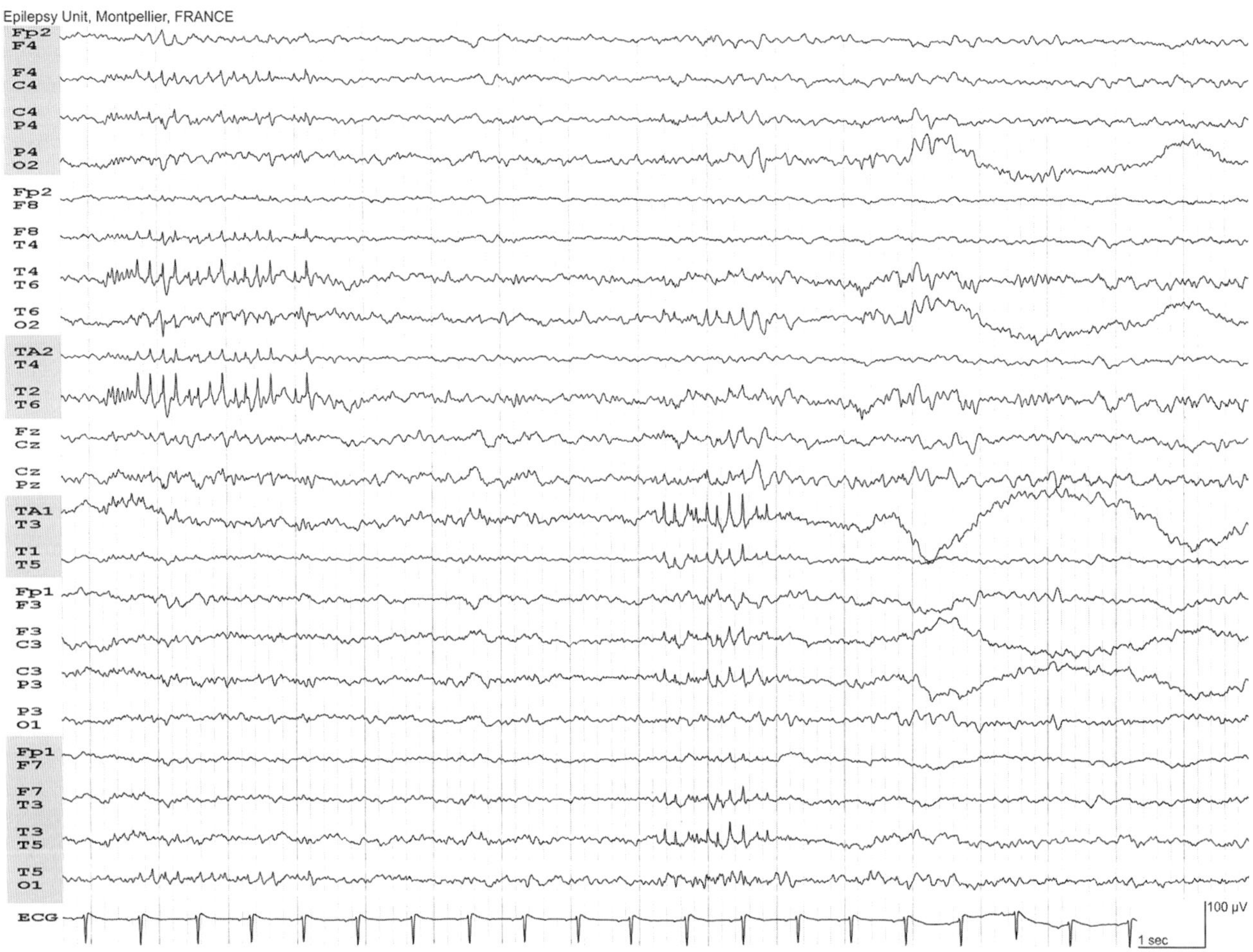

Figure a / Recording at 15 mm/s. Note the occurrence of independent 14- and 6-Hertz positive bursts over the posterior temporal regions.

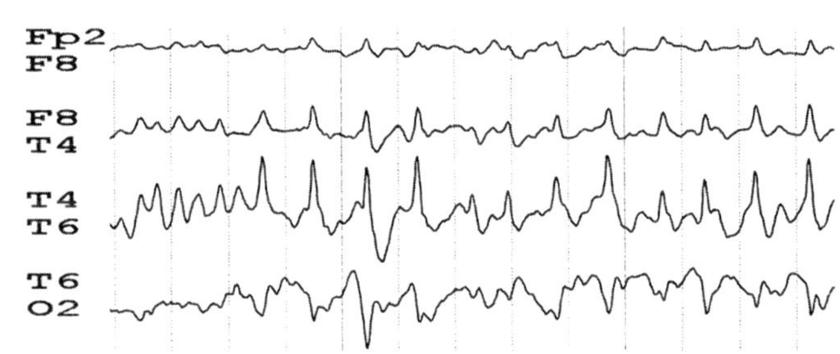

Figure b / 14- and 6-Hz positive burst during REM sleep.

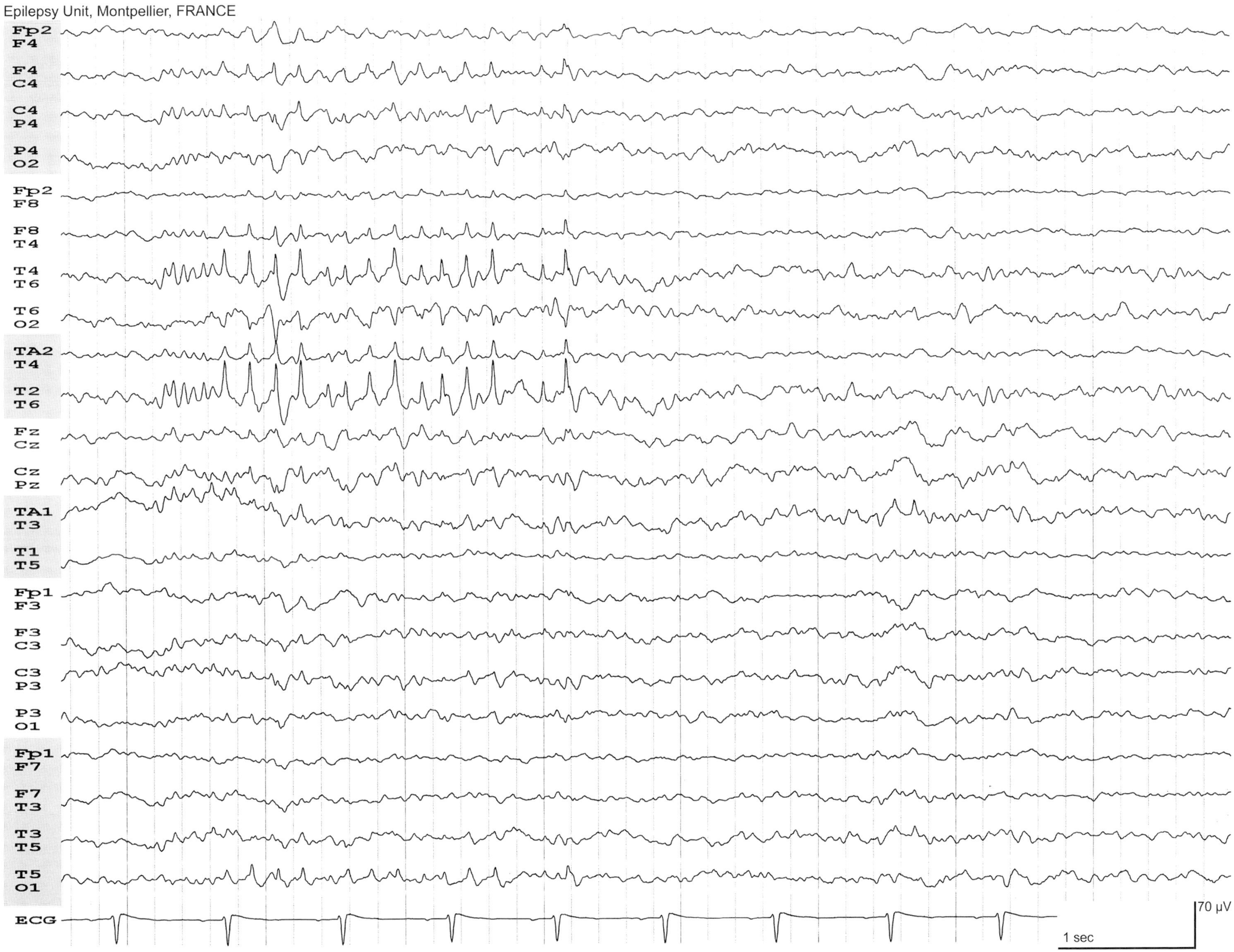
Epilepsy Unit, Montpellier, FRANCE
Fp2 F4
F4 C4
C4 P4
P4 O2
Fp2 F8
F8 T4
T4 T6
T6 O2
TA2 T4
T2 T6
Fz Cz
Cz Pz
TA1 T3
T1 T5
Fp1 F3
F3 C3
C3 P3
P3 O1
Fp1 F7
F7 T3
T3 T5
T5 O1
ECG
70 µV
1 sec

III • 63 Fourteen- and six-Hertz positive bursts during NREM sleep in an adult

Context

18-year-old woman, same patient as on the previous plate.

What to note

Stage N2 sleep, with a K complex. Over the right and the left temporal regions, six-hertz positive burst. Note the asynchrony of some waves between the right and left hemisphere.

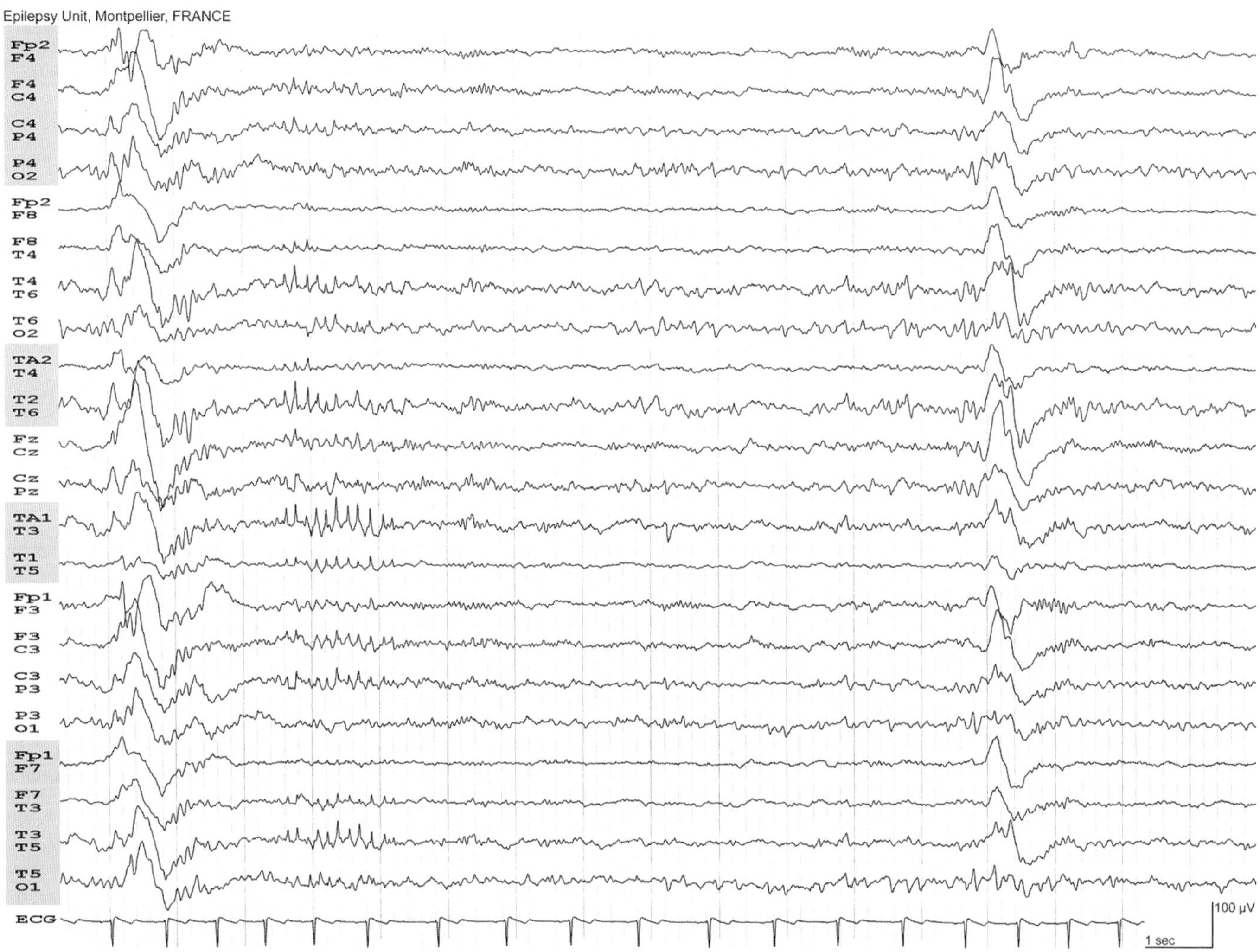

Figure a / Recording at 15 mm/s.

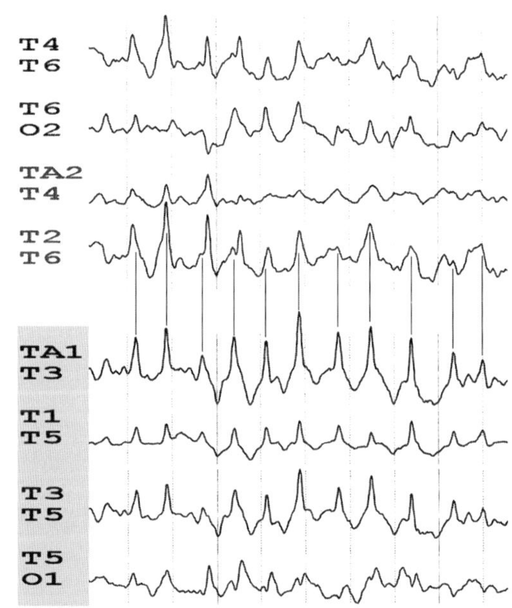

Figure b / 14- and 6-Hz positive burst. Asynchrony of some waves between the left and right hemisphere.

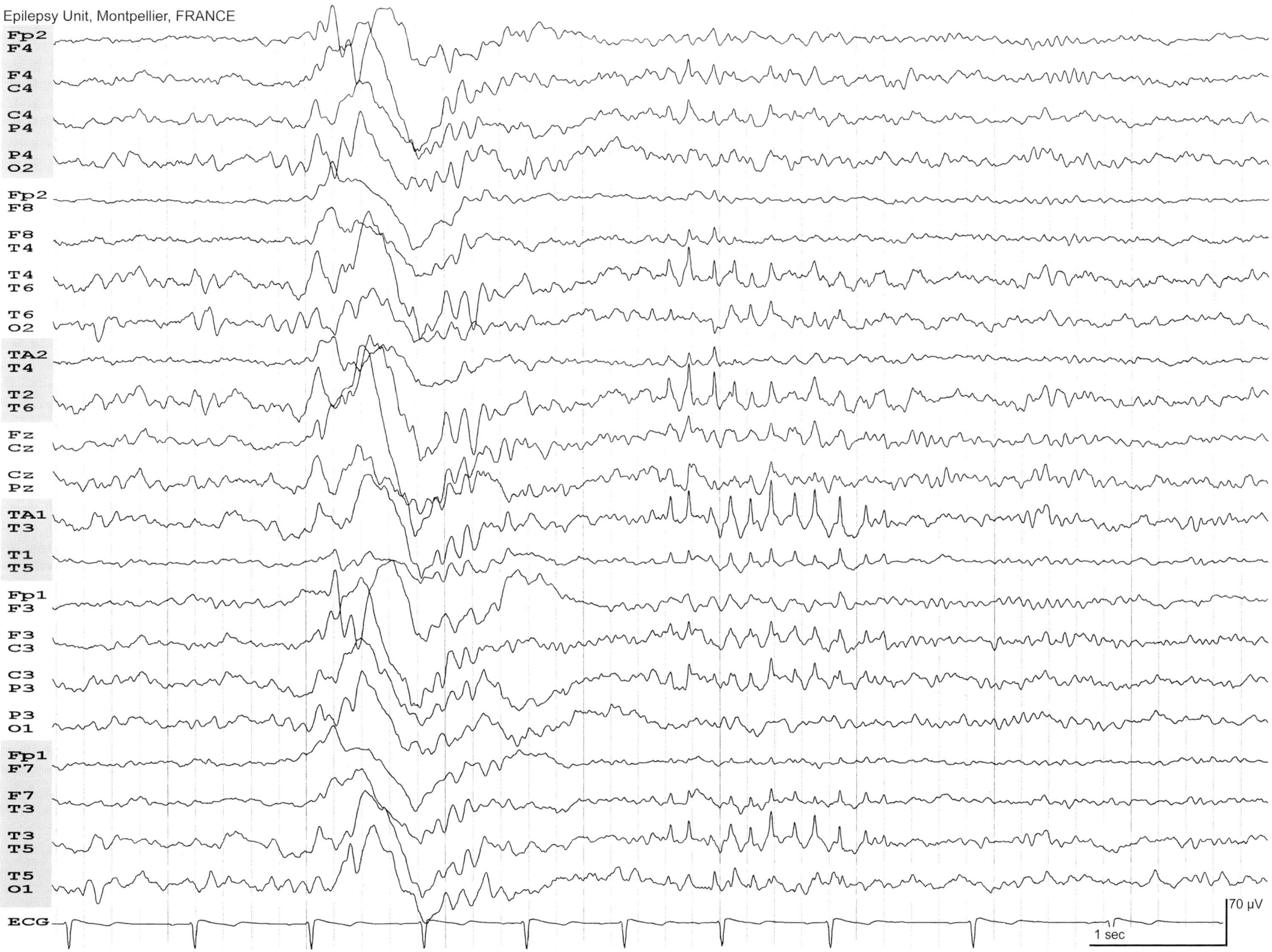
Epilepsy Unit, Montpellier, FRANCE
Fp2 F4
F4 C4
C4 P4
P4 O2
Fp2 F8
F8 T4
T4 T6
T6 O2
TA2 T4
T2 T6
Fz Cz
Cz Pz
TA1 T3
T1 T5
Fp1 F3
F3 C3
C3 P3
P3 O1
Fp1 F7
F7 T3
T3 T5
T5 O1
ECG
70 µV
1 sec

III • 64 Rhythmic midtemporal discharges

Context

18-year-old man with faints later diagnosed as vagal syncopes.

What to note

Eyes closed, relaxed. At the beginning of the plate, the alpha rhythm disappears (drowsiness). A unilateral angular theta activity at 5.5 Hz with a sawtooth-like morphology is observable over the right midtemporal region. This is an unusual non-pathological pattern with a sawtooth-like morphology corresponding to a rhythmic midtemporal discharge. Note an electrode artifact at C3. Prior to this recording, his right midtemporal discharges has been misinterpreted as a right temporal focus and the patient was treated with antiepileptic drugs, which were stopped.

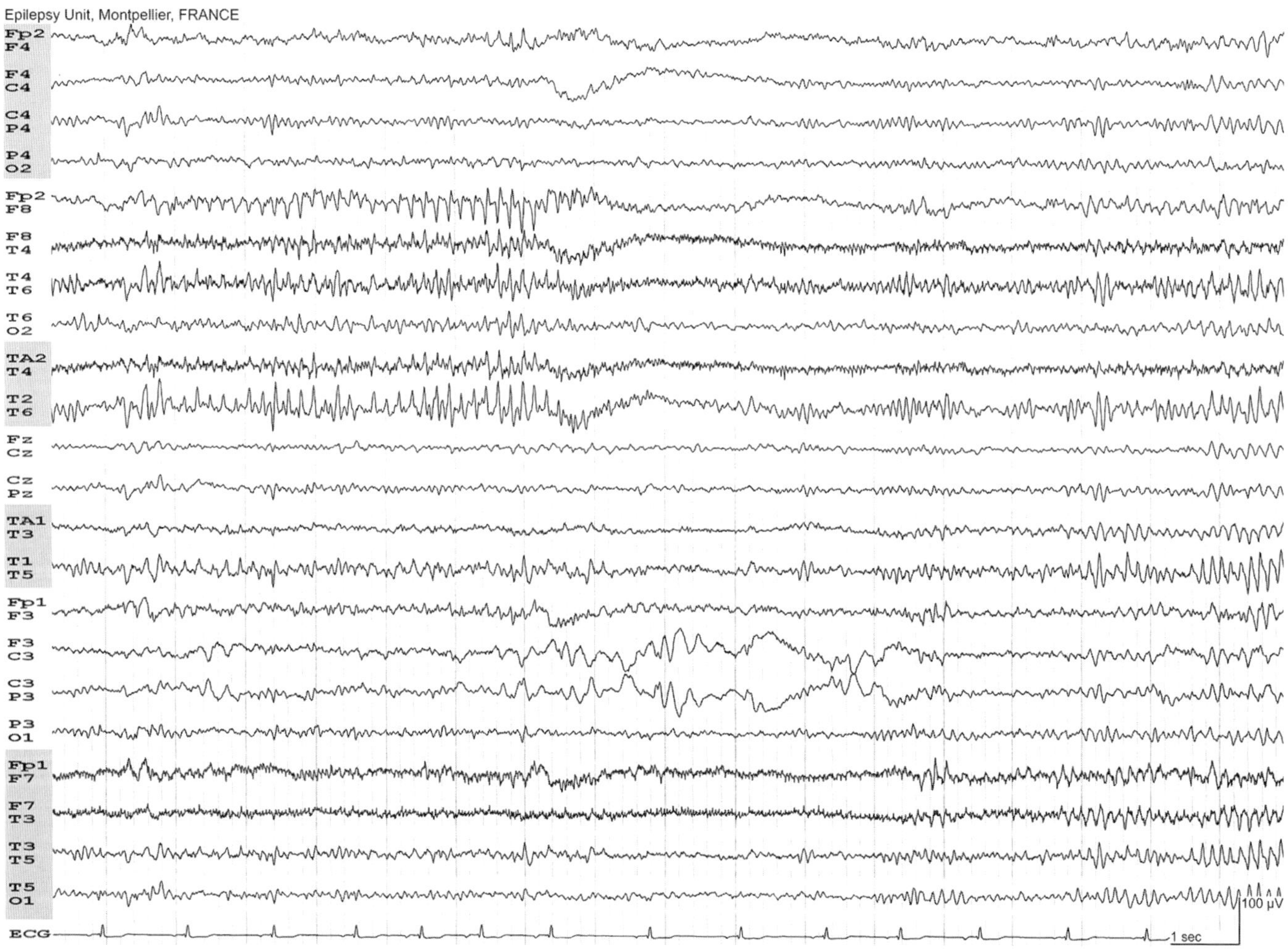

Figure a / Recording at 15 mm/s. Alpha rhythm reappear at the middle of the plate. Electrode artifact at C3.

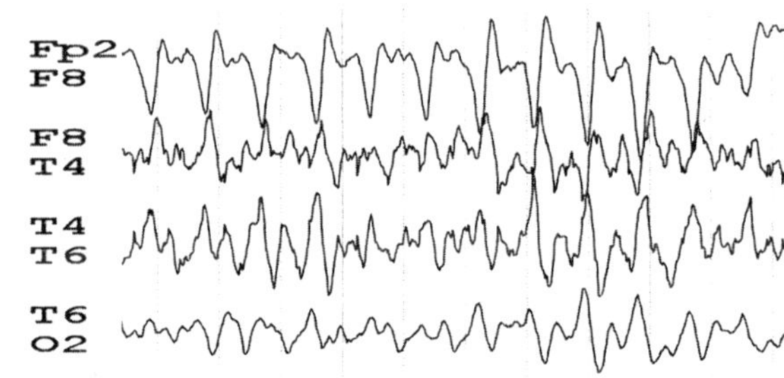

Figure b / Rhythmic midtemporal discharge.

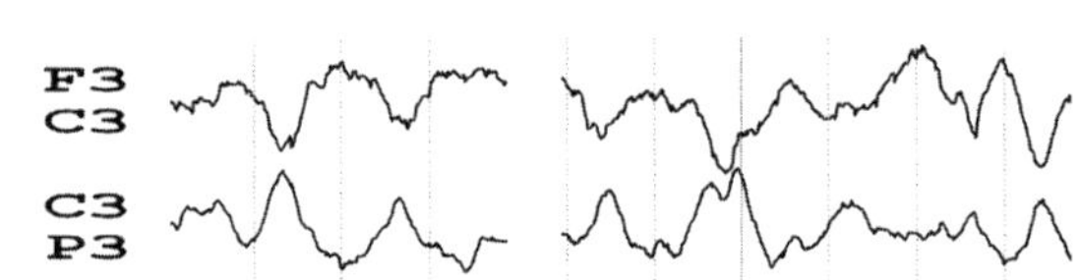

Figure c / Electrode artifact at C3.

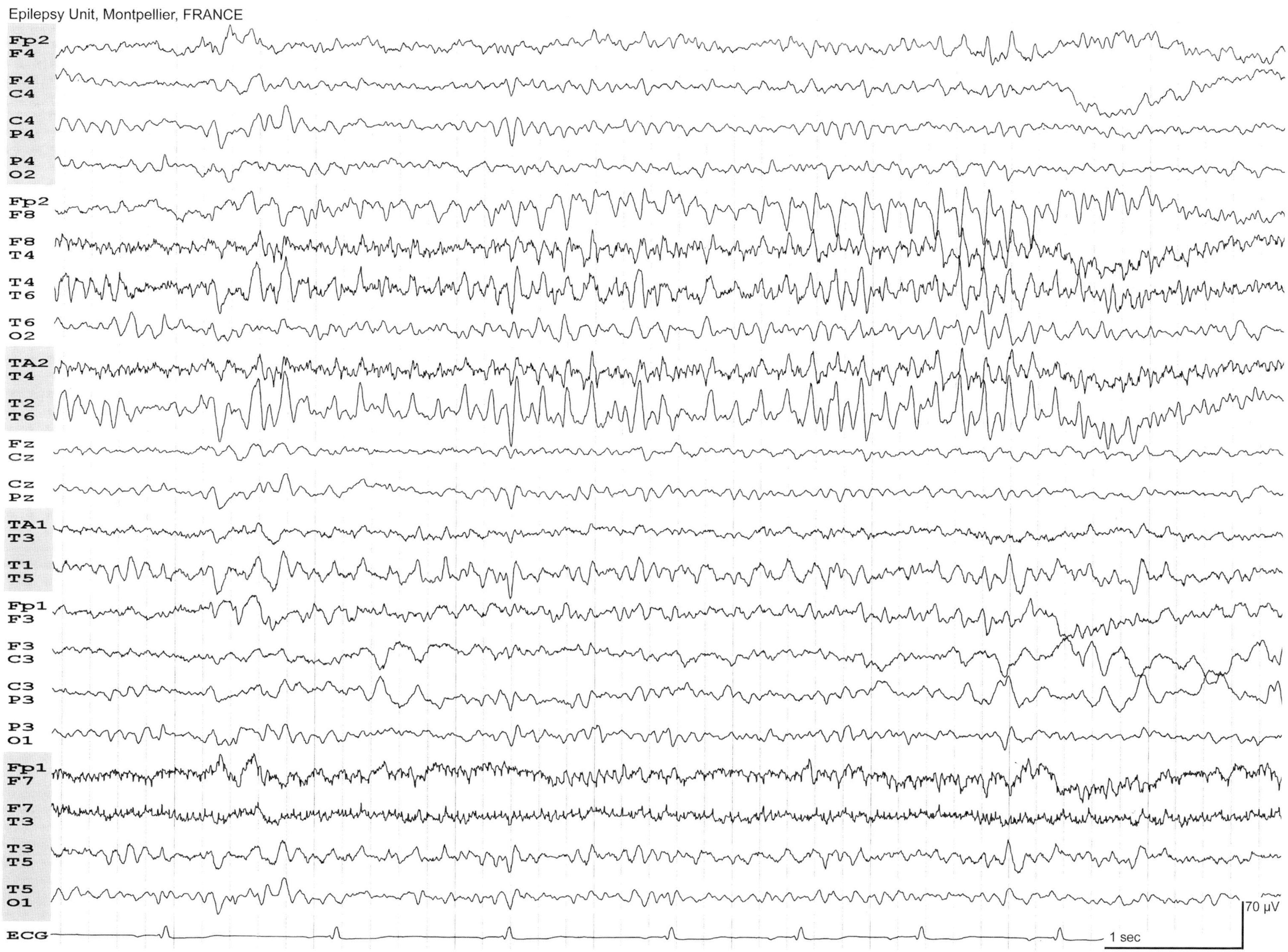
Epilepsy Unit, Montpellier, FRANCE
Fp2 F4
F4 C4
C4 P4
P4 O2
Fp2 F8
F8 T4
T4 T6
T6 O2
TA2 T4
T2 T6
Fz Cz
Cz Pz
TA1 T3
T1 T5
Fp1 F3
F3 C3
C3 P3
P3 O1
Fp1 F7
F7 T3
T3 T5
T5 O1
ECG
70 µV
1 sec

III • 65 Rhythmic midtemporal discharges in a patient with idiopathic generalized epilepsy (1)

Context

16-year-old woman with idiopathic generalized epilepsy.

What to note

Eyes closed, falling asleep. There is no alpha activity. She is in stage N1 sleep with a low-amplitude theta background activity. Theta activity at 5.5 Hz can be observed over the left midtemporal region, developing into a rhythmic discharge corresponding to a rhythmic midtemporal discharge or a rhythmic theta burst of drowsiness. Note the monomorphic character of the discharge. Amplitude remains constant throughout the following plate. Contrary to an epileptic seizure, there is no tendency to spread to adjacent regions.

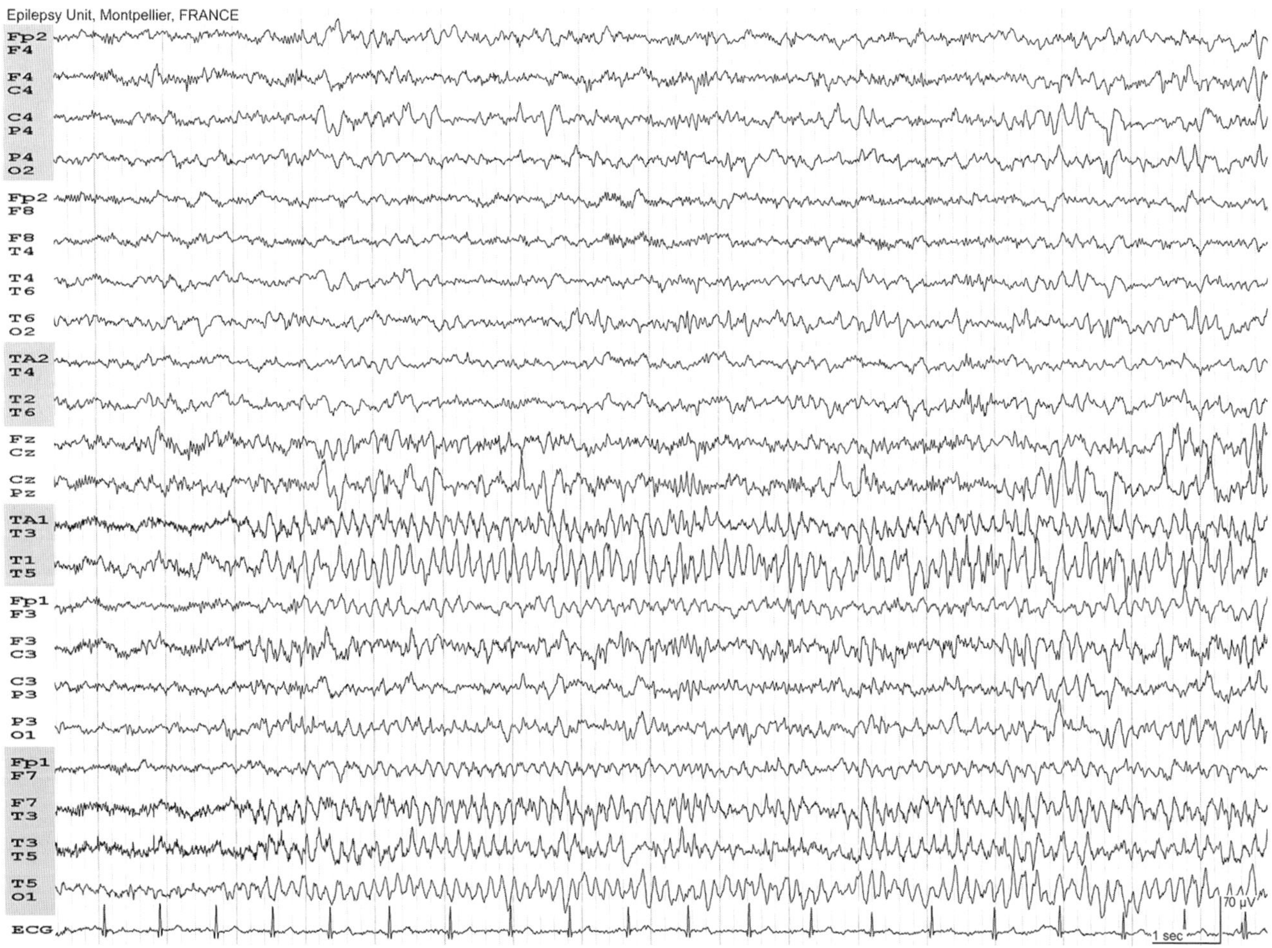

Figure a / Recording at 15 mm/s. Stage N1 sleep. V waves at the end of the plate.

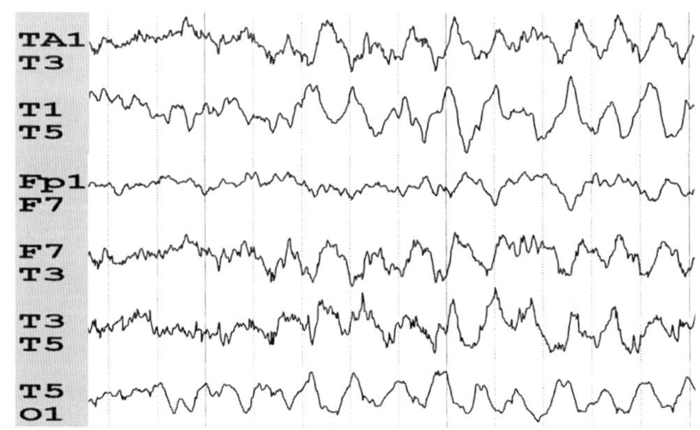

Figure b / Rhythmic monomorphous theta waves over the left midtemporal region.

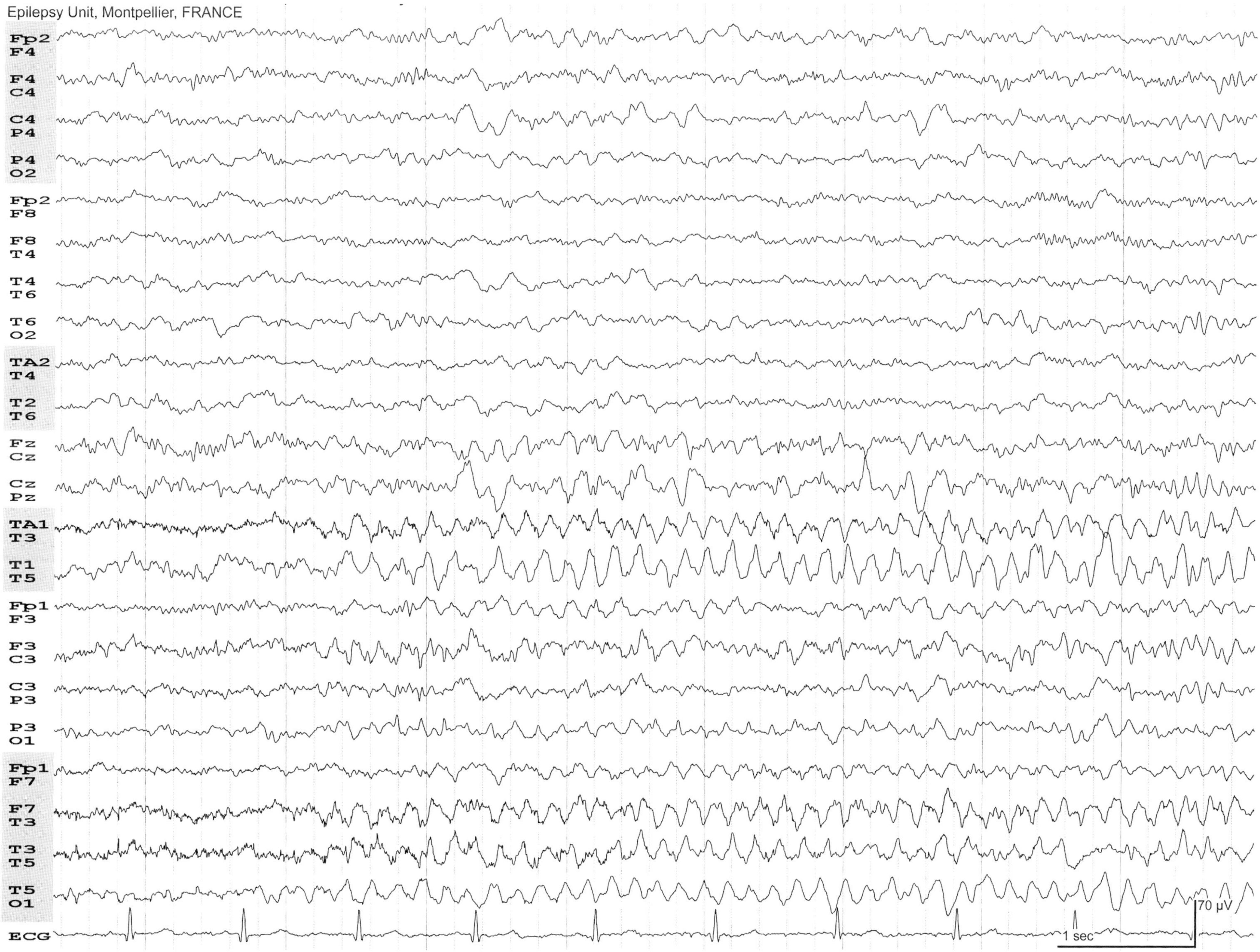
Epilepsy Unit, Montpellier, FRANCE
Fp2 F4
F4 C4
C4 P4
P4 O2
Fp2 F8
F8 T4
T4 T6
T6 O2
TA2 T4
T2 T6
Fz Cz
Cz Pz
TA1 T3
T1 T5
Fp1 F3
F3 C3
C3 P3
P3 O1
Fp1 F7
F7 T3
T3 T5
T5 O1
ECG
70 µV
1 sec

III • 66 Rhythmic midtemporal discharges in a patient with idiopathic generalized epilepsy (2)

Context

16-year-old woman, same patient as on the previous plate.

What to note

Stage N1 sleep with V waves at the end of the plate. Continuation of identical monomorphic theta activity with constant amplitude over the left midtemporal region. It stops suddenly (see below, plate recorded at 15 mm/s). Rhythmic midtemporal discharges are uncommon, non-pathological pattern.

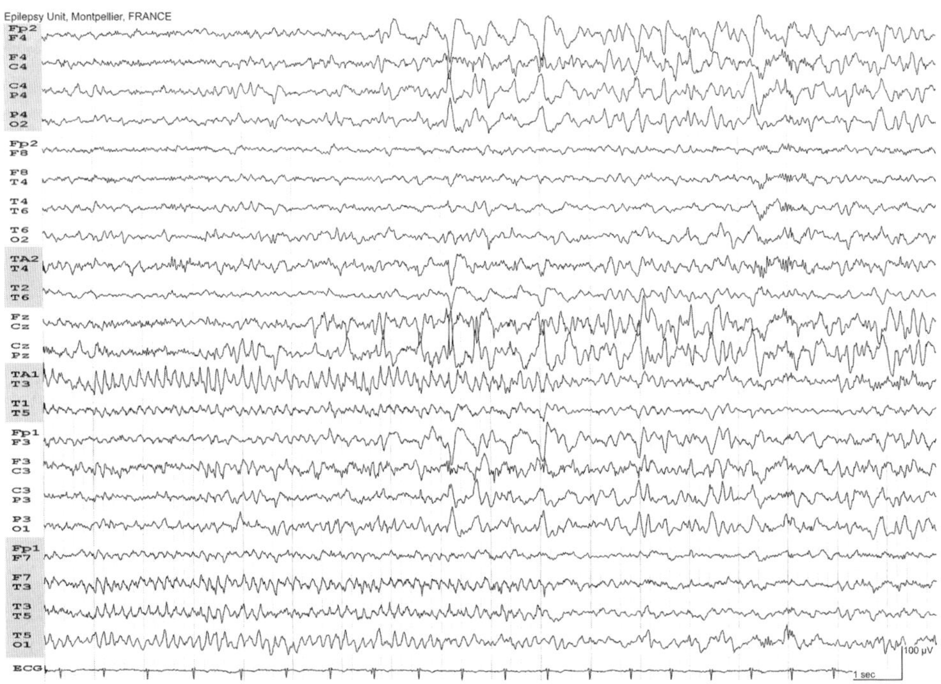

Figure a / Recording at 15 mm/s. The rhythmic midtemporal discharge stops suddenly. V waves spread to the left and right fronto-central regions.

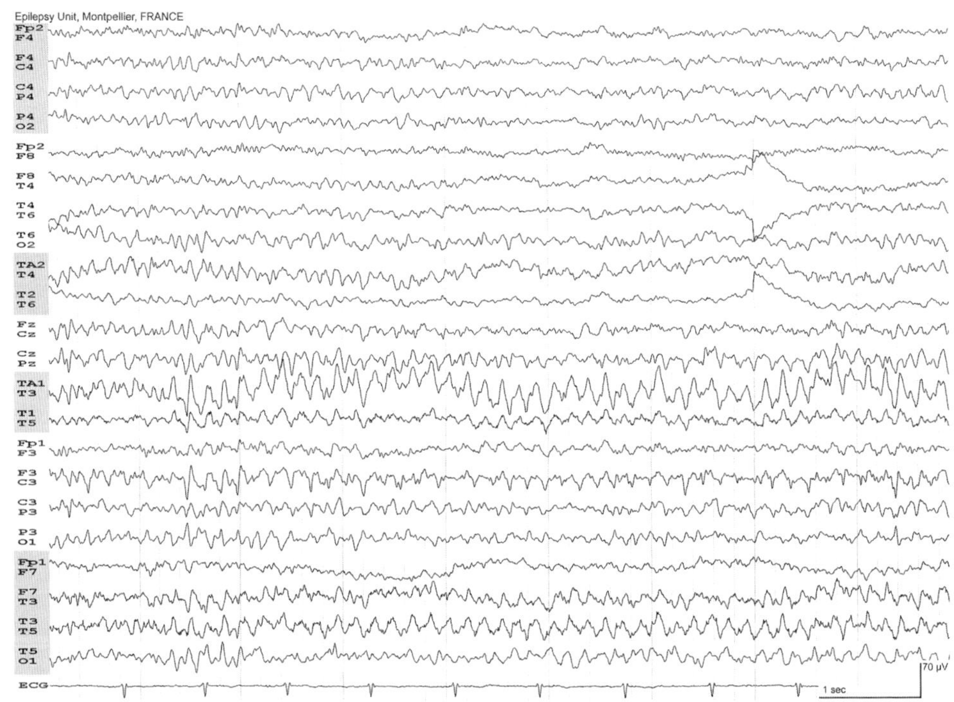

Figure b / Another rhythmic midtemporal discharge in this patient during the same recording.

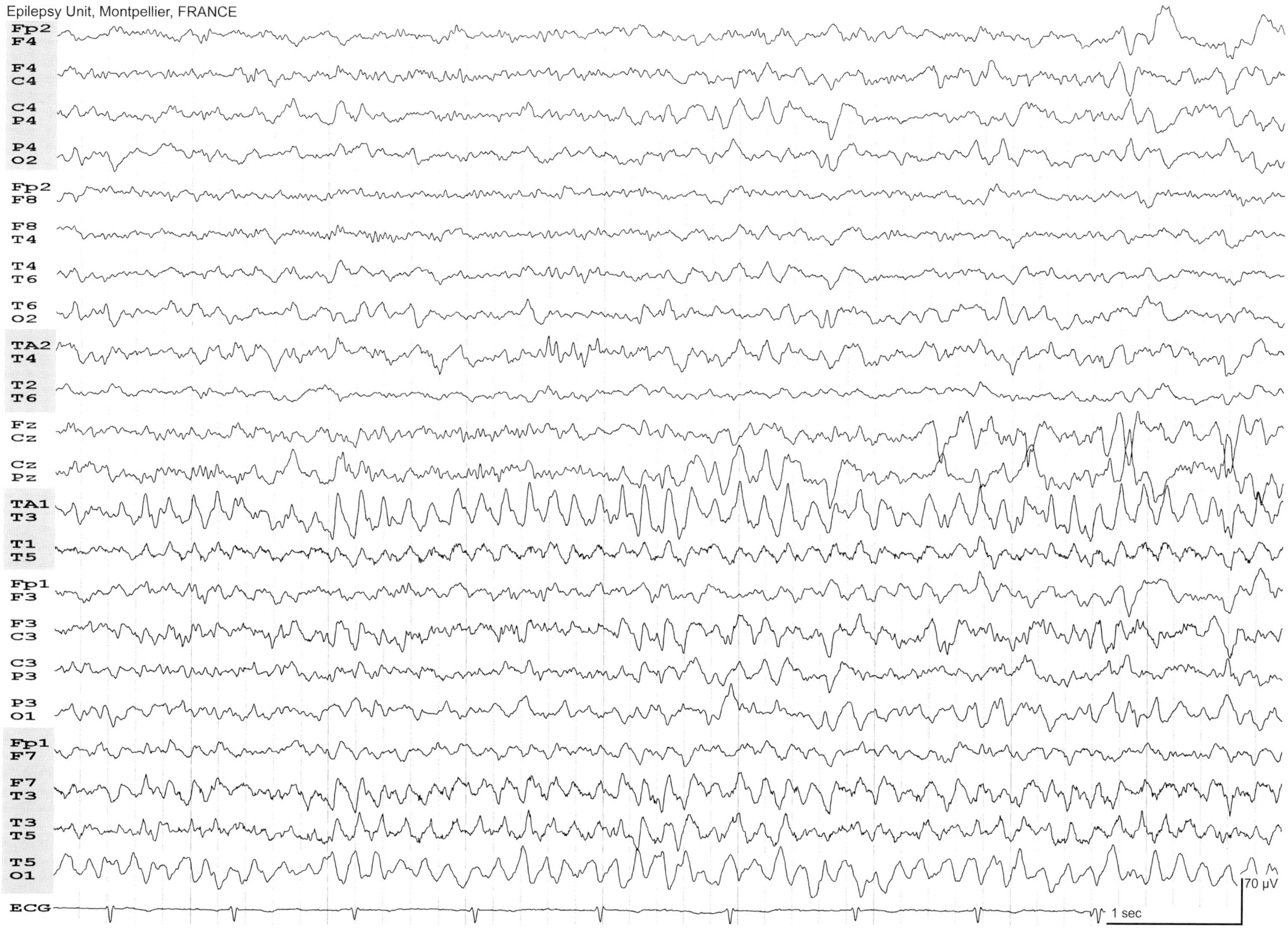
Epilepsy Unit, Montpellier, FRANCE
Fp2 F4
F4 C4
C4 P4
P4 O2
Fp2 F8
F8 T4
T4 T6
T6 O2
TA2 T4
T2 T6
Fz Cz
Cz Pz
TA1 T3
T1 T5
Fp1 F3
F3 C3
C3 P3
P3 O1
Fp1 F7
F7 T3
T3 T5
T5 O1
ECG
70 µV
1 sec

III • 67 Rhythmic midtemporal discharges in a patient with idiopathic generalized epilepsy (3)

Context

17-year-old young woman with juvenile myoclonic epilepsy.

What to note

On the left segment, asleep, then a transient arousal, followed by a 2-second midtemporal discharge with angular theta activities. On the right segment, a generalized polyspike discharge awake while viewing a Japanese cartoon (photoparoxysmal response). Superimposed sharp potentials corresponding to an instrumental environmental artifact (television).

Comment

The presence of a theta activity in the temporal regions could have led to a misdiagnosis of focal epilepsy if visual analysis of the midtemporal discharge had not been accurate. However, there were indication of idiopathic generalized epilepsy (IGE). This example highlights the importance of clinical examinations. EEGs are a necessary tool to confirm hypotheses based on clinical observations, but EEG analysis should not prevail over clinical observations. In this patient, suspicion of IGE epilepsy lead to extensive (and positive) assessment of photosensitivity.

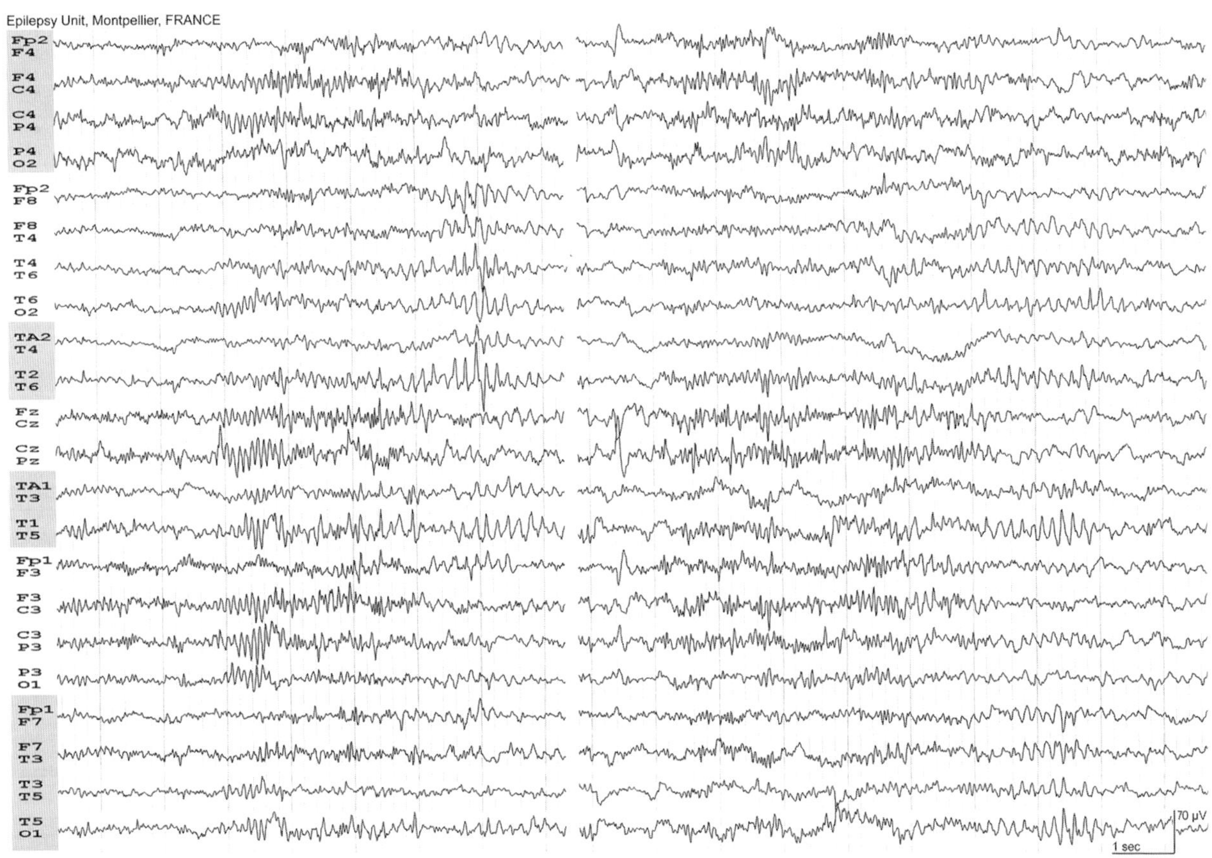

Figure a / Recording at 15 mm/s. Right segment, transient arousal with beta rhythms in 5-second bursts. Then a 2-second midtemporal discharge, more clearly visible on the left temporal region.

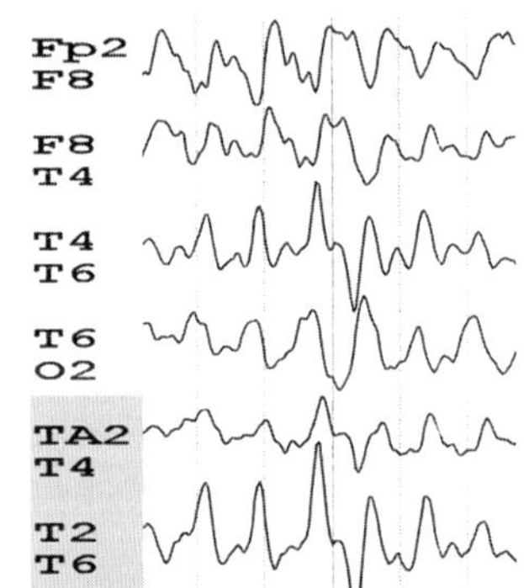

Figure b / Rhythmic midtemporal discharge.

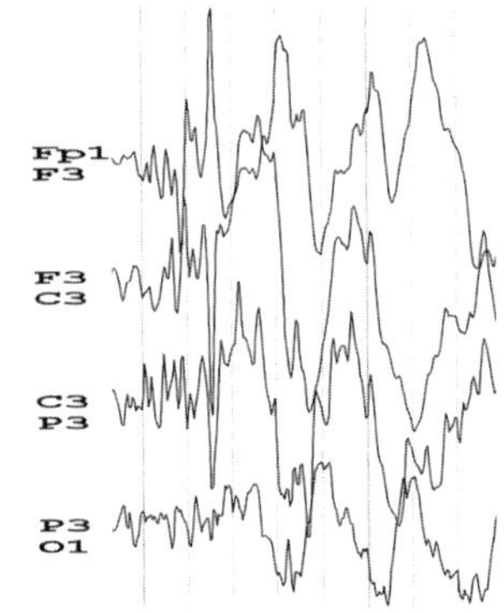

Figure c / Burst of generalized polyspike-waves.

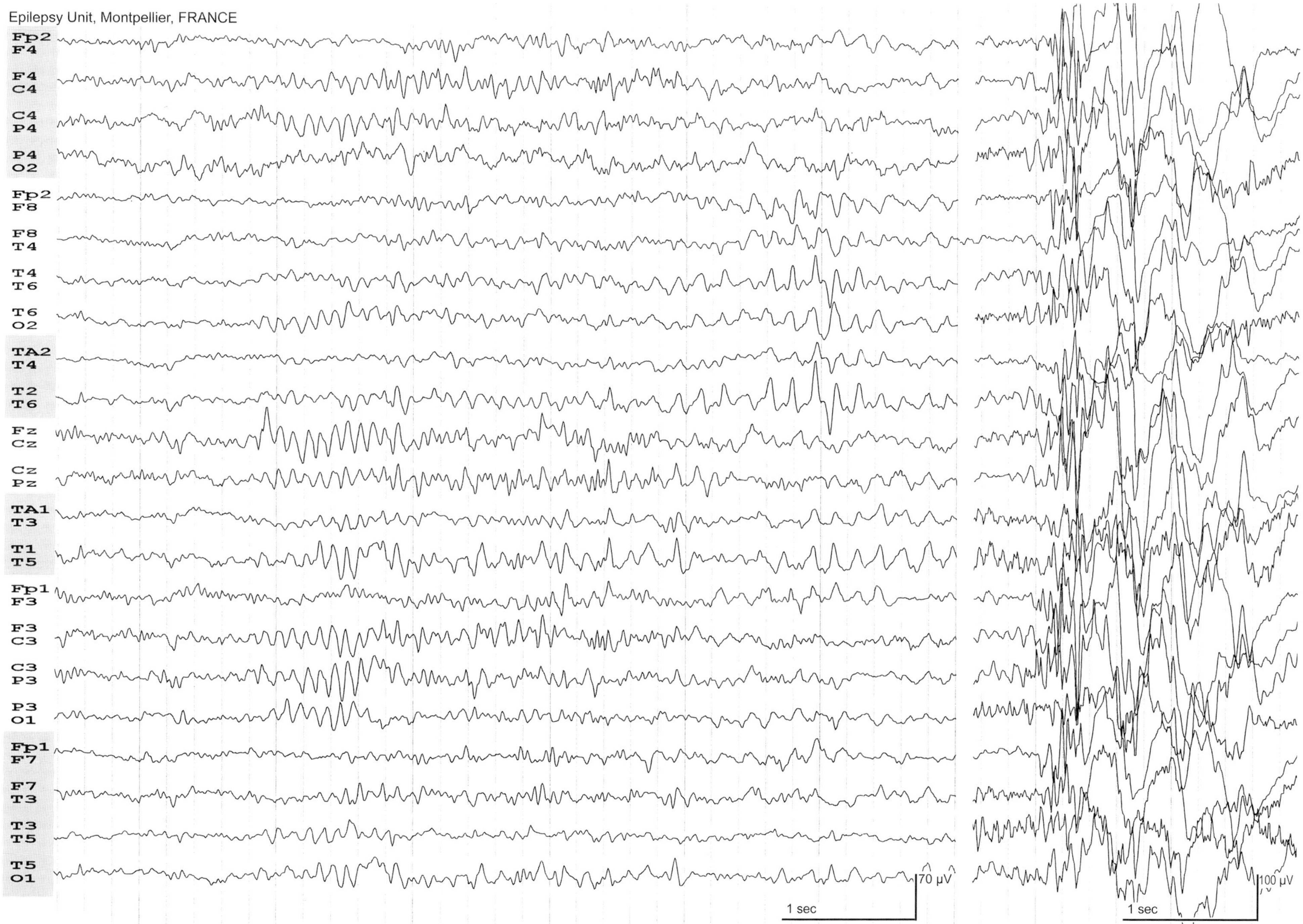
Epilepsy Unit, Montpellier, FRANCE
Fp2 F4
F4 C4
C4 P4
P4 O2
Fp2 F8
F8 T4
T4 T6
T6 O2
TA2 T4
T2 T6
Fz Cz
Cz Pz
TA1 T3
T1 T5
Fp1 F3
F3 C3
C3 P3
P3 O1
Fp1 F7
F7 T3
T3 T5
T5 O1
70 µV
1 sec
100 µV
1 sec

III • 68 Rhythmic midtemporal discharges in a patient with temporal lobe epilepsy

68 Rhythmic midtemporal discharges in a patient with temporal lobe epilepsy

Context

40-year-old woman with cryptogenic left medial temporal lobe epilepsy, presurgical assessment

What to note

Eyes closed and relaxed. Angular theta activities at 5.5 Hz over the right midtemporal region developing into a rhythmic discharge. Note the characteristic sawtooth-like morphology and the phase reversal between Fp2-F8 and T4-T6. Moreover, interictal left temporal lobe abnormalities with diphasic slow waves in phase reversal at F7 can be observed in this patient. The interictal abnormalities are also visible at lower temporal electrodes TA1 and T1. Prior to the presurgical assessment, her right midtemporal discharges had been misinterpreted as a right temporal lobe interictal focus. This woman had been operated for her left medial temporal lobe epilepsy and had been seizure-free for 20 years following the surgical intervention.

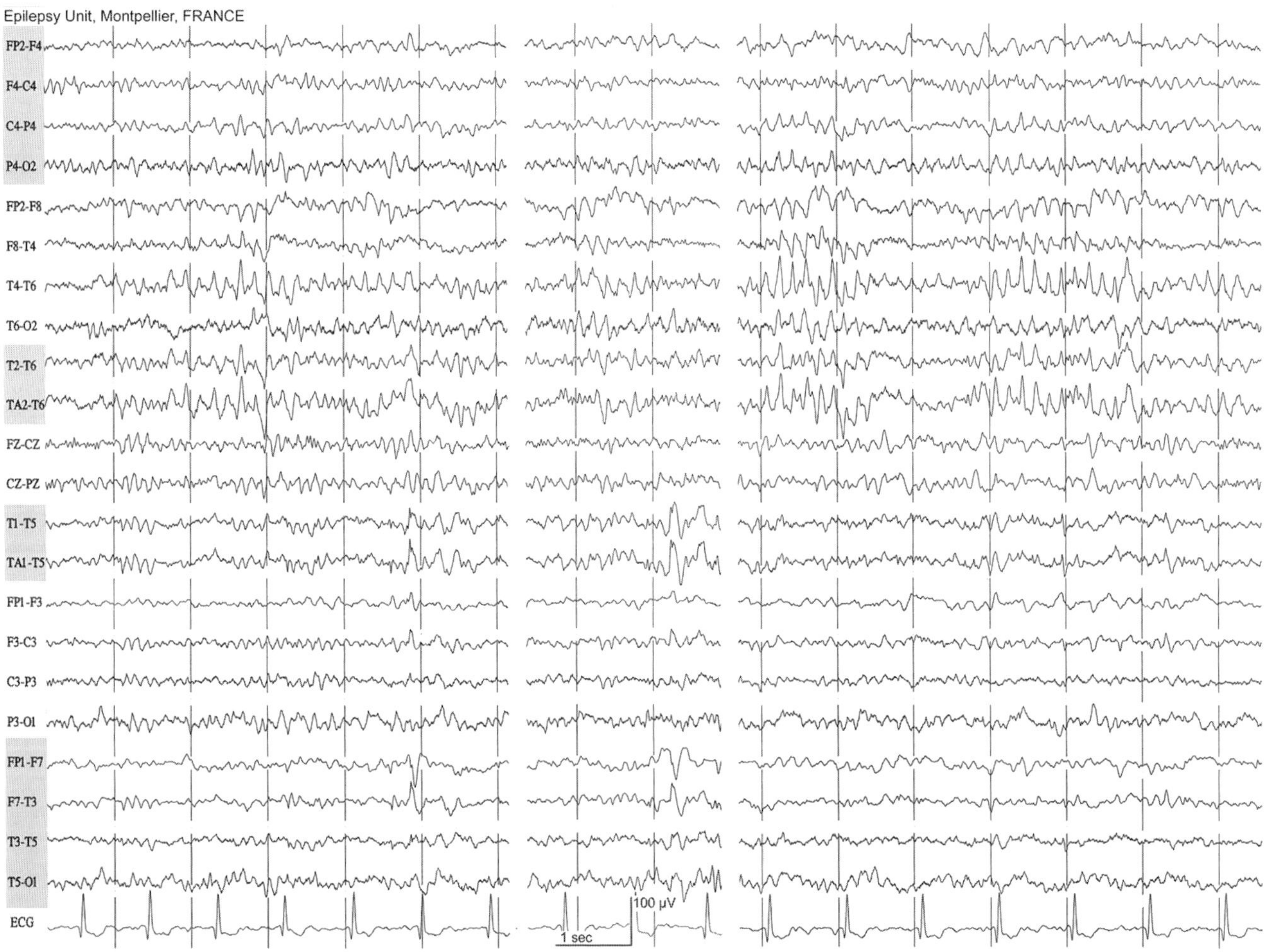

Figure a / Recording at 15 mm/s. Right segment, rhythmic midtemporal discharge over the right temporal region.

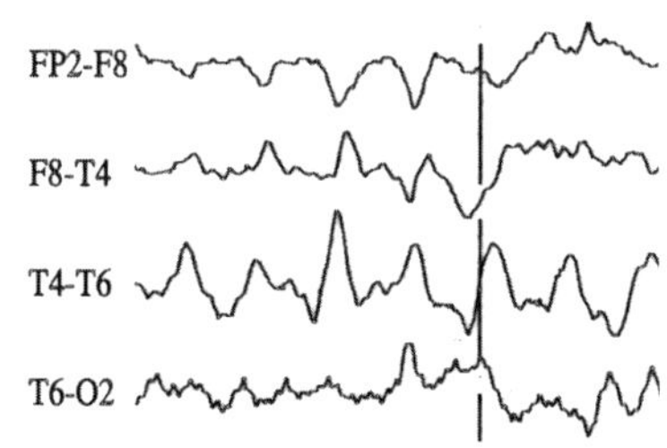

Figure b / Rhythmic midtemporal discharge.

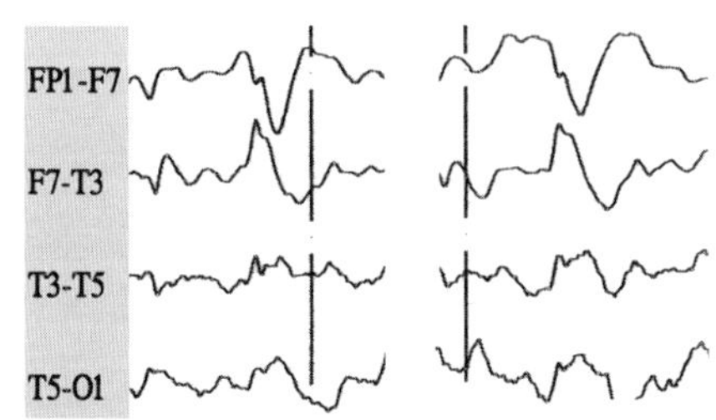

Figure c / Diphasic spike in phase reversal at F7.

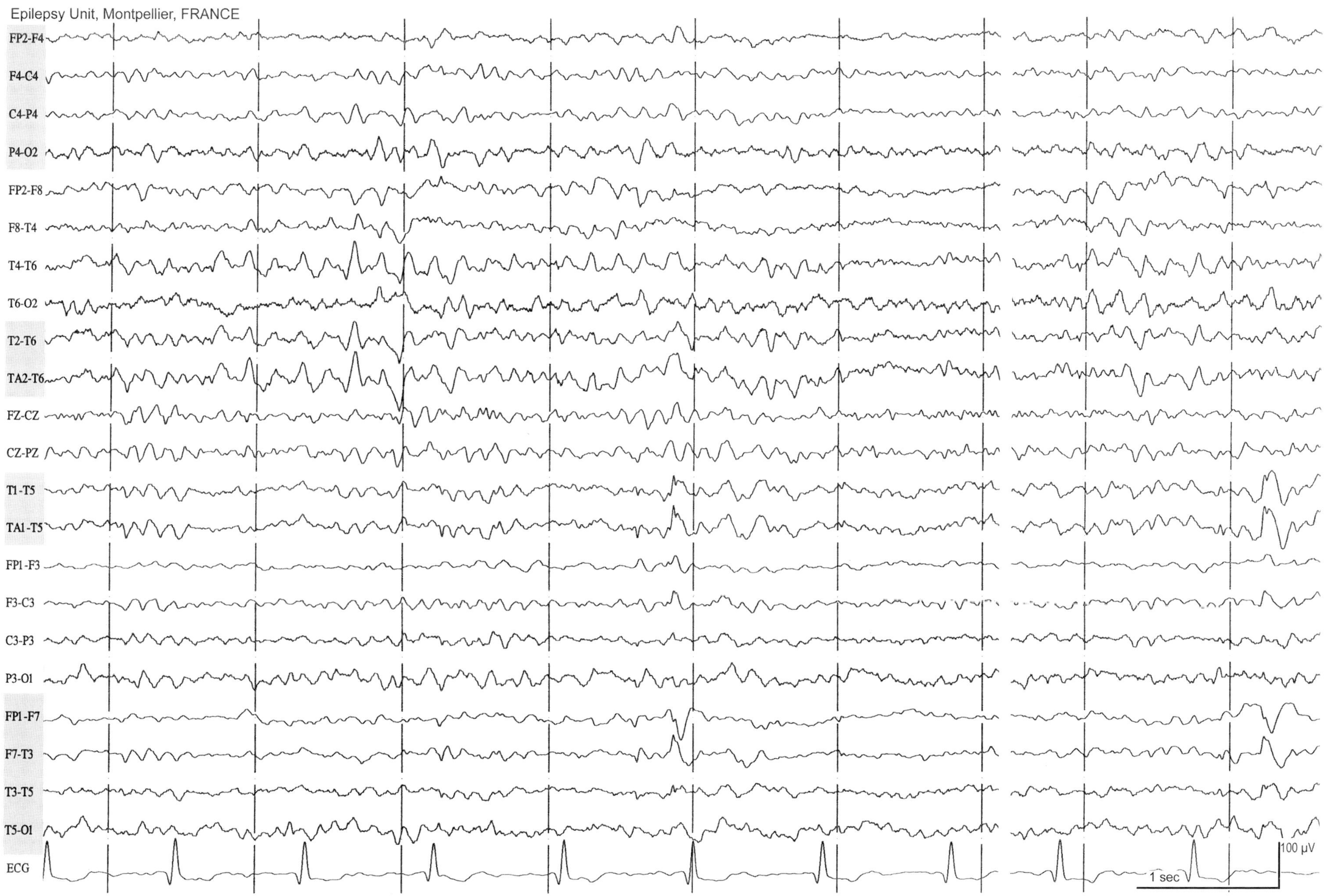
Epilepsy Unit, Montpellier, FRANCE
FP2-F4
F4-C4
C4-P4
P4-O2
FP2-F8
F8-T4
T4-T6
T6-O2
T2-T6
TA2-T6
FZ-CZ
CZ-PZ
T1-T5
TA1-T5
FP1-F3
F3-C3
C3-P3
P3-O1
FP1-F7
F7-T3
T3-T5
T5-O1
ECG
100 µV
1 sec

III • 69 Rhythmic midtemporal discharges in REM Sleep (1)

Context

40-year-old woman, same patient as on the previous plate.

What to note

The theta activity is organized during REM sleep in a monomorphic discharge of theta waveforms with sawtooth-like morphology over the midtemporal region. Compare the morphology with the previous plate. In this patient, this activity was clearly activated during REM sleep (abundant discharges of different durations). The activity was more fragmented in NREM sleep (see figure recorded at 15 mm/s).

Comment

We prefer to employ the term "rhythmic midtemporal discharges" than "rhythmic theta burst of drowsiness". Indeed, rhythmic midtemporal discharges can be observed in drowsiness, but they are observed above all in sleep, especially in REM sleep, as in this patient.

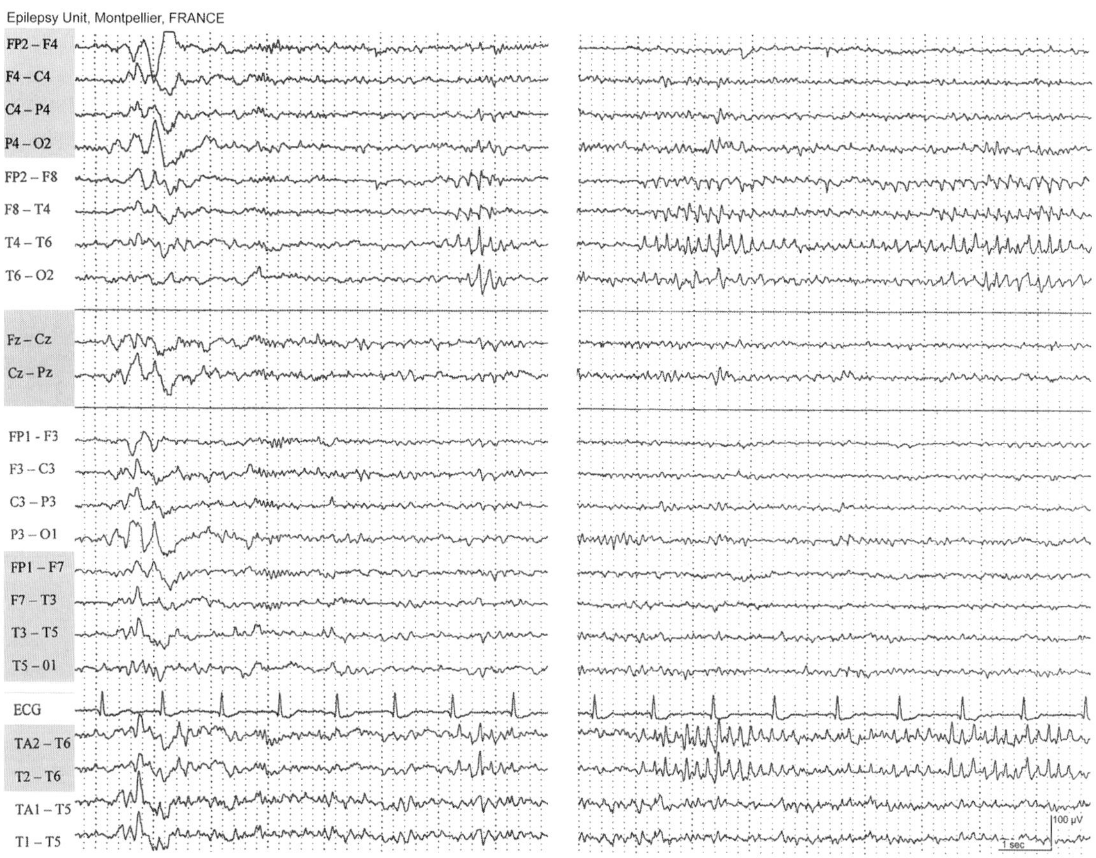

Figure a / Recording at 15 mm/s. On the left, the woman is in stage II sleep (K complex followed by a spindle). A run of rather monomorphic, short lasting, sharp theta waves can be observed over the right midtemporal region. Right segment: REM sleep.

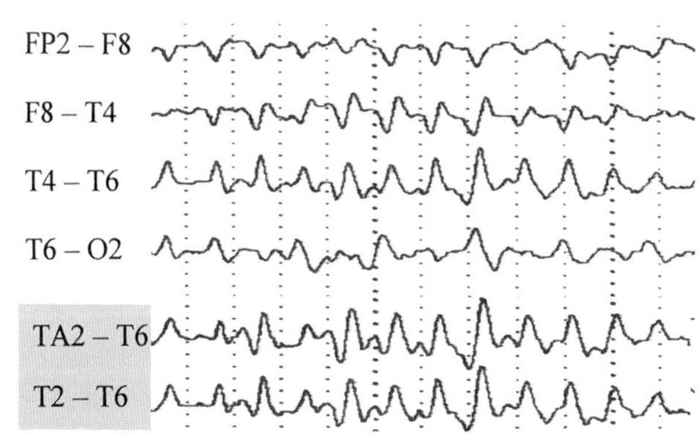

Figure b / Rhythmic midtemporal discharge.

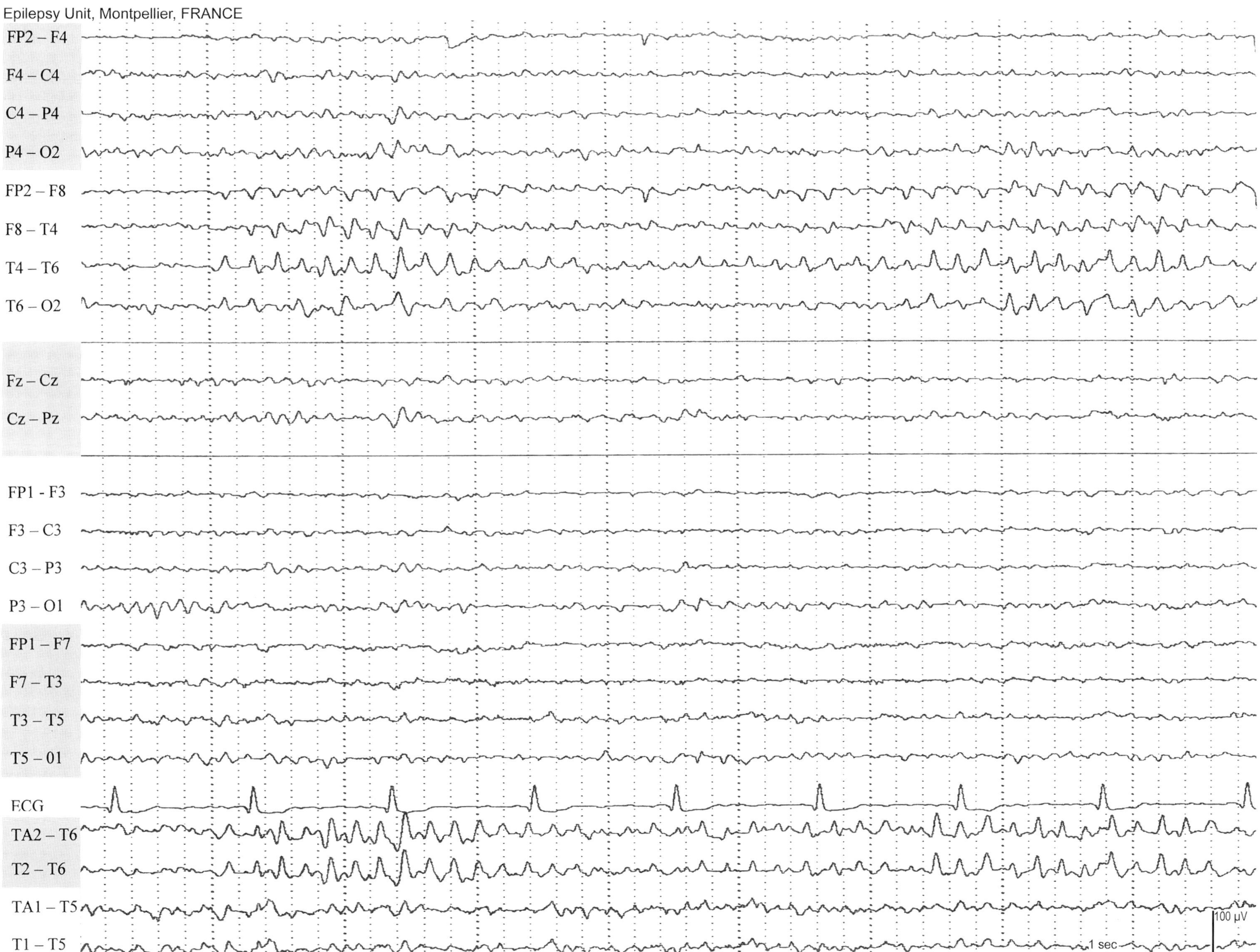
Epilepsy Unit, Montpellier, FRANCE
FP2 – F4
F4 – C4
C4 – P4
P4 – O2
FP2 – F8
F8 – T4
T4 – T6
T6 – O2
Fz – Cz
Cz – Pz
FP1 - F3
F3 – C3
C3 – P3
P3 – O1
FP1 – F7
F7 – T3
T3 – T5
T5 – 01
ECG
TA2 – T6
T2 – T6
TA1 – T5
T1 – T5
100 µV
1 sec

III • 70 Mu rhythm and rhythmic midtemporal discharges in REM Sleep (2)

Context

42-year-old woman referred for temporal lobe epilepsy. Same patient as plates III-32.

What to note

REM sleep. Muscular twitches at the beginning of the plate. Rhythmic midtemporal discharge over the right temporal region. The morphology is typical. Note on this plate, a mu rhythm at F4-C4 and an electrode artifact at F3.

Comment

It may be difficult to differentiate between rhythmic midtemporal discharges and wicket spikes. They may be a continuum between these two patterns. These two patterns are uncommon but mostly paraphysiological. It is more important to determine the physiological nature of the pattern than the exact form. Here the pattern could be mistaken for wicket spikes but the waves are not arch-shaped.

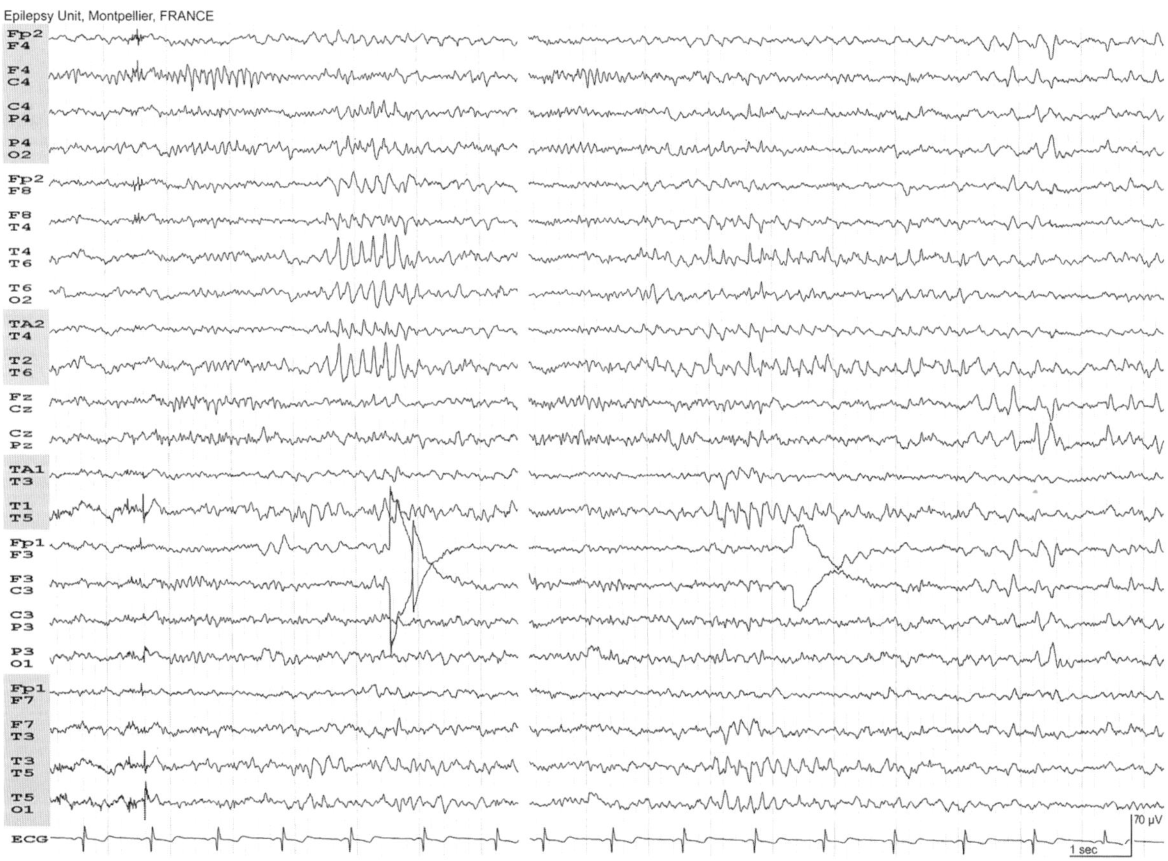

Figure a / Recording at 15 mm/s. Right segment, REM sleep with sawtooth waves on the vertex region and mu rhythm at F4-C4. Rhythmic midtemporal discharge over the right temporal region that spreads to the left midtemporal region. Electrode "pop" artifact at C3.

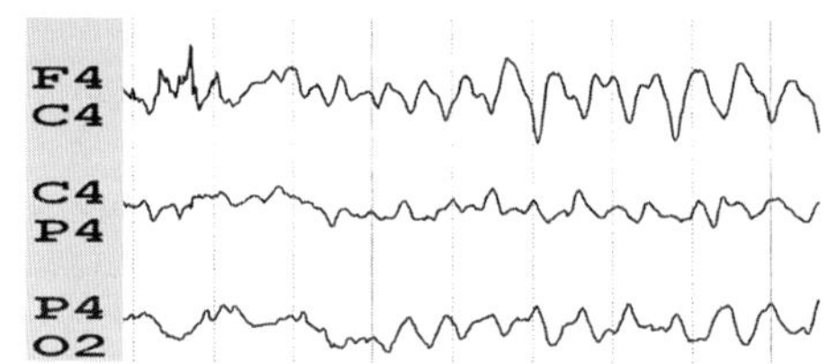

Figure b / Muscular twitch at F4-C4 followed by mu rhythm.

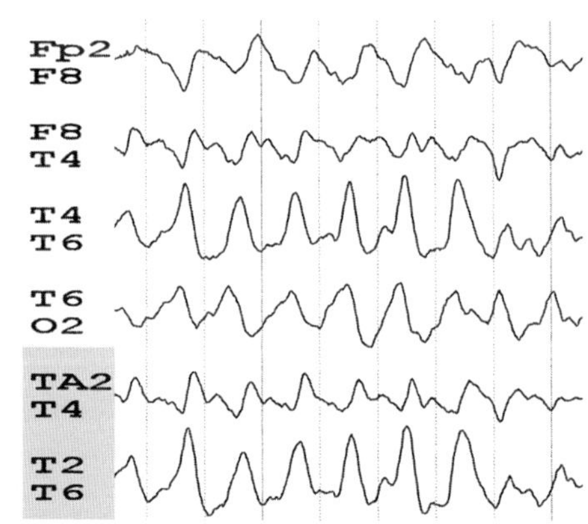

Figure c / Rhythmic midtemporal discharge.

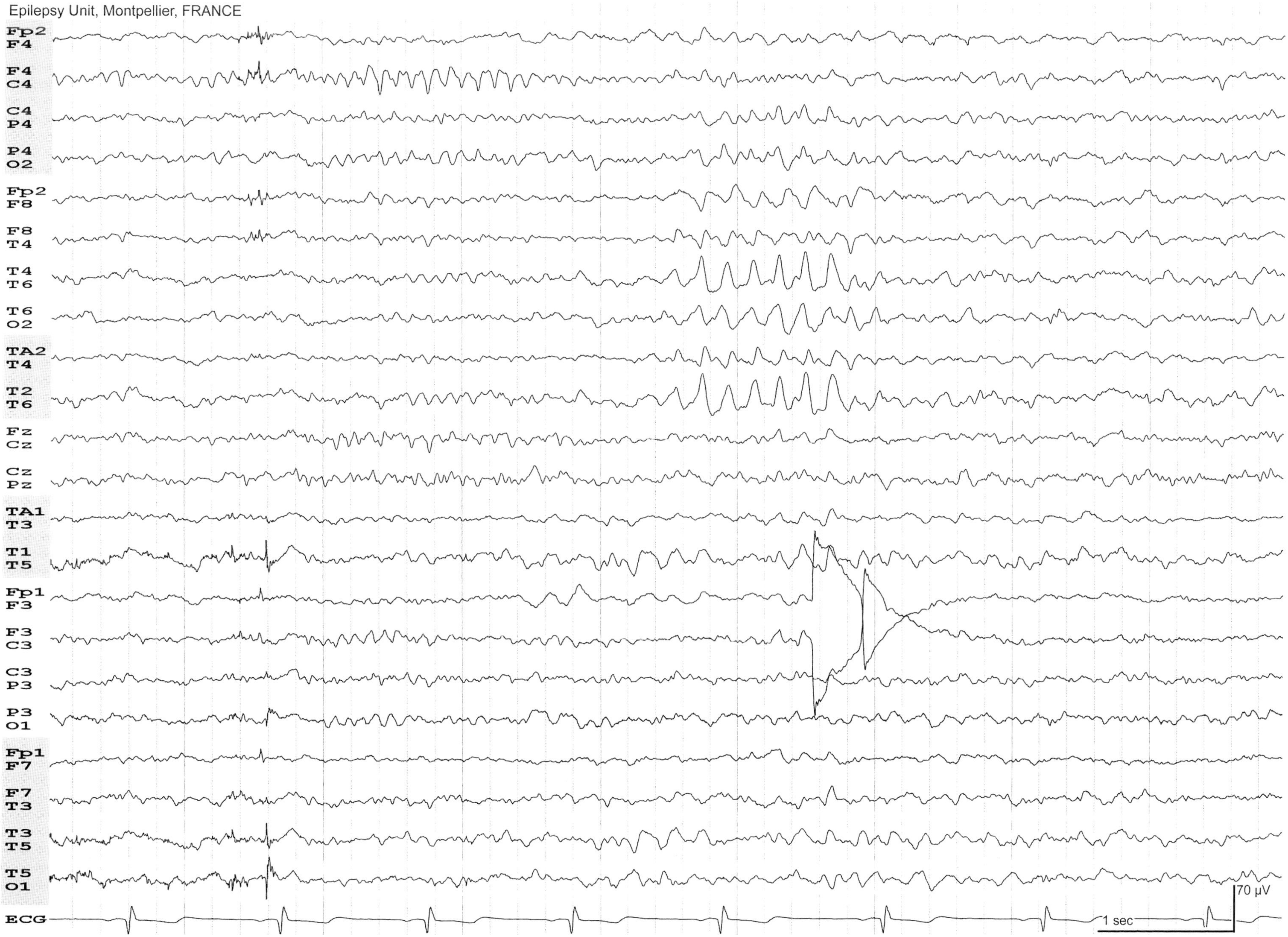
Epilepsy Unit, Montpellier, FRANCE
Fp2 F4
F4 C4
C4 P4
P4 O2
Fp2 F8
F8 T4
T4 T6
T6 O2
TA2 T4
T2 T6
Fz Cz
Cz Pz
TA1 T3
T1 T5
Fp1 F3
F3 C3
C3 P3
P3 O1
Fp1 F7
F7 T3
T3 T5
T5 O1
ECG
70 µV
1 sec

III • 71 Six-Hertz Spike-and-Wave Burst/ Phantom spike-and-wave bursts in drowsiness

Context

19-year-old woman seen after a vasovagal syncope.

What to note

The patient is drowsy. First segment recorded at 15/s and 10 µV/mm. Second segment recorded at 30 mm/s and 70 µV/mm. Two small irregular spike-waves over the posterior regions with predominance on the right hemisphere. These elements do not correspond to a focal occipital lobe epilepsy where the amplitude of the spike-waves is usually higher. These elements observed on this plate correspond to a form of phantom spike-and-wave bursts with posterior distribution found in women, usually referred to as FOLDs (female occipital predominant low amplitude and drowsiness).

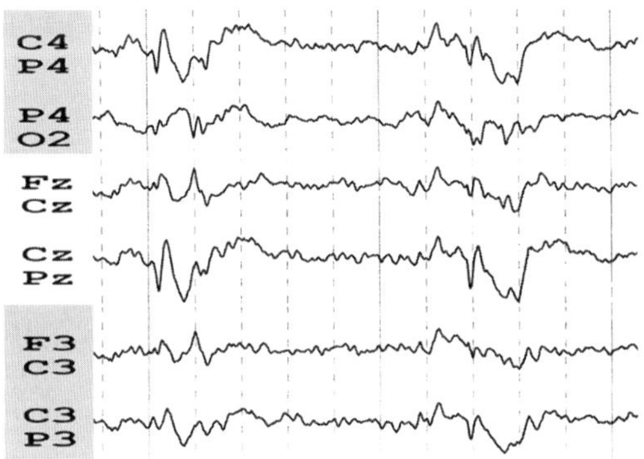

Figure a / Small irregular spike-waves predominating over the posterior regions.

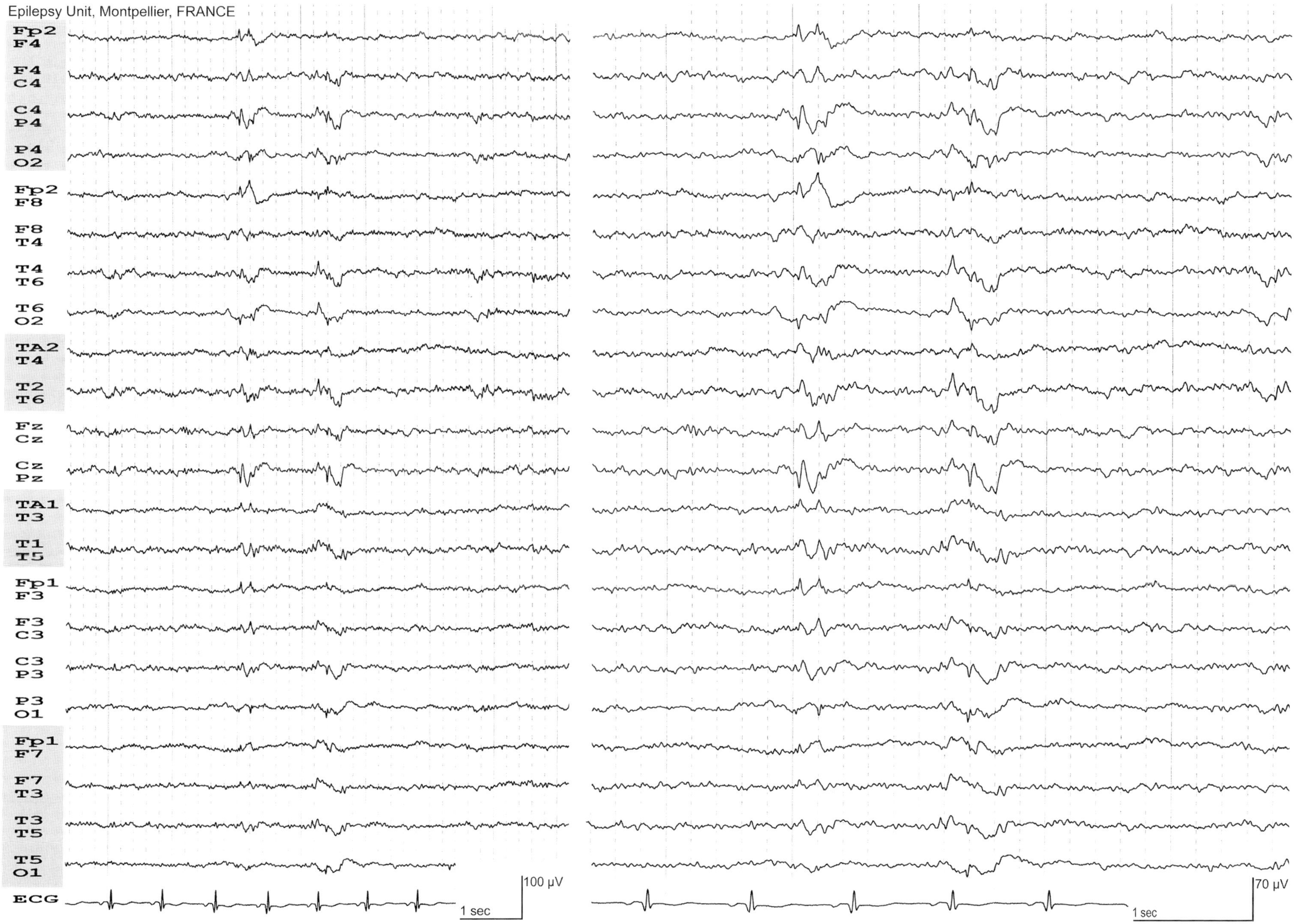
Epilepsy Unit, Montpellier, FRANCE
Fp2 F4
F4 C4
C4 P4
P4 O2
Fp2 F8
F8 T4
T4 T6
T6 O2
TA2 T4
T2 T6
Fz Cz
Cz Pz
TA1 T3
T1 T5
Fp1 F3
F3 C3
C3 P3
P3 O1
Fp1 F7
F7 T3
T3 T5
T5 O1
ECG
100 µV
1 sec
70 µV
1 sec

III • 72 Six-Hertz Spike-and-Wave Burst/ Phantom spike-and-wave bursts in NREM sleep stage 1

Context

16-year-old girl seen after an episode of loss of consciousness.

What to note

Stage N1 sleep. A burst of low-voltage spike-waves at 6 Hz, with a parietal dominant, sharply contoured component, whereas the slow component is more diffuse with anterior spread. These bursts are more ample over Cz-Pz and C4-P4. They correspond to a form of phantom spike-and-wave bursts with posterior distribution found in women, usually referred to as FOLDs (female occipital predominant low amplitude and drowsiness). Posterior dominant phantom spike-and-wave bursts are less often epilepsy-related than anterior dominant phantom spike and wave bursts (WHAMs: wake high amplitude anterior predominance in males) associated with idiopathic generalized epilepsy. Note a pulse artifact at F7.

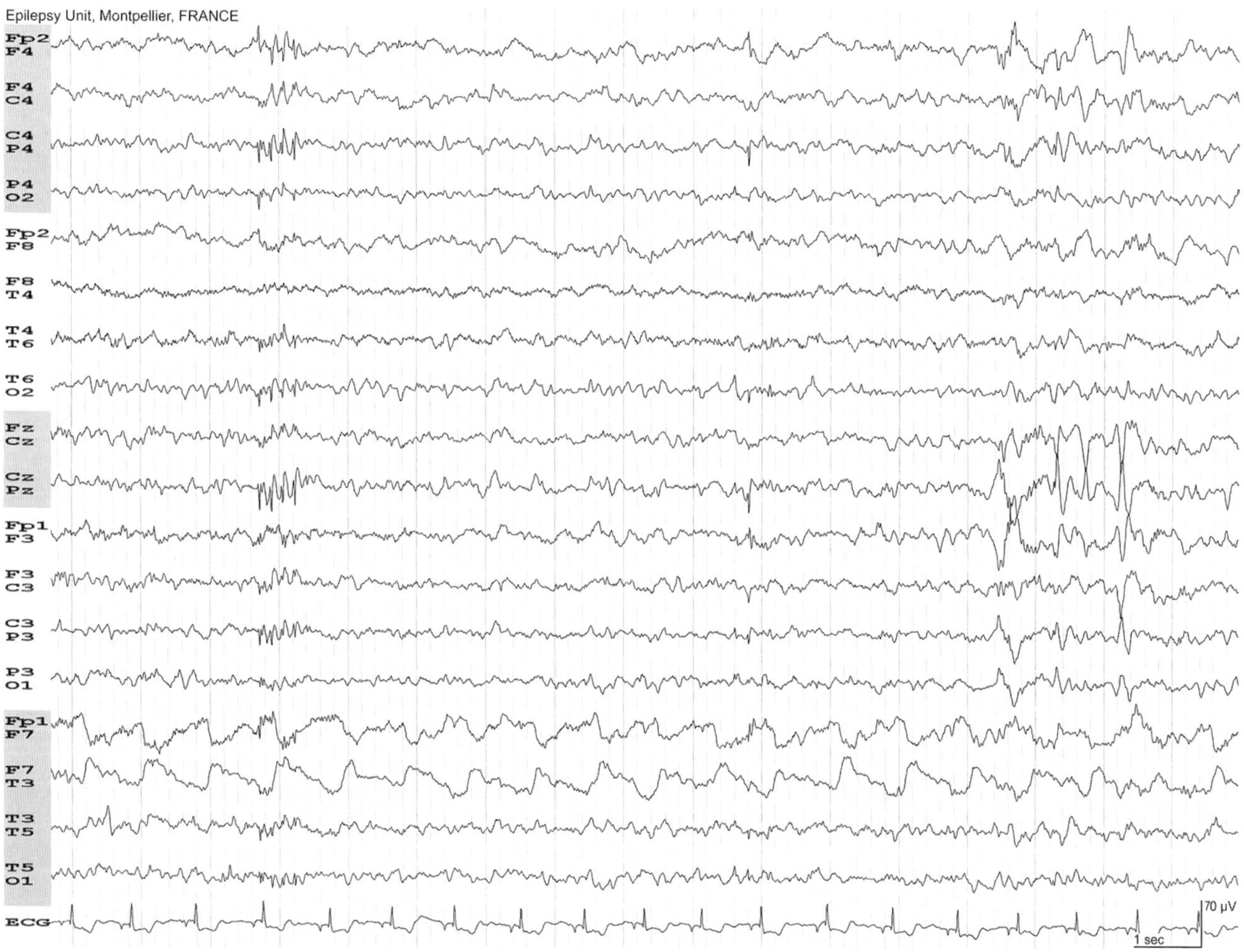

Figure a / Recording at 15 mm/s. Stage N1 sleep with V waves at the end of the plate. In the middle of the plate, an isolated spike can be seen.

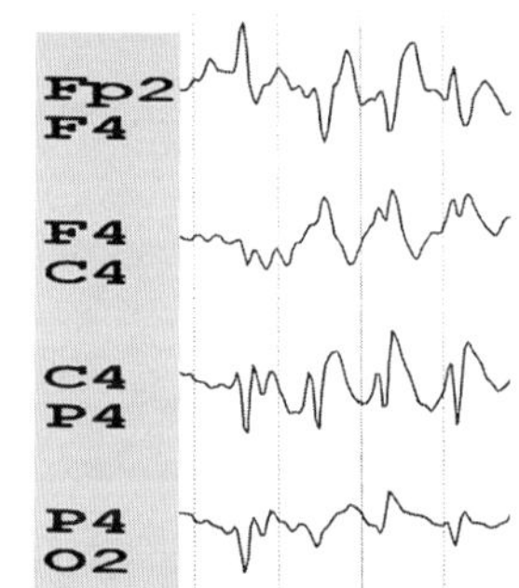

Figure b / Spike-waves at 6 Hz, the sharp component is posterior dominant, with anterior spread of the wave component.

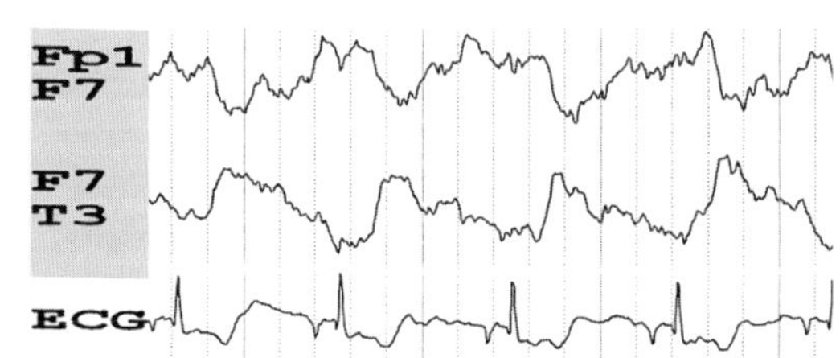

Figure c / Recording at 15 mm//s. Pulse artifact at F7.

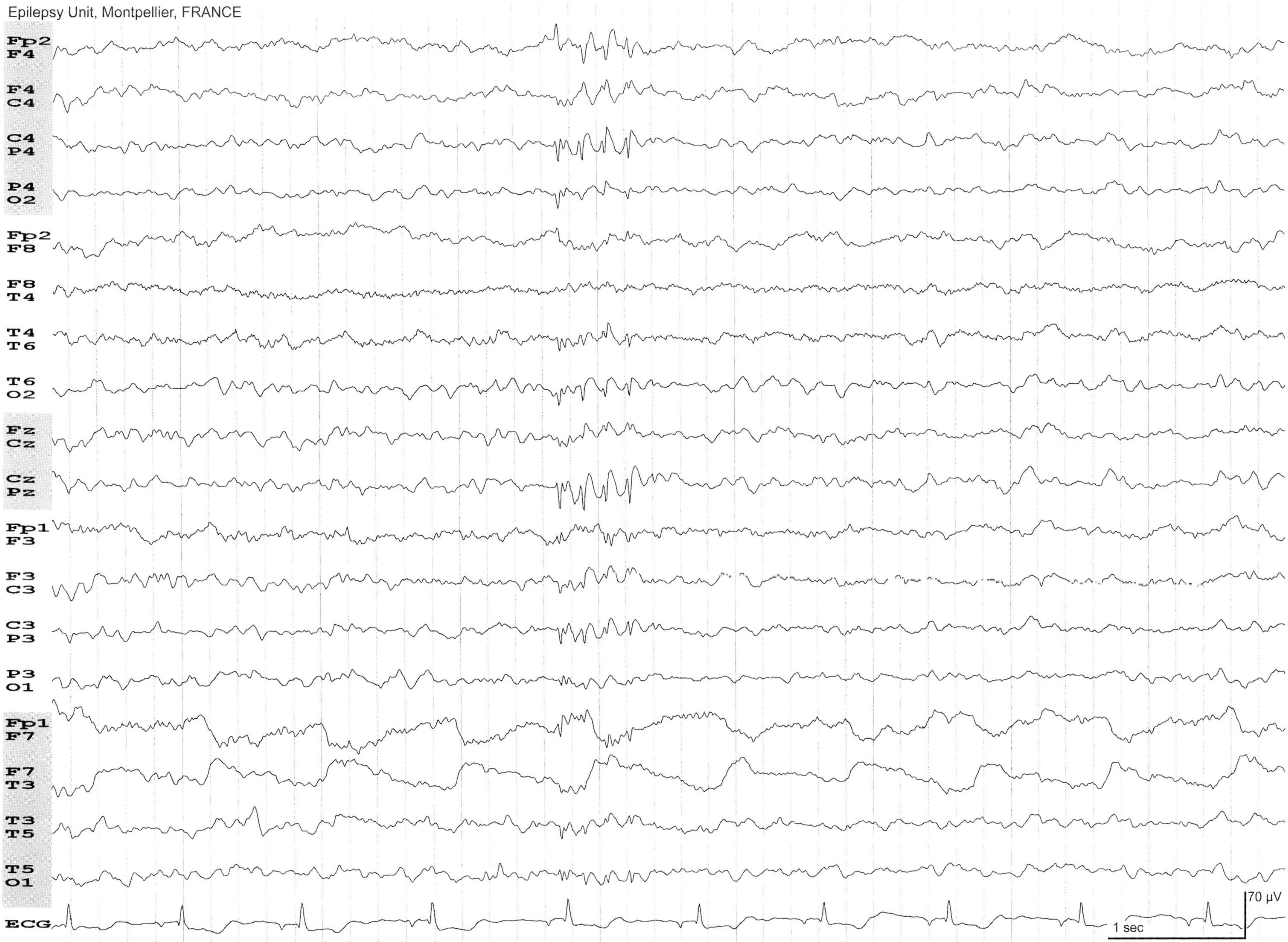
Epilepsy Unit, Montpellier, FRANCE
Fp2 F4
F4 C4
C4 P4
P4 O2
Fp2 F8
F8 T4
T4 T6
T6 O2
Fz Cz
Cz Pz
Fp1 F3
F3 C3
C3 P3
P3 O1
Fp1 F7
F7 T3
T3 T5
T5 O1
ECG
70 µV
1 sec

• 73 Six-Hertz Spike-and-Wave Burst/phantom spike-and-wave bursts in REM sleep

Context

17-year-old woman seen after a brief loss of consciousness: non specific malaise.

What to note

REM sleep with phamtom spike-and-wave bursts (A), sawtooth waves (b) and rapid eye movement (C). The phantom spike-and-waves are more ample over Cz-Pz with a parietal dominance and correspond to a form found in women, referred to as FOLDs (female occipital predominant low amplitude and drowsiness). In this patient, phantom spike-and-waves were present in drowsiness (Figure b). They disappeared in NREM sleep stage 2 but reappeared after transient arousal. The phantom spike-and-waves reappeared with a slight less amplitude in REM sleep.

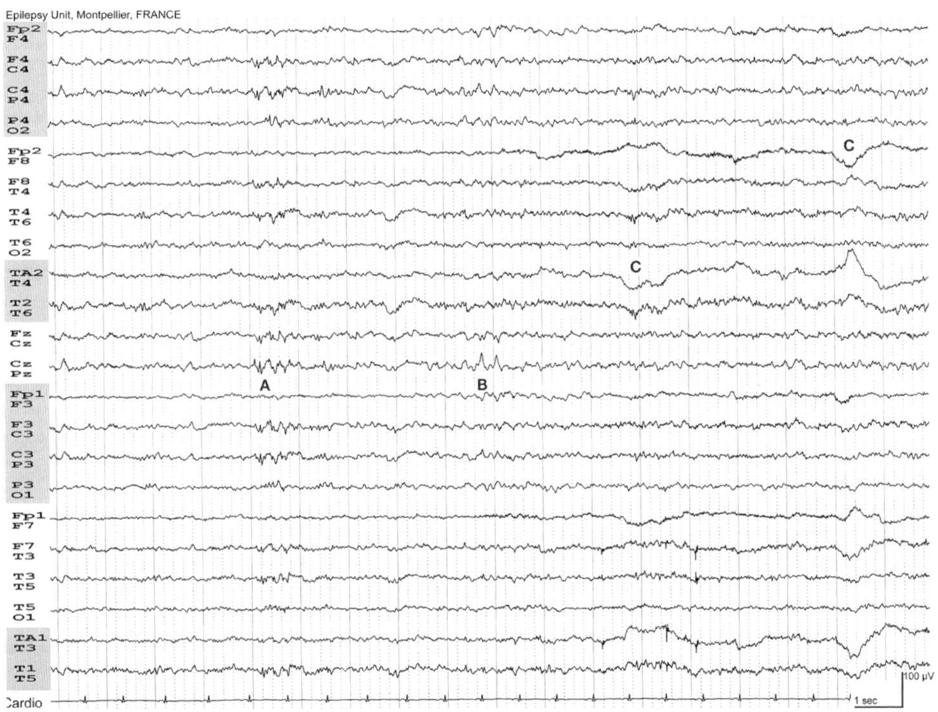

Figure a / Recording at 15 mm/s. REM sleep. A: Phamtom spike-and wave bursts; B: sawtooth waves; C: Rapid eye movements.

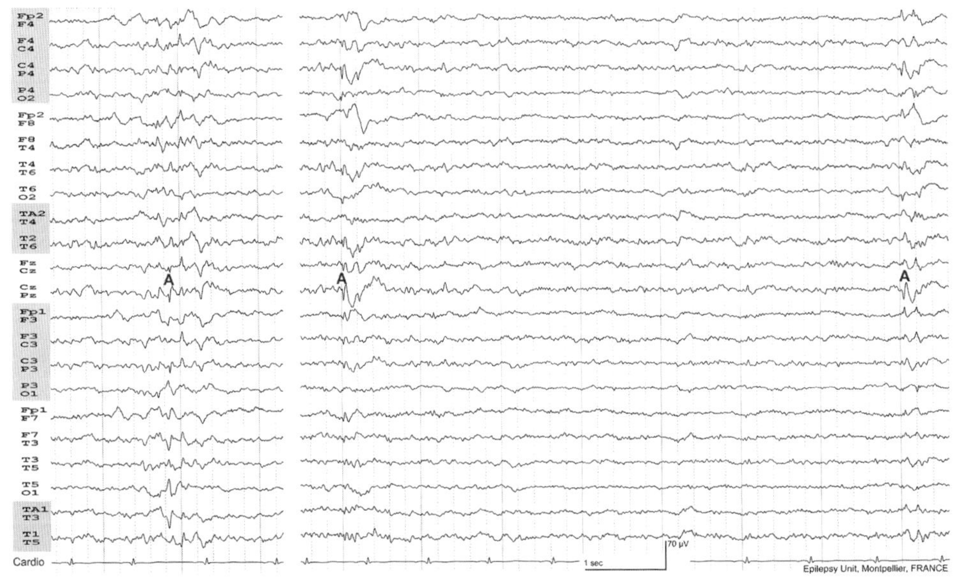

Figure b / Same patient during drowsiness. Posterior phamtom spike-and wave bursts (A).

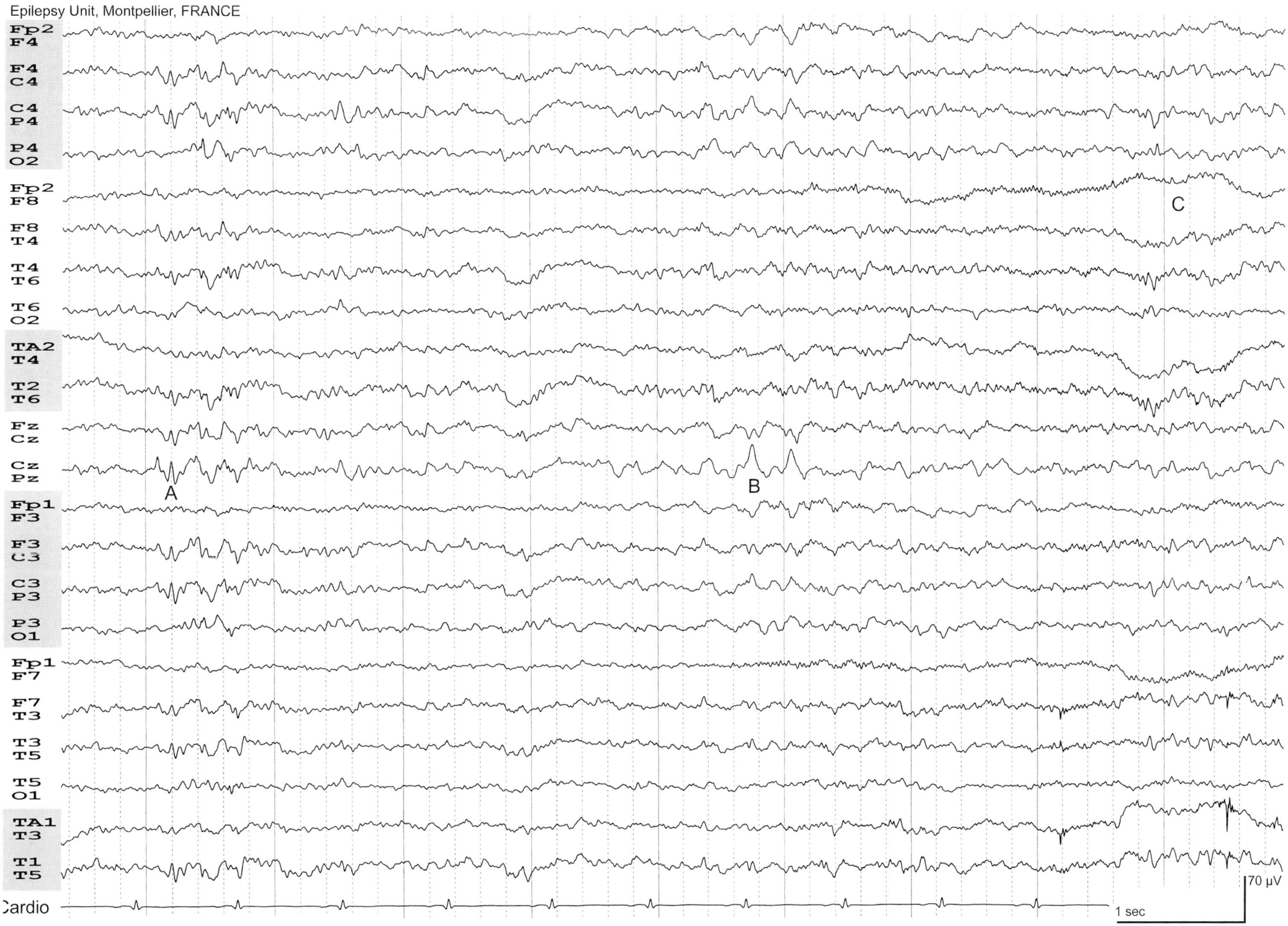
Epilepsy Unit, Montpellier, FRANCE
Fp2 F4
F4 C4
C4 P4
P4 O2
Fp2 F8
F8 T4
T4 T6
T6 O2
TA2 T4
T2 T6
Fz Cz
Cz Pz
Fp1 F3
F3 C3
C3 P3
P3 O1
Fp1 F7
F7 T3
T3 T5
T5 O1
TA1 T3
T1 T5
Cardio
A
B
C
70 µV
1 sec

• 74 SREDA: Transitional phase from NREM stage 2 into REM sleep

Context

39-year-old man seen after two episodes of loss of consciousness. Same patient as plates I.26, I.27.

What to note

Transitional phase from NREM sleep stage 2 into REM sleep. Bilateral slow waves with predominance on the right hemisphere appear on the mid and posterior regions at gradually shorter intervals until there is a theta frequency discharge at 5 Hz (see next plate). Amplitude is maximal from onset and it remains constant, throughout the following plate..

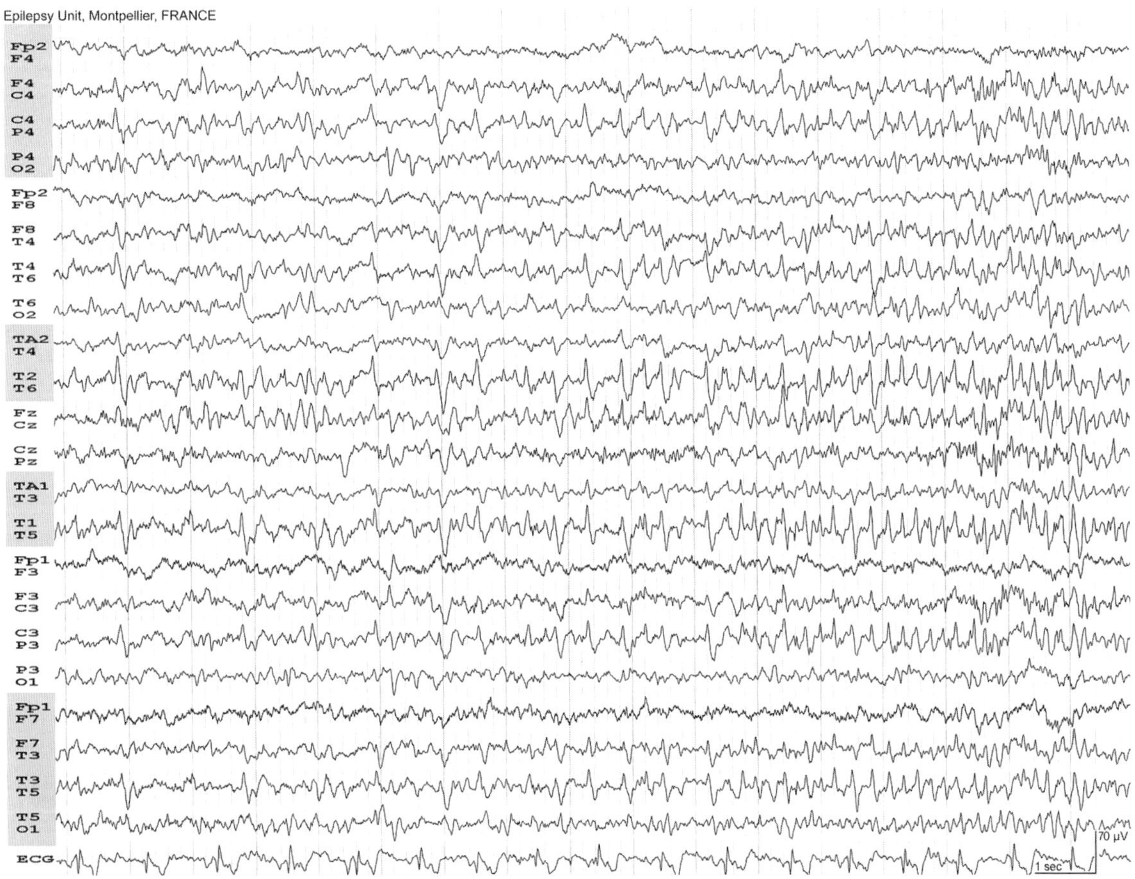

Figure a / Recording at 15 mm/s.

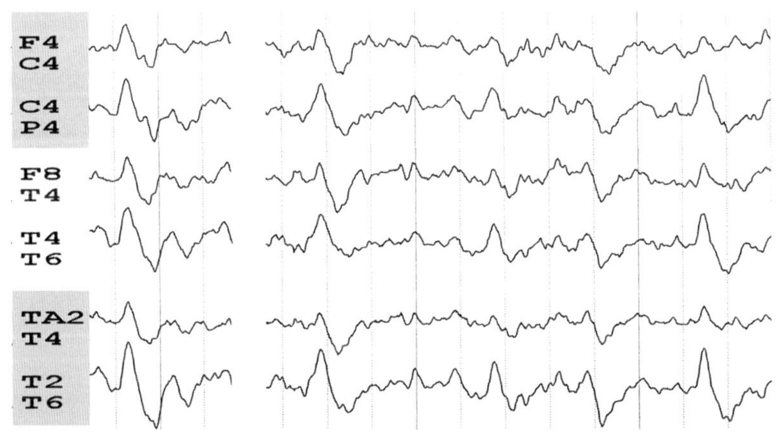

Figure b / Slow waves at gradually shorter intervals.

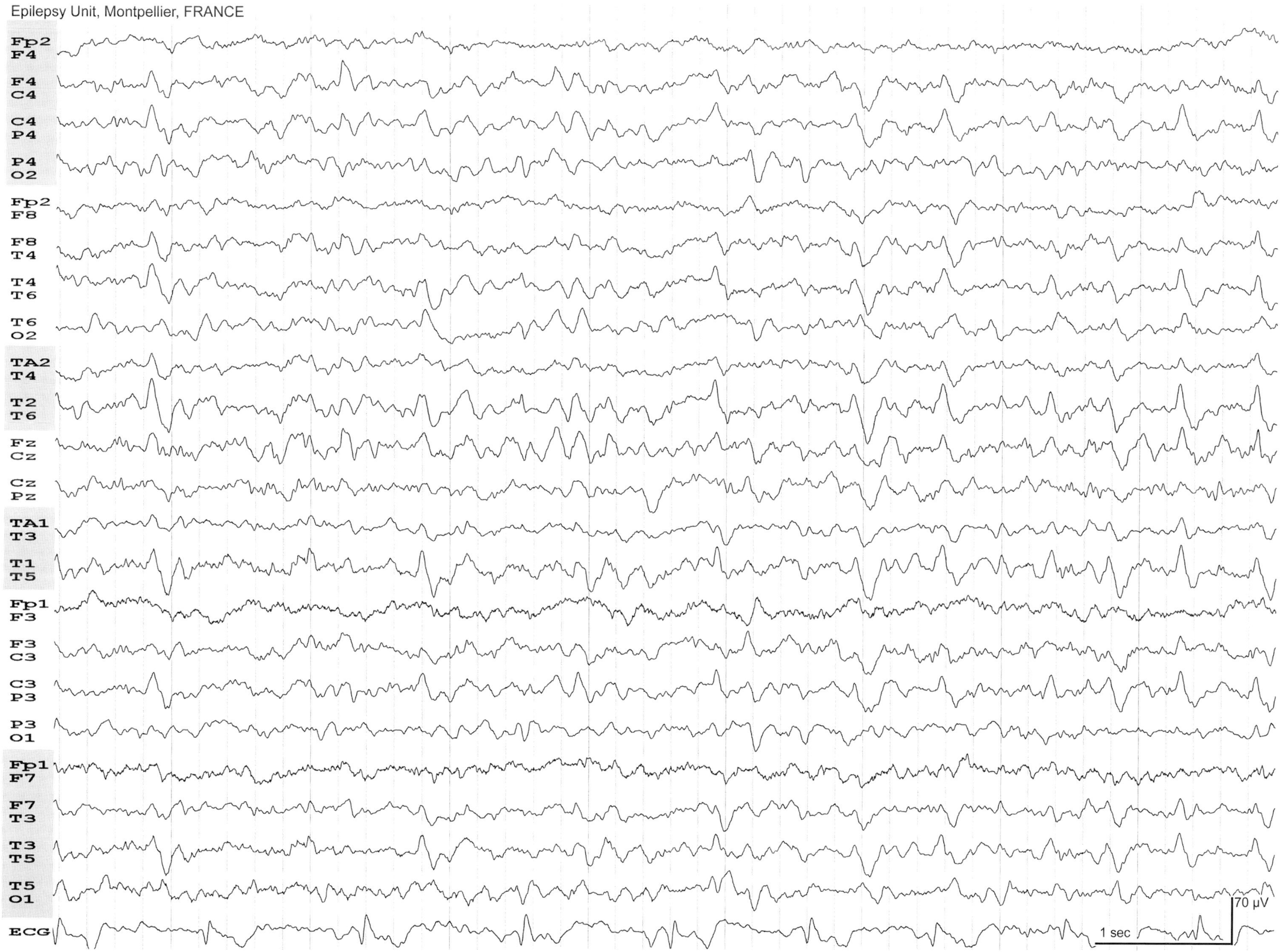
Epilepsy Unit, Montpellier, FRANCE
Fp2 F4
F4 C4
C4 P4
P4 O2
Fp2 F8
F8 T4
T4 T6
T6 O2
TA2 T4
T2 T6
Fz Cz
Cz Pz
TA1 T3
T1 T5
Fp1 F3
F3 C3
C3 P3
P3 O1
Fp1 F7
F7 T3
T3 T5
T5 O1
ECG
70 µV
1 sec

III • 75 SREDA: Transitional phase from NREM stage 2 into REM sleep

Context

39-year-old man, same patient as on III.74, continued.

What to note

Monomorphic theta activity at 5 Hz with constant amplitude. Poorly developed sleep spindles can be seen on the vertex.

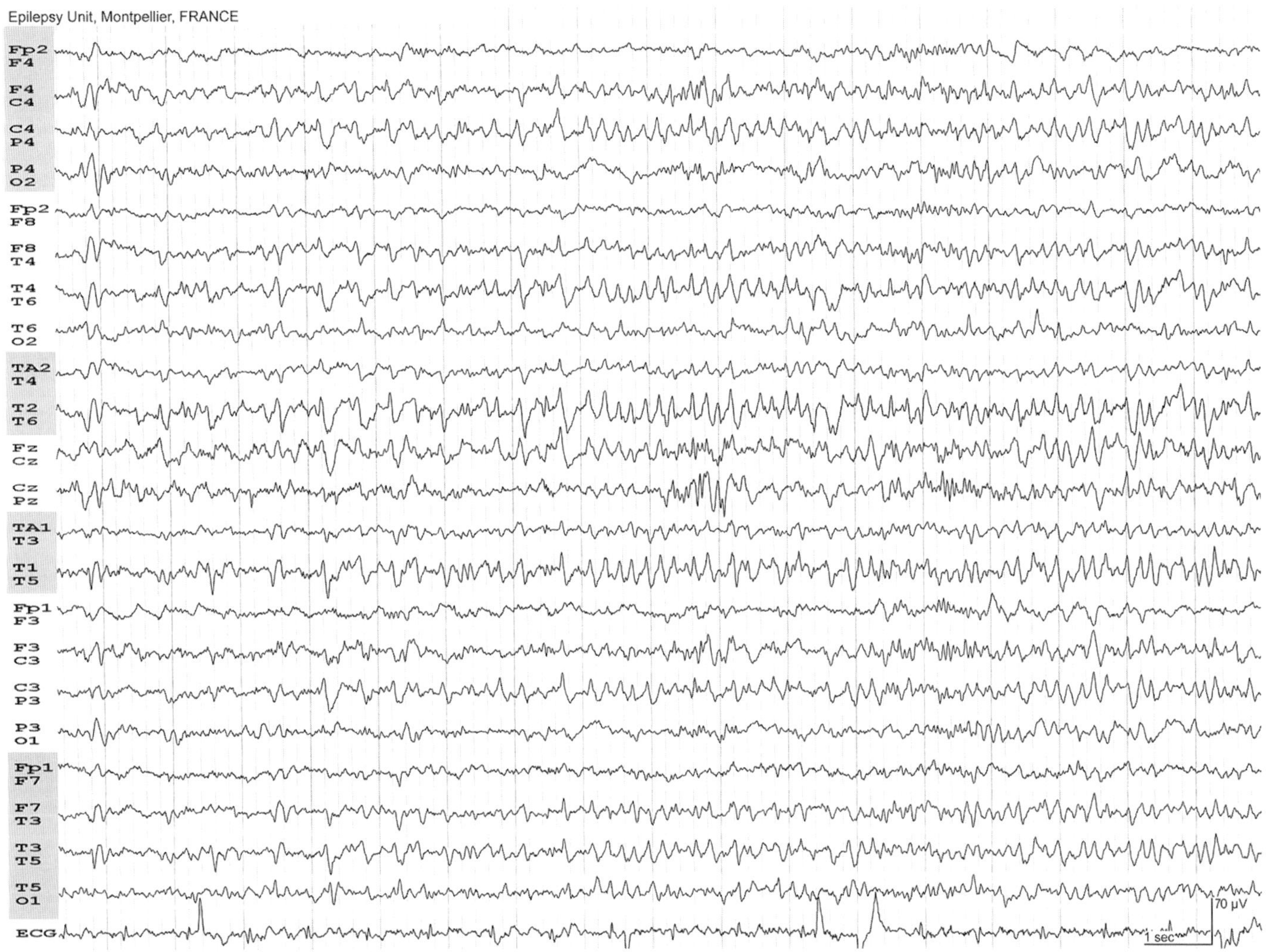

Figure a / Recording at 15 mm/s. Another SREDA in a transitional phase from NREM sleep stage 2 into REM sleep during the same recording. The ECG derivation is partially defective.

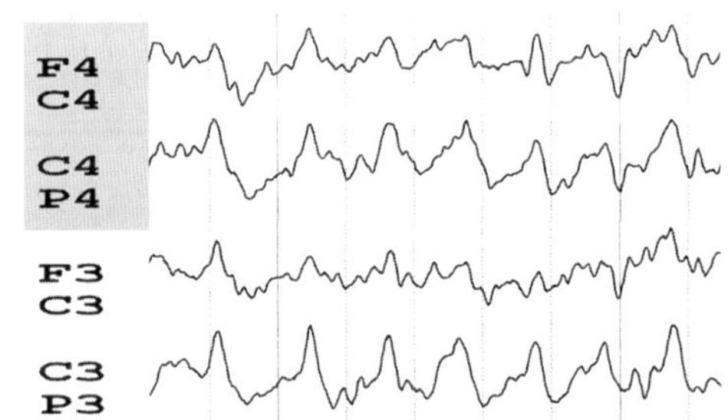

Figure b / Theta waves at 5 Hz.

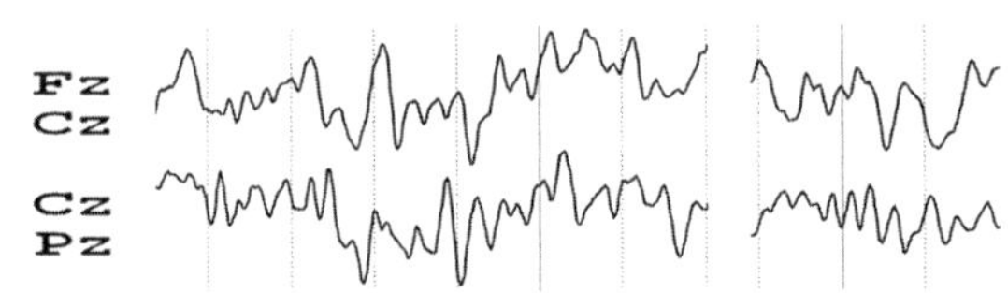

Figure c / Poorly developed sleep spindles.

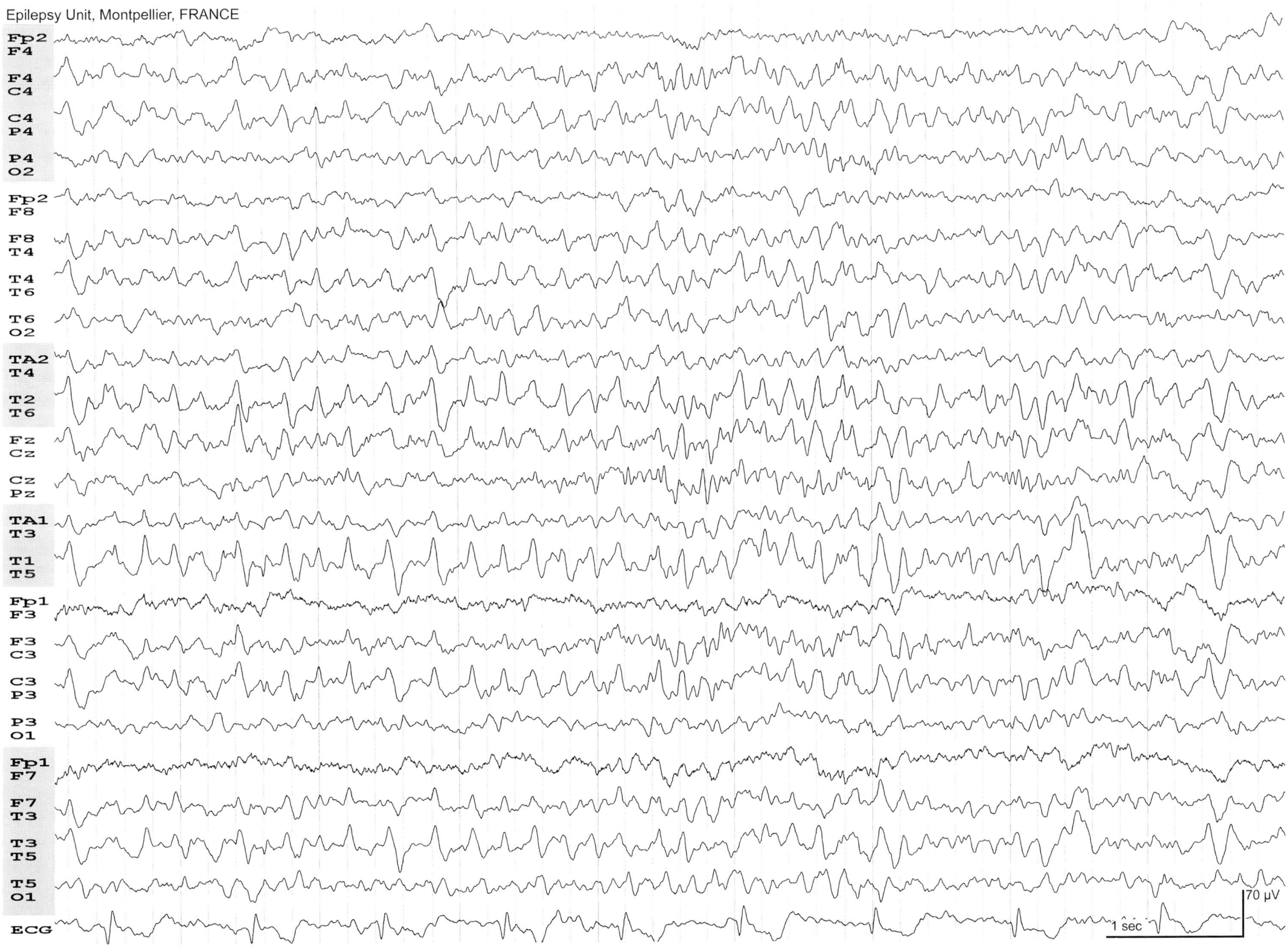
Epilepsy Unit, Montpellier, FRANCE
Fp2 F4
F4 C4
C4 P4
P4 O2
Fp2 F8
F8 T4
T4 T6
T6 O2
TA2 T4
T2 T6
Fz Cz
Cz Pz
TA1 T3
T1 T5
Fp1 F3
F3 C3
C3 P3
P3 O1
Fp1 F7
F7 T3
T3 T5
T5 O1
ECG
70 µV
1 sec

III • 76 Breach rhythm during sleep (1)

Context

48-year-old woman seen 3 years after surgery for right mesial temporal lobe epilepsy.

What to note

Stage N2 sleep with presence of positive occipital sharp transients of sleep (POSTs) clearly detectable over the occipital regions. Left segment, over the right temporal region, monomorphic sharp waves at 8 Hz corresponding to a breach rhythm. Right segment, a very sharply contoured waveform can be observed which, if taken alone, can be mistaken for an "epileptic" spike. But the same element, when seen in longer runs, is clearly an element of breach rhythm.

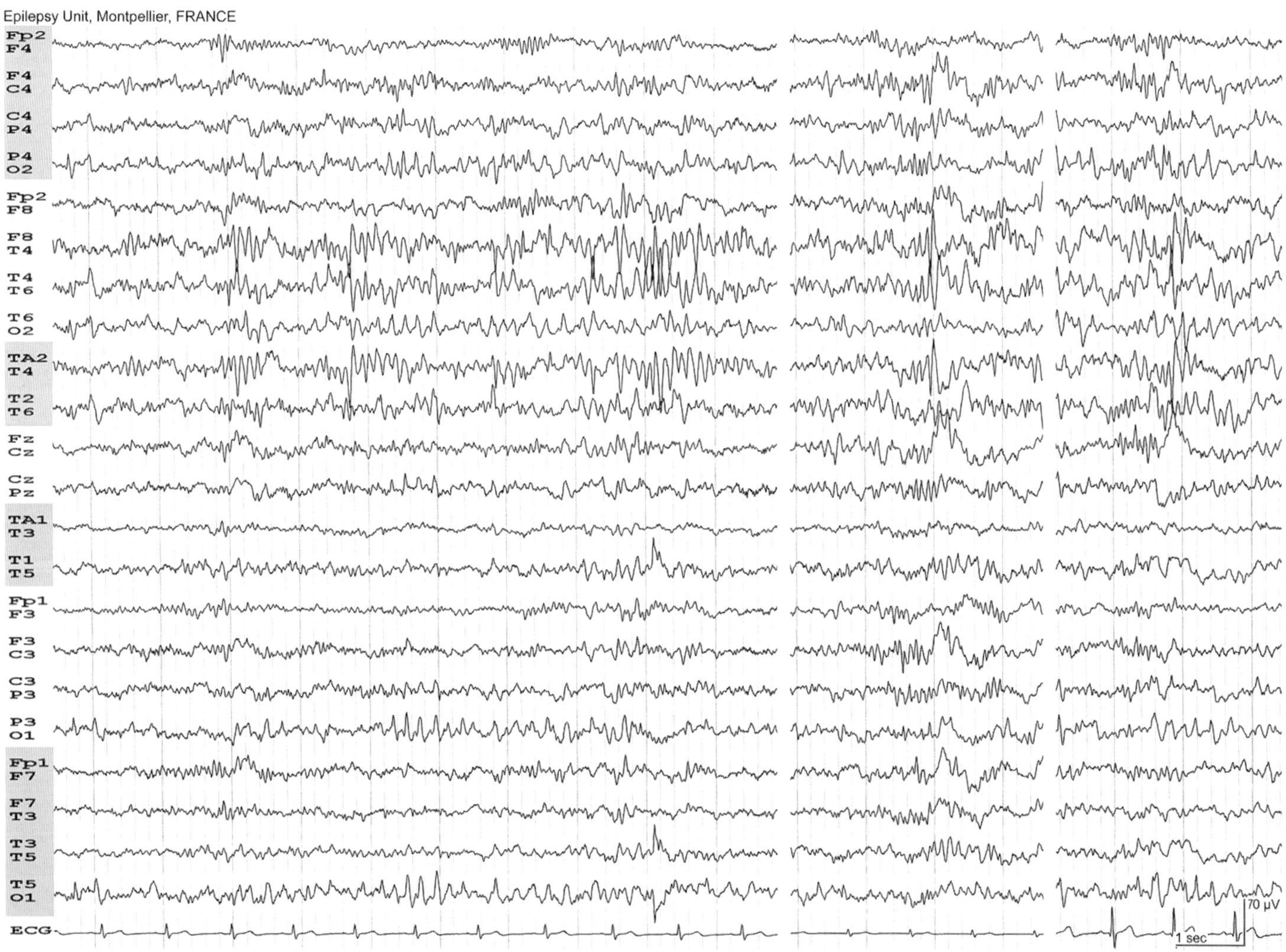

Figure a / Recording at 15 mm/s. Right segment, another example of a very sharply contoured waveform which could have been mistaken for an "epileptic" spike.

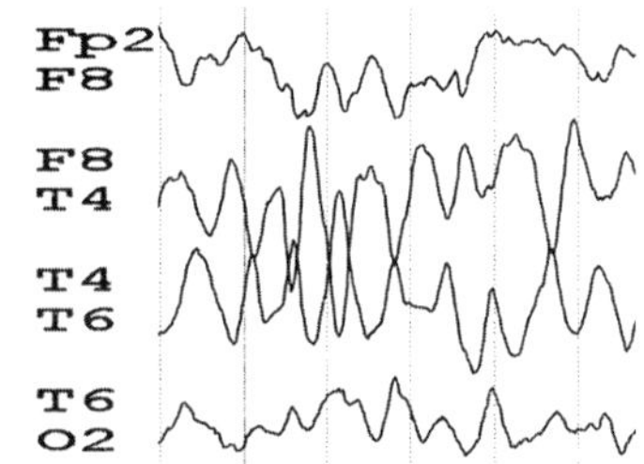

Figure b / Monomorphic sharp waves at 8 Hz corresponding to a breach rhythm.

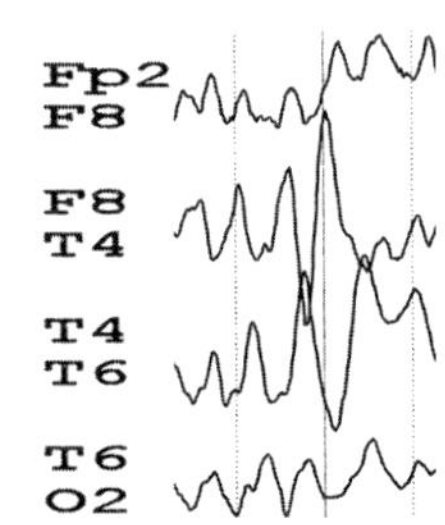

Figure c / Breach rhythm.

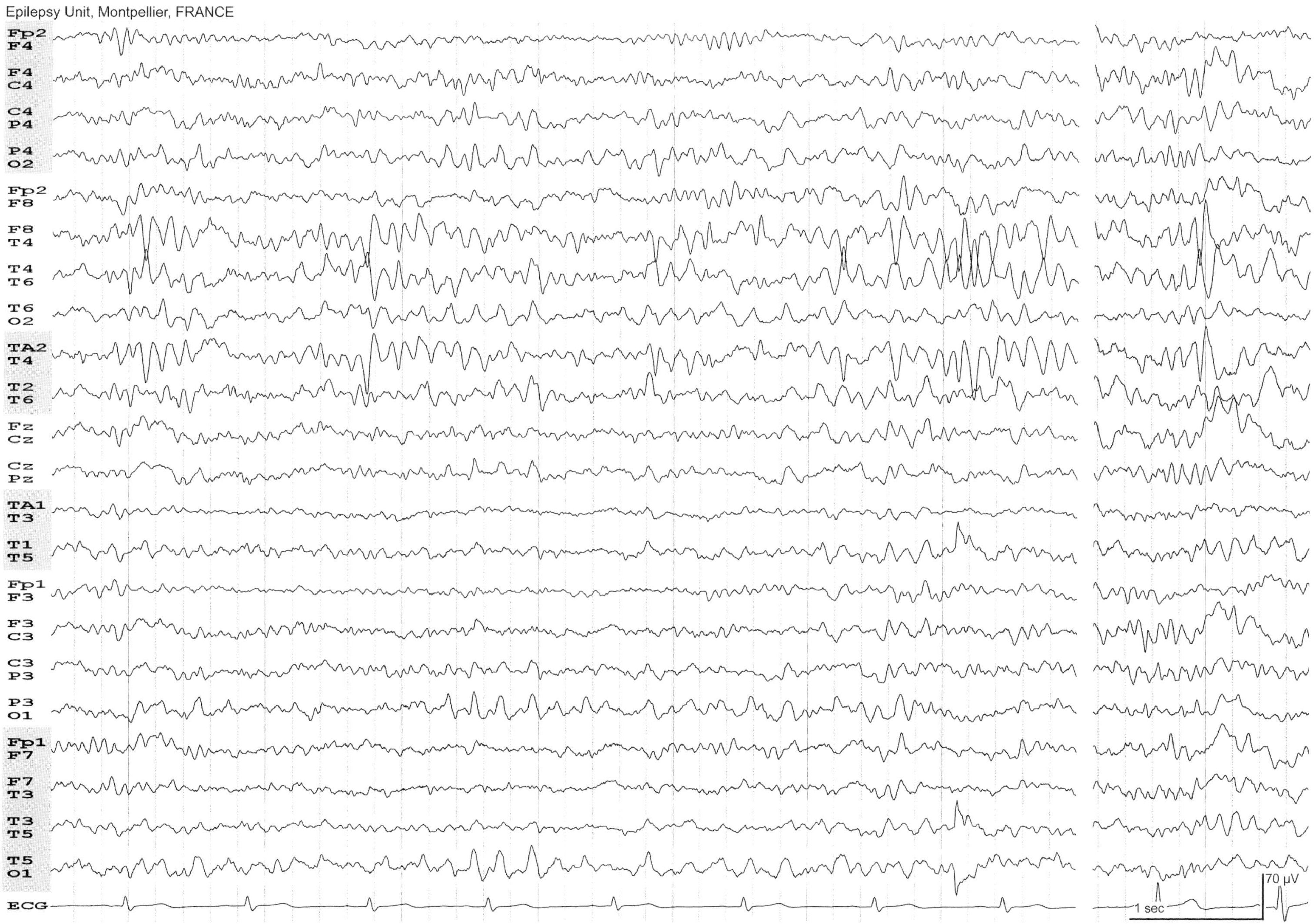
Epilepsy Unit, Montpellier, FRANCE
Fp2 F4
F4 C4
C4 P4
P4 O2
Fp2 F8
F8 T4
T4 T6
T6 O2
TA2 T4
T2 T6
Fz Cz
Cz Pz
TA1 T3
T1 T5
Fp1 F3
F3 C3
C3 P3
P3 O1
Fp1 F7
F7 T3
T3 T5
T5 O1
ECG
70 µV
1 sec

III • 77 Breach rhythm during sleep (2)

Context

50-year-old man with severe right frontal lobe epilepsy following a meningioma operated at age 20 years.

What to note

The man is in NREM stage II sleep with few physiological components. The monomorphic, regular, low-voltage spikes which can be observed at F8 mixed with theta waveforms correspond to a breach rhythm. At the end of the plate recorded at 15 mm/s (at the 16th second), a right fronto-temporal spike-wave of increased amplitude corresponds to interictal abnormalities in this patient.

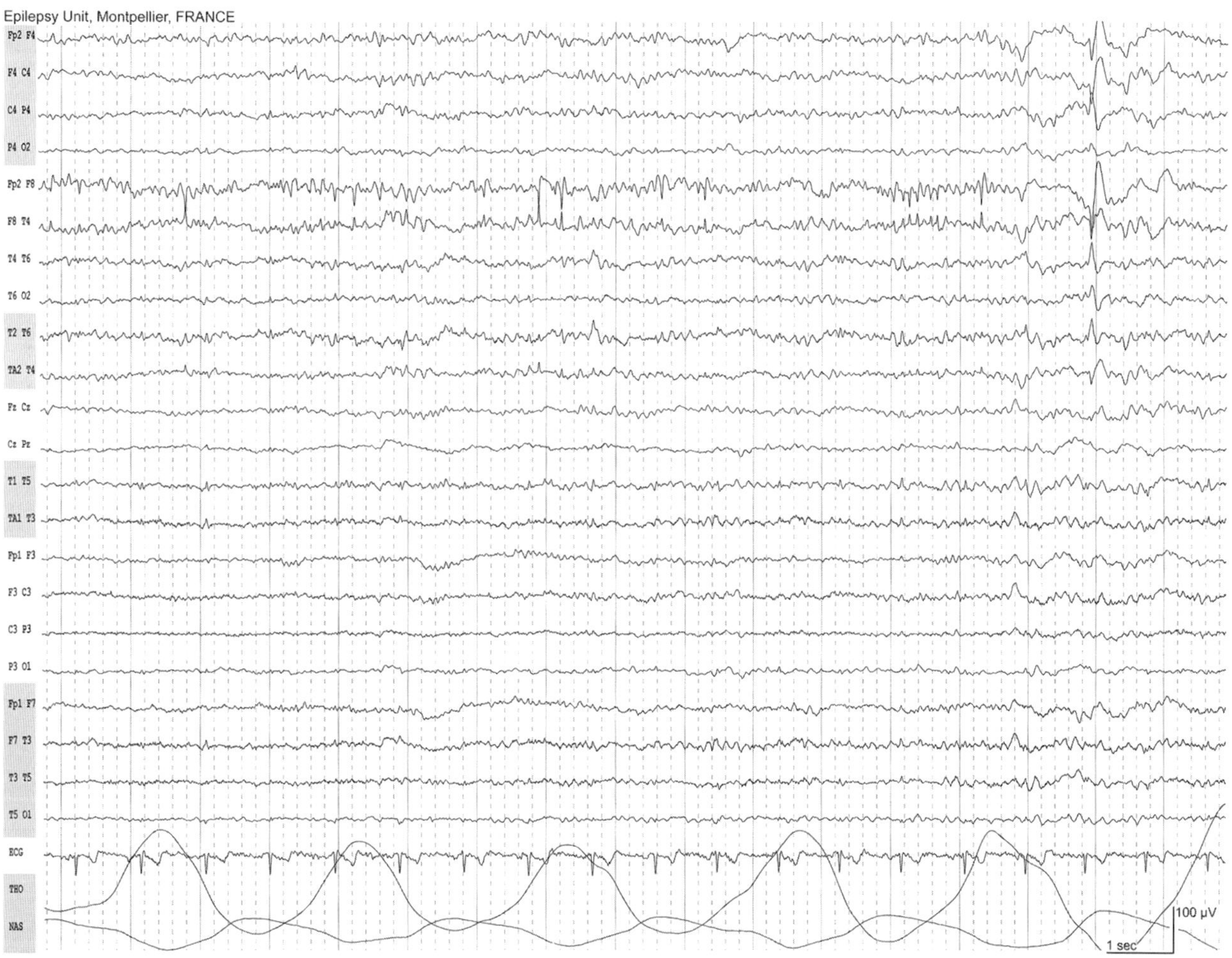

Figure a / Recording at 15 mm/s. At the 16th second, a right fronto-temporal interictal spike-wave.

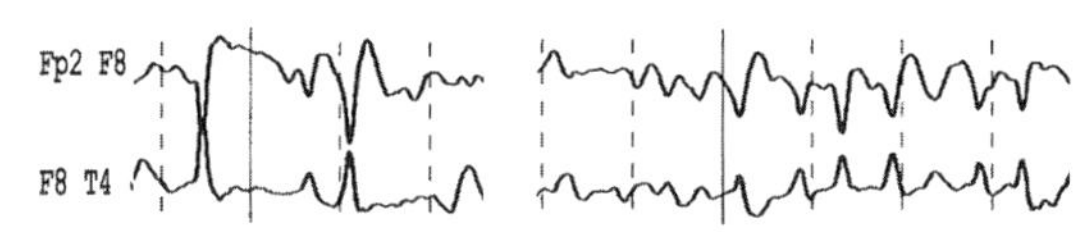

Figure b / Presence of monomorphic, regular, low-voltage spikes at F8 mixed with theta waveforms corresponding to a breach rhythm.

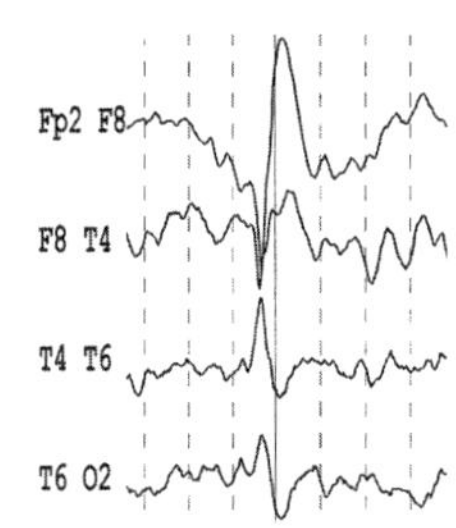

Figure c / Recording at 15 mm/s. Interictal fronto-temporal spike-wave.

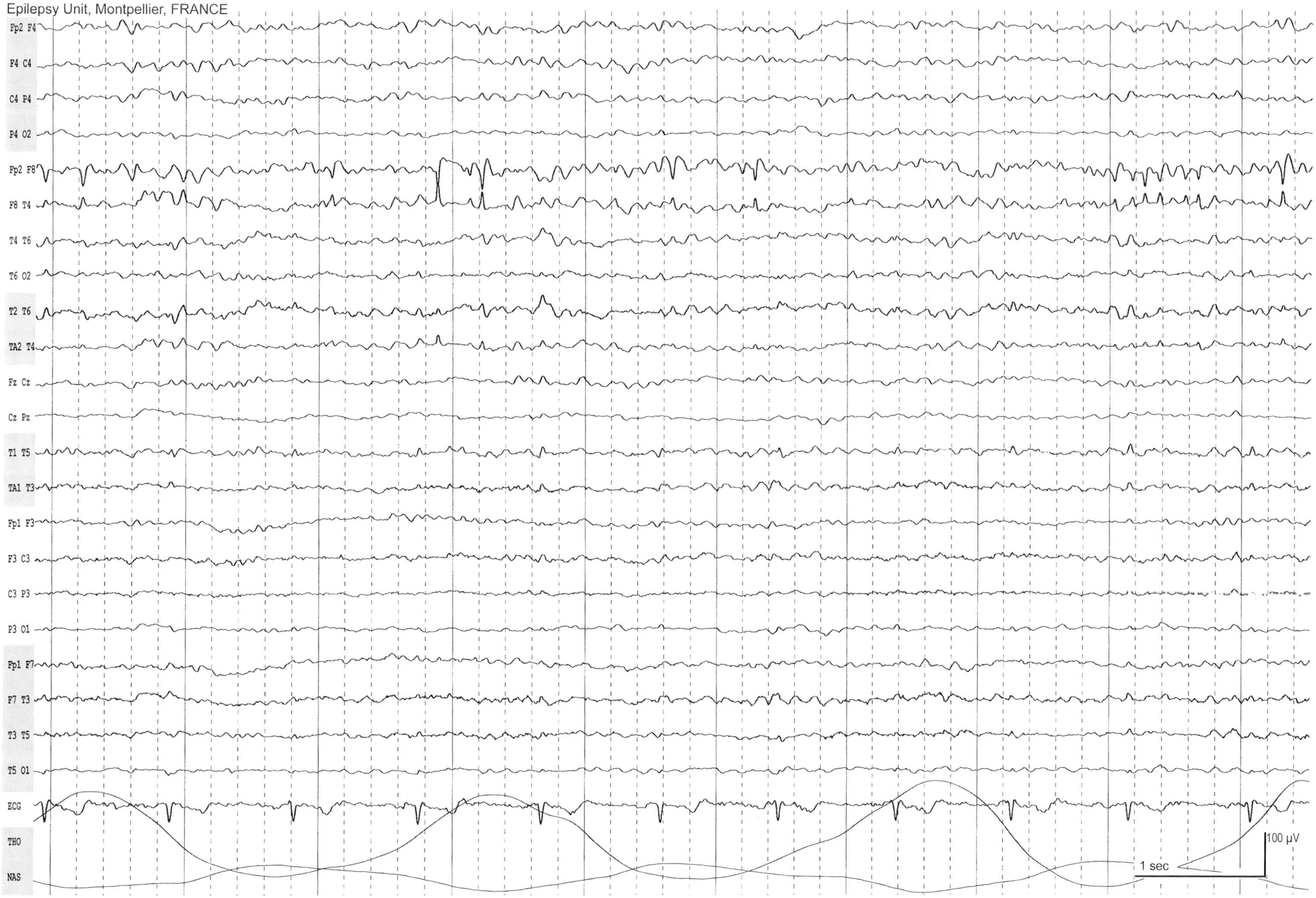
Epilepsy Unit, Montpellier, FRANCE
Fp2 F4
F4 C4
C4 P4
P4 O2
Fp2 F8
F8 T4
T4 T6
T6 O2
T2 T6
TA2 T4
Fz Cz
Cz Pz
T1 T5
TA1 T3
Fp1 F3
F3 C3
C3 P3
P3 O1
Fp1 F7
F7 T3
T3 T5
T5 O1
ECG
THO
NAS
100 µV
1 sec

III • 78 When the EEG complicates the situation! Benign spikes in children without epilepsy

Context

Left segment, 8-year-old child see after a faint. Right segment, 6-year-old child seen for learning difficulties.

What to note

The two children are in stage N2 sleep (K complex followed by onset of a spindle at the end of the right segment). On the left segment, diphasic spike-waves over the left parietal region with spread to the right. On the right segment, two left central spike-waves with some spread over the left temporal region. Neither of these two children had epilepsy. The morphology of these waveforms is similar to rolandic spikes seen in benign partial epilepsy of childhood with centro-temporal spikes (BECTS) but without its activation profile (strong increase during sleep) or distribution. These waveforms are age dependent and will disappear by puberty (maturation of the central nervous system). Note the electrode artifact on the left at F7 and on the right at Fp1 due to poor impedance (lack of electrolytic gel). On the right segment, there is no high-pass filter. On the left segment, the EEG was filtered at 30 Hz, therefore conveying a less typical impression of this artifact.

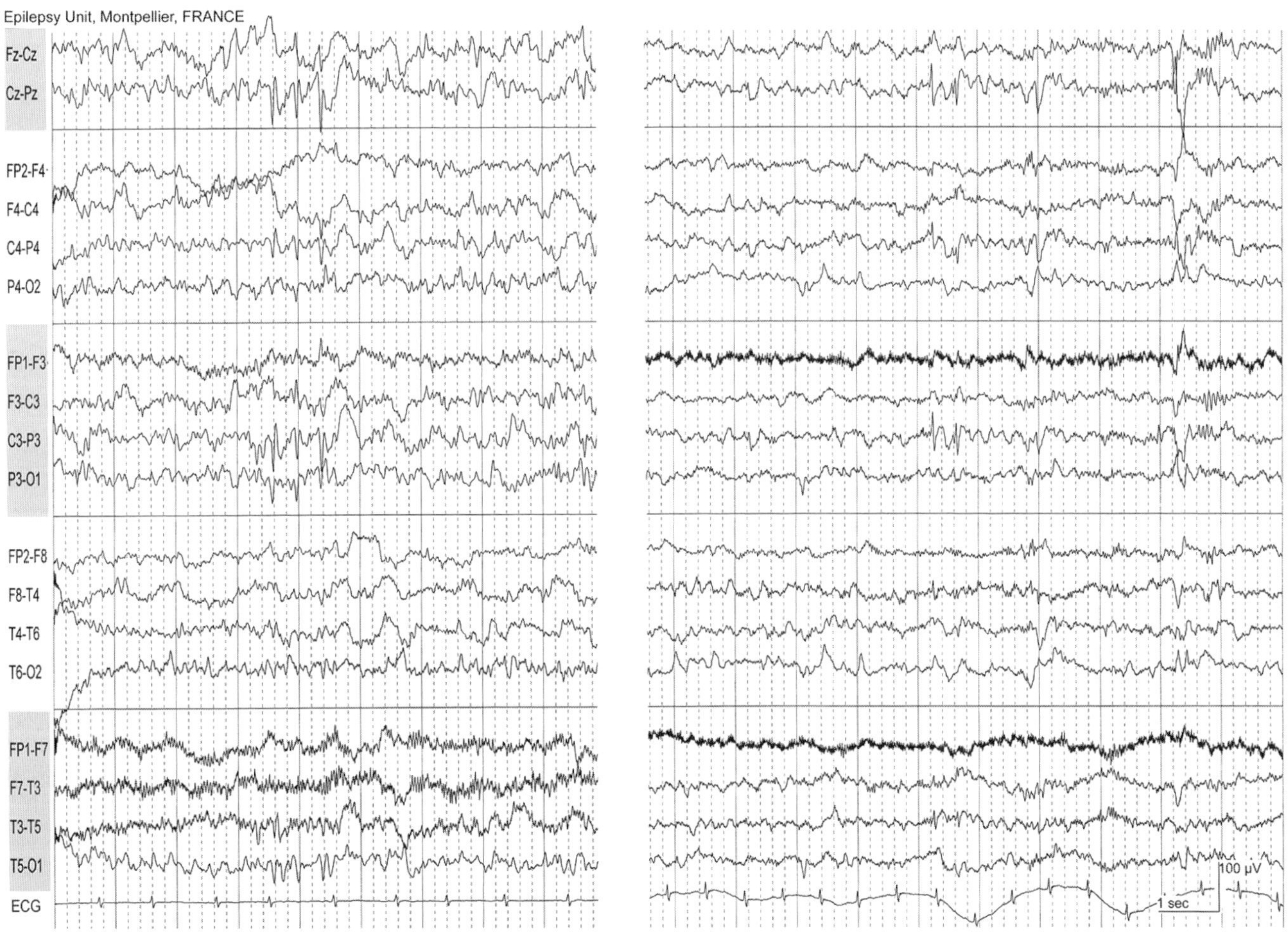

Figure a / Recording at 15 mm/s.

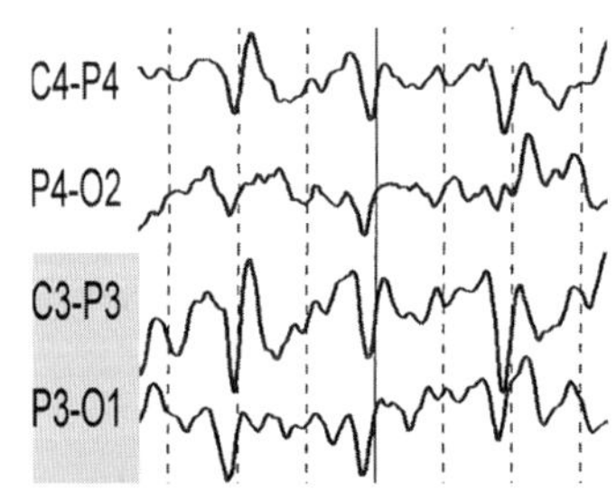

Figure b / Diphasic spike-waves dominant at P3.

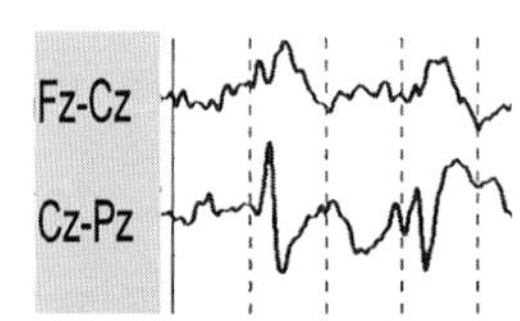

Figure c / Diphasic spike-waves at Cz-Pz.

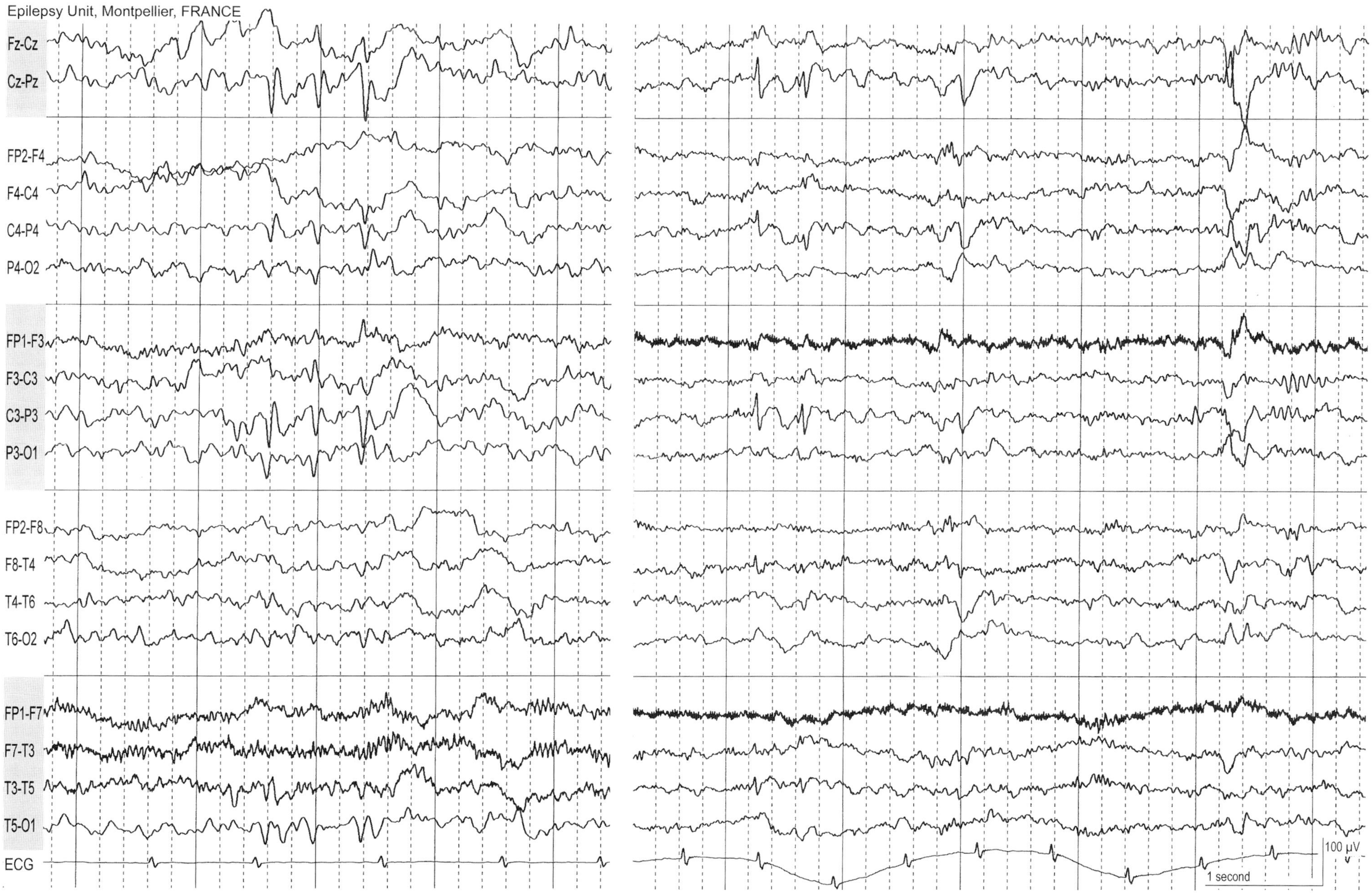
Epilepsy Unit, Montpellier, FRANCE
Fz-Cz
Cz-Pz
FP2-F4
F4-C4
C4-P4
P4-O2
FP1-F3
F3-C3
C3-P3
P3-O1
FP2-F8
F8-T4
T4-T6
T6-O2
FP1-F7
F7-T3
T3-T5
T5-O1
ECG
100 µV
1 second

Artifacts

CHAPITRE IV

The recording of an EEG is often made complex by the presence of a variety of artifacts. Artifactual activity can be quite difficult to identify and may result in misinterpreting artifacts as pathological activity. Some are easily identified, others not so easily. The use of polygraphy is often very helpful for the recognition of artifacts and their sources, in particular the ECG, breathing plethysmography and the EMG. Concomitant video monitoring is particularly helpful in identifying movement artifacts.

In this chapter, we will present the most common artifacts as well as several unusual ones. We do not claim to be exhaustive, as the range of non-physiological and physiological artifacts is very wide. One of the major goals of the technologist is to provide skilled detailed observation of the patient, thereby providing evidence whenever the activity is not of cerebral origin. The technologist must always try to correct the artifact, and this is not feasible, he should indicate exactly what the patient was doing at that particular moment. The better the tracing, the more relevant the analysis of the EEG will be.

IV • 1 Electrodermogram (sweat artifact)

Context

Full-term neonate, 1 month old, admitted for a head trauma. EEG performed in the pediatric intensive care unit.

What to note

Note the very high amplitude activity at a frequency of 0.5 Hz in all derivations. Its identical appearance in all derivations identifies it as a perspiration artifact (electrodermogram). These activities will disappear gradually when the baby is fanned to eliminate perspiration (see below).

What to do

To reduce perspiration artifacts, it is important to carry out recordings at a room temperature below 20° C, using air conditioning if necessary. Otherwise, it is always possible to use a fan or a sheet of paper, provided this is done gently to avoid displacement of the electrode wires. Also reassure the patient about the test he is undergoing to relieve anxiety.

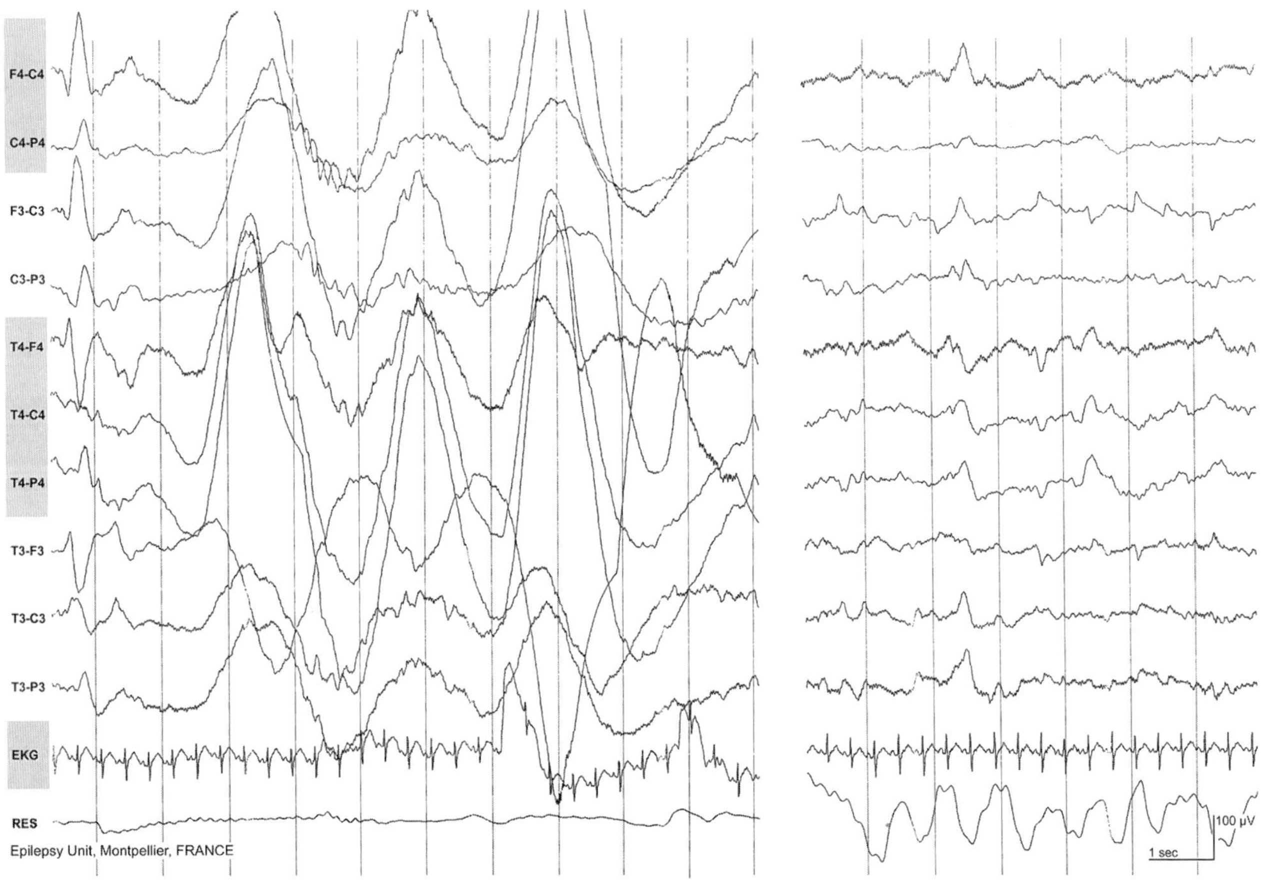

Figure a / Recording at 15 mm/s. Right segment, offset of slow waves after ventilation of the infant.

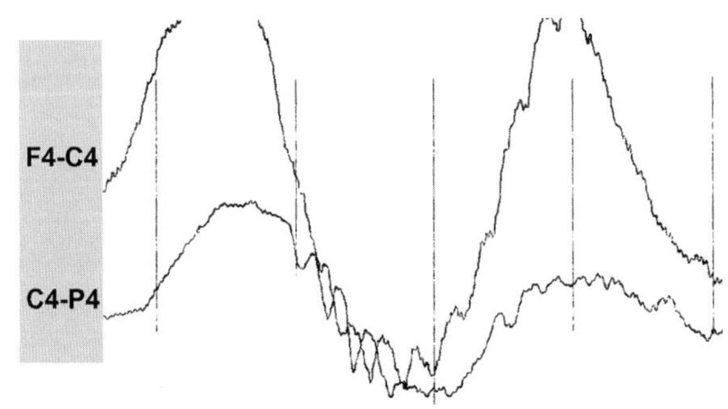

Figure b / Recording at 15 mm/s. High-amplitude delta waves corresponding to an electrodermogram.

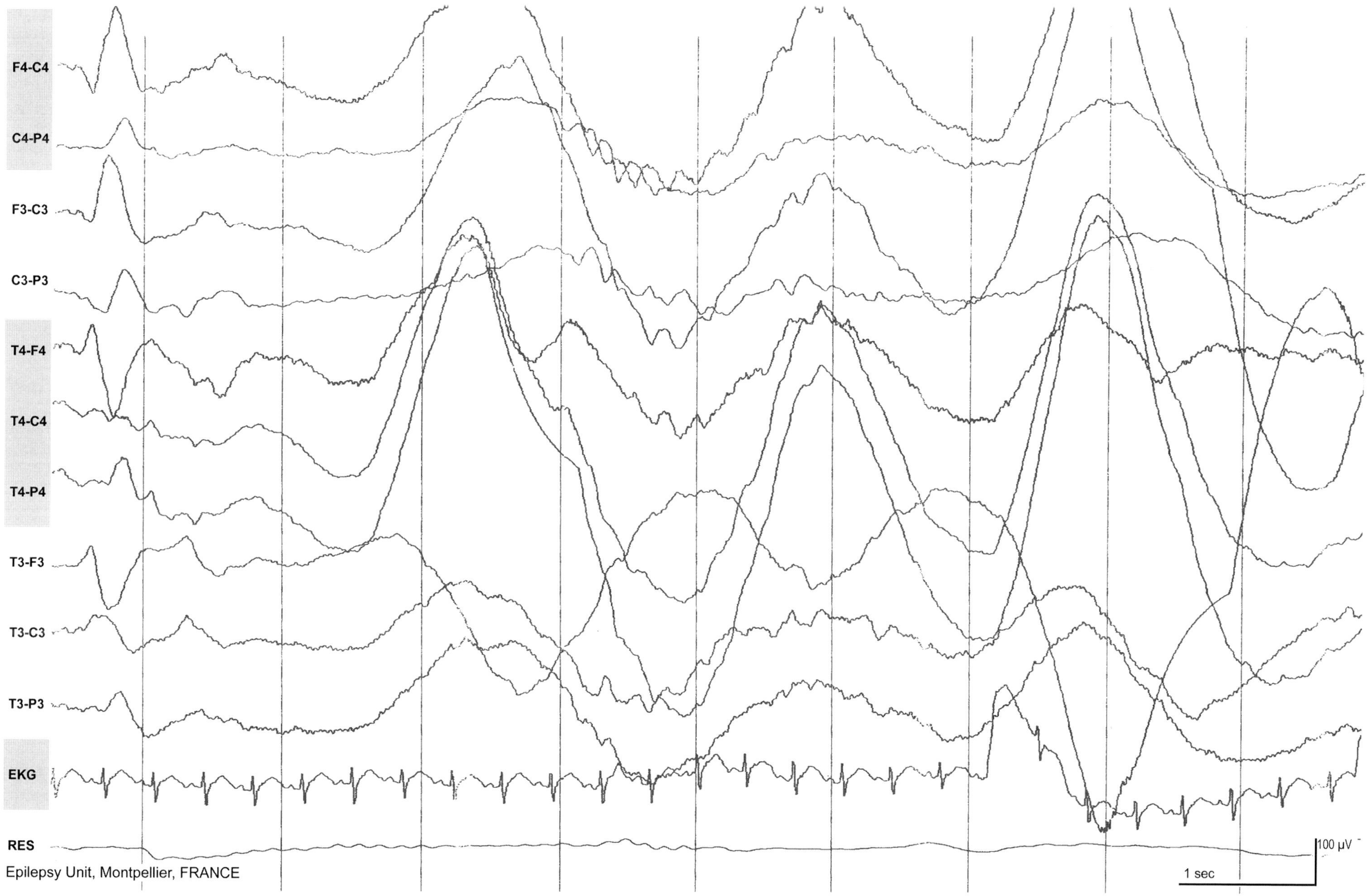
F4-C4
C4-P4
F3-C3
C3-P3
T4-F4
T4-C4
T4-P4
T3-F3
T3-C3
T3-P3
EKG
RES
Epilepsy Unit, Montpellier, FRANCE
100 µV
1 sec

IV • 2 ECG and electrodermogram artifacts

Context

45-year-old man with right mesio-temporal epilepsy, presurgical assessment.

What to note

The man is in non-REM sleep with a poor organization and sparse physiological sleep transients. Isolated low-voltage spikes over the two hemispheres which are time locked to the QRS complex of the ECG. At the 5th second, note the presence of three ventricular extrasystoles which create the false impression of a burst of sharp waves, clearly detectable at T6 and T5. Also note the presence of a fluctuation at T4-T6, T6-O2, Fp1-F3, F3-C3 corresponding to a perspiration artifact (electrodermogram).

What to do

Always check whether each ECG artifact is time locked to a QRS. To attenuate or eliminate these artifacts, check impedances, the ground electrode and put it on the right side of the patient. Also check whether the patient is leaning on the electrodes which express the ECG artifact.

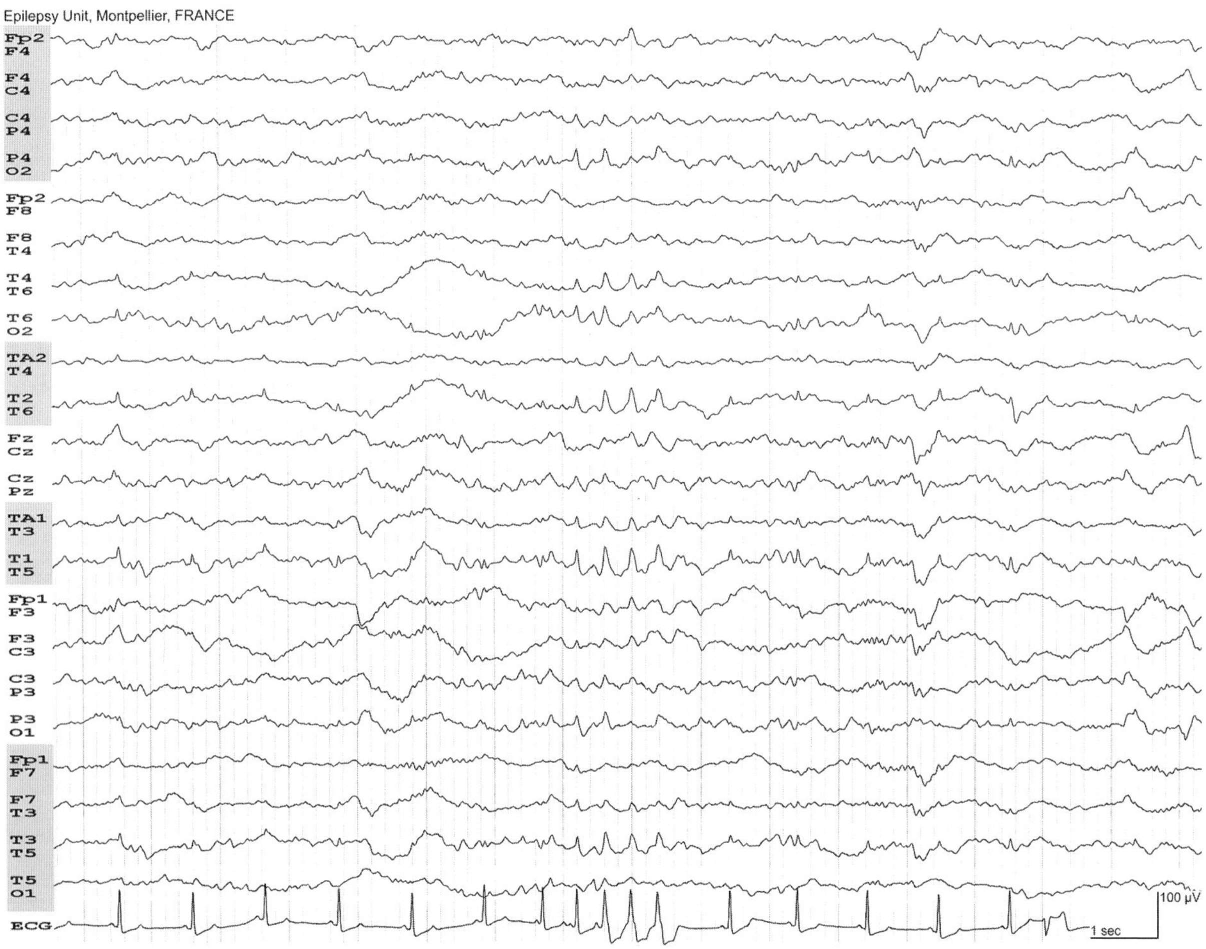

Figure a / Recording at 15 mm/s.

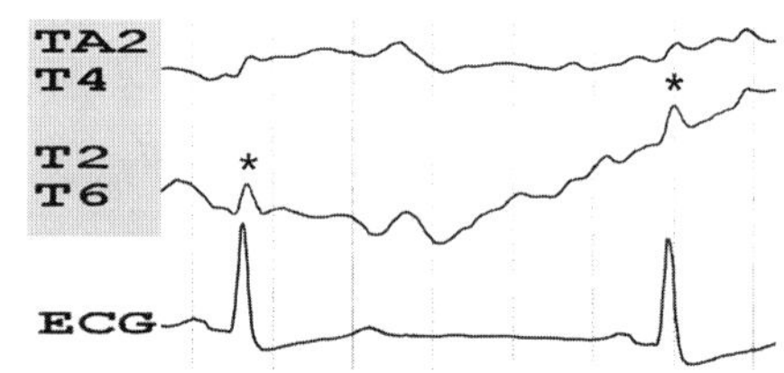

Figure b / Small sharp waves corresponding to an ECG artifact (*). Fluctuating tracings due to perspiration.

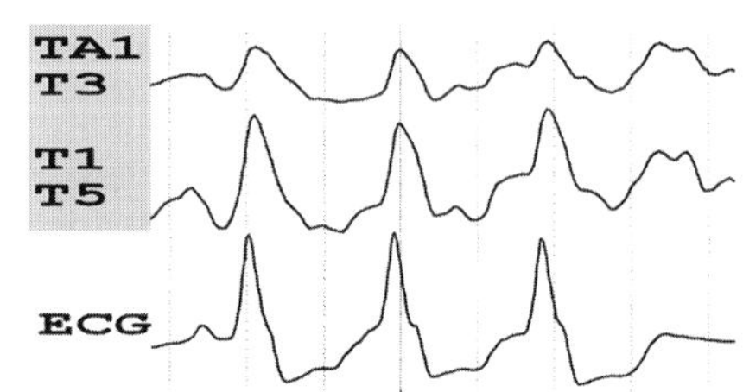

Figure c / Ventricular extrasystoles creating the false impression of a burst of sharp waves.

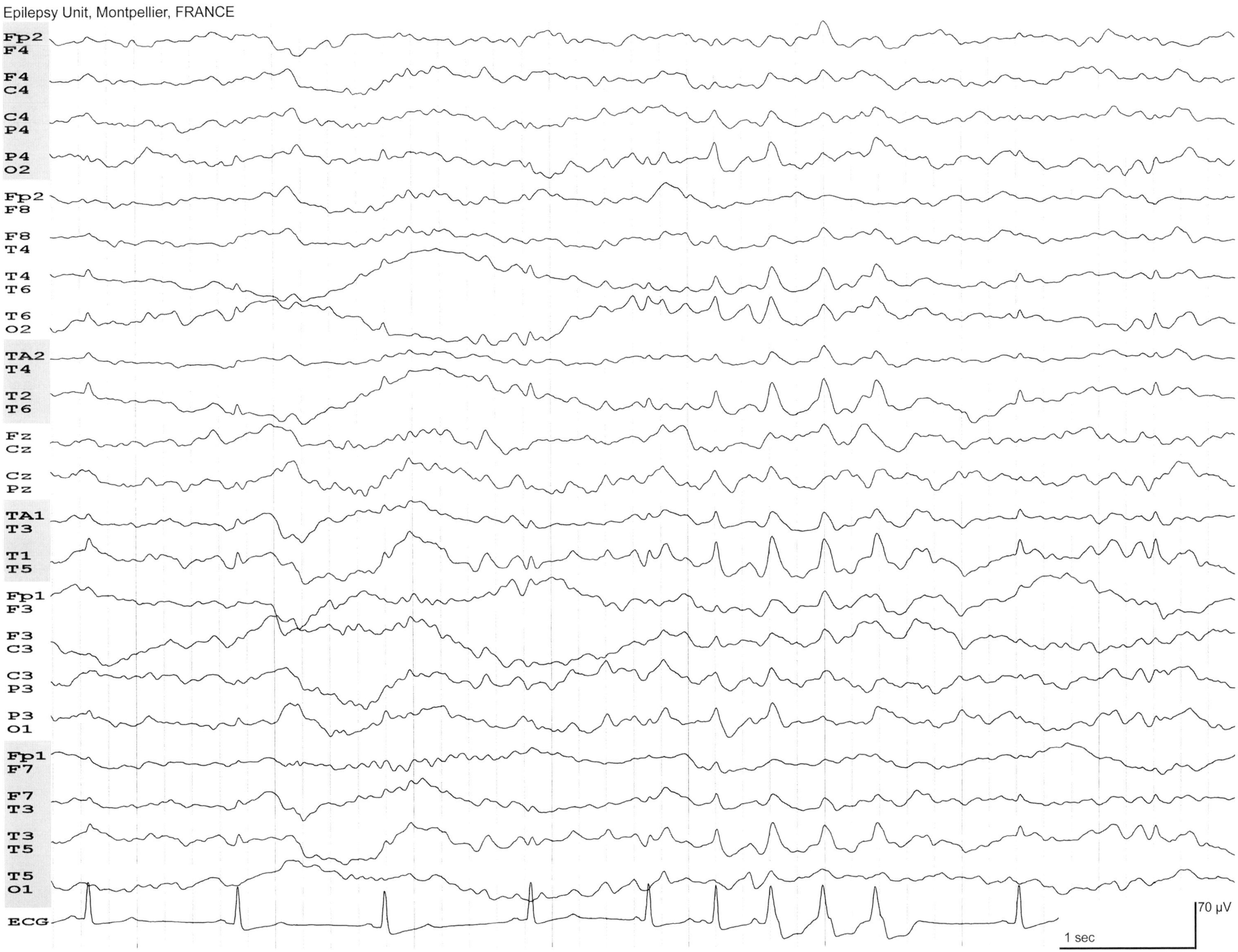
Epilepsy Unit, Montpellier, FRANCE
Fp2 F4
F4 C4
C4 P4
P4 O2
Fp2 F8
F8 T4
T4 T6
T6 O2
TA2 T4
T2 T6
Fz Cz
Cz Pz
TA1 T3
T1 T5
Fp1 F3
F3 C3
C3 P3
P3 O1
Fp1 F7
F7 T3
T3 T5
T5 O1
ECG
70 µV
1 sec

IV • 3 ECG artifacts

Context

49-year-old man with cryptogenic focal epilepsy.

What to note

REM sleep with low voltage activity. Isolated low-voltage spikes over the two hemispheres, which are time locked to the QRS complex of the ECG. This patient has numerous ventricular extrasystoles creating a false impression of diffuse and periodic sharp waves.

Comment

ECG artifacts are often seen in overweight individuals, in patients with a very-low-voltage tracing, and in REM sleep. It is usually observed over the left hemisphere. In brain death (absence of cerebral activity), only cardiac activity can be seen on the recording, so an ECG derivation is required in this case to provide evidence of its artifactual origin.

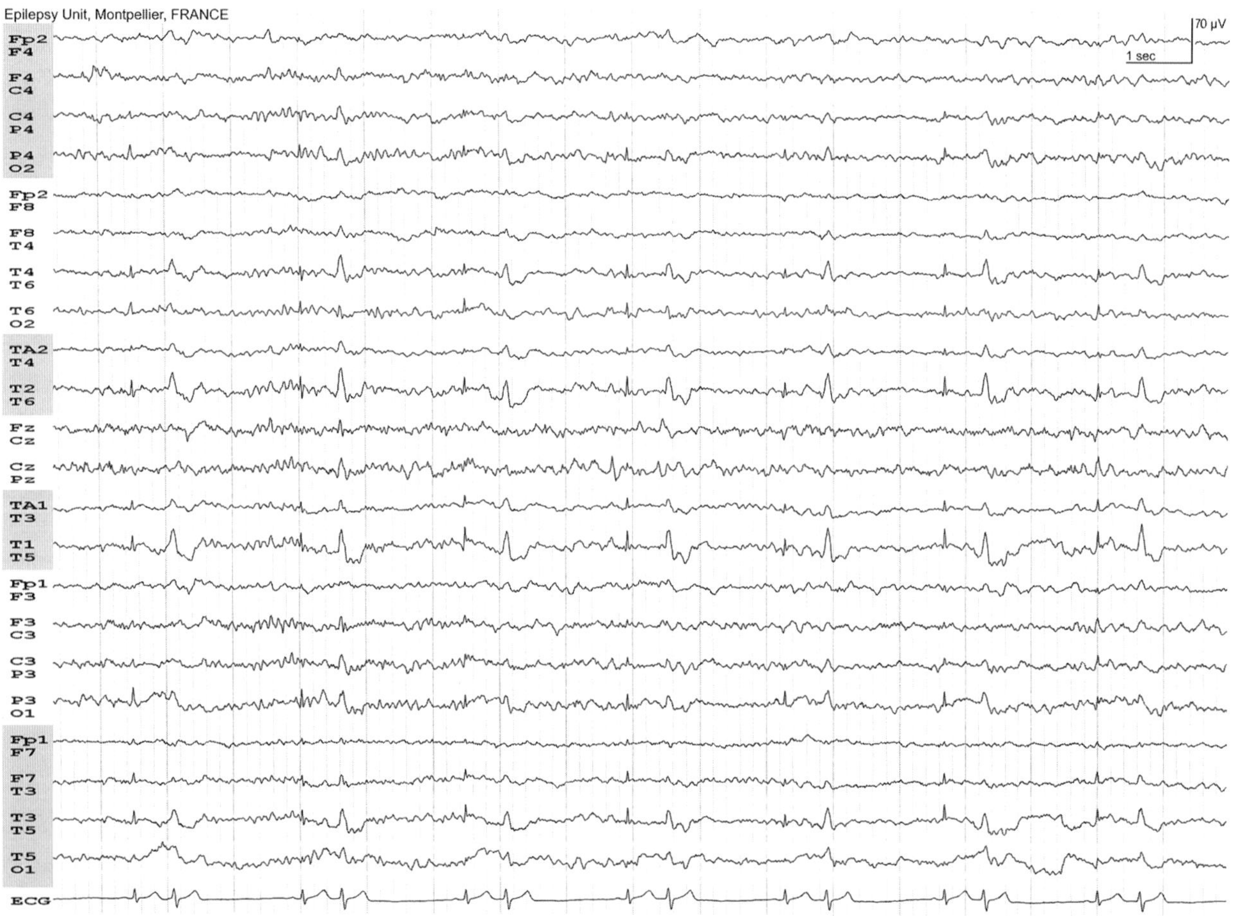

Figure a / Recording at 15 mm/s.

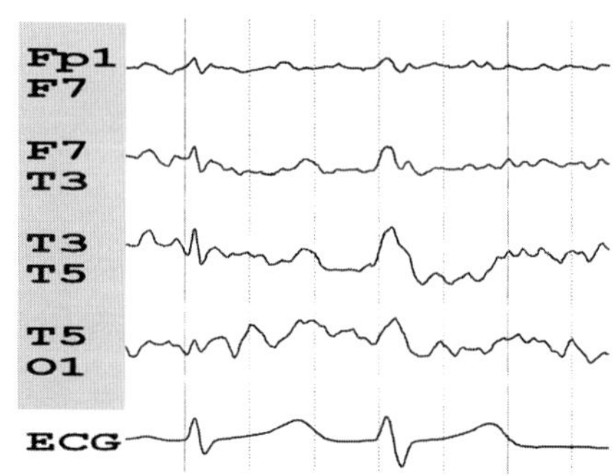

Figure b / A small spike (ECG artifact) followed by a sharp wave (extrasystole).

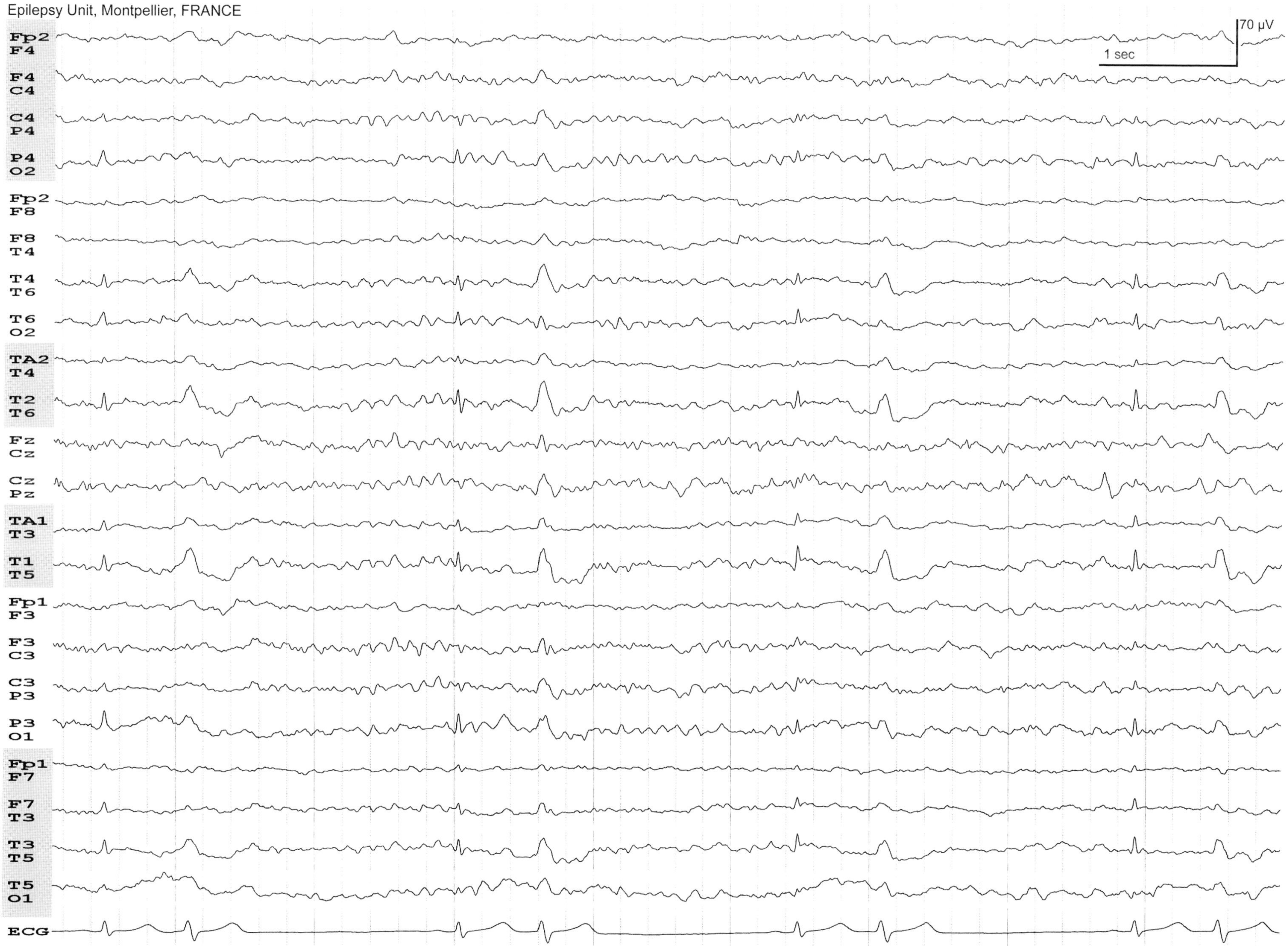
Epilepsy Unit, Montpellier, FRANCE
70 µV
1 sec
Fp2 F4
F4 C4
C4 P4
P4 O2
Fp2 F8
F8 T4
T4 T6
T6 O2
TA2 T4
T2 T6
Fz Cz
Cz Pz
TA1 T3
T1 T5
Fp1 F3
F3 C3
C3 P3
P3 O1
Fp1 F7
F7 T3
T3 T5
T5 O1
ECG

IV • 4 Pulse artifact in a child

Context

6-year-old child referred for a first generalized tonic-clonic seizure.

What to note

The pulse artifact under F4 is in phase with the ECG (sinusal tachycardia at 135/min). Furthermore, the pulse artifact preceded by an ECG artifact can be seen at Fp1-F7 (small spikes) and, to a lesser extent, at Fp2-F8. ECG artifacts correspond to direct recording of cardiac contractions. Hence, the ECG artifact is time locked with the QRS (very-low-voltage spikes).

What to do

To avoid pulse artifact, the electrode must be reapplied so that it is no longer placed over superficial arteries.

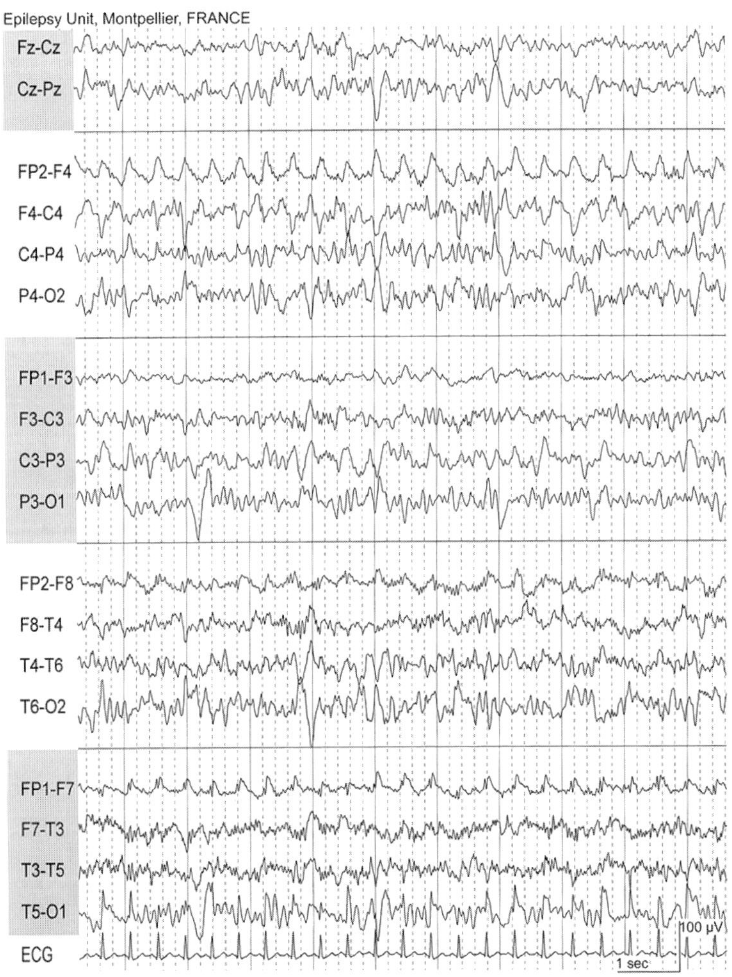

Figure a / Recording at 15 mm/s.

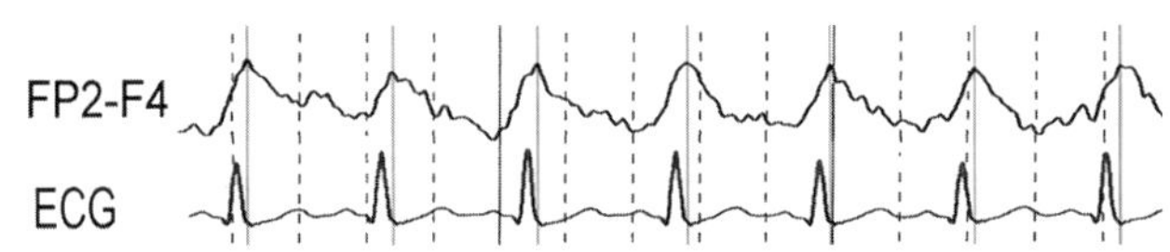

Figure b / Pulse artifact at F4 (grey lines). Note the periodicity, the peak at F4 follows the QRS complex.

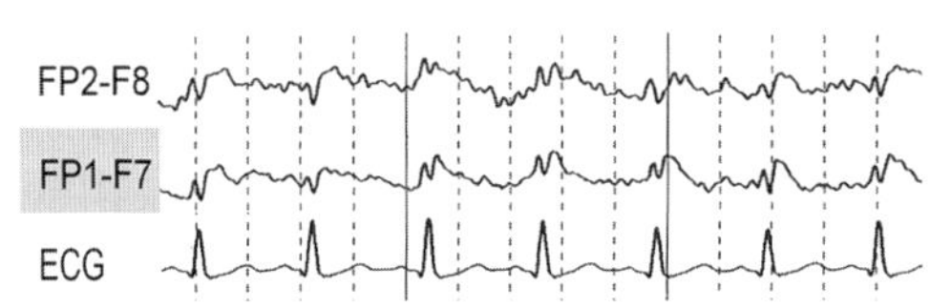

Figure c / QRS artifact at Fp1-F7 and to a lesser extent at Fp2-F8.

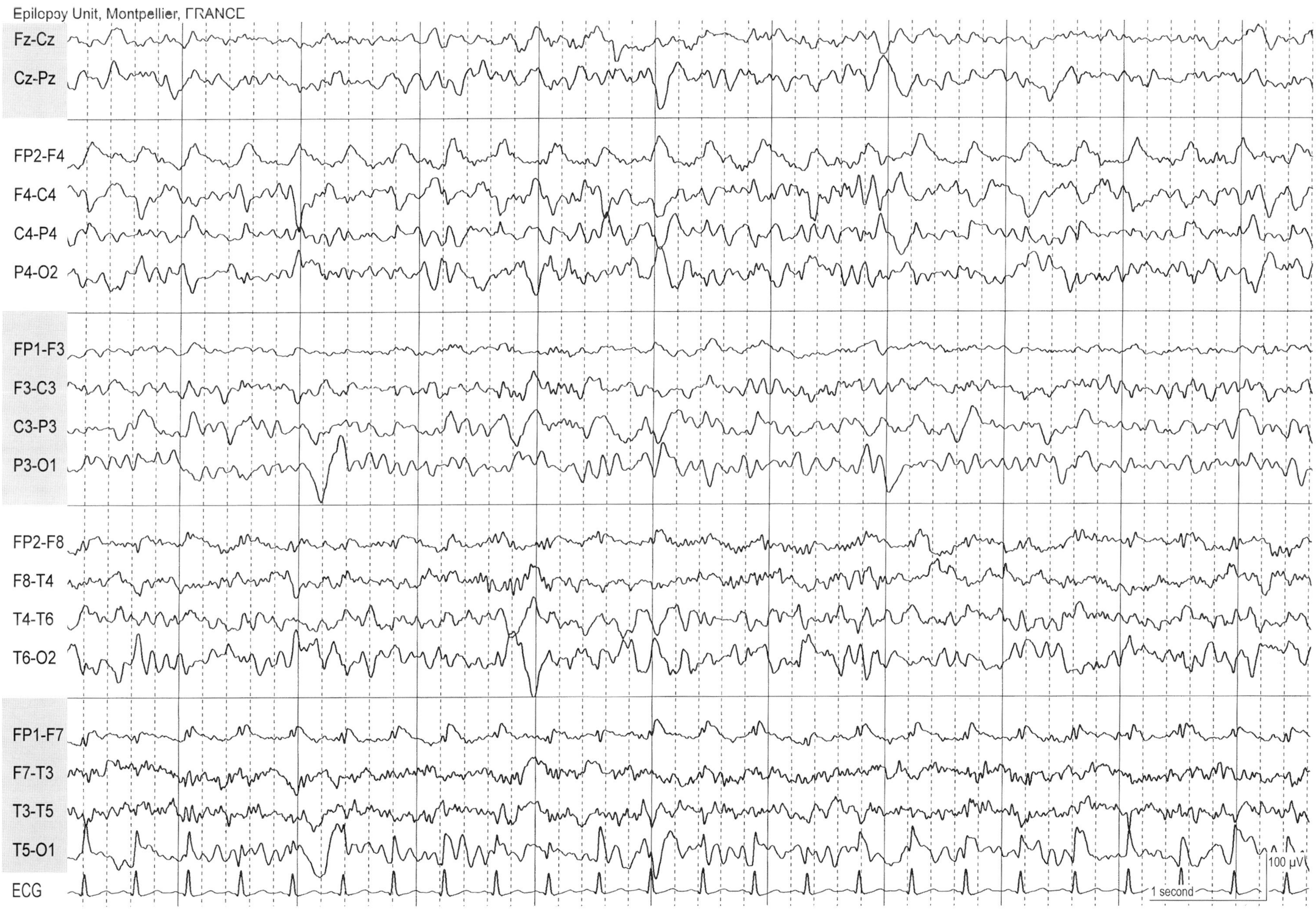
Epilepsy Unit, Montpellier, FRANCE
Fz-Cz
Cz-Pz
FP2-F4
F4-C4
C4-P4
P4-O2
FP1-F3
F3-C3
C3-P3
P3-O1
FP2-F8
F8-T4
T4-T6
T6-O2
FP1-F7
F7-T3
T3-T5
T5-O1
ECG
100 µV
1 second

IV • 5 Pulse artifact in an adult (1)

Context

21-year-old man with left medial temporal lobe epilepsy, presurgical assessment.

What to note

Stage N2 sleep with sleep spindles. The periodic fluctuating activity under F8 corresponds to a pulse artifact at the same frequency as the ECG rhythm due to contact of the F8 electrode with an artery. The activity recorded corresponds to a pulse. The peak of each waveform and the QRS complex are not time locked (transmission of the systolic contractions). Note the electrode artifact at T5 due to poor impedance and an ECG artifact at T3.

Comment

Pulses are commonly recorded in patients with hypertension, in bald patients, and in EEGs immediately following head trauma.

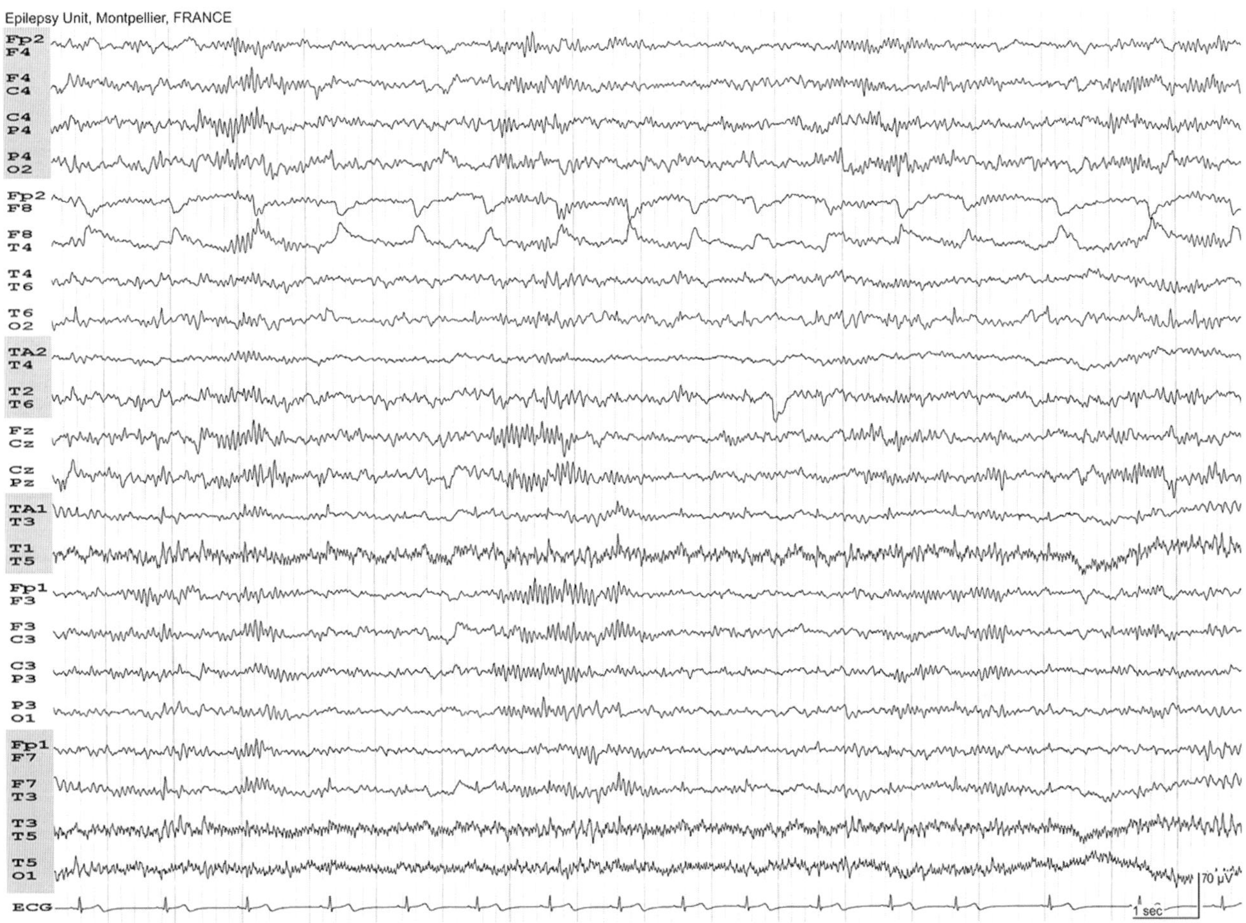

Figure a / Recording at 15 mm/s.

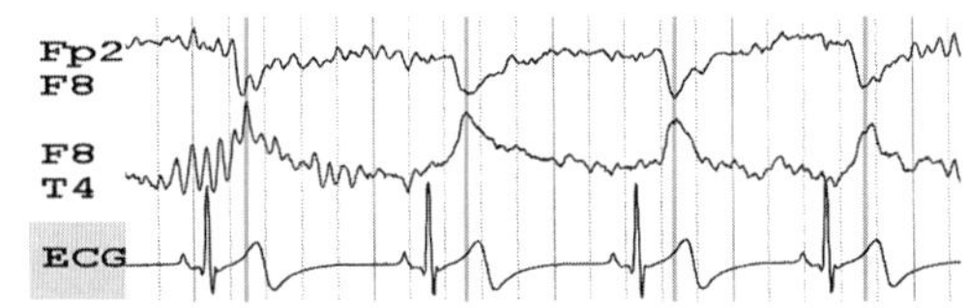

Figure b / Recording at 15 mm/s.
Pulse artifact (grey lines) at F8.
Note the periodicity, the peak at F8 follows the QRS complex.

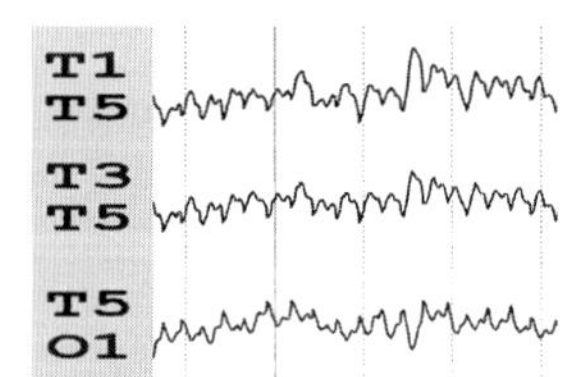

Figure c / Electrode artifact at T5.

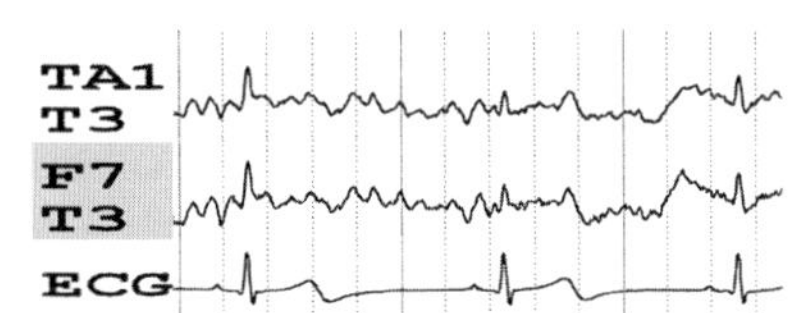

Figure d / Recording at 15 mm/s.
ECG artifact at T3.

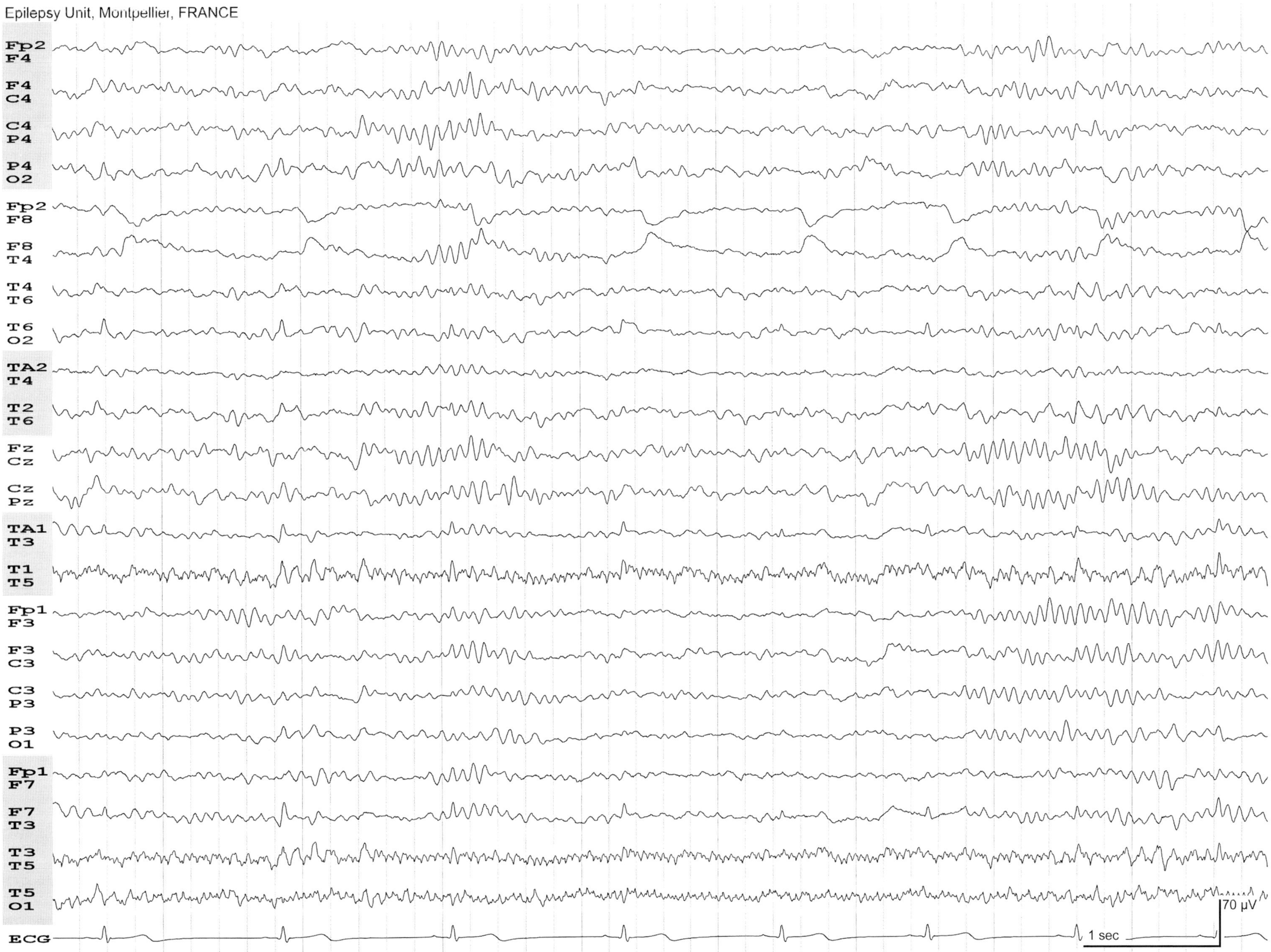
Epilepsy Unit, Montpellier, FRANCE
Fp2 F4
F4 C4
C4 P4
P4 O2
Fp2 F8
F8 T4
T4 T6
T6 O2
TA2 T4
T2 T6
Fz Cz
Cz Pz
TA1 T3
T1 T5
Fp1 F3
F3 C3
C3 P3
P3 O1
Fp1 F7
F7 T3
T3 T5
T5 O1
ECG
70 µV
1 sec

IV • 6 Pulse artifact in an adult (2)

Context

30-year-old man with cryptogenic frontal lobe epilepsy.

What to note

The patient's eyes are closed. Low-amplitude alpha background activity with superimposed abundant rapid pharmacological rhythms (benzodiazepines and barbiturates) over the anterior regions. Slow activity can be seen at C3-P3 and at P3-O1 with periodical sharp waves in phase reversal at P3. This corresponds to a pulse artifact. This activity is confined to a single electrode, P3, and it is time locked with the ECG. Had there been a slow focus or some epileptiform activity, there would have been some spread to adjoining electrodes. When confronted with this type of activity, the technologist must always try to correct the electrode placement (see below plate recording at 15 mm/s).

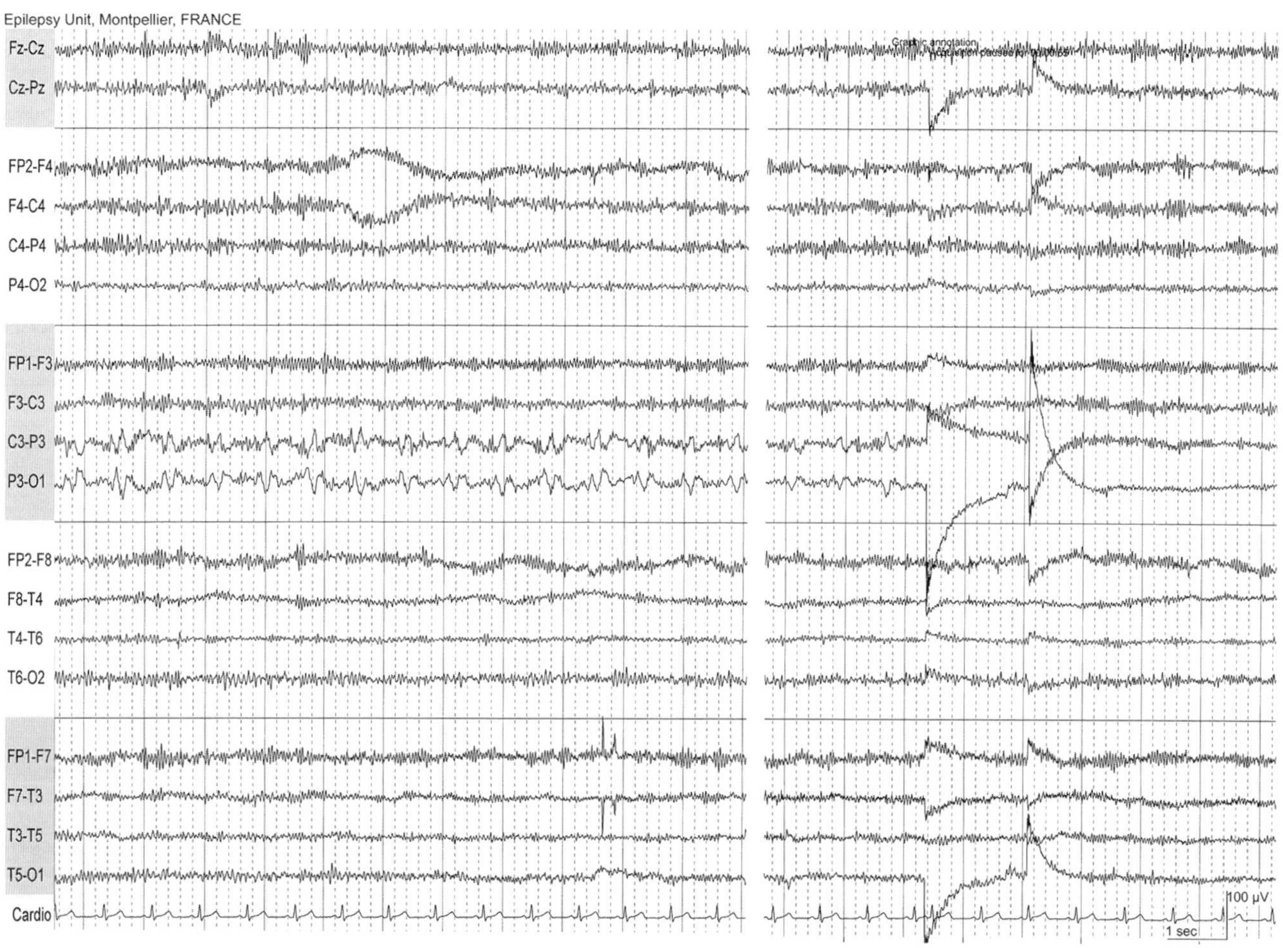

Figure a / Recording at 15 mm/s. On the right, the electrode artifact is still present at P3 during the first two seconds, but it ceases as soon as the electrode lead is reapplied. Note the "pop" electrode artifact during electrode readjustment.

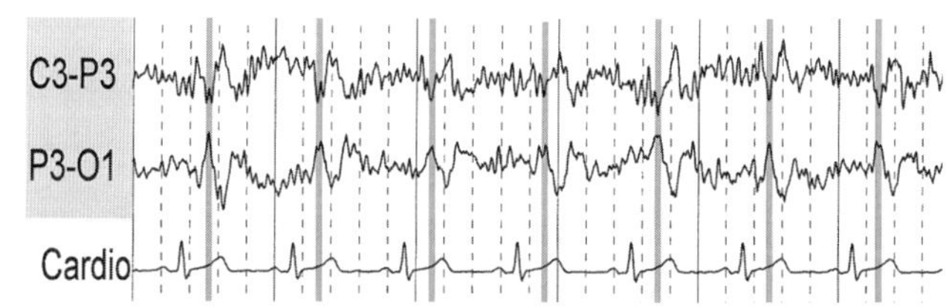

Figure b / Recording at 15 mm/s. Periodical activity at P3 (grey lines). Note the periodicity, the peak at P3 follows the QRS complex.

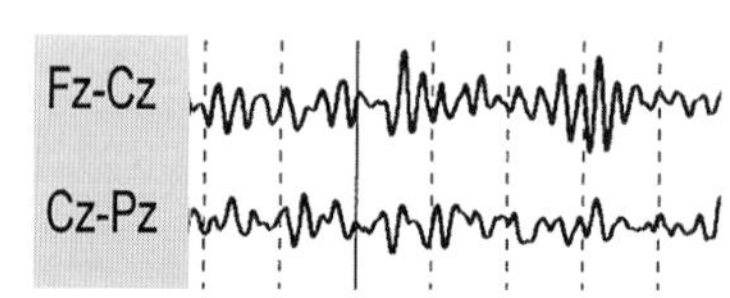

Figure c / Pharmacological beta rhythm.

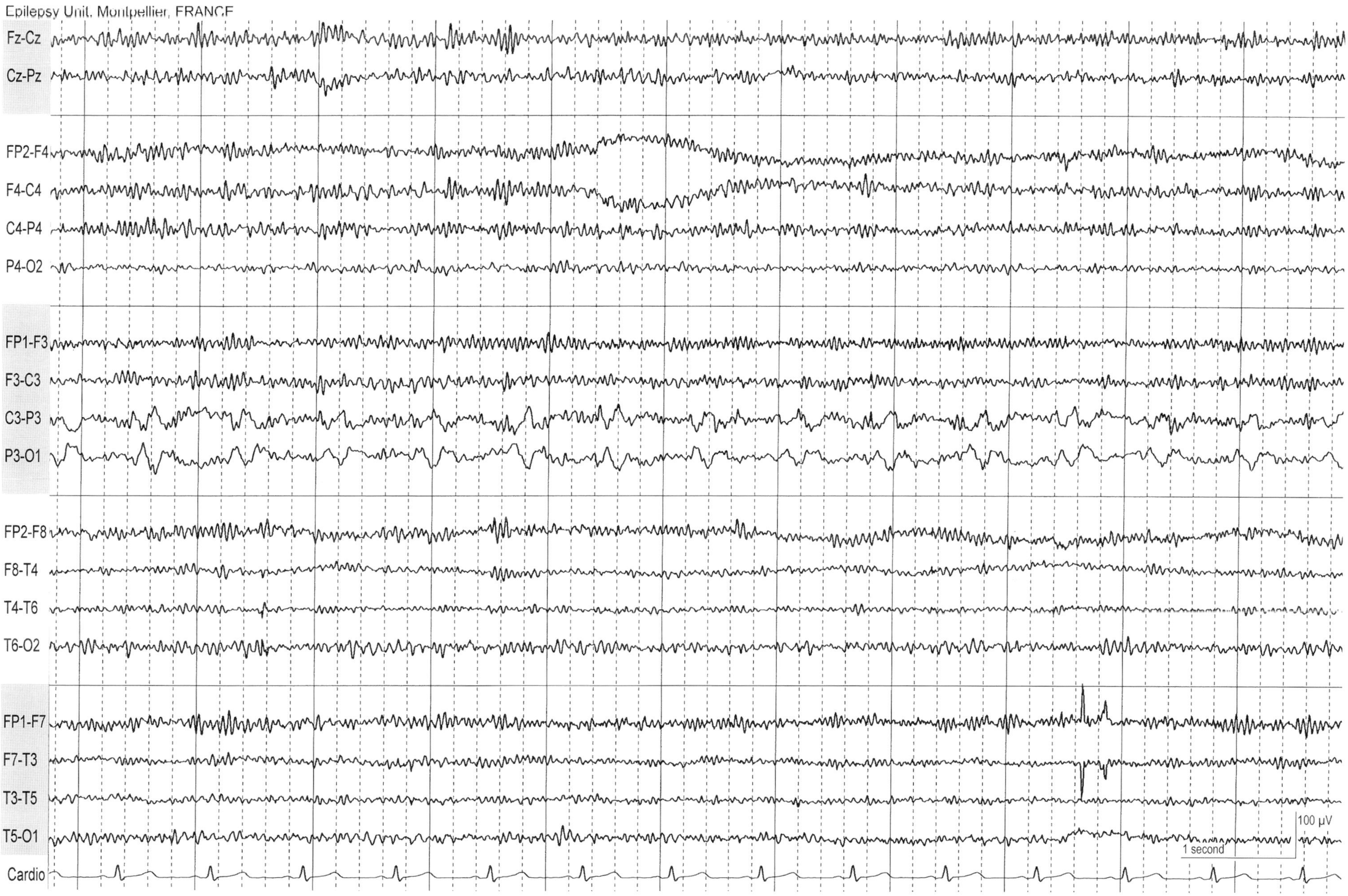
Epilepsy Unit, Montpellier, FRANCE
Fz-Cz
Cz-Pz
FP2-F4
F4-C4
C4-P4
P4-O2
FP1-F3
F3-C3
C3-P3
P3-O1
FP2-F8
F8-T4
T4-T6
T6-O2
FP1-F7
F7-T3
T3-T5
T5-O1
Cardio
100 µV
1 second

IV • 7 Eye flutter artifact

Context

46-year-old woman seen after a faint.

What to note

The woman is very anxious about her EEG. The rhythmic activity at a frequency of 7 Hz on the frontal polar derivations ceases when she is asked to open her eyes and stare at a point. At the end of the plate, an eye opening artifact with upward eyelid blinking can be seen, the patient stares at a point and keeps her eyes open for 3 seconds, then closes them again (downward eyelid blinking artifact) (see below plate recorded at 15 mm/s). During these 3 seconds, the eyelid flutter artifact disappears. Compared to typical eyelid blinking, flutter artifact has a lower amplitude. At the right and left temporal derivations, the rapid low-amplitude activity corresponding to muscle activity is filtered at 35 Hz. This clenched jaws activity also produces muscle activity recorded at the occipital electrodes.

What to do

Reassure patients about their EEG in order to relieve their anxiety and help them relax. Ask them to unclench their jaws and keep their mouth slightly open. Hyperventilation can also help patients relax.

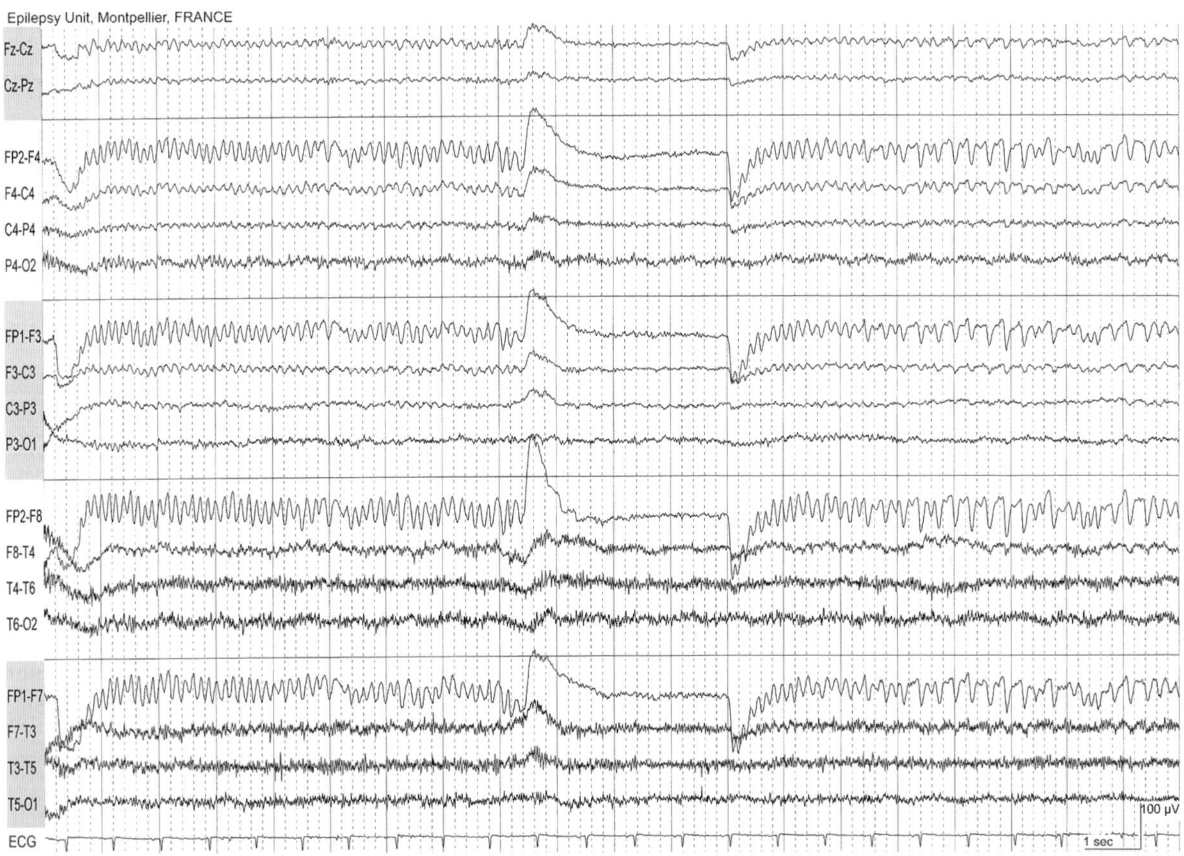

Figure a / Recording at 15 mm/s. Upon closure of eyes, continuous blinking of the woman's eyelids starts again but the artifacts are not as fast or ample.

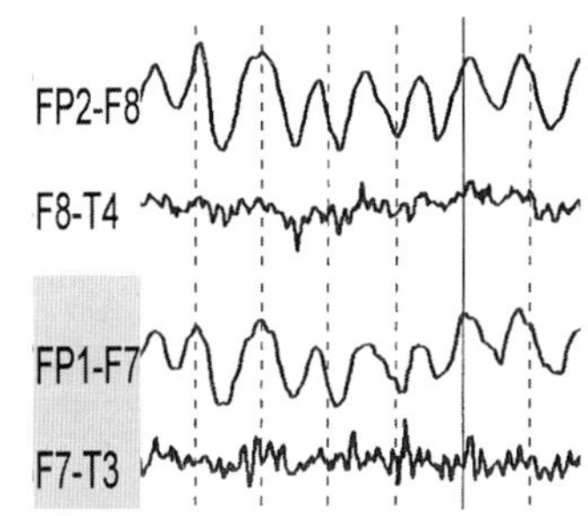

Figure b / Very rapid eyelid blinking (flutter).

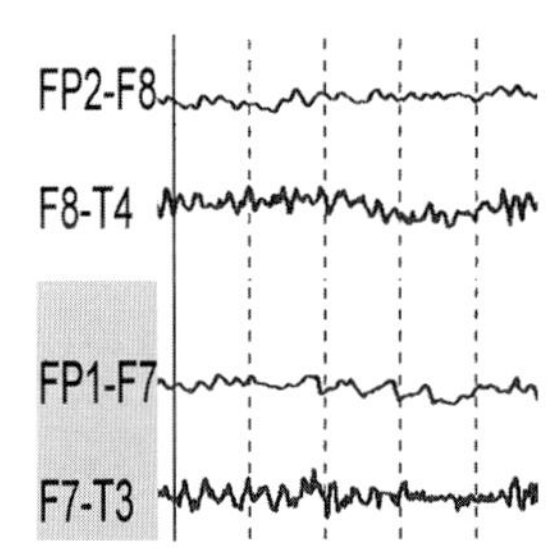

Figure c / Offset of eyelid blinking. Muscle activity at temporal derivations.

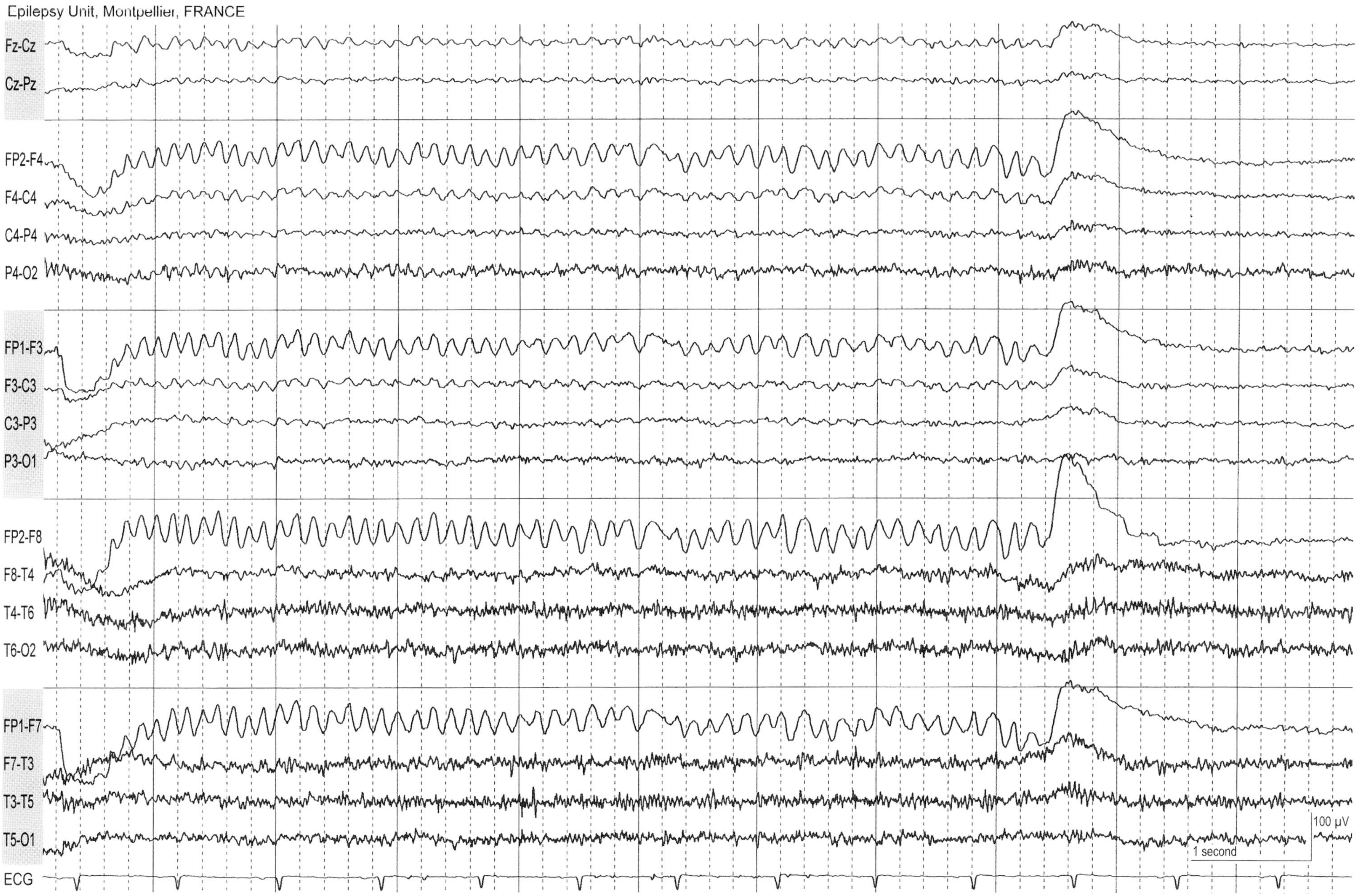
Epilepsy Unit, Montpellier, FRANCE
Fz-Cz
Cz-Pz
FP2-F4
F4-C4
C4-P4
P4-O2
FP1-F3
F3-C3
C3-P3
P3-O1
FP2-F8
F8-T4
T4-T6
T6-O2
FP1-F7
F7-T3
T3-T5
T5-O1
ECG
100 µV
1 second

IV • 8 Eye movements in a child

Context

8-year-old boy referred for cryptogenic focal epilepsy.

What to note

Awake, eyes closed. Posterior alpha at 9 Hz mixed with slower theta waves. At the frontal polar derivations, irregular rhythmic waves at a frequency of 3-4 Hz with spreading over the adjacent regions. This activity corresponds to rather rapid eye movements. In the last 3 seconds of the plate, when the child spontaneously interrupts eye movements, these rhythmic slow waves disappear. Also note the presence over the right parietal regions (P4 and Pz) of very fine interictal spike-waves. These very spike-waves are not artifactual because they involve several electrodes and the same morphology can be seen at all the concerned electrodes. Mild sinusal cardiac arrhythmia.

What to do

Ask the patient to keep his eyes still and to imagine he is staring at a point. In presence of rhythmic activity over the anterior regions, put hands gently over the eyes whenever in doubt so as to interrupt the eye movements and provide evidence that it is artifactual.

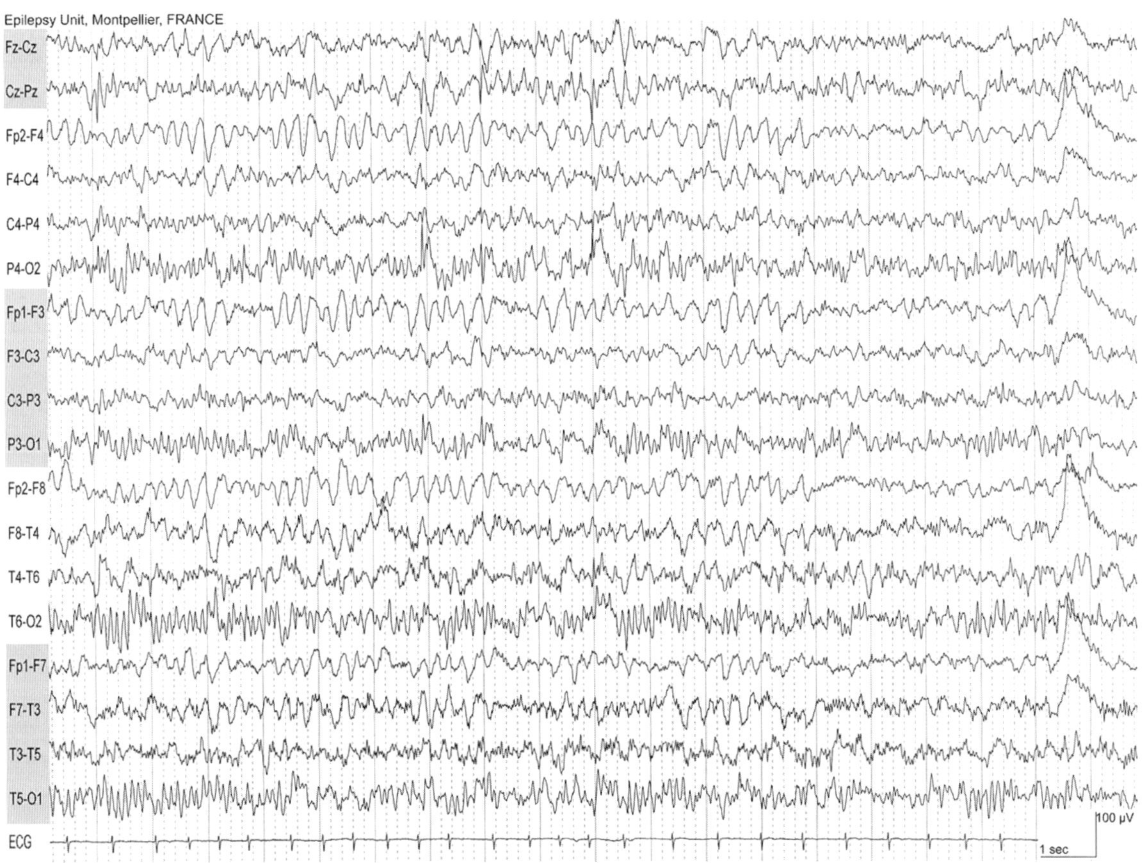

Figure a / Recording at 15 mm/s.

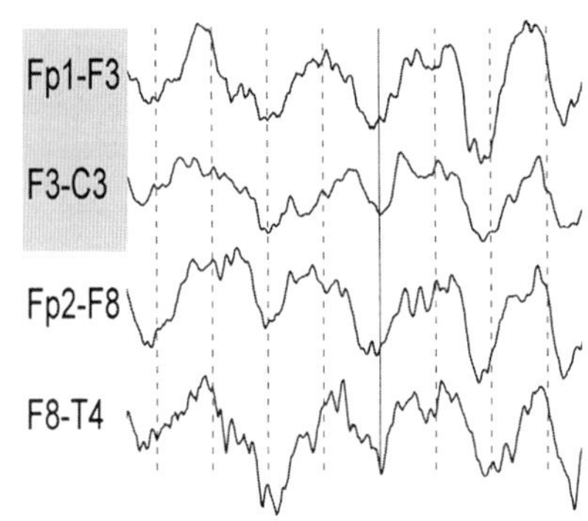

Figure b / Rhythmic activity at the frontal polar derivations (eye movements).

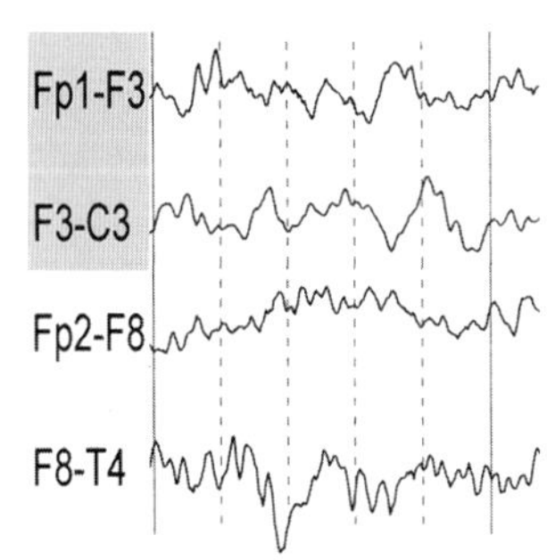

Figure c / Spontaneous offset of the delta activity.

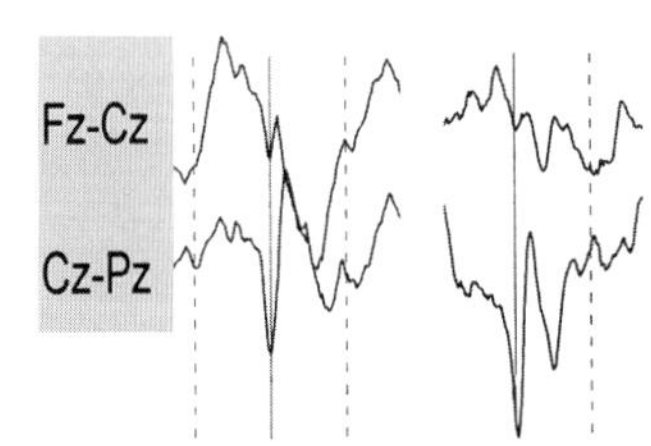

Figure d / Spike-waves.

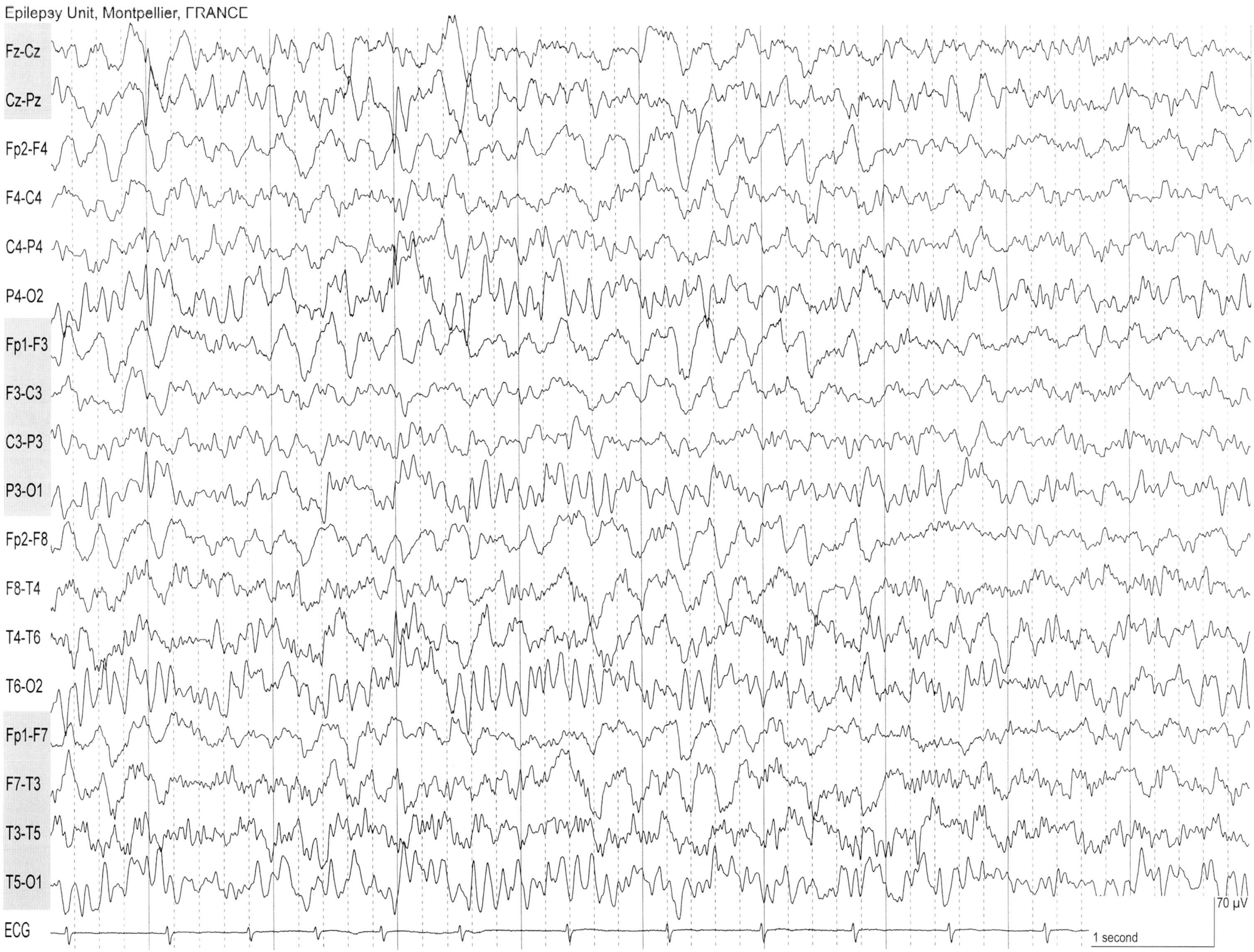
Epilepsy Unit, Montpellier, FRANCE
Fz-Cz
Cz-Pz
Fp2-F4
F4-C4
C4-P4
P4-O2
Fp1-F3
F3-C3
C3-P3
P3-O1
Fp2-F8
F8-T4
T4-T6
T6-O2
Fp1-F7
F7-T3
T3-T5
T5-O1
ECG
70 µV
1 second

IV • 9 Eye movements in an adult, a "pop" electrode artifact

Context

37-year-old man seen after a faint.

What to note

Eyes closed, posterior alpha at 11 Hz. At the frontal polar derivations, rhythmic activity at 2-3 Hz which ceases as soon as the eye movements are stopped. At the 5th second, a "pop" electrode artifact at Cz, corresponding to faulty contact between the electrode and the wire, then a similar but more ample artifact at P4 one second later. At P4-O2 and T6-O2, the lines move when the head moves.

What to do

Put hands gently over the eyes whenever in doubt so as to interrupt eye movements. Check for poorly attached electrodes.

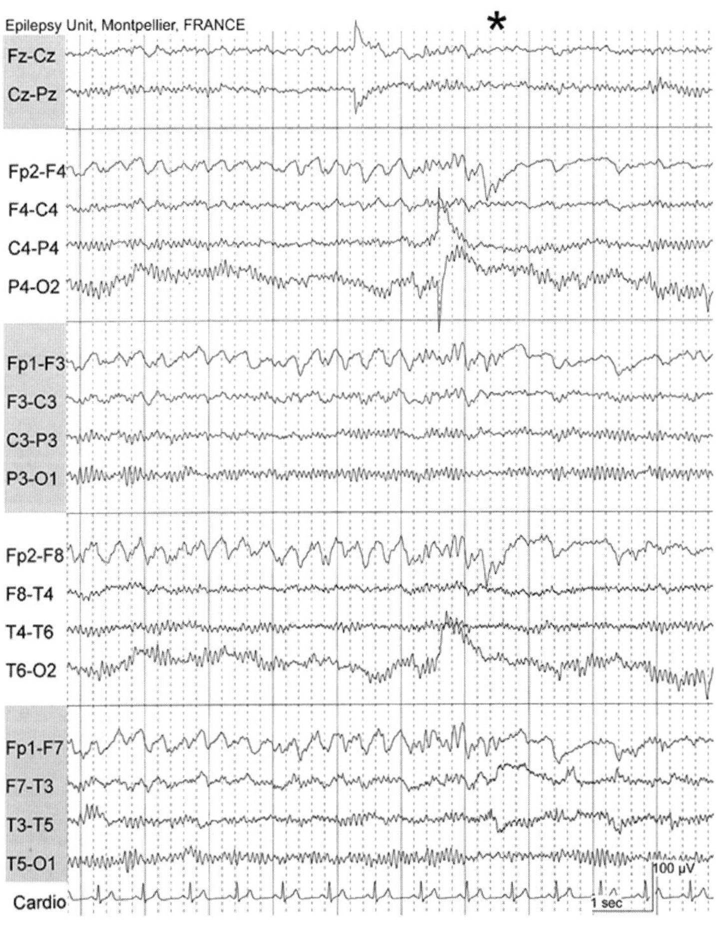

Figure a / Recording at 15 mm/s.

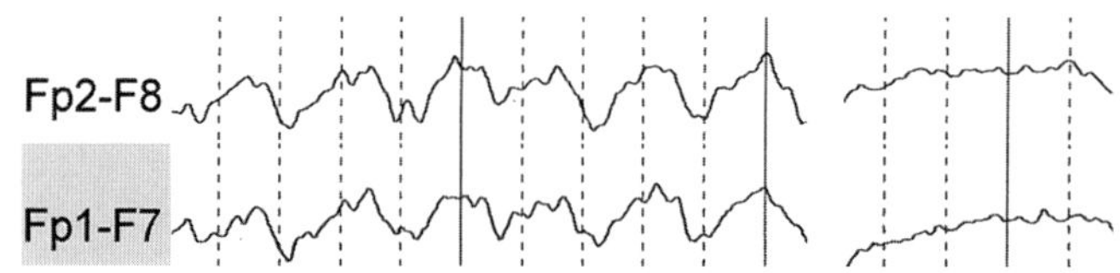

Figure b / Eye movements at the frontal polar derivations, which cease when eyes are held still.

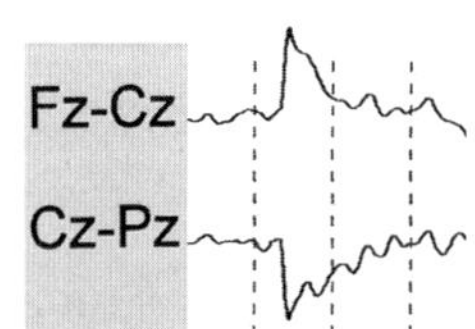

Figure c / "Pop" electrode artifacts at Cz.

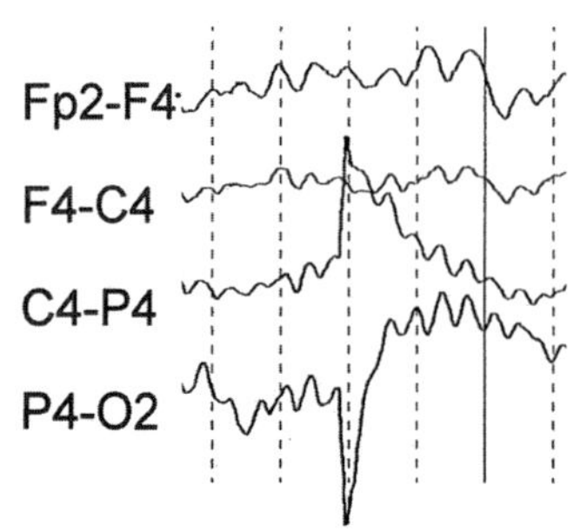

Figure d / "Pop" electrode artifacts at P4.

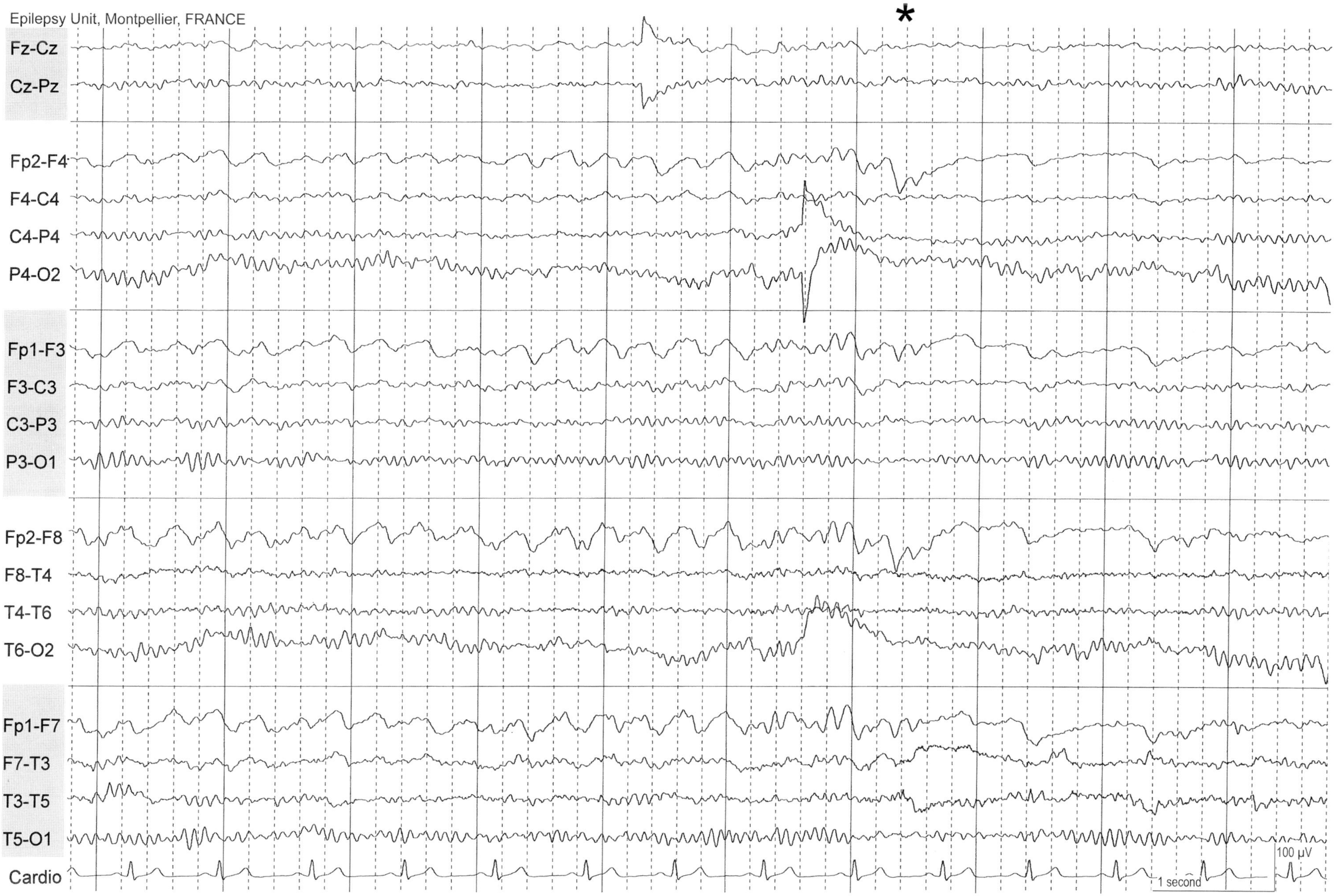
Epilepsy Unit, Montpellier, FRANCE
*
Fz-Cz
Cz-Pz
Fp2-F4
F4-C4
C4-P4
P4-O2
Fp1-F3
F3-C3
C3-P3
P3-O1
Fp2-F8
F8-T4
T4-T6
T6-O2
Fp1-F7
F7-T3
T3-T5
T5-O1
Cardio
100 µV
1 second

IV • 10 Saccadic eye movements and lateral rectus spike

Context

26-year-old woman with idiopathic generalized epilepsy.

What to note

The patient is awake, eyes open. At the anterior temporal and frontal polar derivations, the EEG signal has a square-shaped morphology. The patient has rapid lateral eye movements. There are also fast potentials over the frontal anterior regions (phase reversal at F7 and F8) corresponding to contraction of the lateral rectus muscle. This muscle artifact is termed a lateral rectus spike. Note the presence of lambda waves on the occipital regions.

What to do

Ask the patient to keep his eyes still, tell him to imagine he is staring at a point.

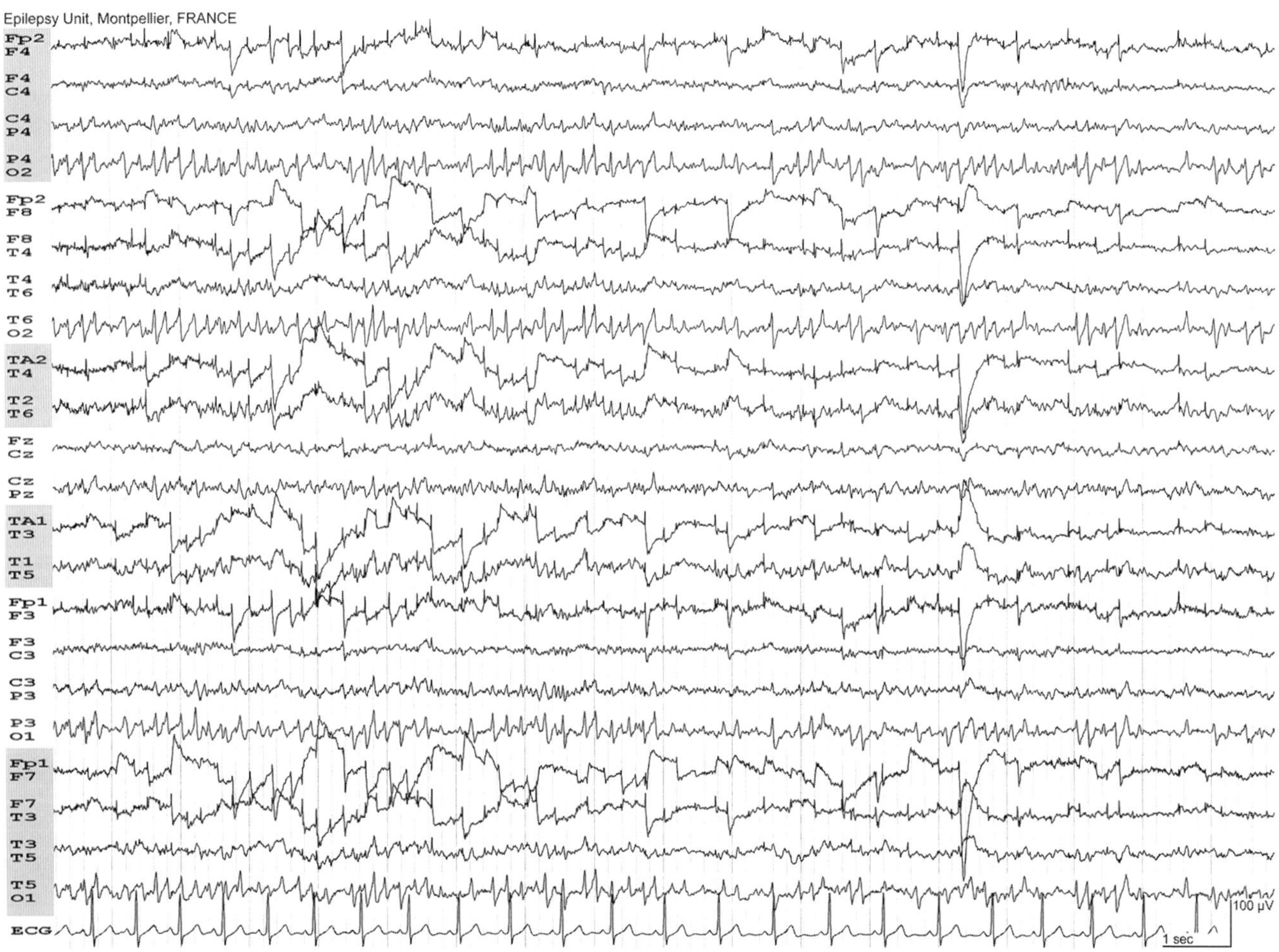

Figure a / Recording at 15 mm/s.

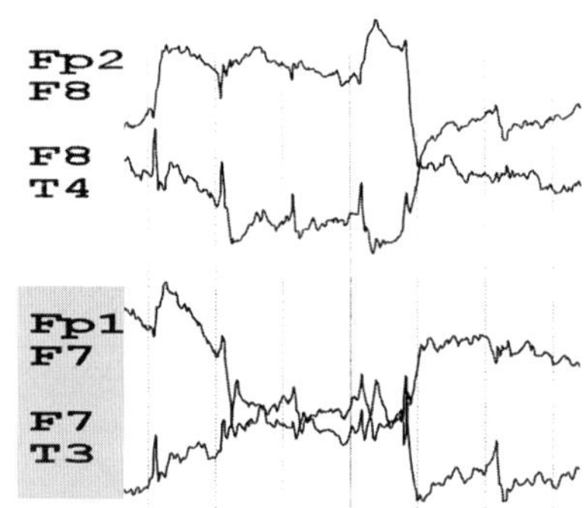

Figure b / Saccadic eye movements and lateral rectus spike.

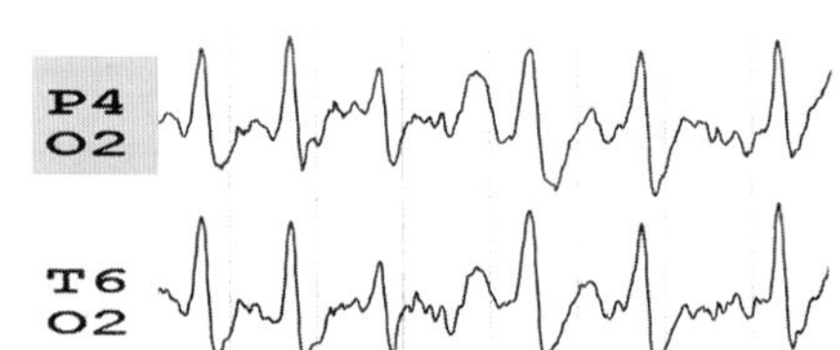

Figure c / Lambda waves.

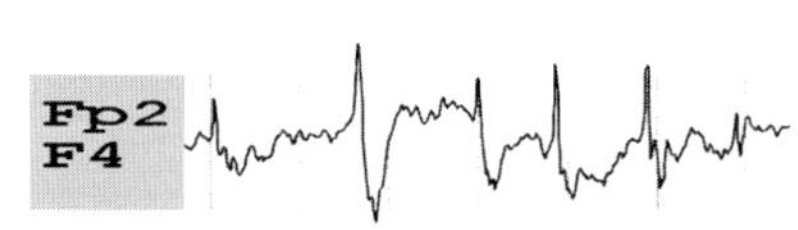

Figure d / Lateral rectus spike.

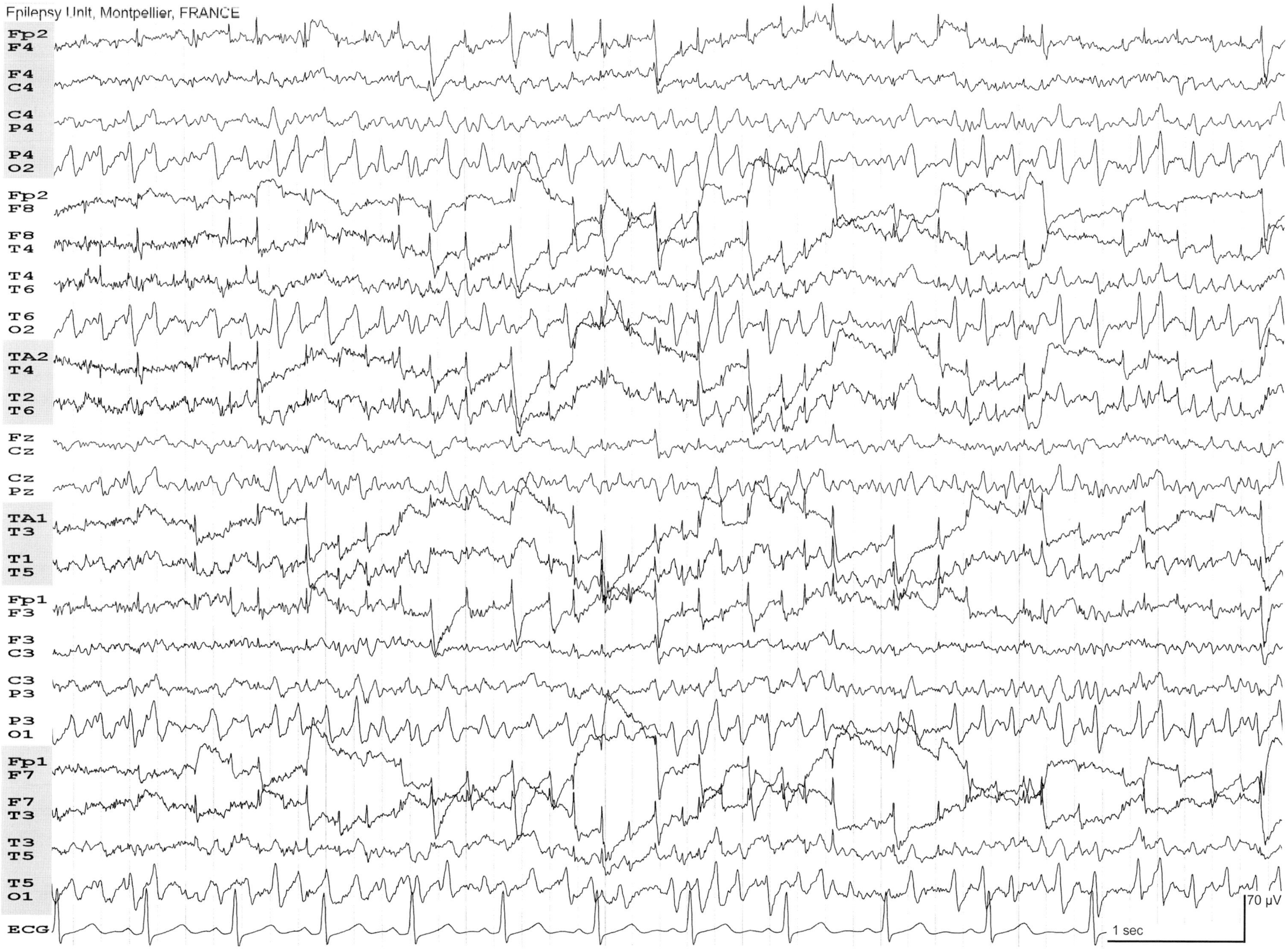
Epilepsy Unit, Montpellier, FRANCE
Fp2 F4
F4 C4
C4 P4
P4 O2
Fp2 F8
F8 T4
T4 T6
T6 O2
TA2 T4
T2 T6
Fz Cz
Cz Pz
TA1 T3
T1 T5
Fp1 F3
F3 C3
C3 P3
P3 O1
Fp1 F7
F7 T3
T3 T5
T5 O1
ECG
70 µV
1 sec

IV • 11 Asymmetric saccadic eye movements and eyelid artifacts, muscular activity

Context

54-year-old man with focal epilepsy.

What to note

The patient's eyes are open. Asymmetric eyelid movement artifacts and also some saccadic eye movements over the right hemisphere (patient had a left enucleation and prosthetic eye replacement). Muscular activity on the left temporal region (contraction of the left masseter).

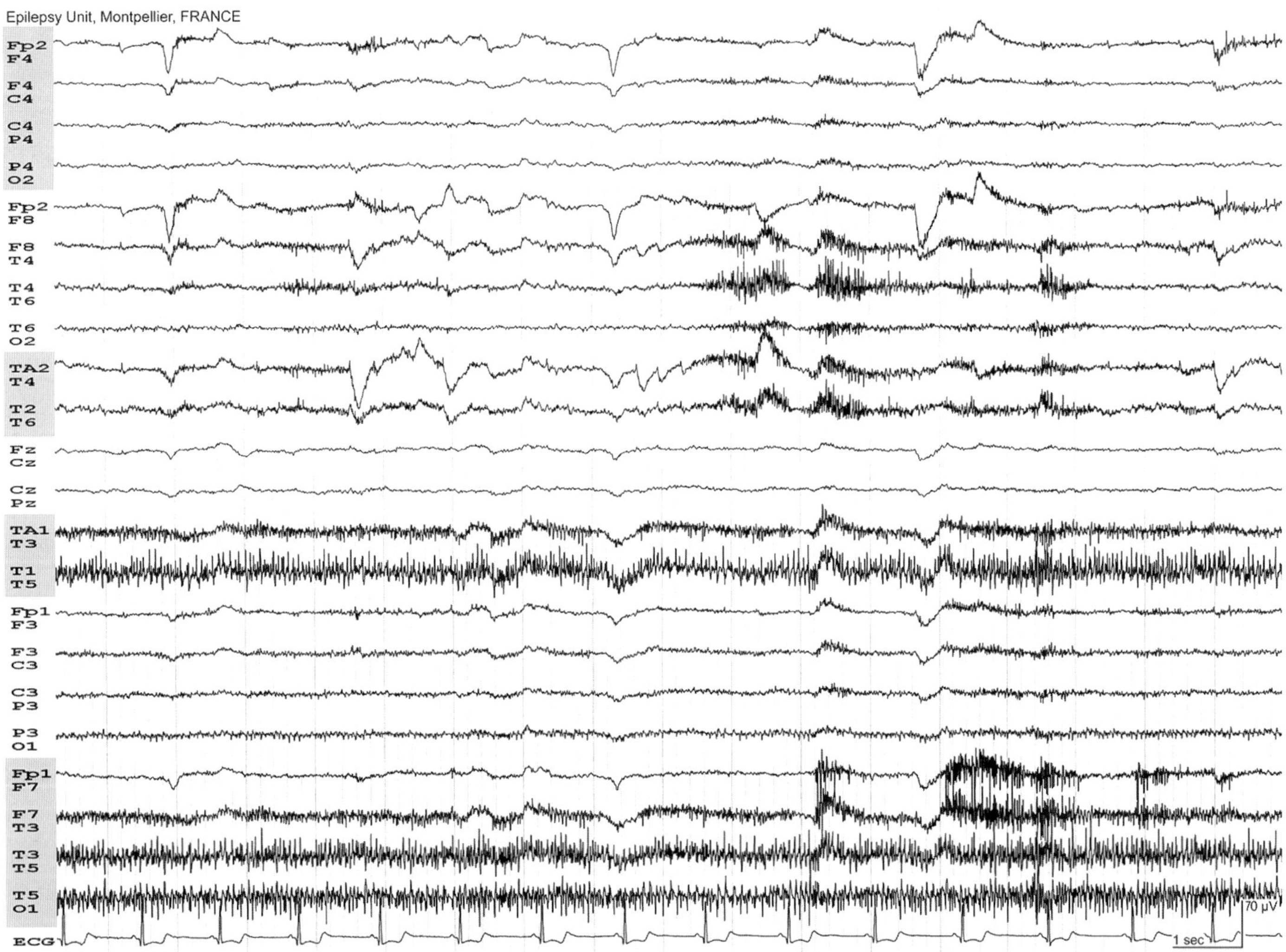

Figure a / Recording at 15 mm/s.

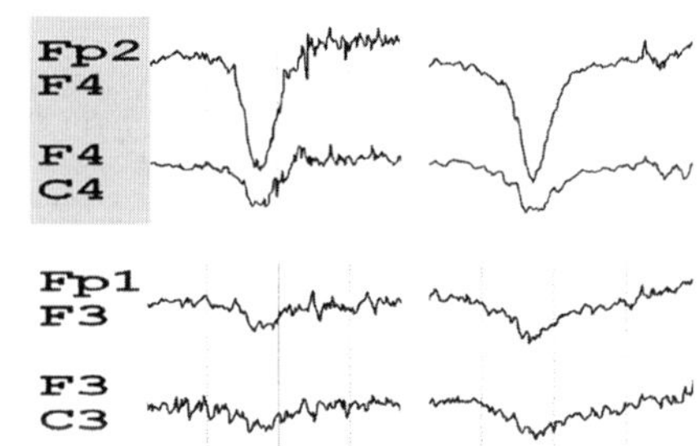

Figure b / Asymmetric eyelid movement artifact.

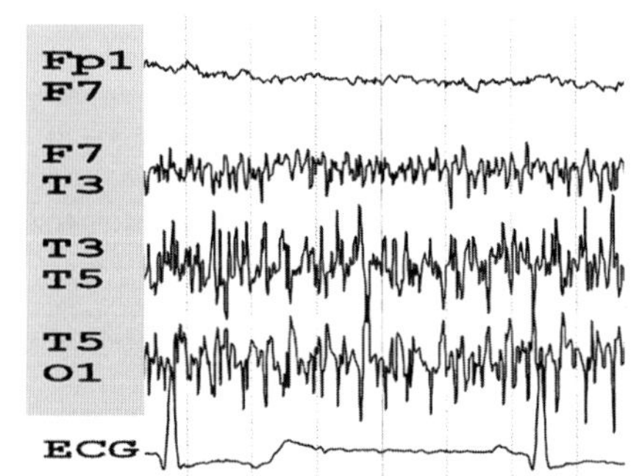

Figure c / Fast activity corresponding to a muscle activity (contraction of the left masseter muscle).

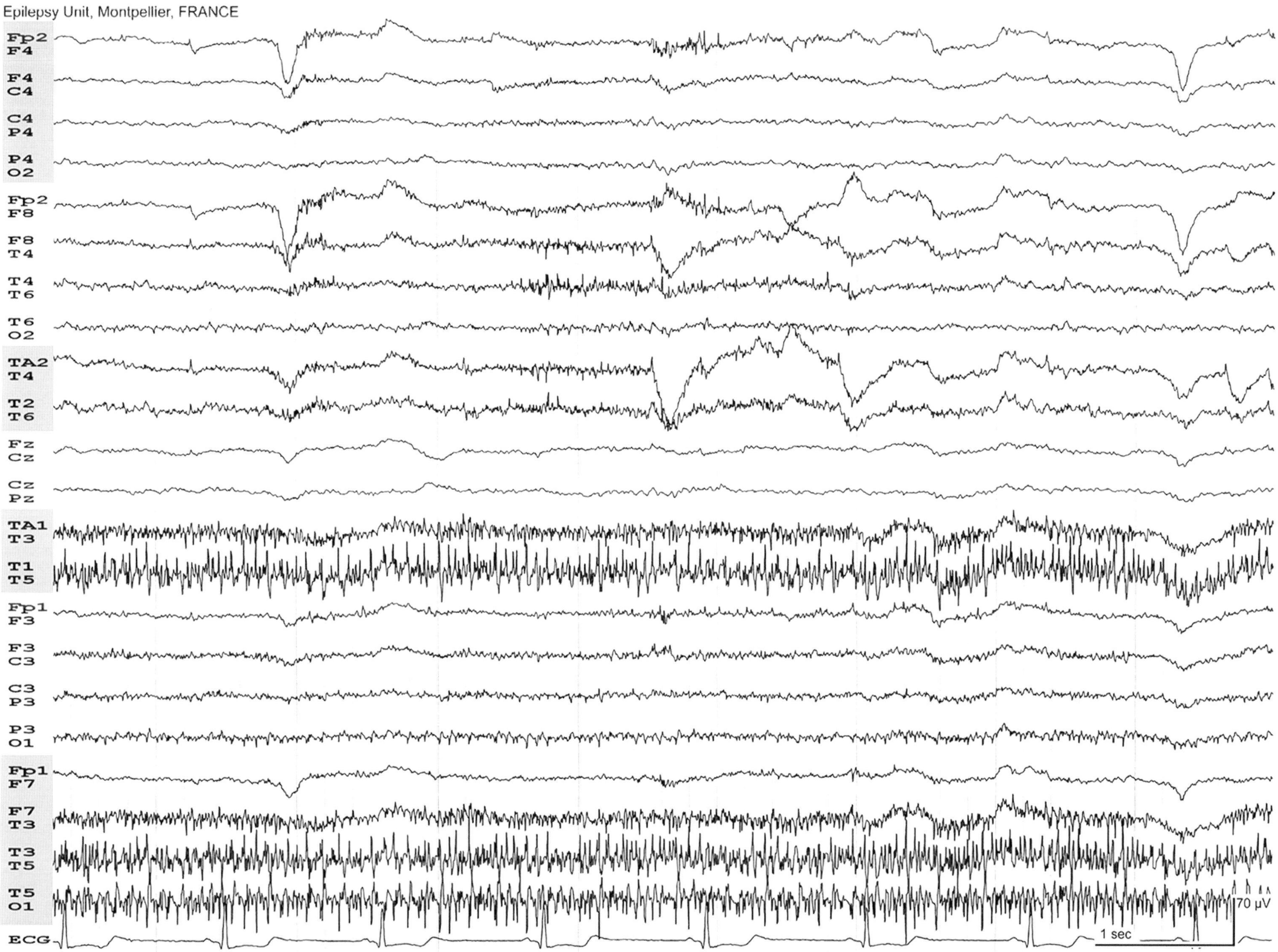
Epilepsy Unit, Montpellier, FRANCE
Fp2 F4
F4 C4
C4 P4
P4 O2
Fp2 F8
F8 T4
T4 T6
T6 O2
TA2 T4
T2 T6
Fz Cz
Cz Pz
TA1 T3
T1 T5
Fp1 F3
F3 C3
C3 P3
P3 O1
Fp1 F7
F7 T3
T3 T5
T5 O1
ECG
70 µV
1 sec

IV • 12 Asymmetric rapid eye movements in REM sleep

Context

19-year-old man with post-traumatic epilepsy.

What to note

REM sleep with asymmetric rapid eye movements clearly predominating over the right hemisphere. Severe orbital fractures with enopthalmos of the left eye.

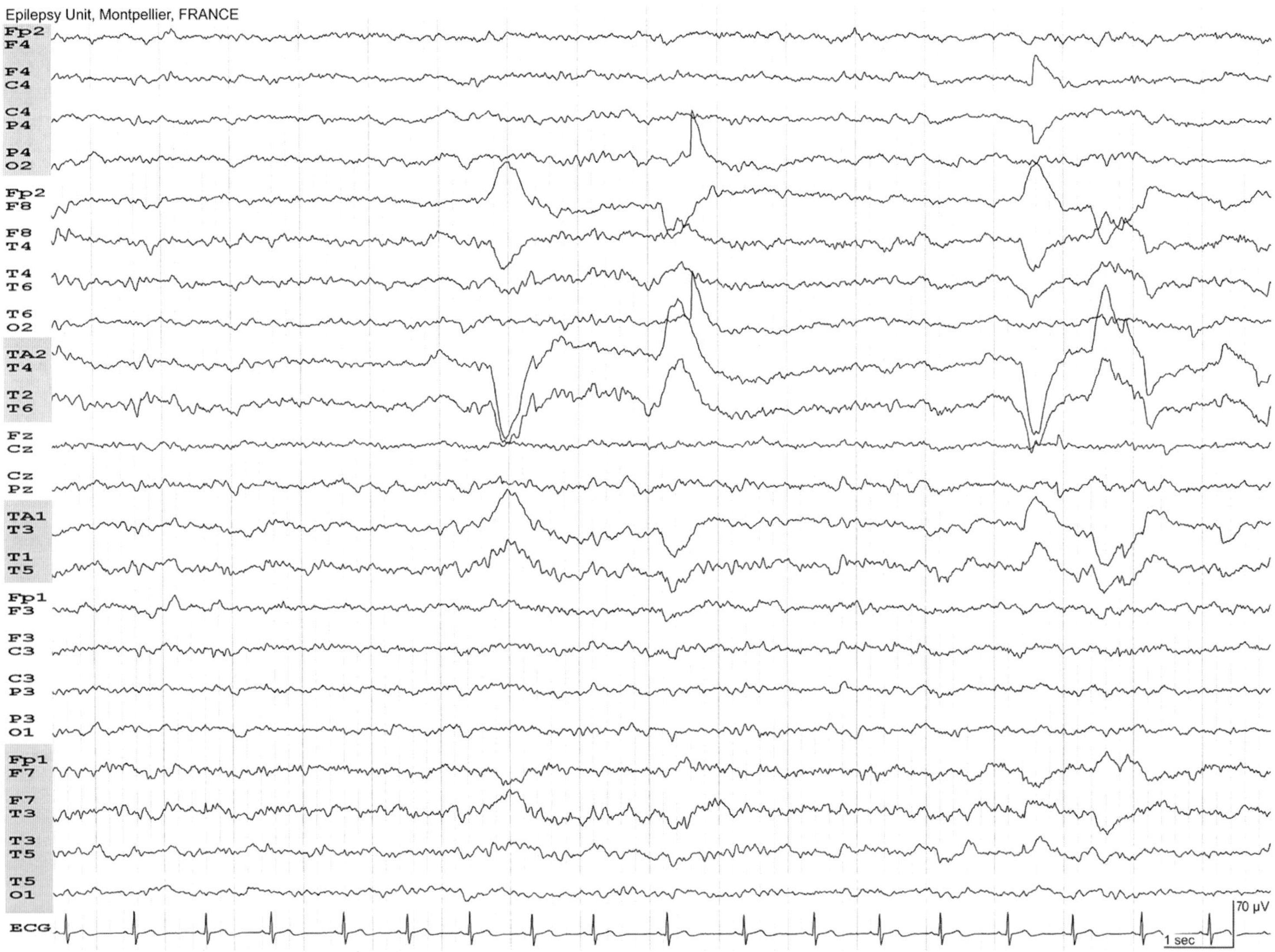

Figure a / Recording at 15 mm/s.

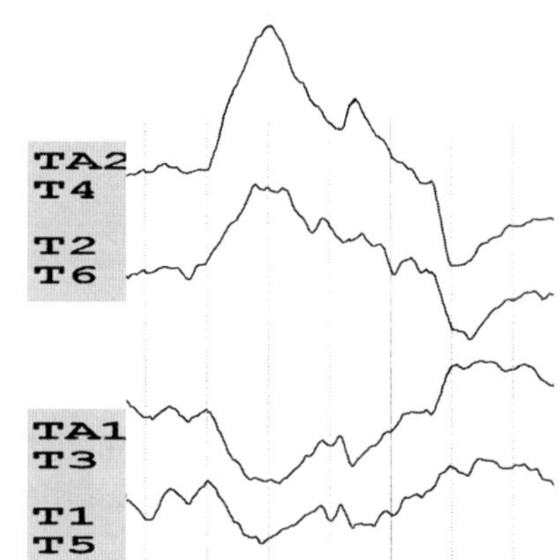

Figure b / Clearly asymmetric rapid eye movements.

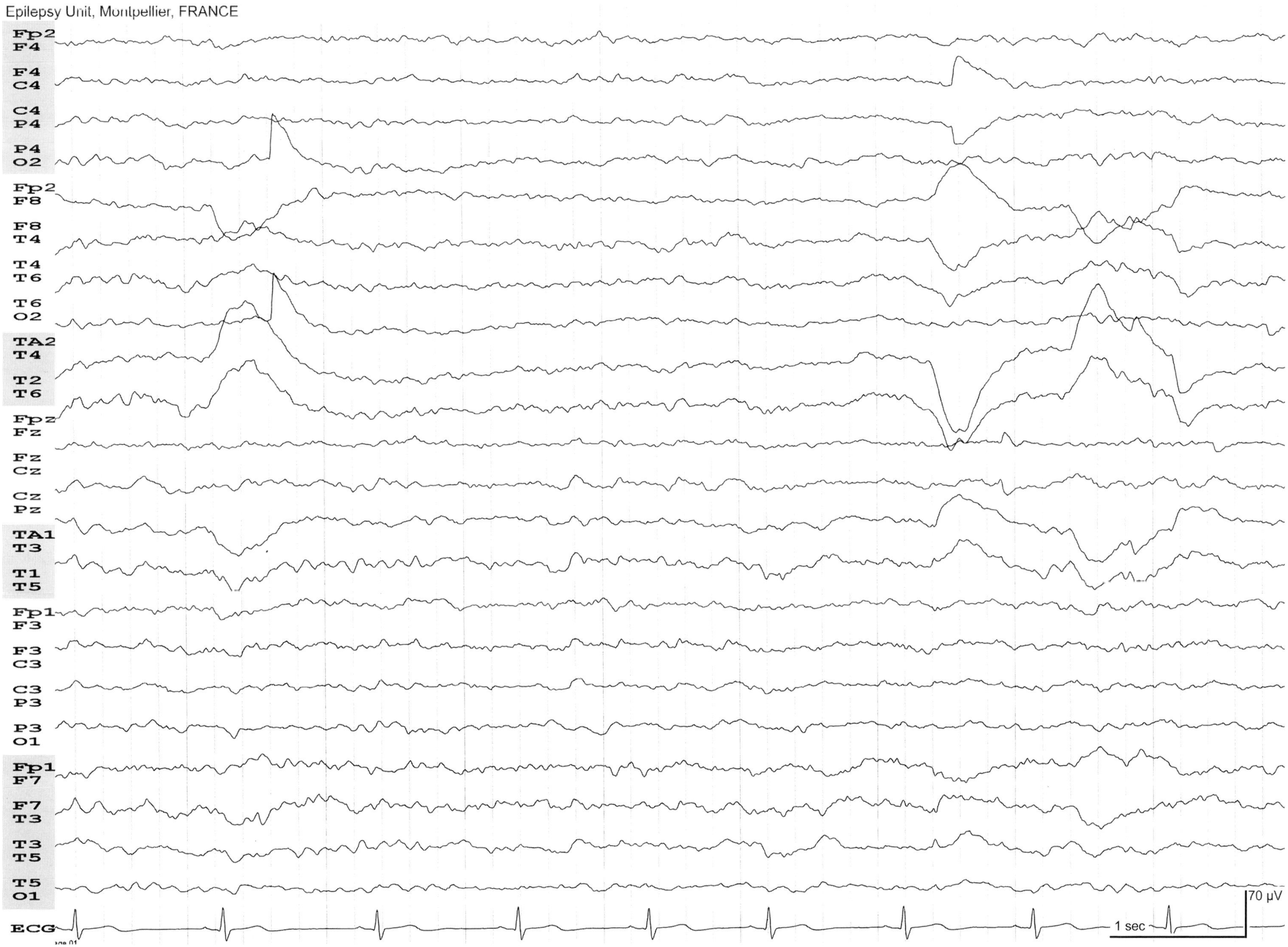
Epilepsy Unit, Montpellier, FRANCE
Fp2 F4
F4 C4
C4 P4
P4 O2
Fp2 F8
F8 T4
T4 T6
T6 O2
TA2 T4
T2 T6
Fpz Fz
Fz Cz
Cz Pz
TA1 T3
T1 T5
Fp1 F3
F3 C3
C3 P3
P3 O1
Fp1 F7
F7 T3
T3 T5
T5 O1
ECG
70 µV
1 sec

IV • 13 Isoelectric line and eye movements in an adult

Context
34-year-old man with idiopathic generalized epilepsy.

What to note
The patient's eyes are closed. Background alpha activity at 9 Hz. Presence of eye movements at the frontal polar and anterior temporal derivations. The artifacts spread to the frontal derivations. The Cz-Pz derivation is very-low-voltage (isoelectric line) compared with other derivations due to excess electrode gel between Cz and Pz.

What to do
Put hands gently over the eyes whenever in doubt so as to interrupt the eye movements. Wipe off excess electrode gel.

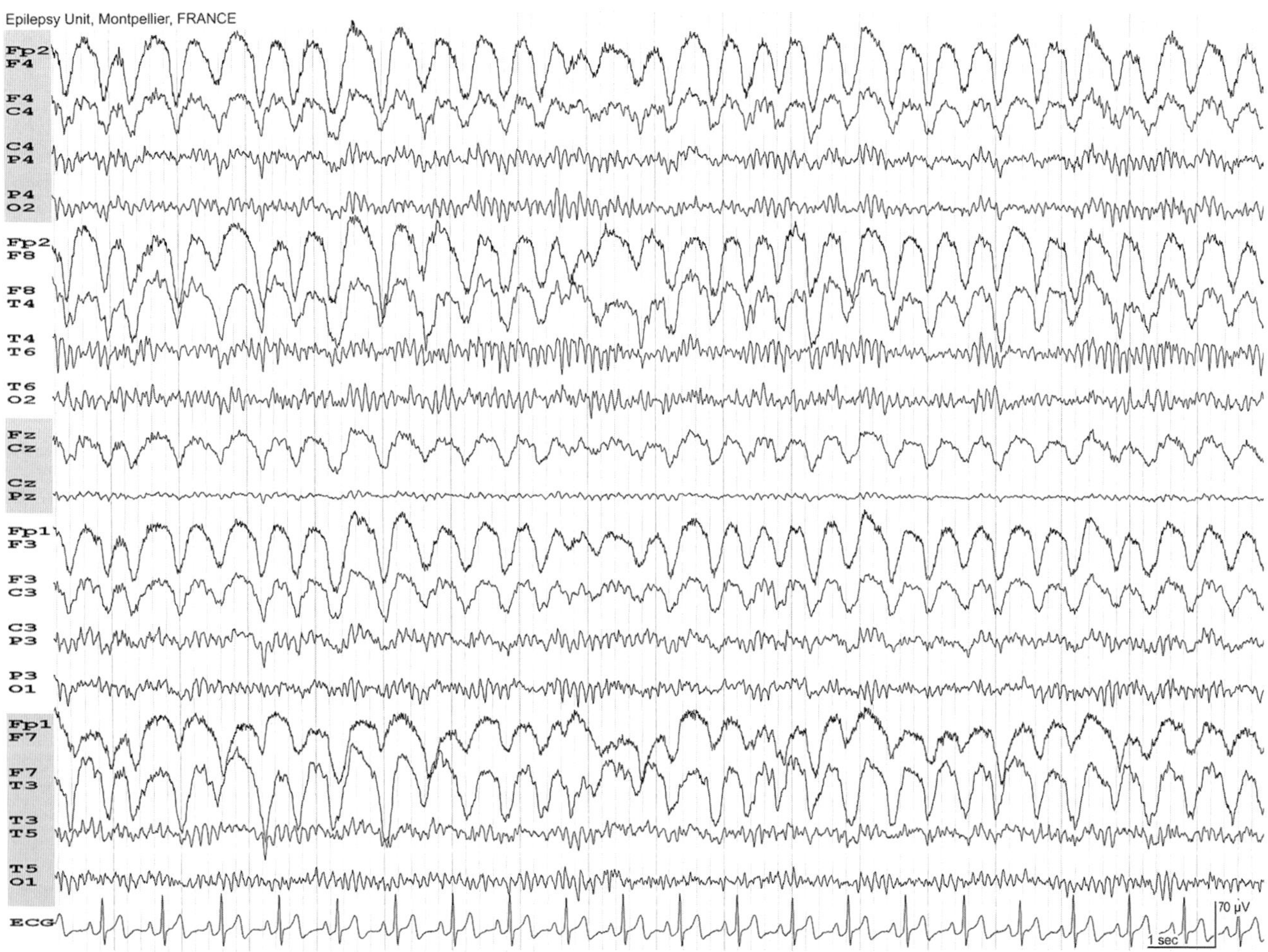

Figure a / Recording at 15 mm/s.

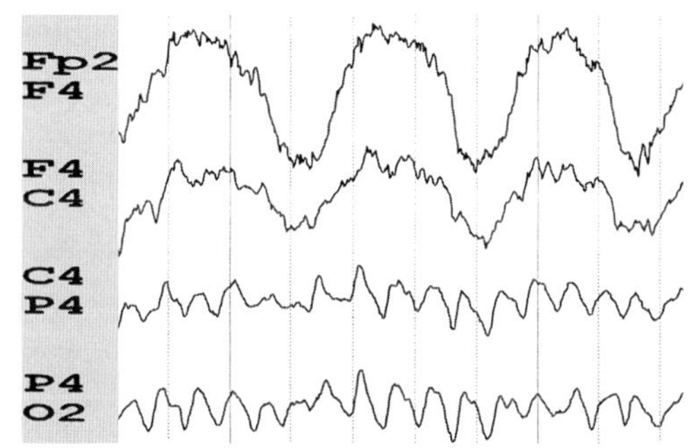

Figure b / Eye movement artifacts on the frontal derivations. Alpha rhythm over the posterior derivations.

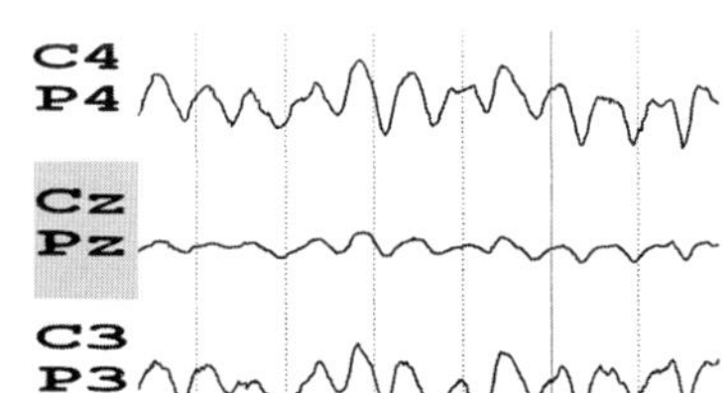

Figure c / Excess electrode gel between Cz and Pz.

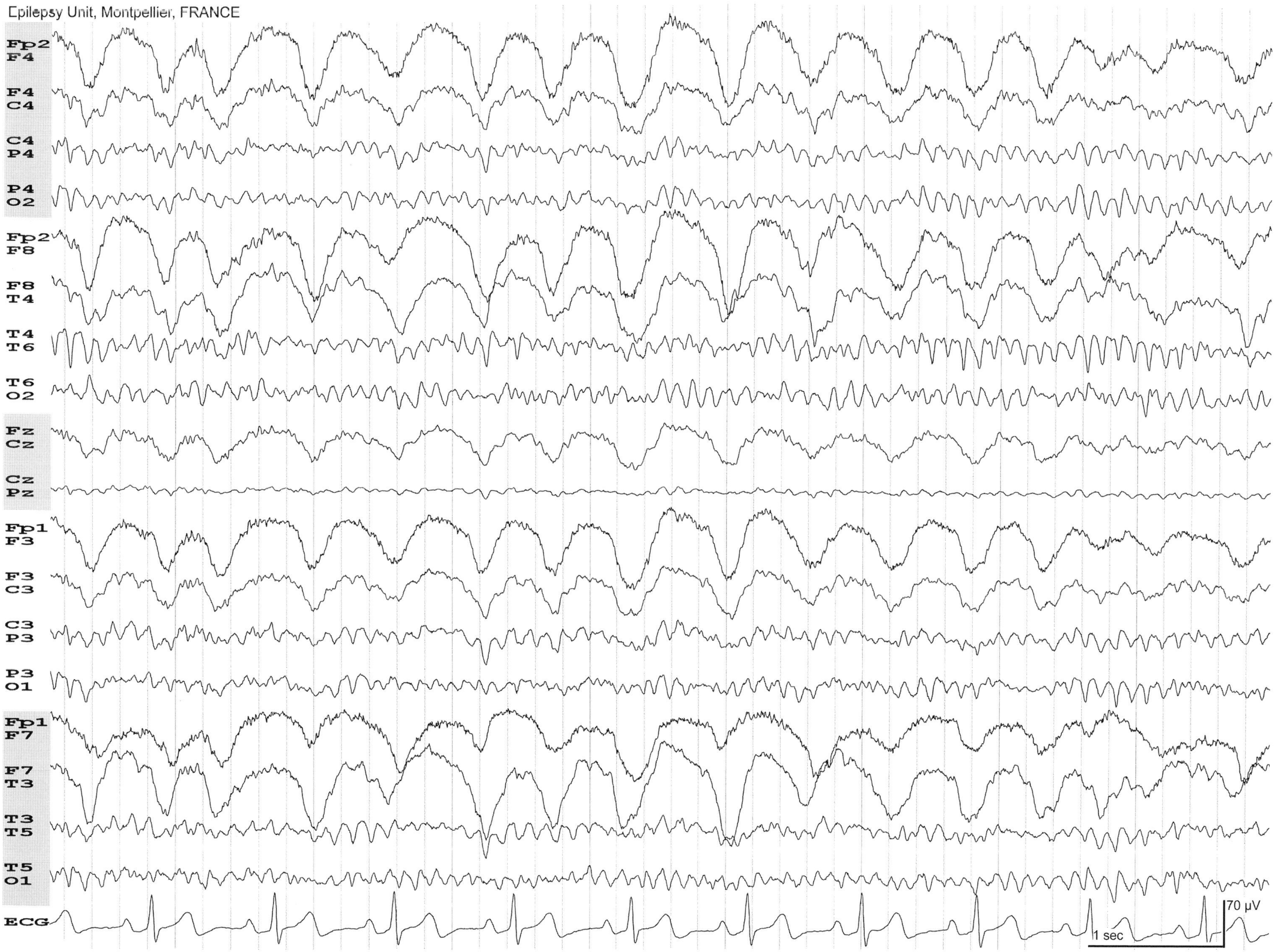
Epilepsy Unit, Montpellier, FRANCE
Fp2 F4
F4 C4
C4 P4
P4 O2
Fp2 F8
F8 T4
T4 T6
T6 O2
Fz Cz
Cz Pz
Fp1 F3
F3 C3
C3 P3
P3 O1
Fp1 F7
F7 T3
T3 T5
T5 O1
ECG
1 sec
70 µV

IV • 14 Muscle and movement artifact

Context

19-year-old man, EEG for pilot licence.

What to note

Stage N2 sleep. On the left segment, burst of muscular potentials over the right temporal region followed by a head movement artifact. The patient had a myoclonic jerk of the neck. This muscle activity and the artifact of movement create the false impression of a polyspike-wave discharge. On the right plate, another example of myoclonic jerk. After the myoclonic jerk, there is a transient arousal.

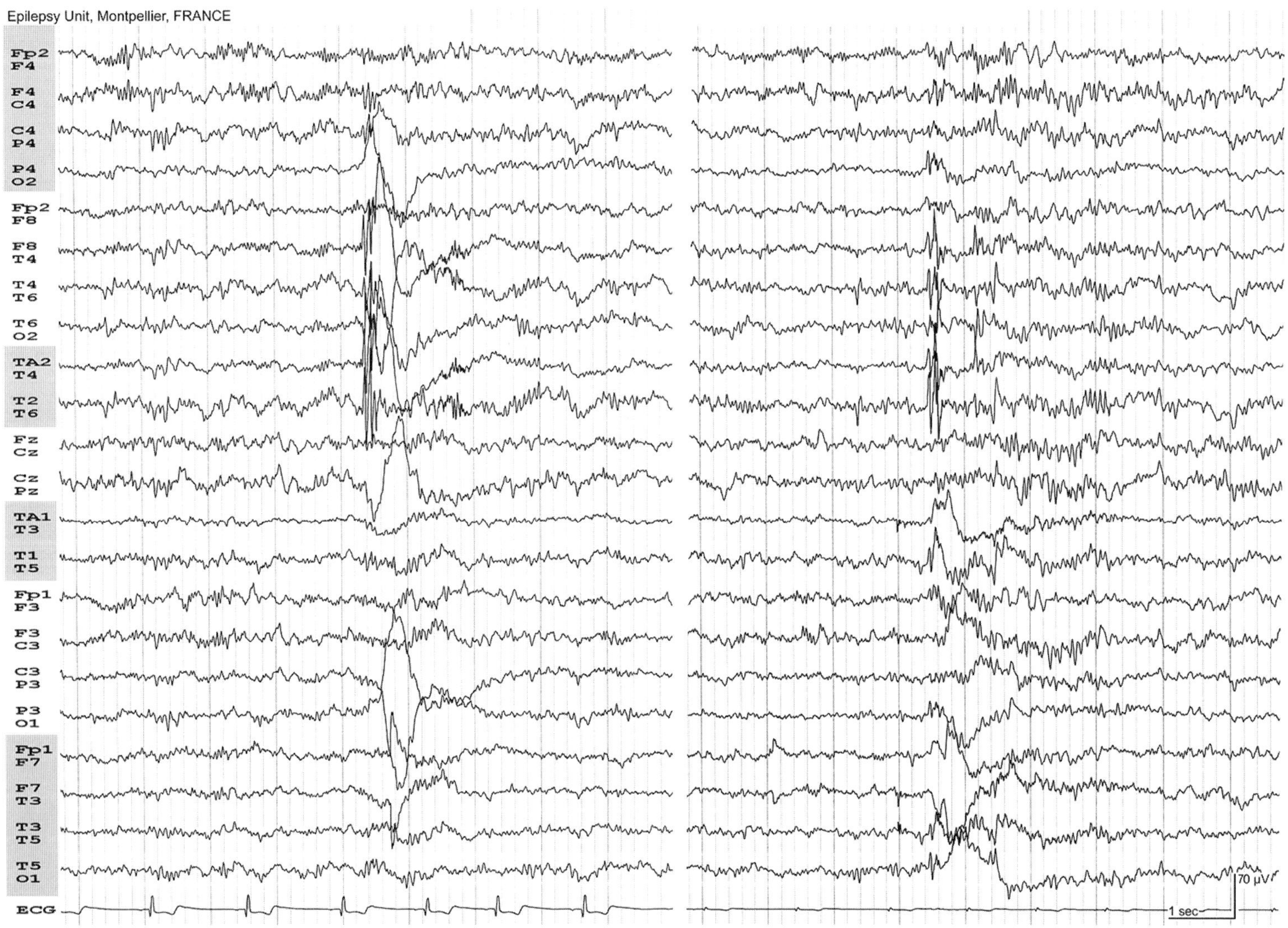

Figure a / Recording at 15 mm/s.

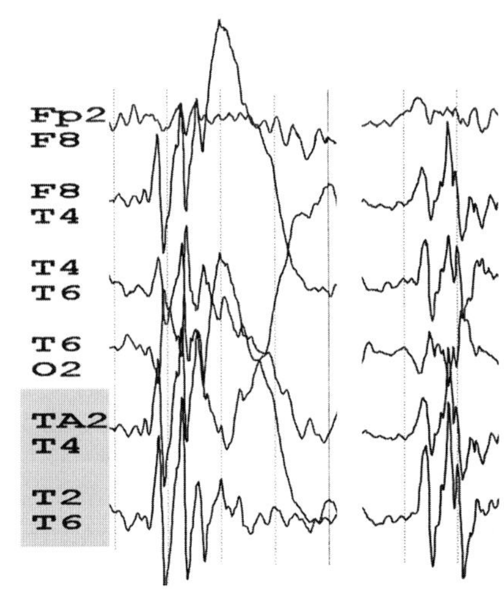

Figure b / Artifact.

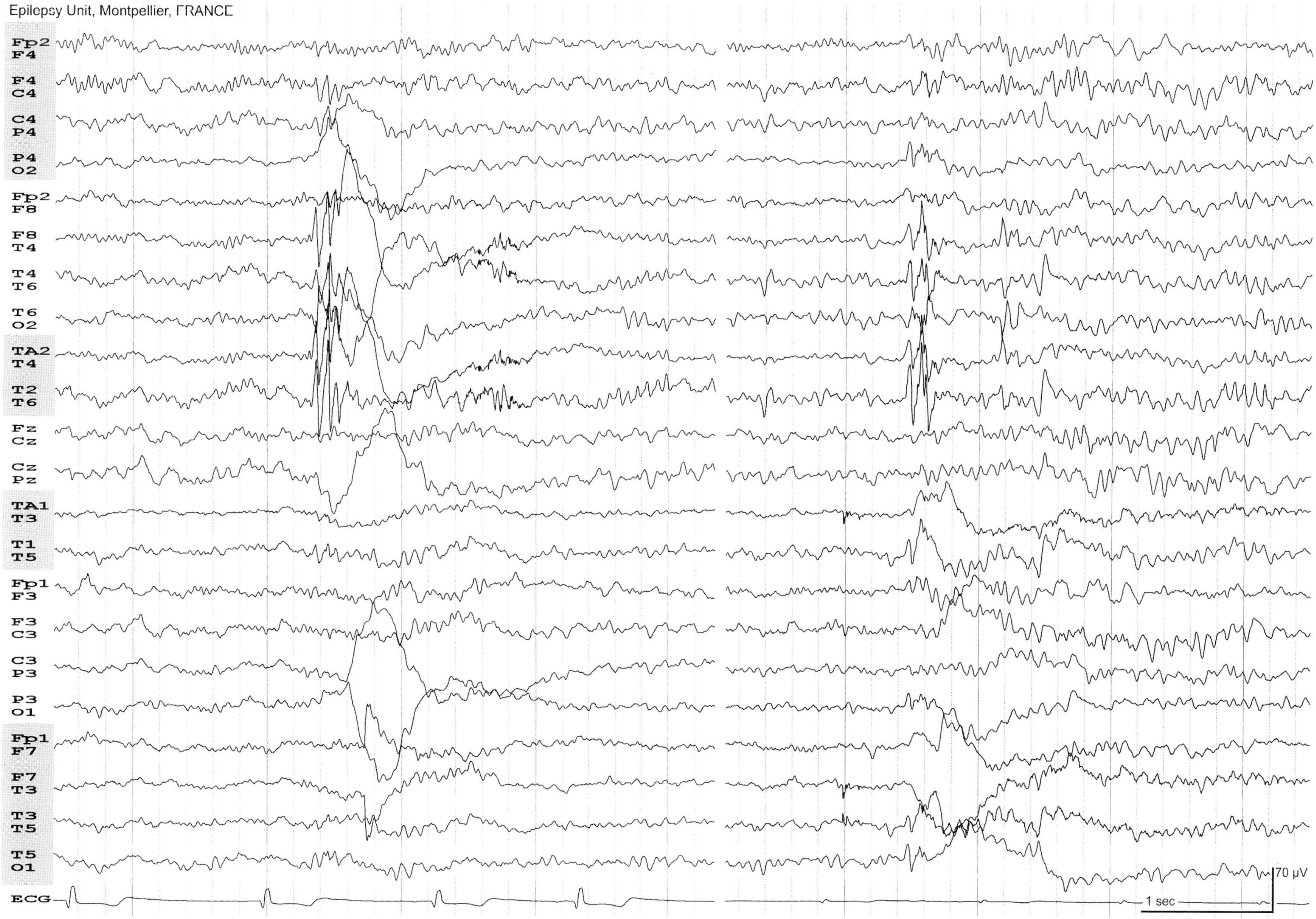
Epilepsy Unit, Montpellier, FRANCE
Fp2 F4
F4 C4
C4 P4
P4 O2
Fp2 F8
F8 T4
T4 T6
T6 O2
TA2 T4
T2 T6
Fz Cz
Cz Pz
TA1 T3
T1 T5
Fp1 F3
F3 C3
C3 P3
P3 O1
Fp1 F7
F7 T3
T3 T5
T5 O1
ECG
70 µV
1 sec

• 15 Rhythmic movements: body rocking (1)

Context

28-year-old man with idiopathic generalized epilepsy.

What to note

Drowsiness. Rhythmic delta waves at 2.5 Hz over the left posterior temporal region and the vertex region. These slow waves can also be seen over the left suprasylvian region but they are not as prominent. This rhythmic activity does not correspond to an epileptic seizure. Indeed, the rhythm is very regular, maximal from onset and then with decreasing amplitude (which would be the opposite in an epileptic seizure). Furthermore, the cerebral distribution, with activity over the left posterior temporal region and the vertex region simultaneously, would not be logical. Body rocking, a rhythm found in drowsiness, is clearly detectable on the video. The patient is rocking himself to sleep. There is also a *jactatio capitis*, easily diagnosed with the EEG, given the abundance of the artifacts generated by lateral movements of the head. There is muscle generated rapid low-voltage activity at F4 as well.

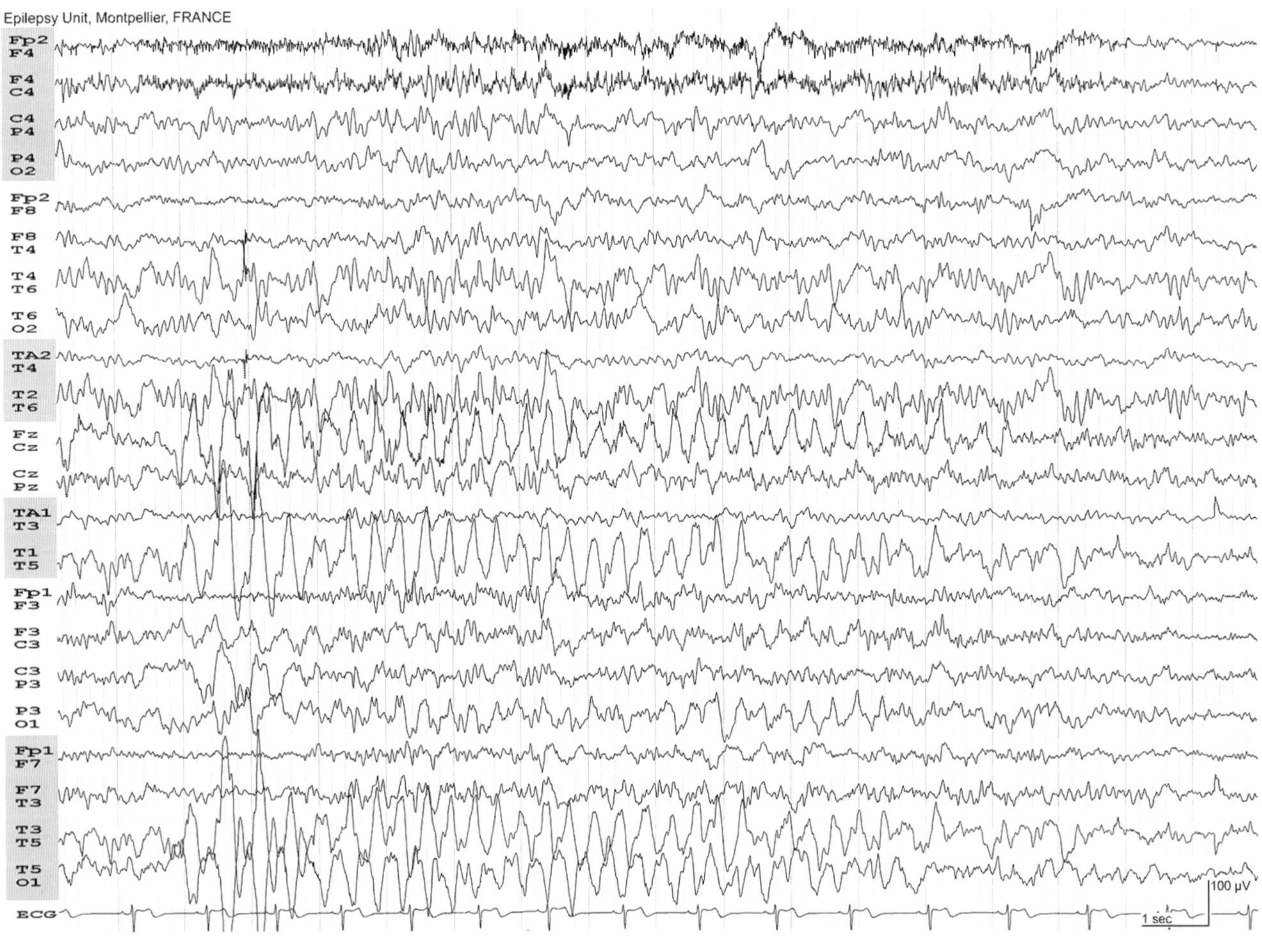

Figure a / At the 5th second, rhythmic delta waves over the left posterior temporal region and the vertex region.

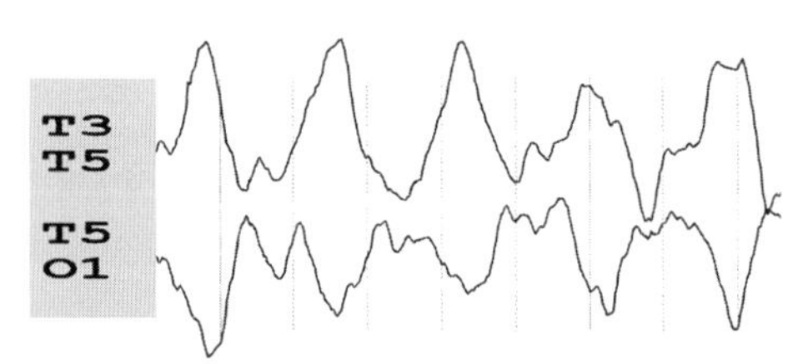

Figure b / Artifact generated by body rocking at T5.

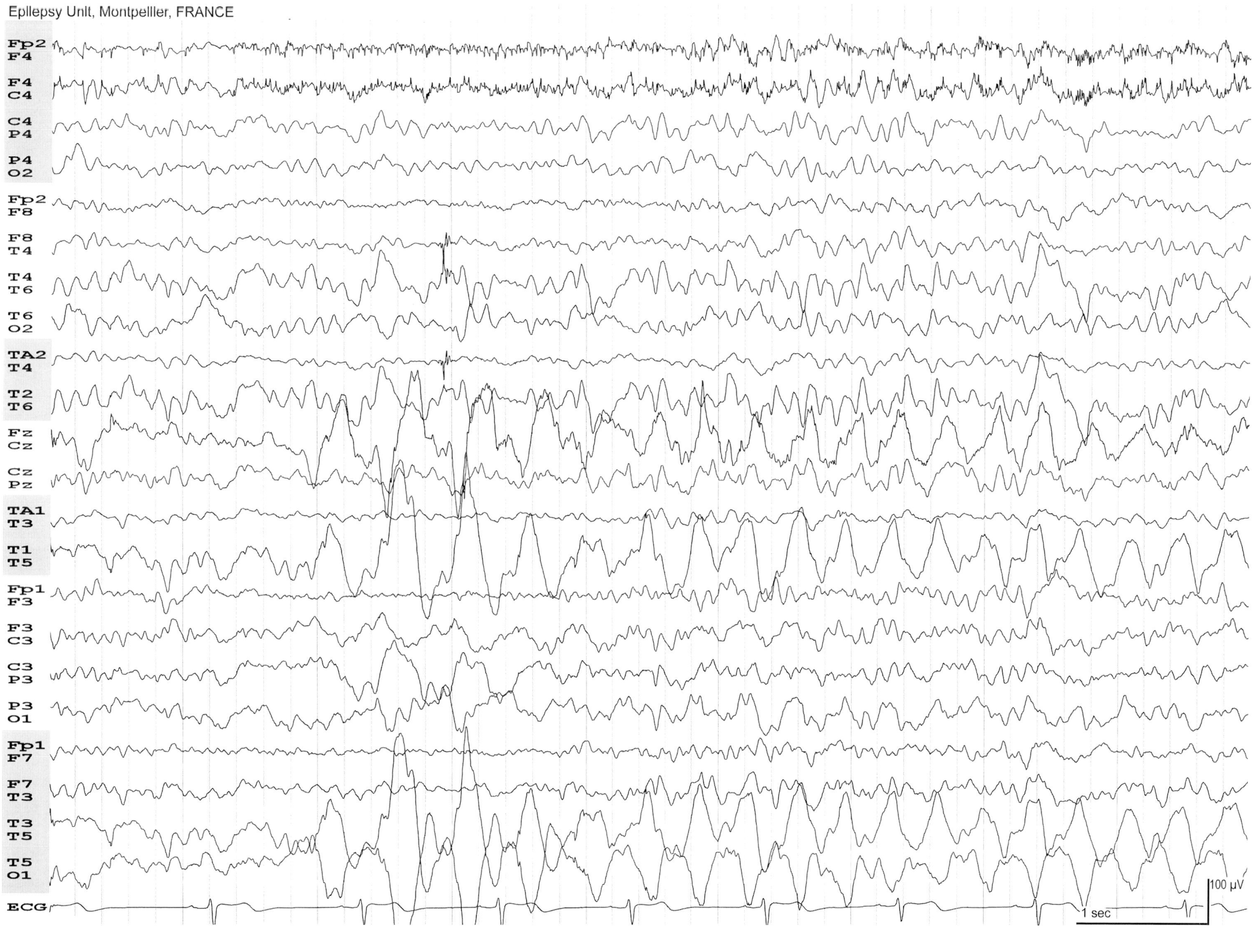
Epilepsy Unit, Montpellier, FRANCE
Fp2 F4
F4 C4
C4 P4
P4 O2
Fp2 F8
F8 T4
T4 T6
T6 O2
TA2 T4
T2 T6
Fz Cz
Cz Pz
TA1 T3
T1 T5
Fp1 F3
F3 C3
C3 P3
P3 O1
Fp1 F7
F7 T3
T3 T5
T5 O1
ECG
100 µV
1 sec

• 16 Rhythmic movements: head tremor (2)

Context

83-year-old woman seen after a faint and a fall.

What to note

Over the right anterior temporal region (T4), the rhythmic theta activity at a frequency of 5-6 Hz spreads toward the right central region. This activity corresponds to a head tremor artifact with predominance on the right temporal region. Note that, contrary to a seizure or unusual physiological rhythms such as rhythmic midtemporal discharge, the amplitude of this activity is more variable and its development is more sinusoidal. This type of artifact is usually seen with muscle activities, only slightly detectable on this tracing over the frontal polar and the left suprasylvian region due to the use of a high-pass muscle activity filter at 35 Hz. Note an arrhythmia at the ECG derivation.

What to do

The technologist plays a crucial role in cases such as this one by providing evidence that this activity is a tremor artifact.

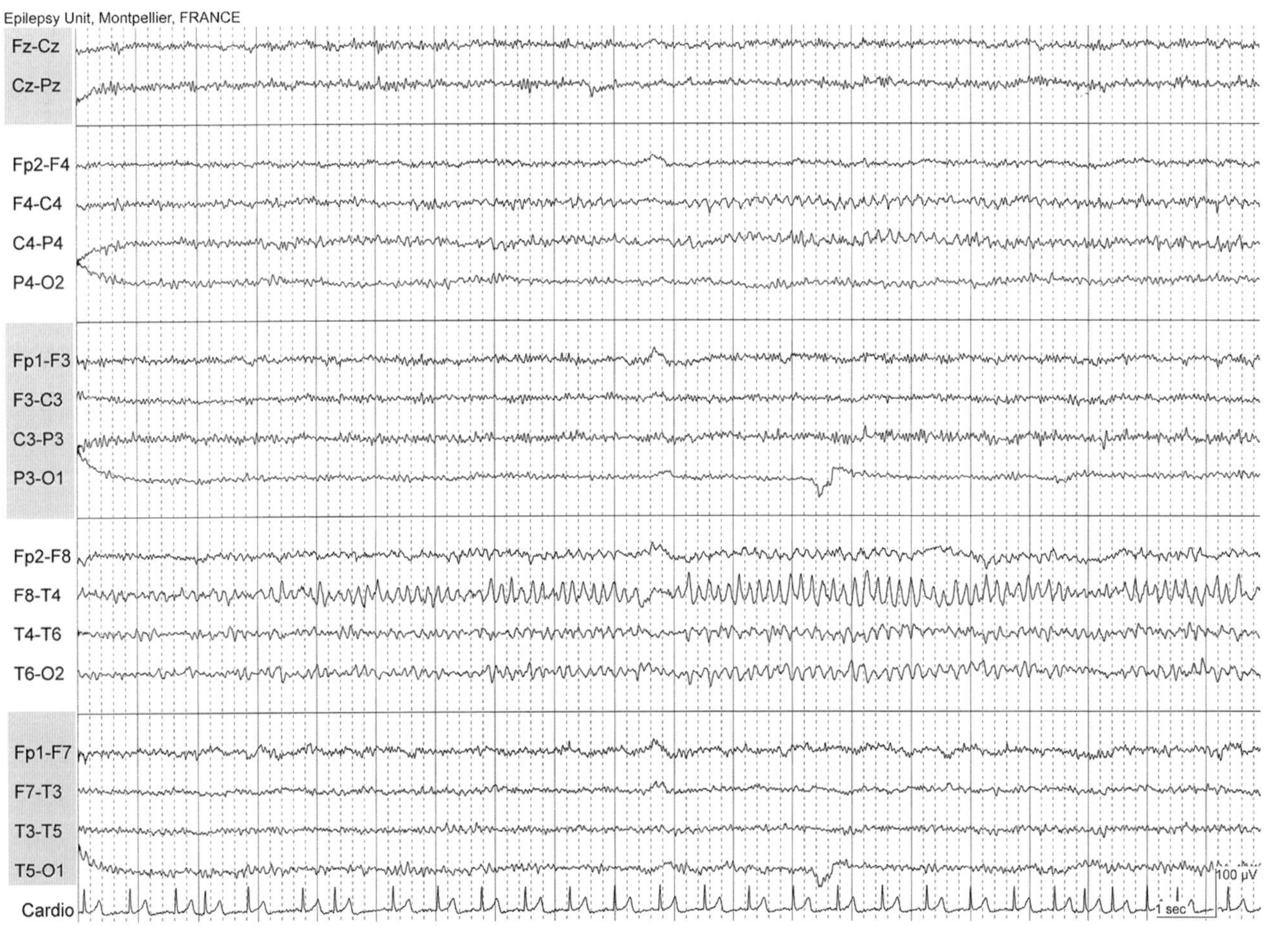

Figure a / Recording at 15 mm/s.

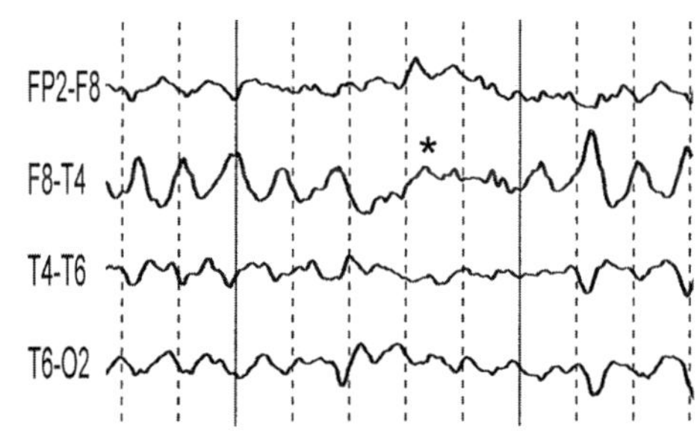

Figure b / Rhythmic theta activity generated by a tremor. Offset (*) then resumption of the activity.

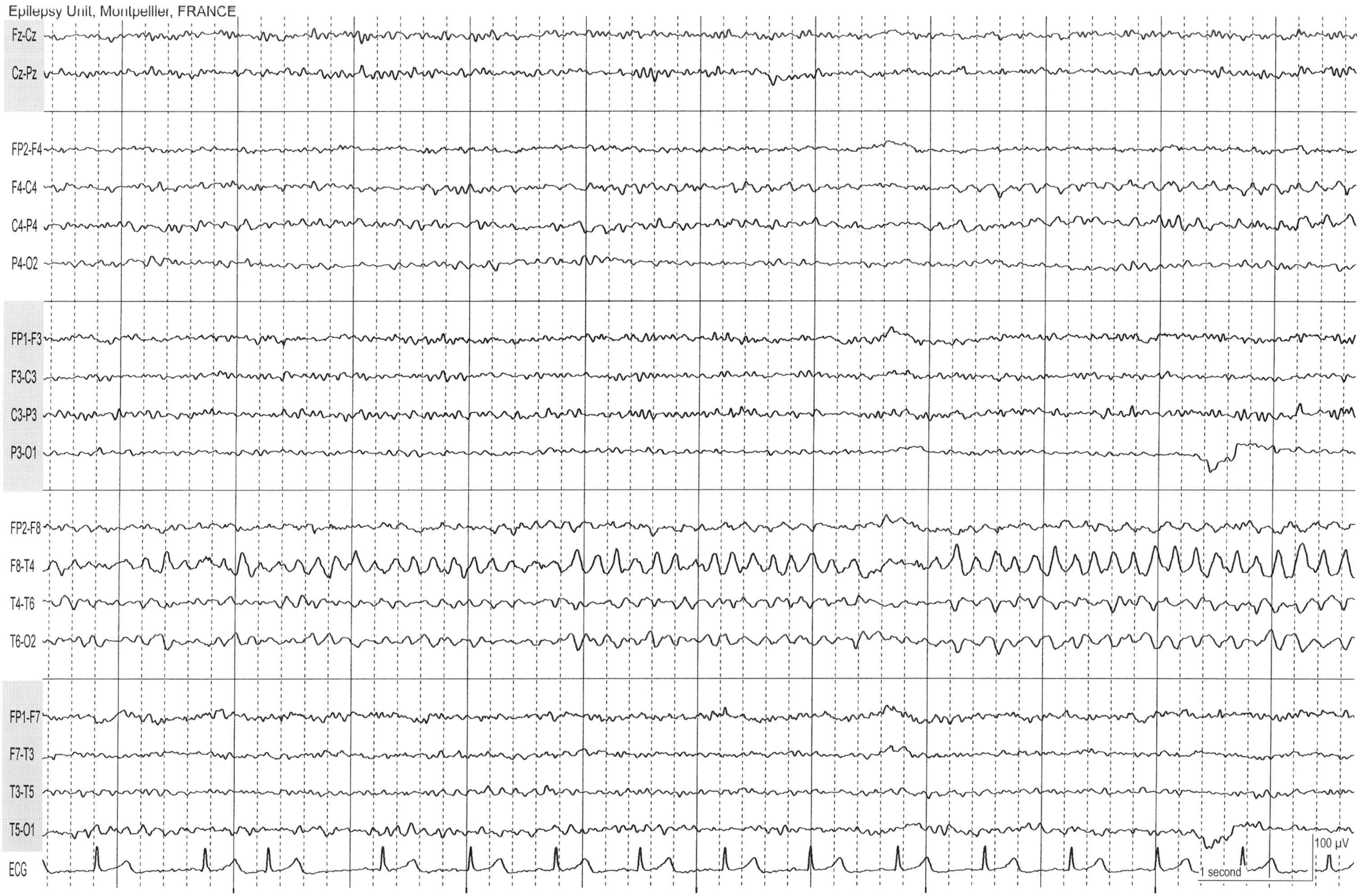
Epilepsy Unit, Montpellier, FRANCE
Fz-Cz
Cz-Pz
FP2-F4
F4-C4
C4-P4
P4-O2
FP1-F3
F3-C3
C3-P3
P3-O1
FP2-F8
F8-T4
T4-T6
T6-O2
FP1-F7
F7-T3
T3-T5
T5-O1
ECG
100 µV
1 second

IV • 17 Rhythmic movements: head tremor (3)

Context

20-year-old woman with left mesio-temporal lobe epilepsy, presurgical assessment.

What to note

The patient's eyes are open. Eyelid movement artifact at the beginning of the plate followed by muscle activities over the fronto-polar derivations. Theta discharge at 4.5 Hz on the left temporal region lasting 6.5 seconds. This corresponds to a head tremor artifact: rhythmic activity of the right deltoid with propagation of the tremor to the head.

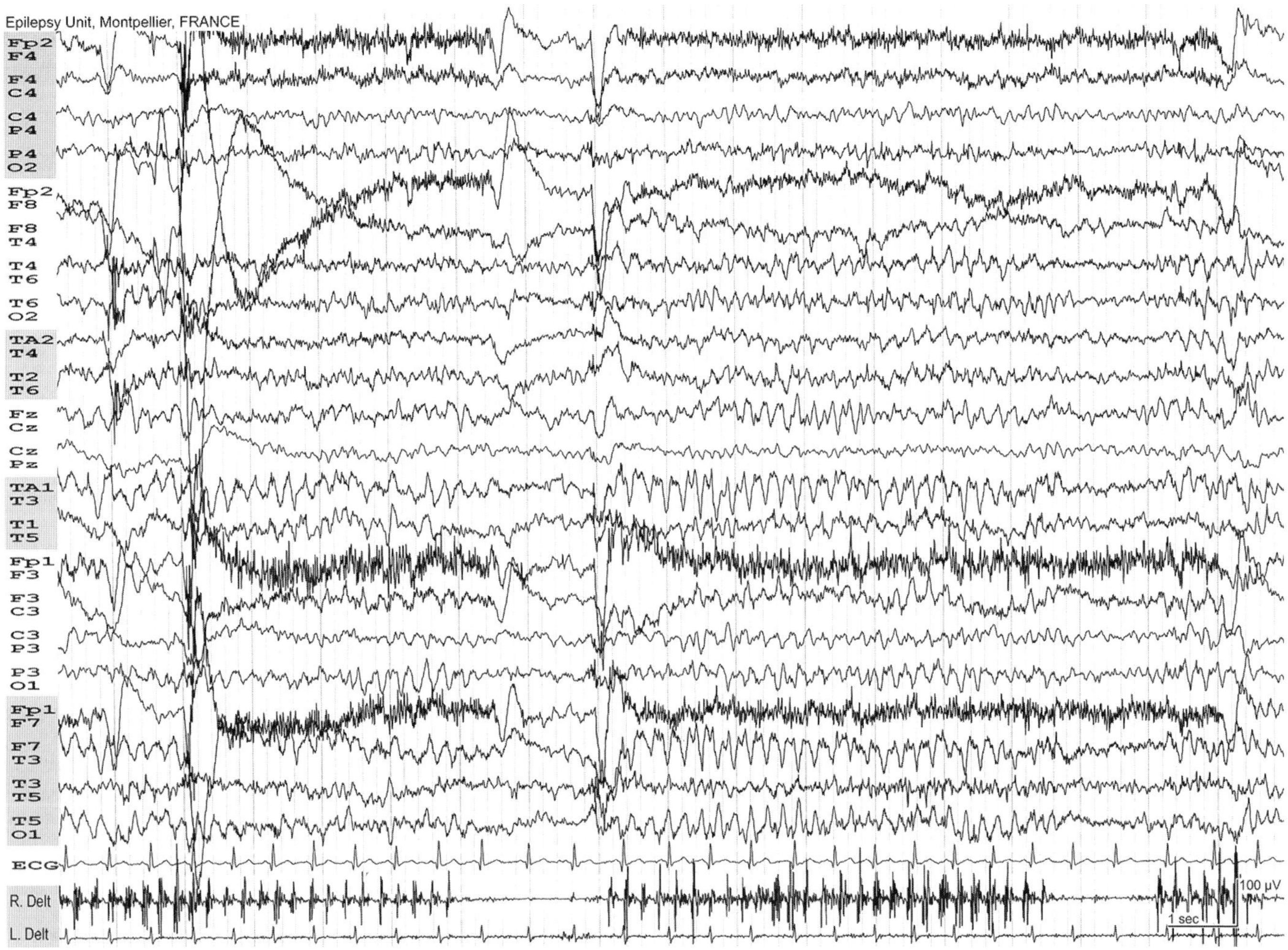

Figure a / Recording at 15 mm/s.

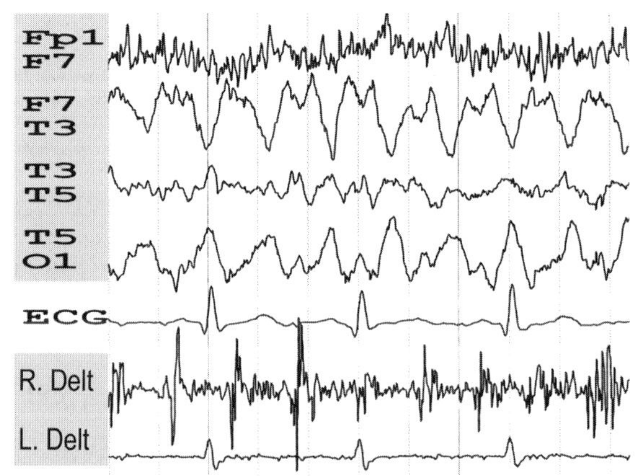

Figure b / Theta activity on the left temporal region corresponding to a rhythmical activity of the right deltoid.

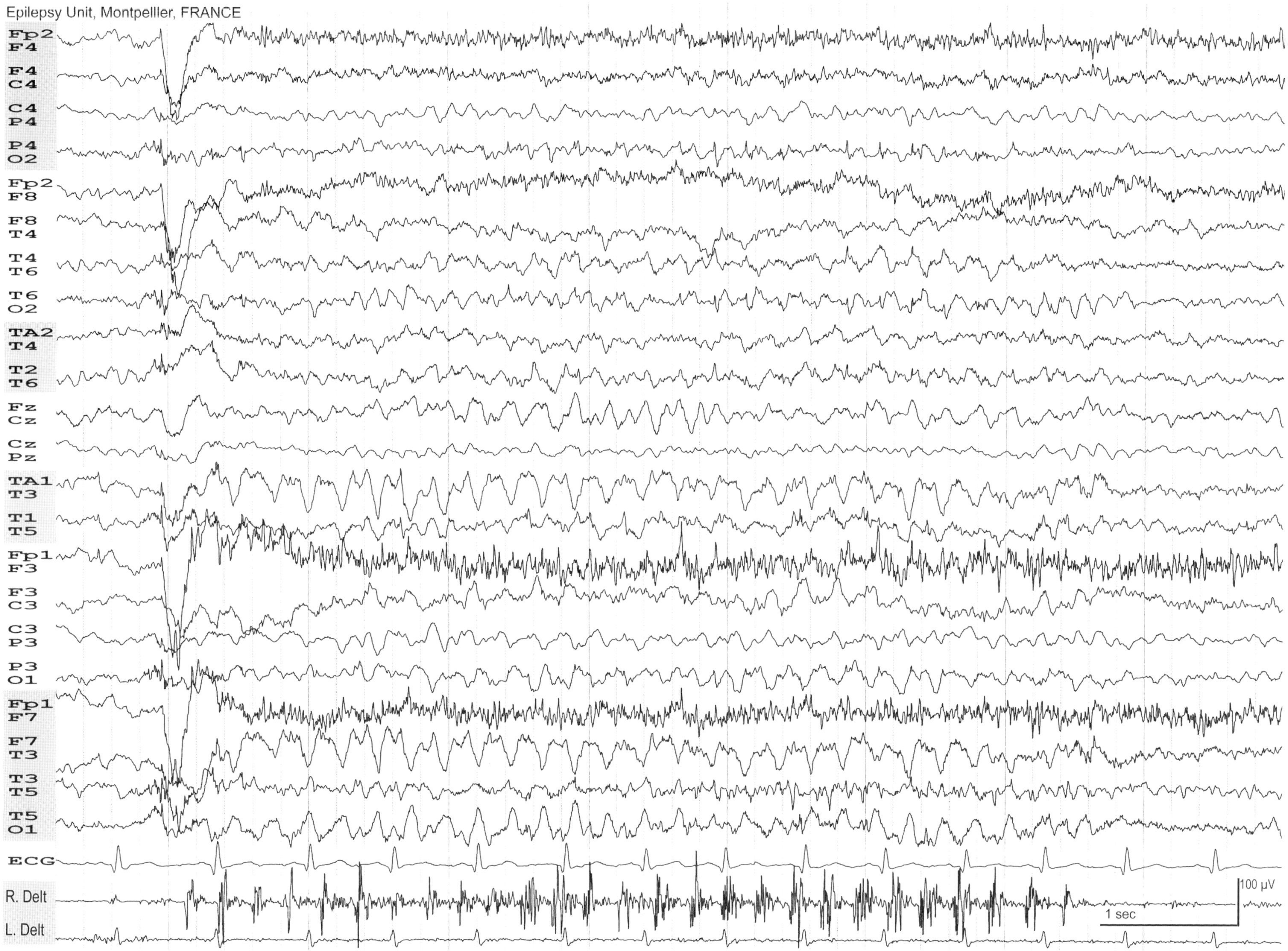
Epilepsy Unit, Montpellier, FRANCE
Fp2 F4
F4 C4
C4 P4
P4 O2
Fp2 F8
F8 T4
T4 T6
T6 O2
TA2 T4
T2 T6
Fz Cz
Cz Pz
TA1 T3
T1 T5
Fp1 F3
F3 C3
C3 P3
P3 O1
Fp1 F7
F7 T3
T3 T5
T5 O1
ECG
R. Delt
L. Delt
100 µV
1 sec

• 18 Rhythmic movements: head tremor (4)

Context

40-year-old man with severe psychomotor retardation with worsening of epilepsy.

What to note

The patient's eyes are open. Some small eyelid movement artifacts at the beginning of the plate. Rhythmic sharp theta waves over the occipital regions, especially on the right. The amplitude gradually builds up then decreases progressively (see plates below). Note the sinusoidal aspect on these plates. This activity corresponds to a tremor of the head. The sinusoidal aspect does not evoke a seizure.

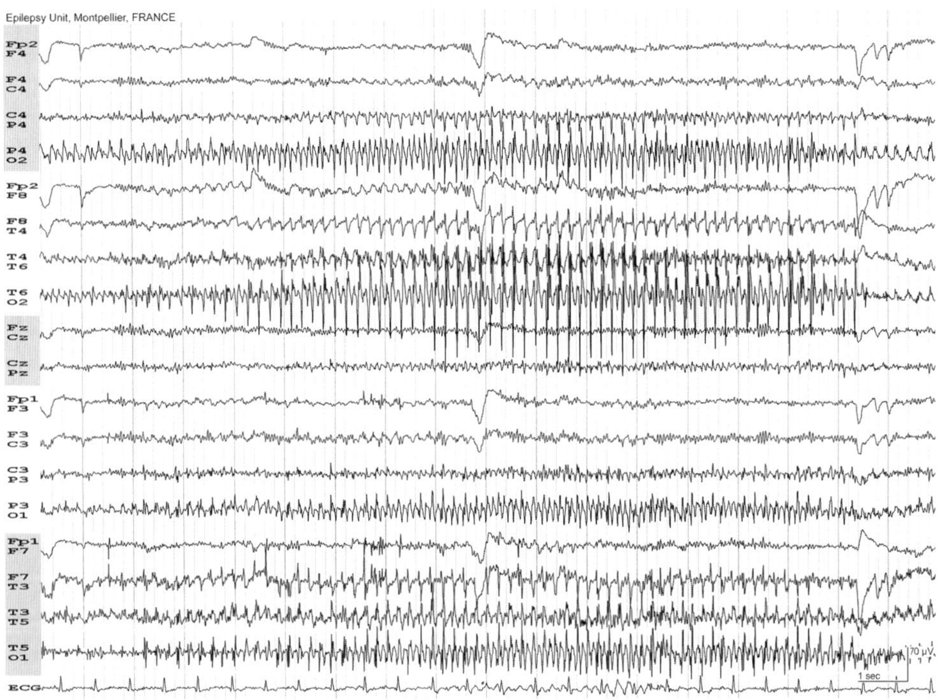

Figure a / Recording at 15 mm/s. Note the sinusoidal aspect.

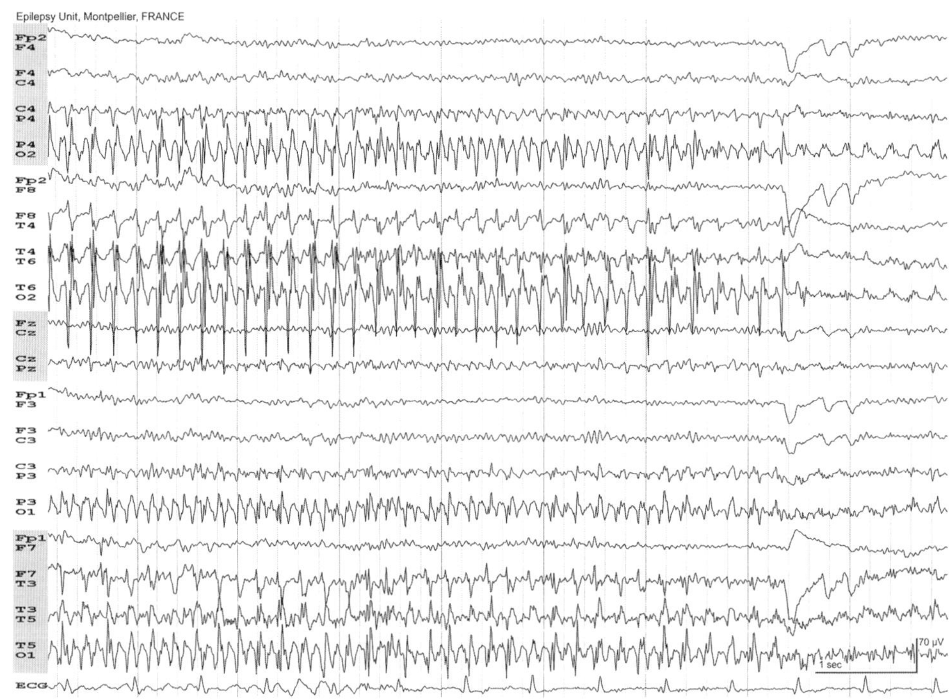

Figure b / End of the tremor. The activity decreases progressively and stops at the end of the plate.

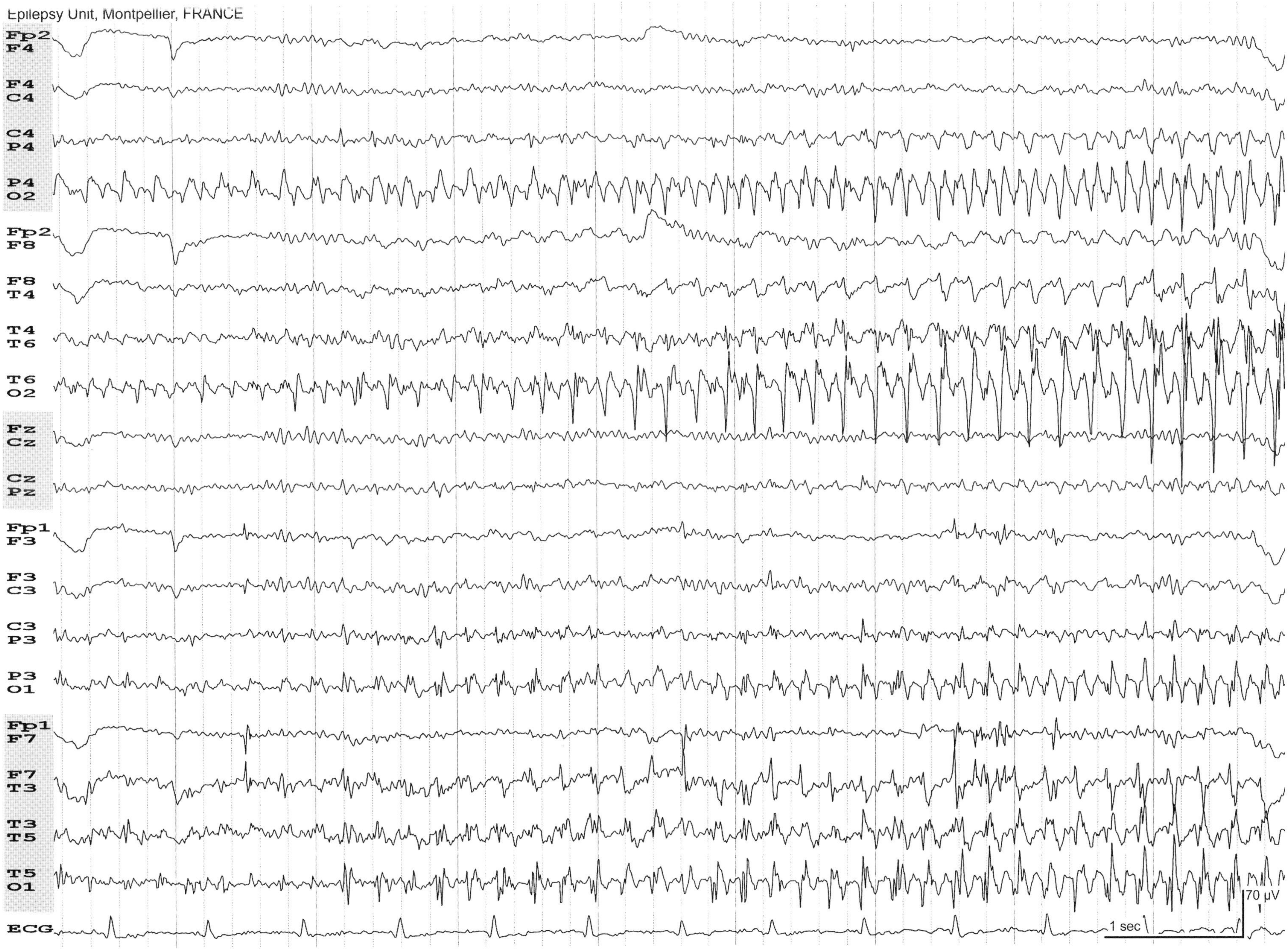
Epilepsy Unit, Montpellier, FRANCE
Fp2 F4
F4 C4
C4 P4
P4 O2
Fp2 F8
F8 T4
T4 T6
T6 O2
Fz Cz
Cz Pz
Fp1 F3
F3 C3
C3 P3
P3 O1
Fp1 F7
F7 T3
T3 T5
T5 O1
ECG
70 µV
1 sec

IV • 19 Rhythmic movements: head movements (5)

Context

76-year-old man with dementia.

What to note

Over the right occipital region, rhythmic slow waves at 5 Hz corresponding to oscillating movements of the head are observed. Over the left central region, slow theta waves also correspond most likely to these movements of the head. The fact that these activities are only observed at O2 and C3 argues in favor of an artifact. Given the agitated state of the patient, this EEG is difficult to interpret. It is therefore not possible to confirm a suspicion of focal slowing. Over the frontal polar regions, artifacts involving eye and eyelid movements mixed with muscle activities at fluctuating amplitudes (see plate recorded at 15 mm/s). The highest amplitude muscle potentials correspond to contractions of the periorbital muscles. The ECG derivation is partially defective here.

Comment

Rocking artifact in an infant produces a similar activity with rhythmic posterior slow waves whose frequency is time locked to the rocking frequency.

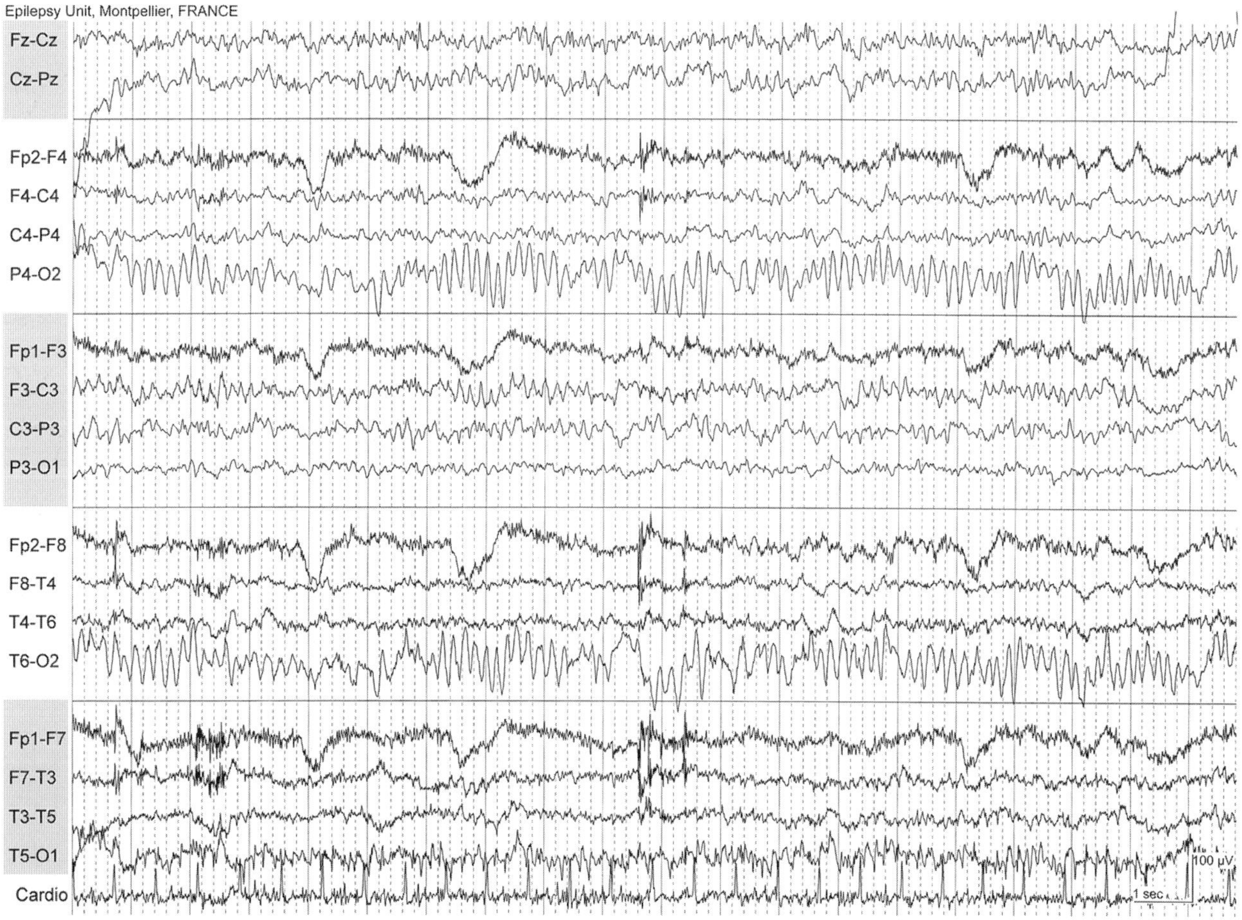

Figure a / Recording at 15 mm/s.

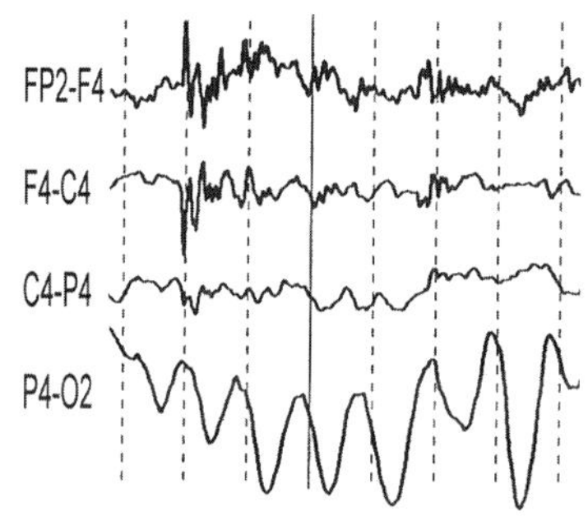

Figure b / Rhythmic activity at O2 corresponding to a head tremor. Muscular activities corresponding to knit brow.

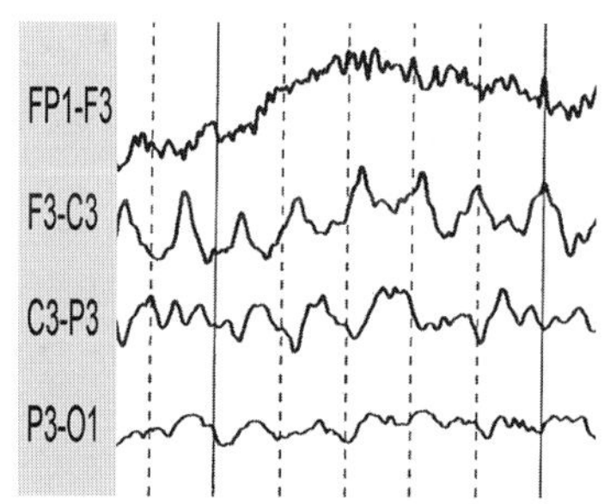

Figure c / Rhythmic activity at C3 corresponding to a head tremor.

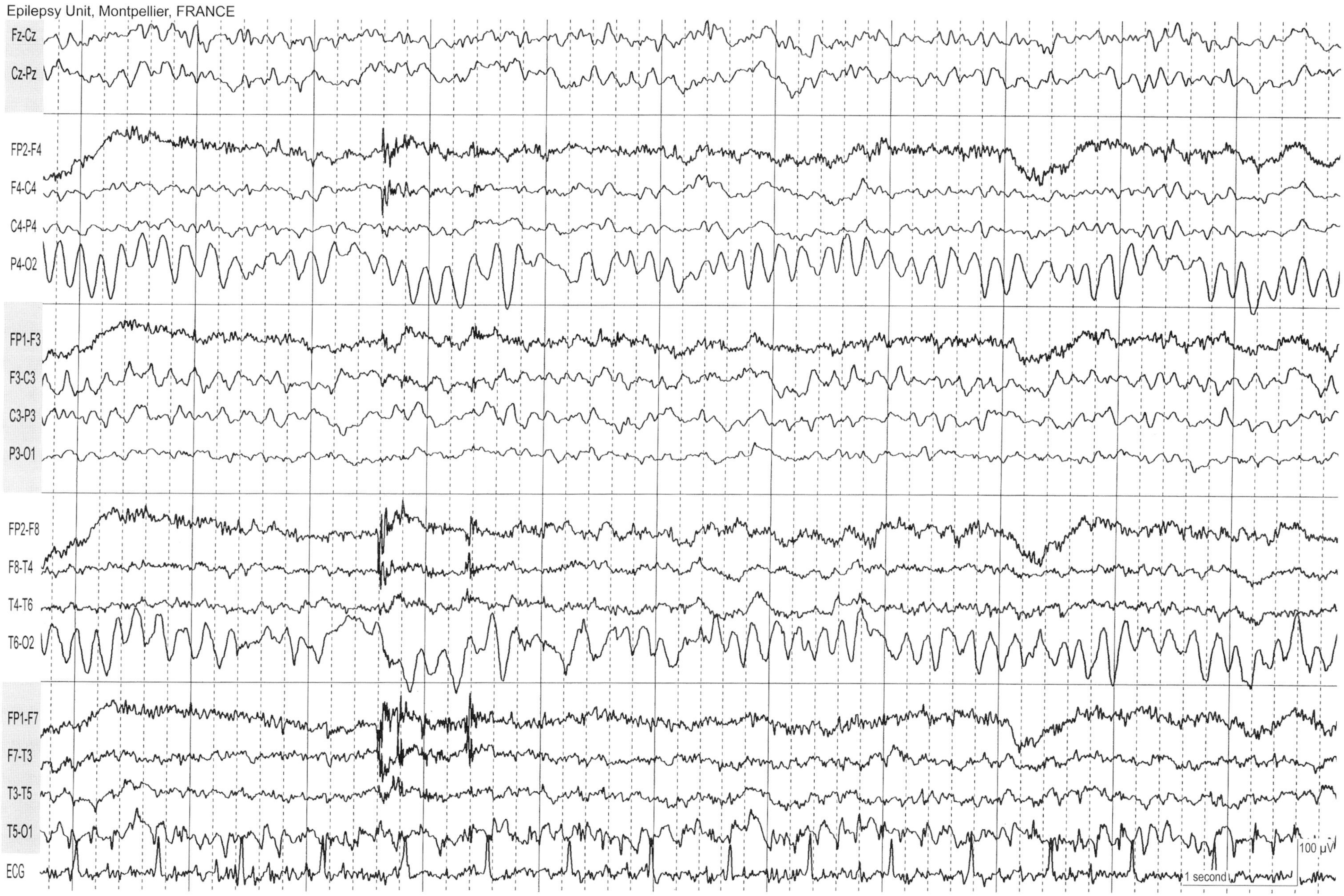
Epilepsy Unit, Montpellier, FRANCE
Fz-Cz
Cz-Pz
FP2-F4
F4-C4
C4-P4
P4-O2
FP1-F3
F3-C3
C3-P3
P3-O1
FP2-F8
F8-T4
T4-T6
T6-O2
FP1-F7
F7-T3
T3-T5
T5-O1
ECG
100 µV
1 second

IV • 20 Rhythmic movements: head movements (6)

Context

78-year-old man with a dementia.

What to note

At Fz and C3 but also at a lesser degree over the temporal regions, rhythmic sharp theta activity. The amplitude gradually builds up. The activity recorded at C3 stops suddenly but not at Fz (see plate recorded at 15 mm/s). These activities correspond to rapid head movements.

What to do

Ask the patient to stay still, keep the patient from leaning on the electrodes or try to maintain his head. This may eliminate the movement artifact but not the muscle artifacts because the patient can become even more agitated when he does not understand. The EEG technician must mention that the artifact corresponds to rhythmic movements of the head. It is quite difficult to perform an EEG in demented patients.

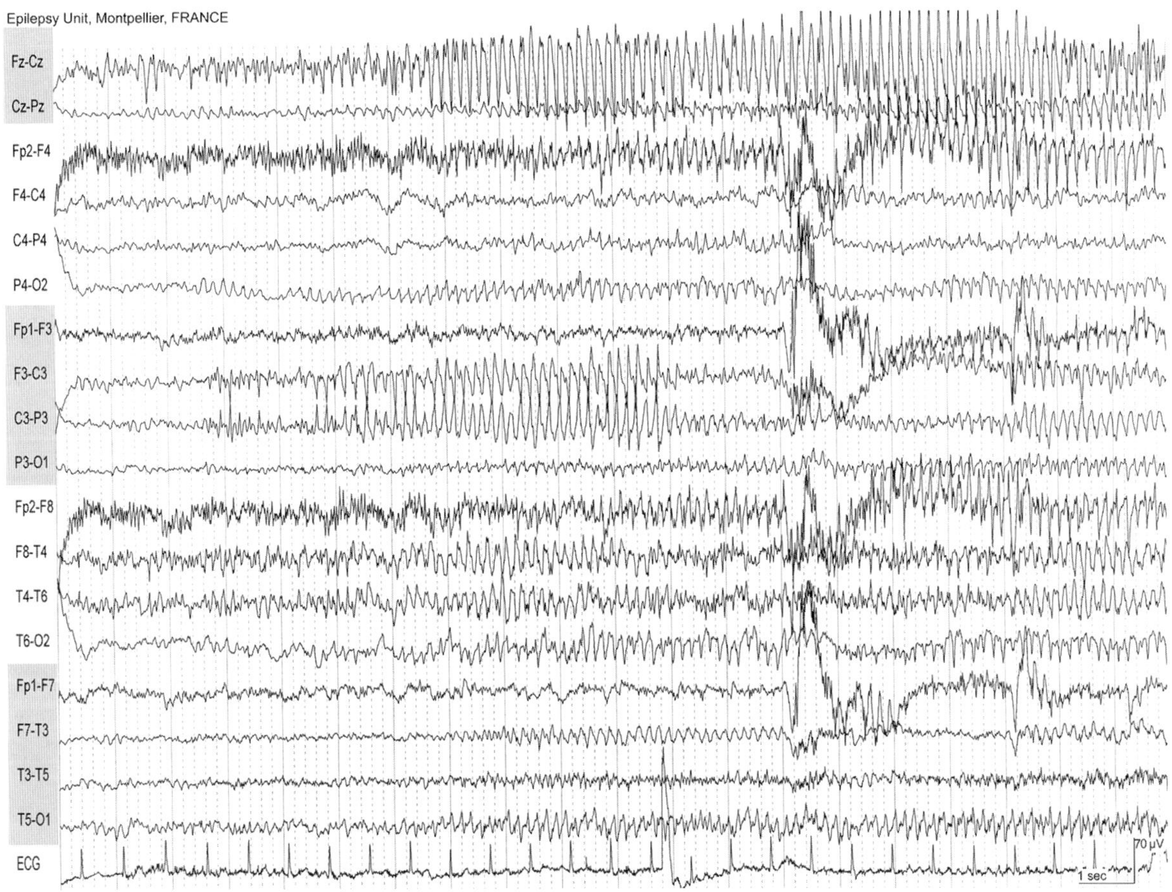

Figure a / Recording at 15 mm/s. The amplitude at Fz builds up then progressively decreases at the end of the plate when head movements decrease.

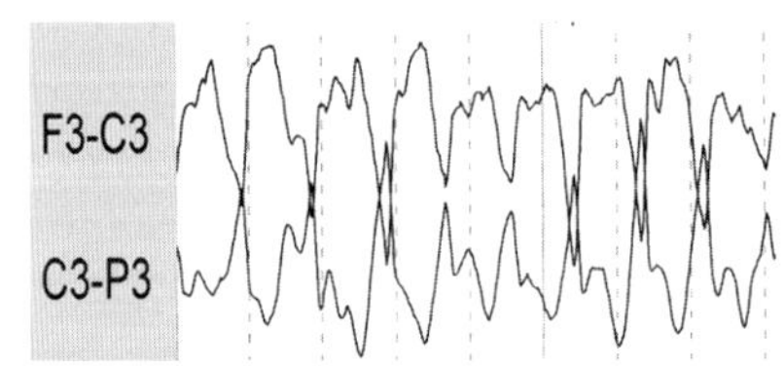

Figure b / Sharp theta activity at C3.

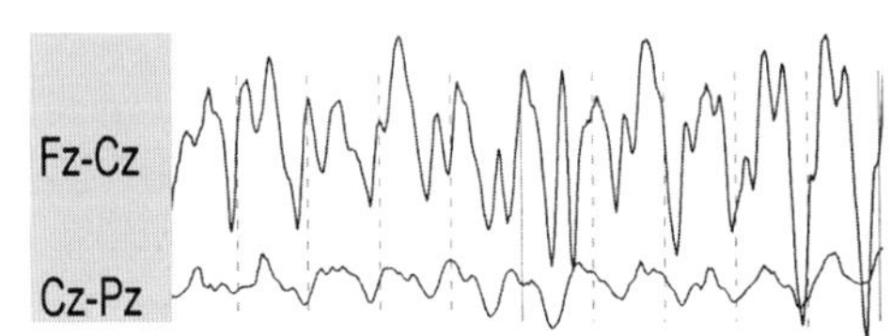

Figure c / Sharp theta activity at Fz.

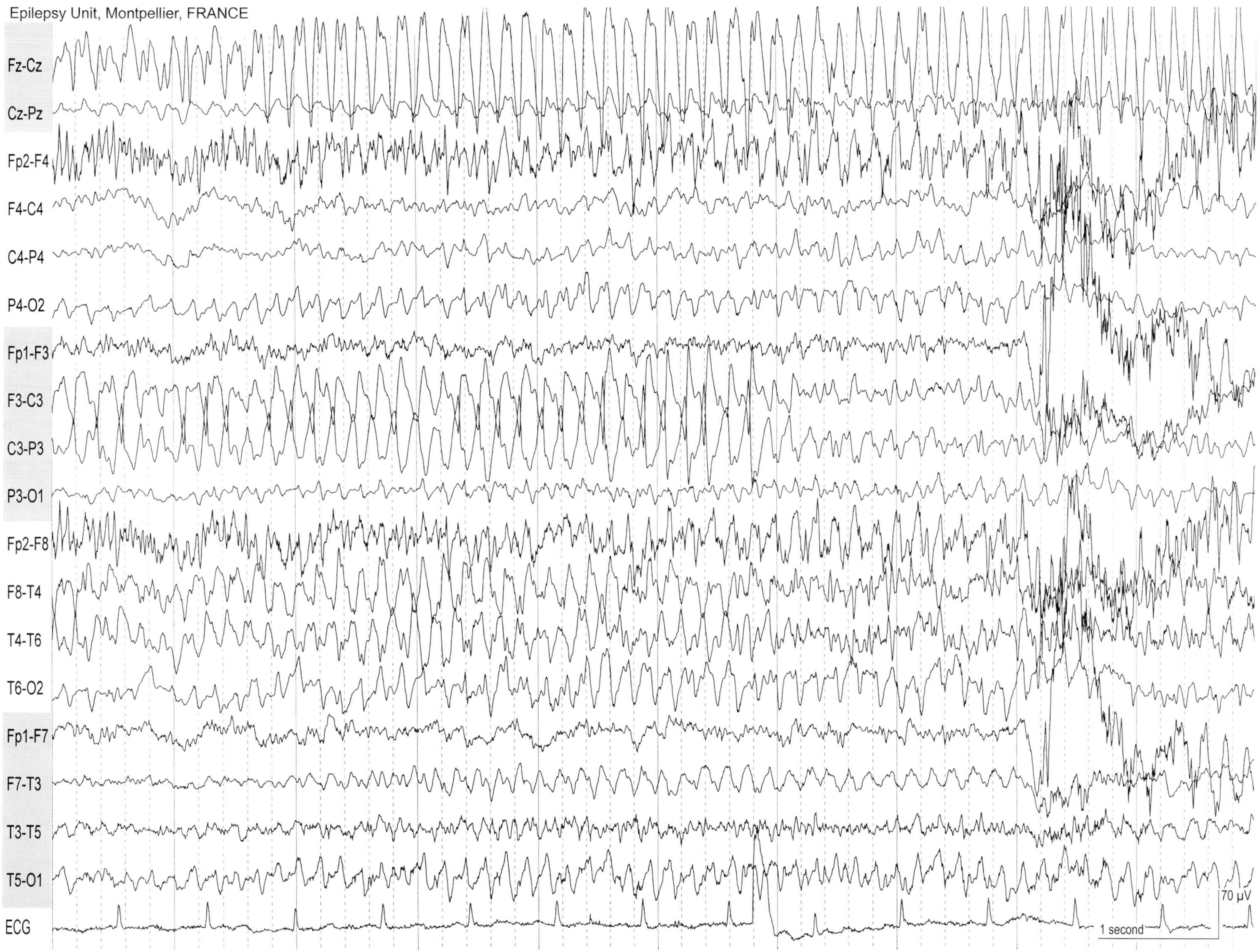
Epilepsy Unit, Montpellier, FRANCE
Fz-Cz
Cz-Pz
Fp2-F4
F4-C4
C4-P4
P4-O2
Fp1-F3
F3-C3
C3-P3
P3-O1
Fp2-F8
F8-T4
T4-T6
T6-O2
Fp1-F7
F7-T3
T3-T5
T5-O1
ECG
70 µV
1 second

IV • 21 Rhythmic movements: tremor in Parkinson's disease and dyskinesias (7)

Context

40-year-old man with Parkinson's disease.

What to note

The tracing is superimposed with muscle activities. Over the right occipital region, theta waves (5 Hz) with a somewhat sinusoidal pattern correspond to a tremor artifact. Over the left occipital region, ample sharp electrographic elements, sometimes occurring in repetitive bursts, correspond to muscle artifacts due to abnormal movements (dyskinesias).

Comment

The technician must indicate all abnormal movements of the patient during the recording. EEG is no longer a common indication in parkinsonian syndromes. The most usual artifacts are eyelid flutter and theta activity at 6 Hz (resting tremor) with or without muscle activity.

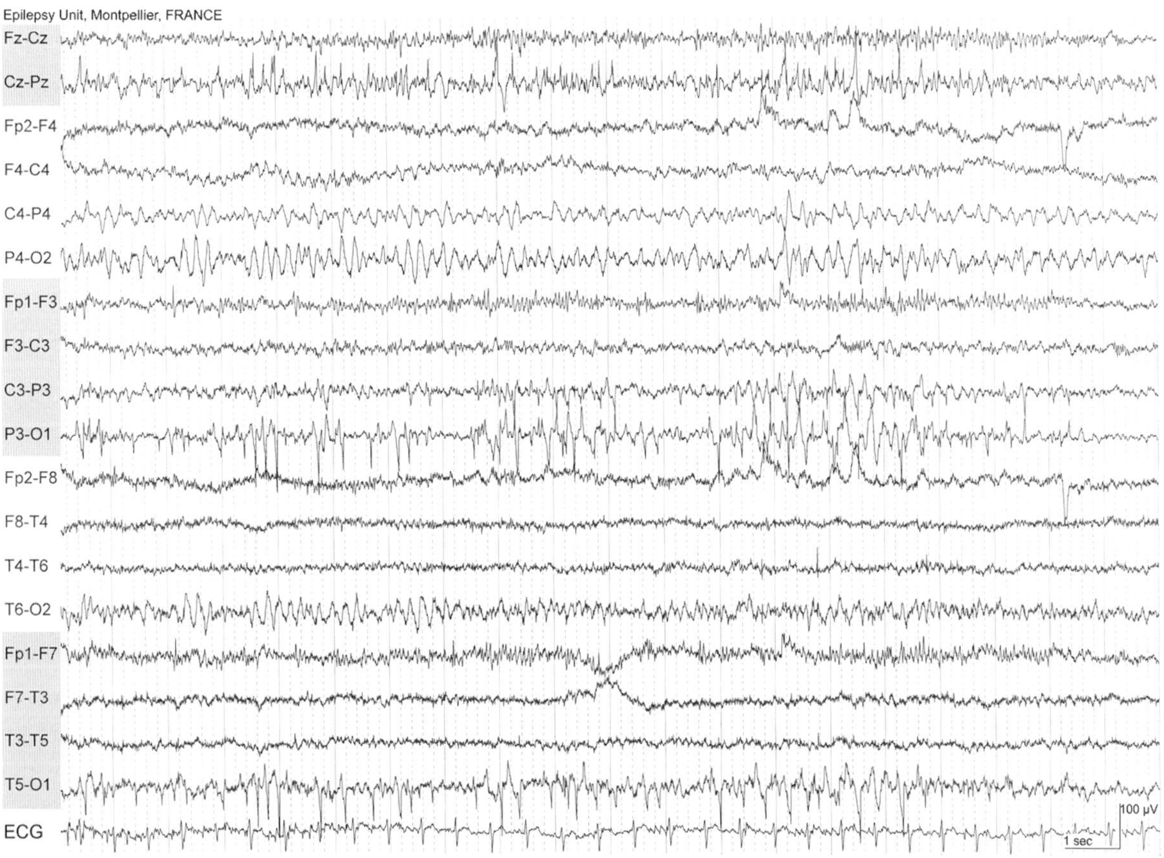

Figure a / Recording at 15 mm/s.

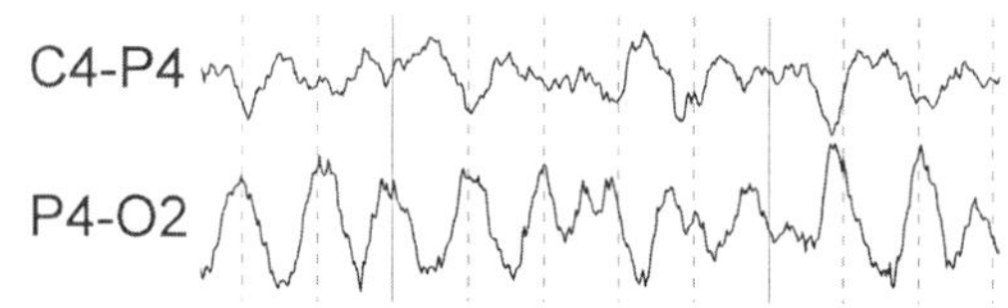

Figure b / Rhythmic theta activity recorded over the right occipital region (tremor).

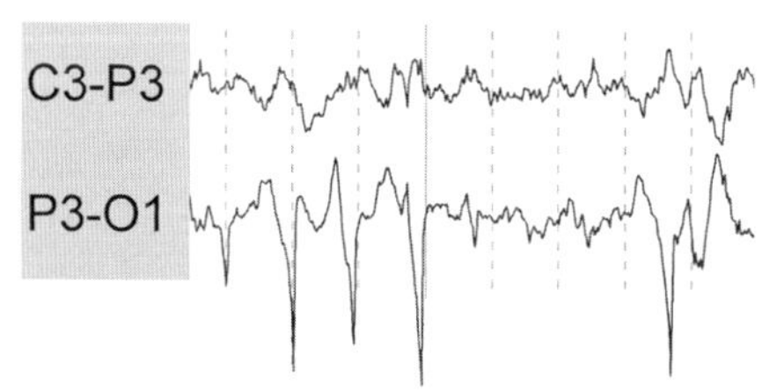

Figure c / Muscle potentials conveying an impression of very sharp waveforms (dyskinesias).

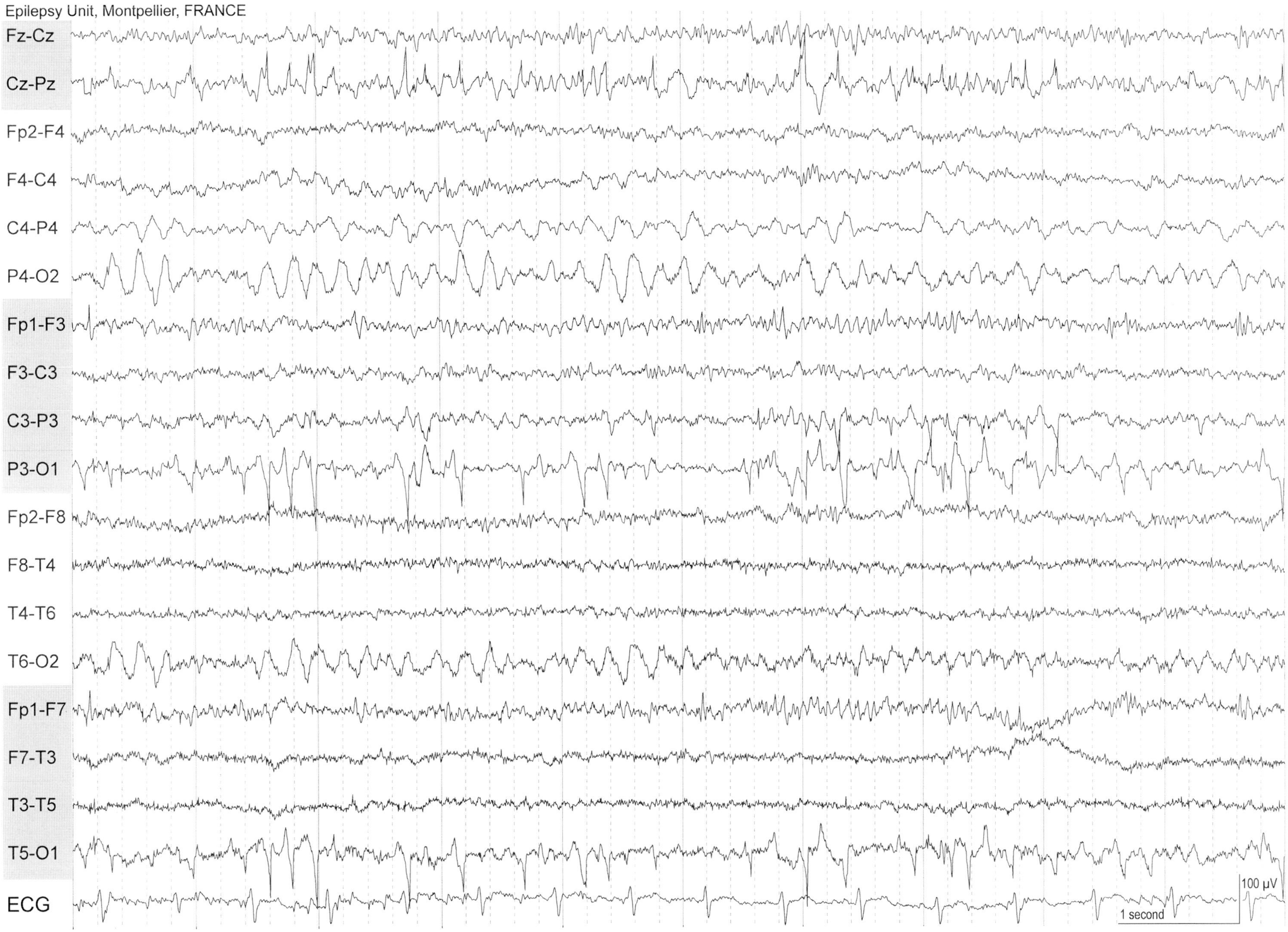
Epilepsy Unit, Montpellier, FRANCE
Fz-Cz
Cz-Pz
Fp2-F4
F4-C4
C4-P4
P4-O2
Fp1-F3
F3-C3
C3-P3
P3-O1
Fp2-F8
F8-T4
T4-T6
T6-O2
Fp1-F7
F7-T3
T3-T5
T5-O1
ECG
100 µV
1 second

IV • 22 Rhythmic movements: tremor and electrode artifact (8)

Context

50-year-old man with left temporal lobe epilepsy.

What to note

Superimposed muscle activities, especially over the left temporal region. Rhythmic polyphasic activity at 7 Hz corresponding to oscillating movements of the head at T6. This activity spreads to the occipital regions. On the Cz-Pz derivation theta/delta waves. Some waves have a square morphology. Other waves mimic spikes. This is an electrode artifact because the waves only involve one electrode (Pz). The Fz-Cz derivation is low-voltage compared with the others due to excess electrode gel between Fz and Cz.

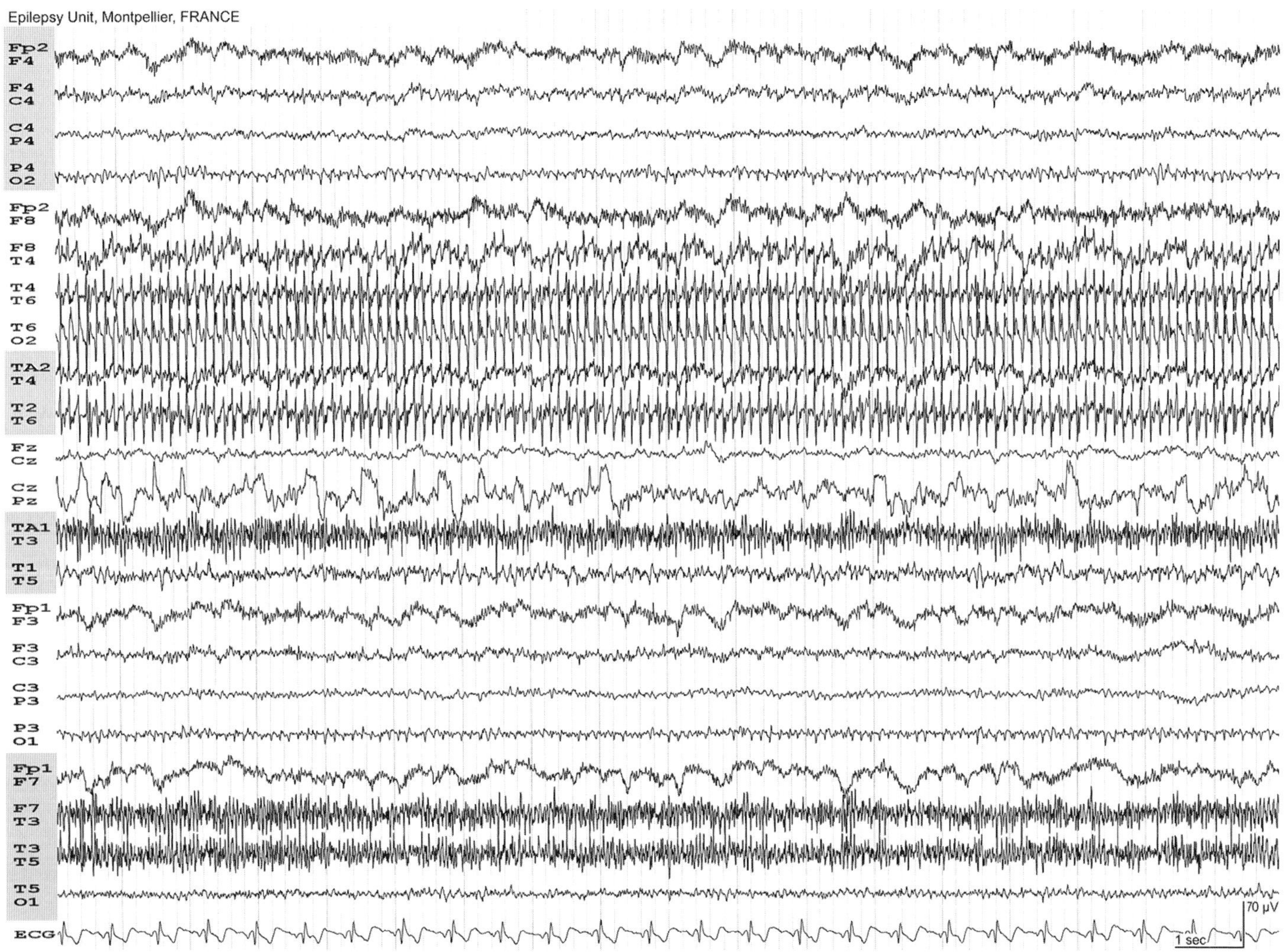

Figure a / Recording at 15 mm/s.

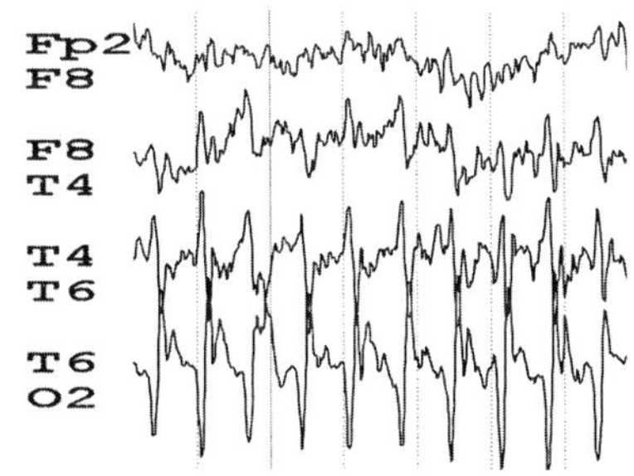

Figure b / Artifact of tremor at T6.

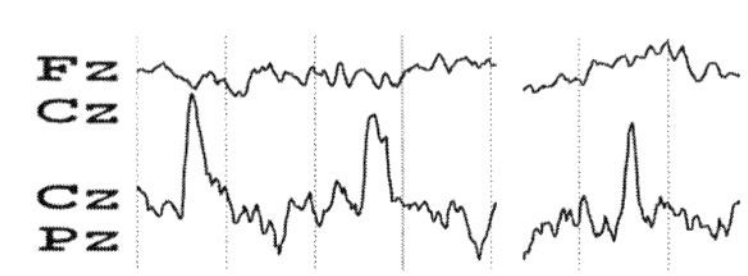

Figure c / Electrode artifacts that mimic spikes.

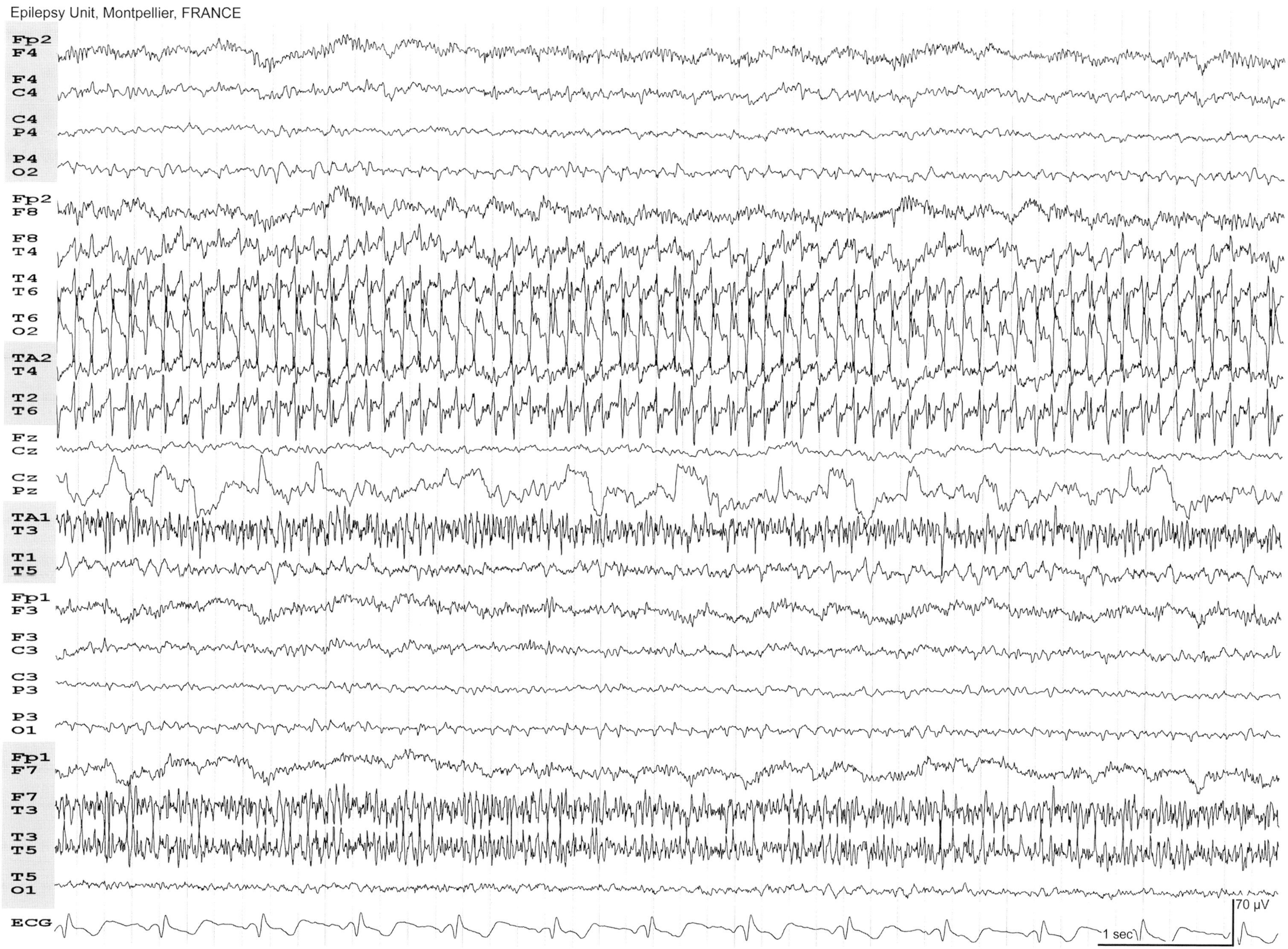
Epilepsy Unit, Montpellier, FRANCE
Fp2 F4
F4 C4
C4 P4
P4 O2
Fp2 F8
F8 T4
T4 T6
T6 O2
TA2 T4
T2 T6
Fz Cz
Cz Pz
TA1 T3
T1 T5
Fp1 F3
F3 C3
C3 P3
P3 O1
Fp1 F7
F7 T3
T3 T5
T5 O1
ECG
70 µV
1 sec

IV • 23 Electrode artifacts (1)

Context

30-year-old woman referred after a first generalized tonic-clonic seizure. After recurrence of seizures, a diagnosis of juvenile myoclonic epilepsy was made.

What to note

The patient's eyes are closed. Background activity with 10 Hz alpha rhythm. On the left temporal region, sharp theta/delta waves. This is an electrode artifact because the waves only involve one electrode (T3). Interictal abnormalities spread to the adjacent region and are not limited to one electrode. Correction of T3 led to cessation of the slow activity (see below plate recorded at 15 mm/s).

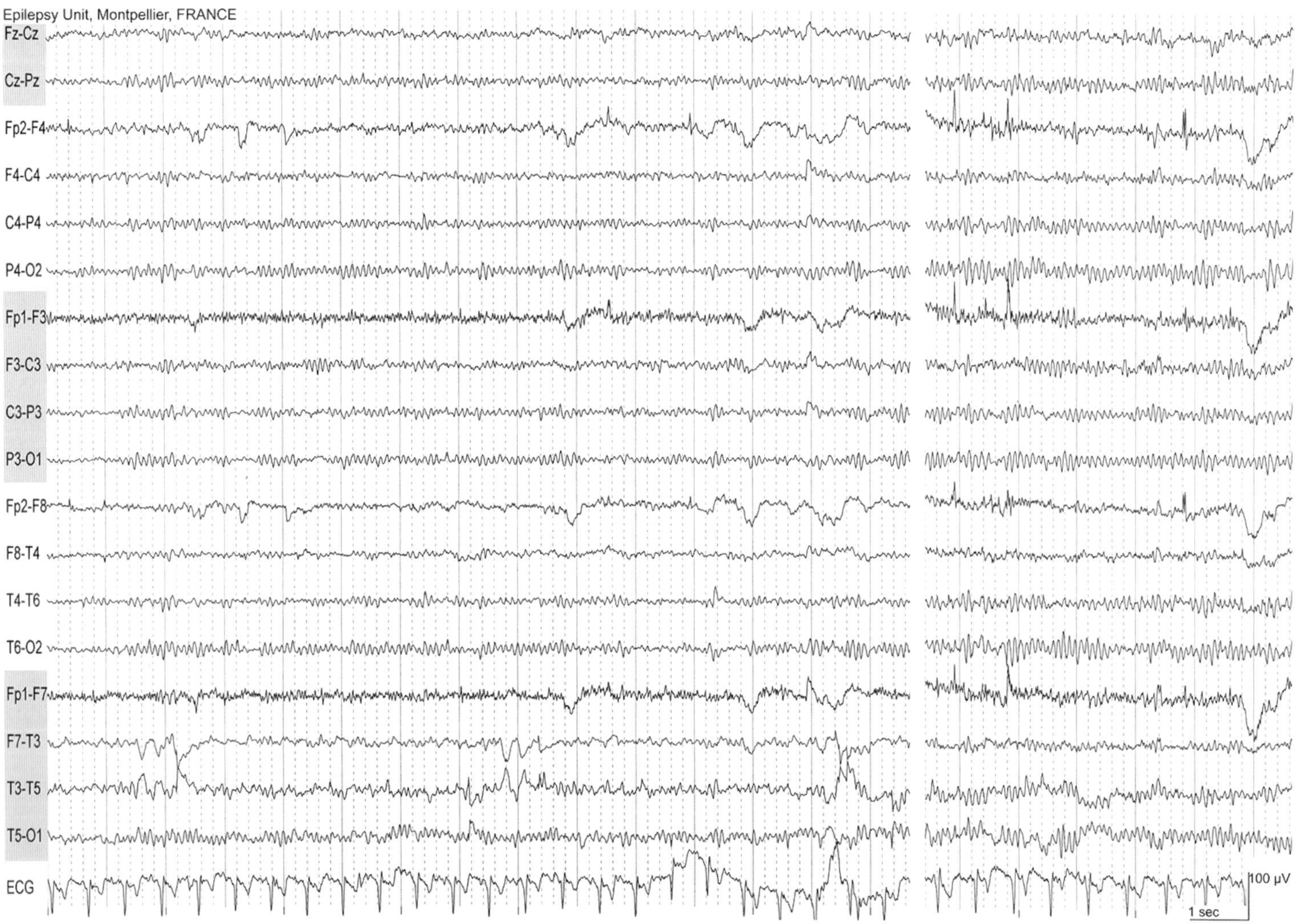

Figure a / Recording at 15 mm/s. Correction of T3 led to cessation of the slow activity (right plate).

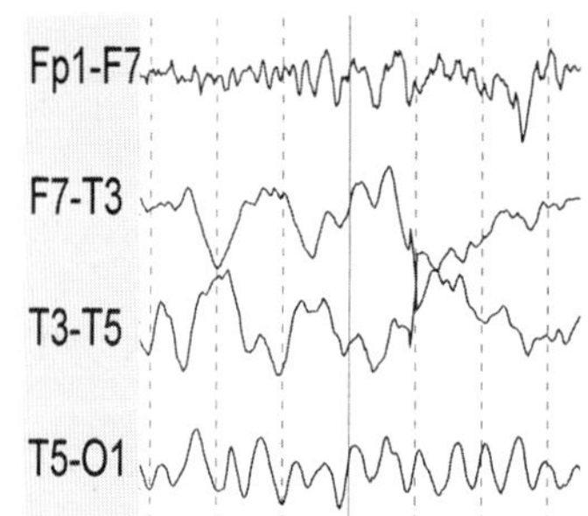

Figure b / Electrode artifact at T3. Muscle activity at Fp1-F7.

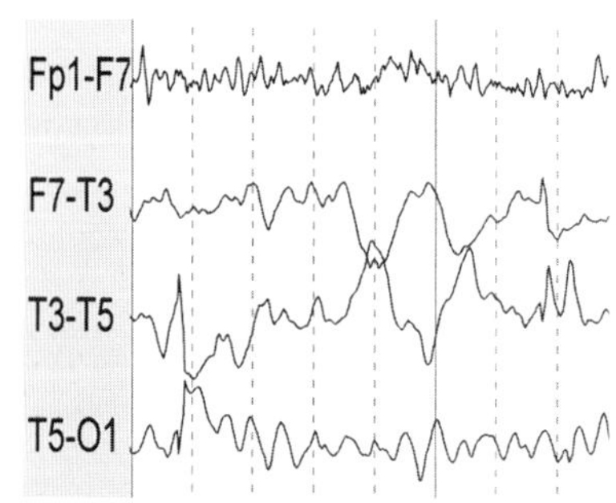

Figure c / Electrode artifact at T3. Muscle activity at Fp1-F7.

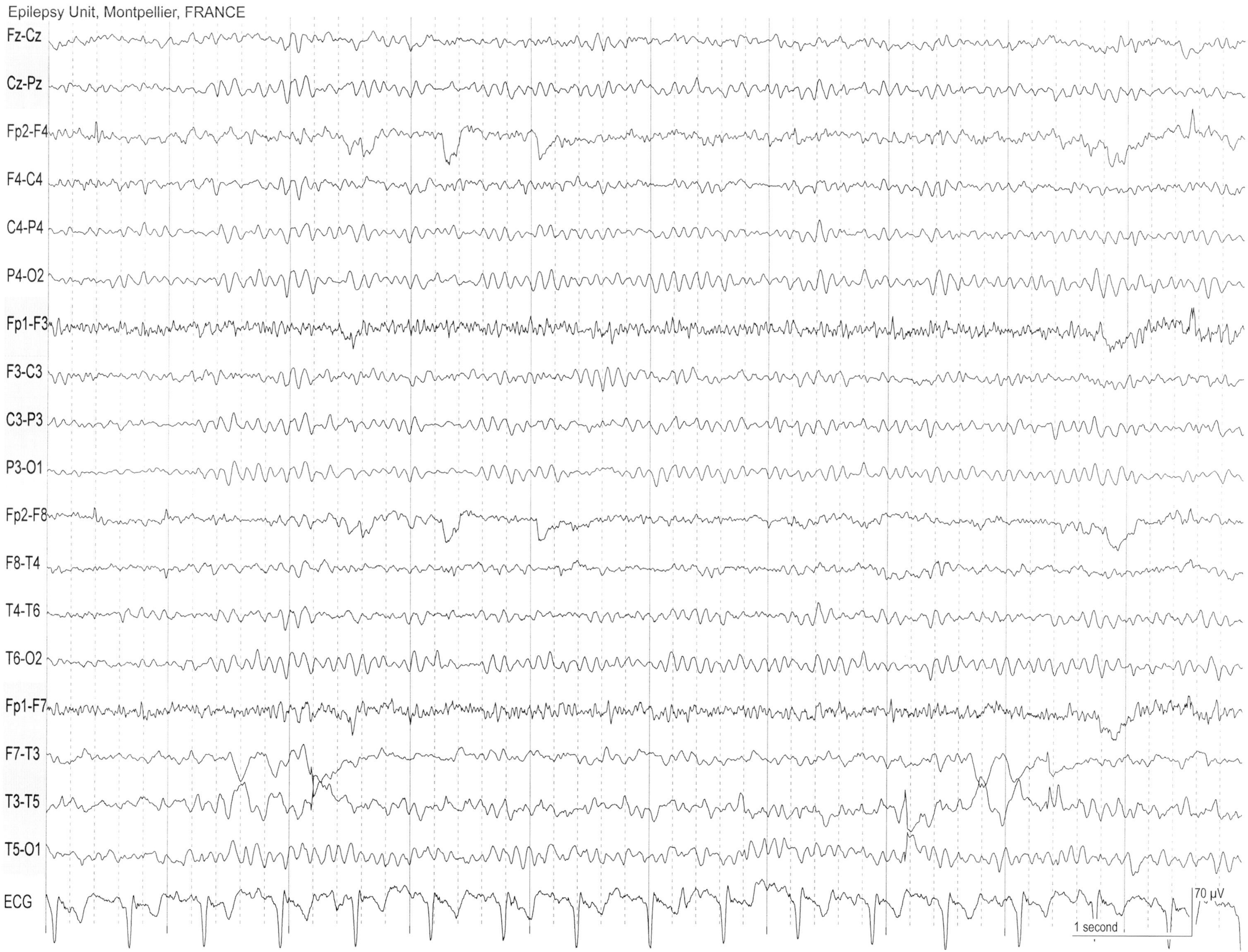
Epilepsy Unit, Montpellier, FRANCE
Fz-Cz
Cz-Pz
Fp2-F4
F4-C4
C4-P4
P4-O2
Fp1-F3
F3-C3
C3-P3
P3-O1
Fp2-F8
F8-T4
T4-T6
T6-O2
Fp1-F7
F7-T3
T3-T5
T5-O1
ECG
70 µV
1 second

IV • 24 Electrode artifacts (2)

Context

39-year-old man with cryptococcosis and neuromeningeal complications and several faints, one causing a car crash.

What to note

The patient's eyes are open. Continuous slow irregular activity (4 to 5 Hz) at O1. This electrode artifact is caused by poor lead-scalp interface. Had there been a slow focus, several electrodes would have been involved. Correction of O1 led to cessation of the slow activity (see below, plate recorded at 15 mm/s). A "pop" electrode artefact can also be seen at F8.

What to do

Identify an electrode artifact whenever the activity is clearly confined to a single electrode and always attempt to correct it. First lead-scalp interface should be examined, after which the impedances should be examined if necessary. Also check whether the patient is leaning on O1.

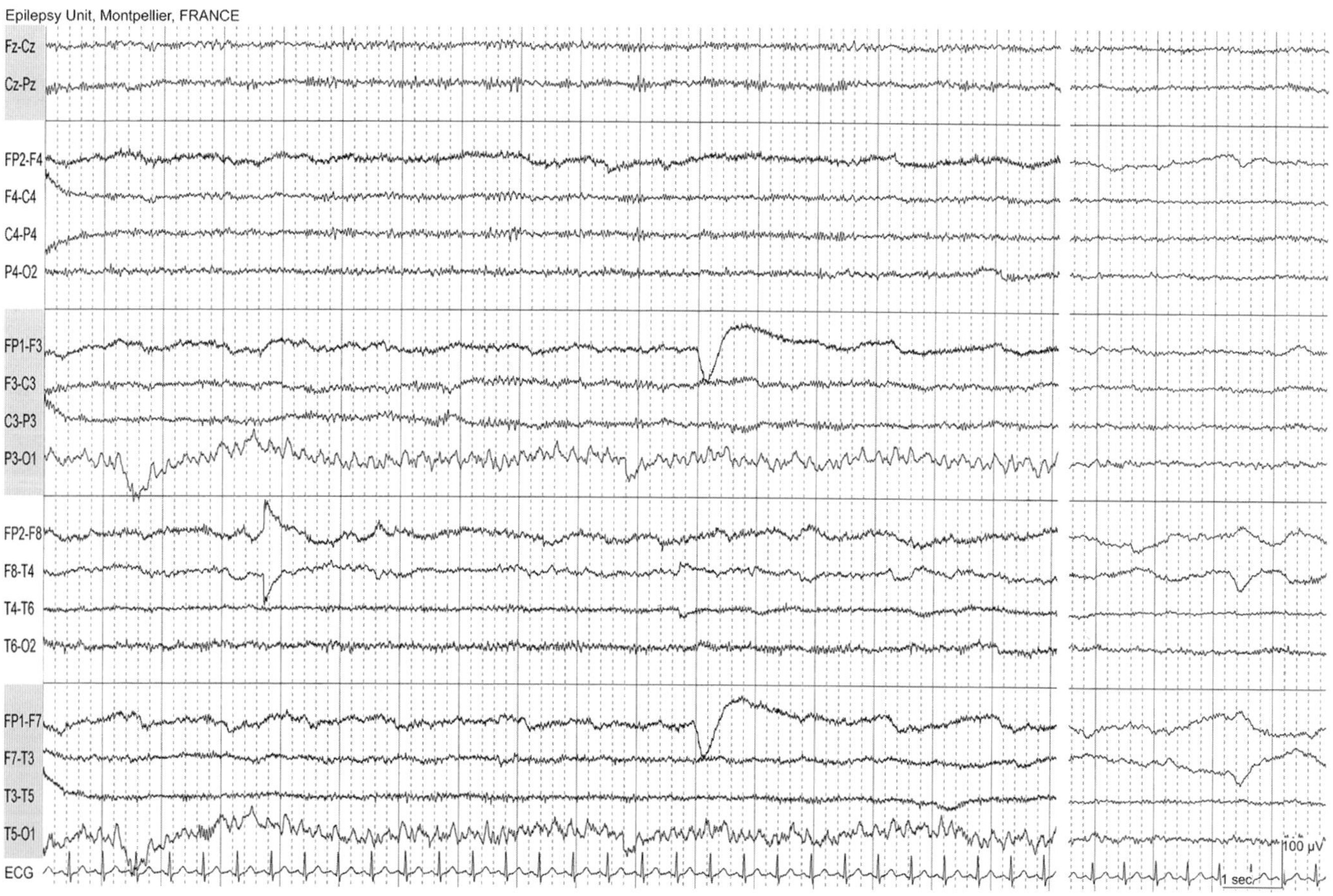

Figure a / Recording at 15 mm/s. Right plate, cessation of the artifact at O1 after correction of the electrode. Muscle activities can be seen on the left plate, but not on the right plate when the patient is more relaxed.

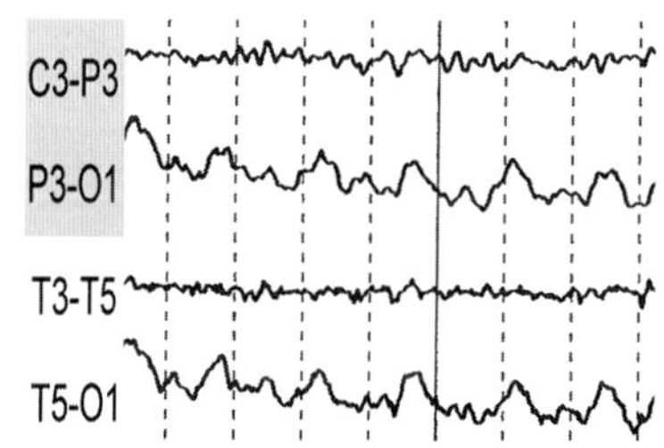

Figure b / Electrode artifact at O1.

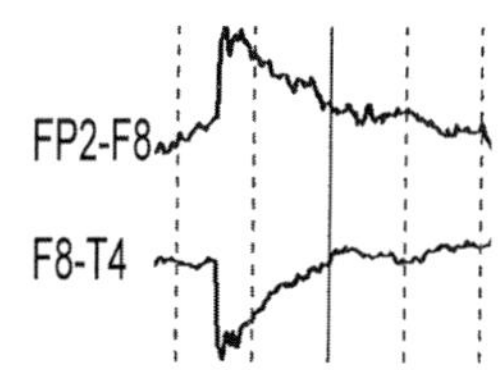

Figure c / "Pop" electrode artifact (F8).

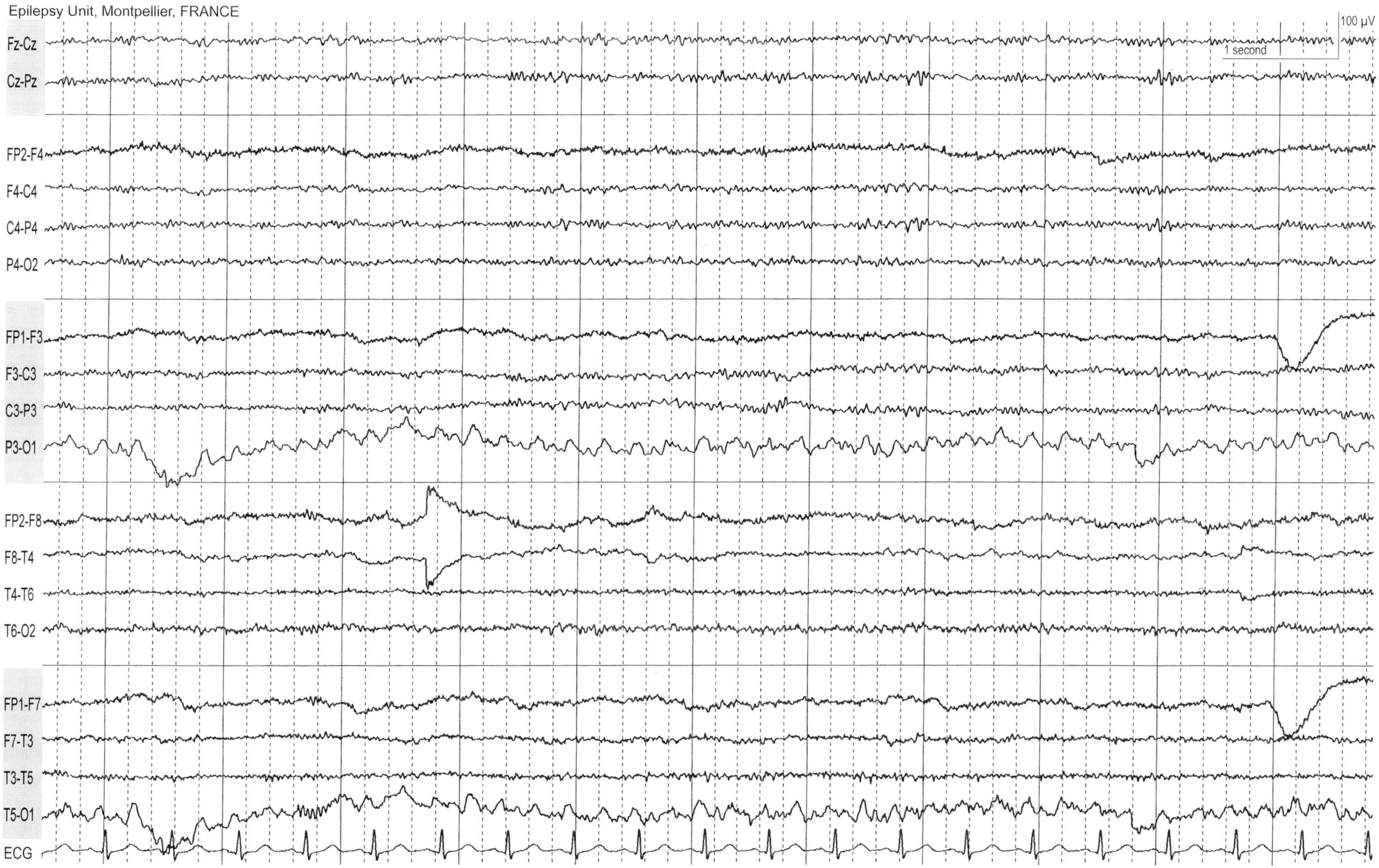
Epilepsy Unit, Montpellier, FRANCE
100 µV
1 second
Fz-Cz
Cz-Pz
FP2-F4
F4-C4
C4-P4
P4-O2
FP1-F3
F3-C3
C3-P3
P3-O1
FP2-F8
F8-T4
T4-T6
T6-O2
FP1-F7
F7-T3
T3-T5
T5-O1
ECG

IV • 25 Hiccup artifact and 50 Hz interference

Context

Premature infant, born at 32 weeks.

What to note

Slow high-amplitude diphasic pseudoperiodical complexes over the two hemispheres and on the ECG: hiccup artifact. There is also a 50 Hz interference involving all derivations but above all the left supra-sylvian derivations. This artifact is modified due to the presence of a low-pass 30 Hz filter used along with notch filter (50 Hz). The respiration channel is partially defective here

What to do

Make detailed note on the tracing whenever hiccups occurs. To eliminate the 50 or 60 Hz interference, use the notch filter which only filters the 50 or 60 Hz frequency. Then check impedances, the ground electrode, and make sure no wires are broken. And if the artifact is still not eliminated, look for other sources: electric appliance or device, outlet without ground, contact between wires or between the headbox and a metal object, etc.

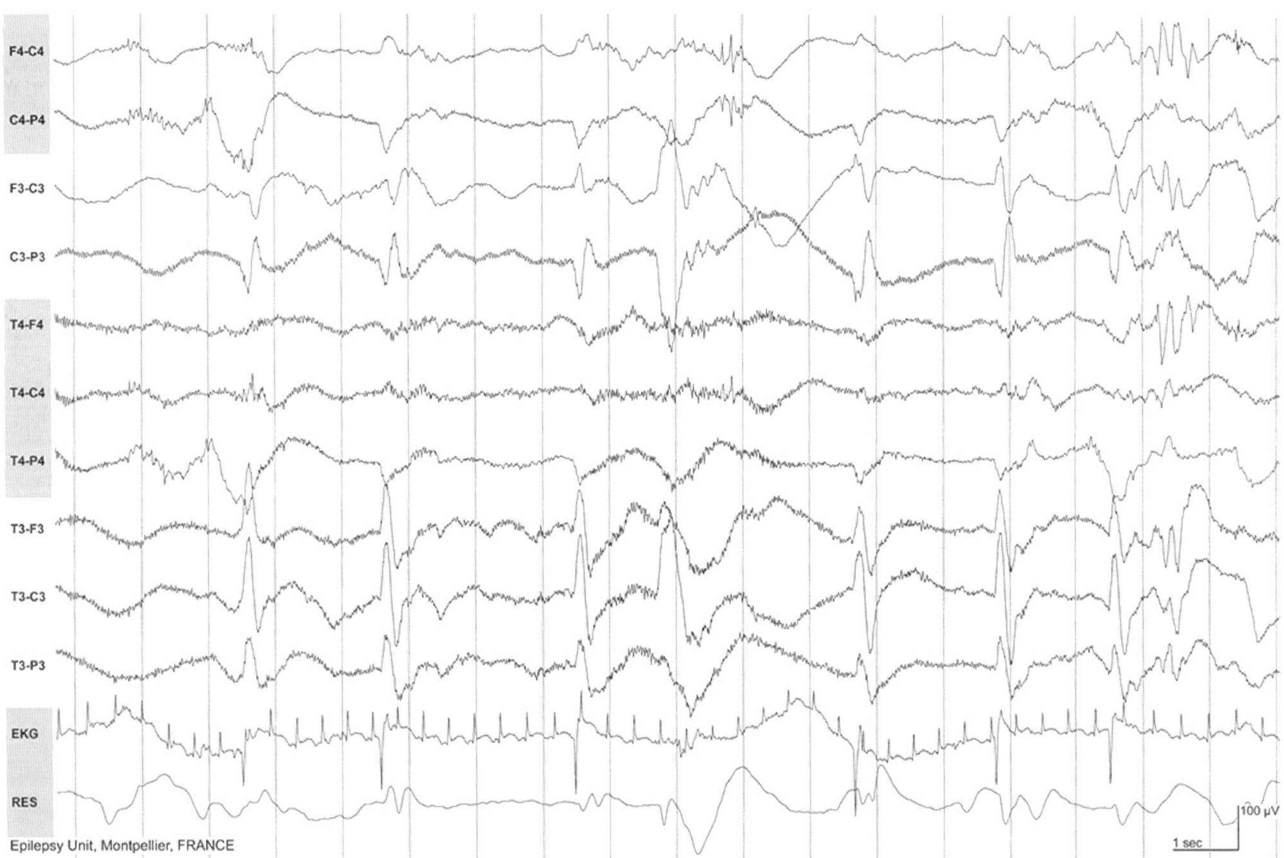

Figure a / Recording at 15 mm/s.

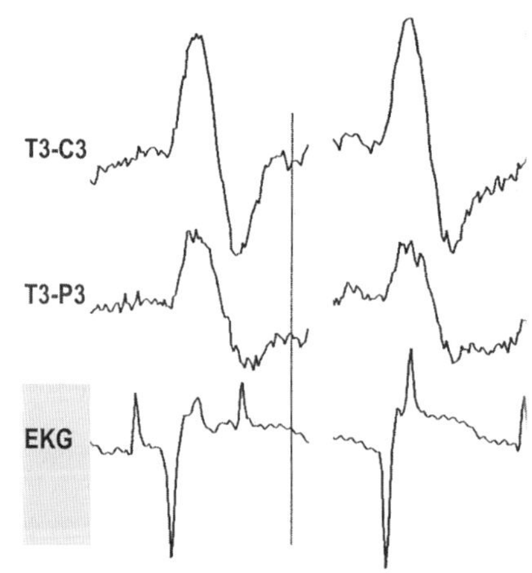

Figure b / High-voltage slow complexes corresponding to a hiccup artifact, also visible on the ECG.

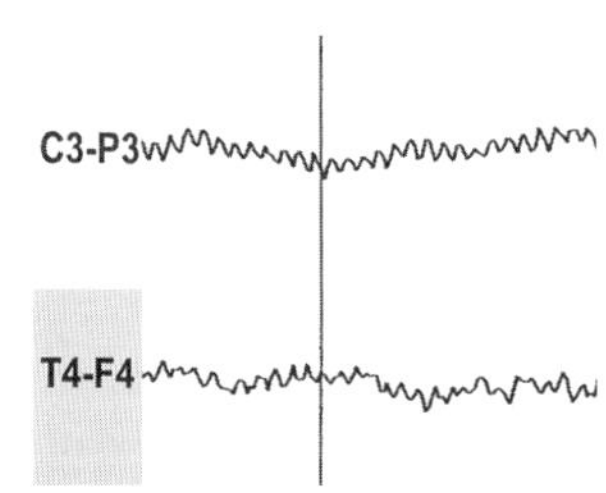

Figure c / A 50 Hz interference filtered with a low pass 30 Hz filter.

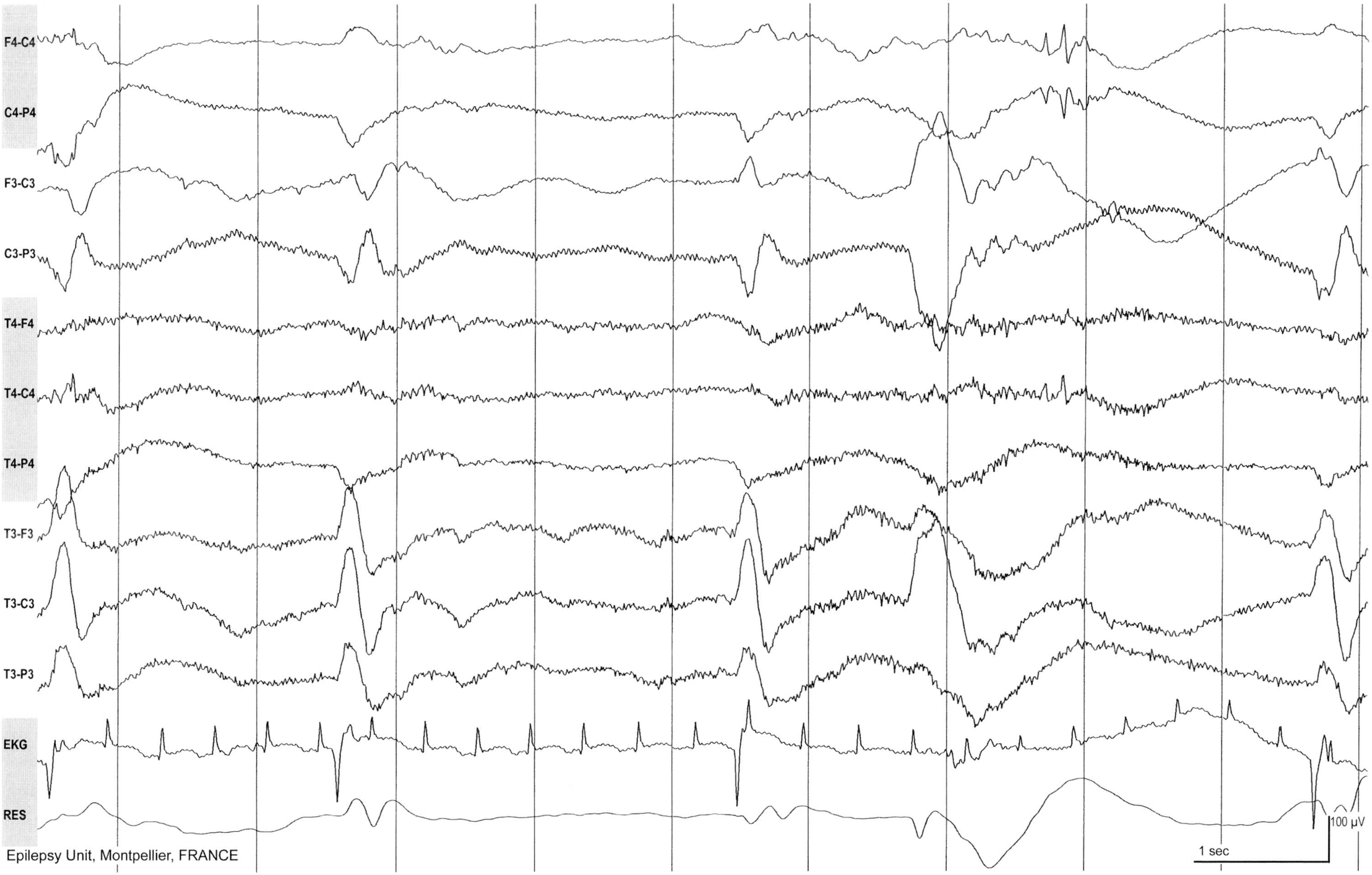
F4-C4
C4-P4
F3-C3
C3-P3
T4-F4
T4-C4
T4-P4
T3-F3
T3-C3
T3-P3
EKG
RES
Epilepsy Unit, Montpellier, FRANCE
1 sec
100 µV

IV • 26 Instrumental and environmental artifacts: incubators

Context

Premature neonate.

What to note

Fast potentials of very low amplitude in bursts mainly over the right temporal region. These potentials cease when the incubator is turned off (right side of the plate).

What to do

Identify the origin interfering with the EEG signal so as to eliminate it. Instrumental/environmental artifacts can be very troublesome especially in intensive care units. The technician should try plugging the EEG into another socket, request interruption if possible of other devices, switch off the neon lights. Impedances, ground electrode, wires and lead-scalp interfaces must also be systematically verified.

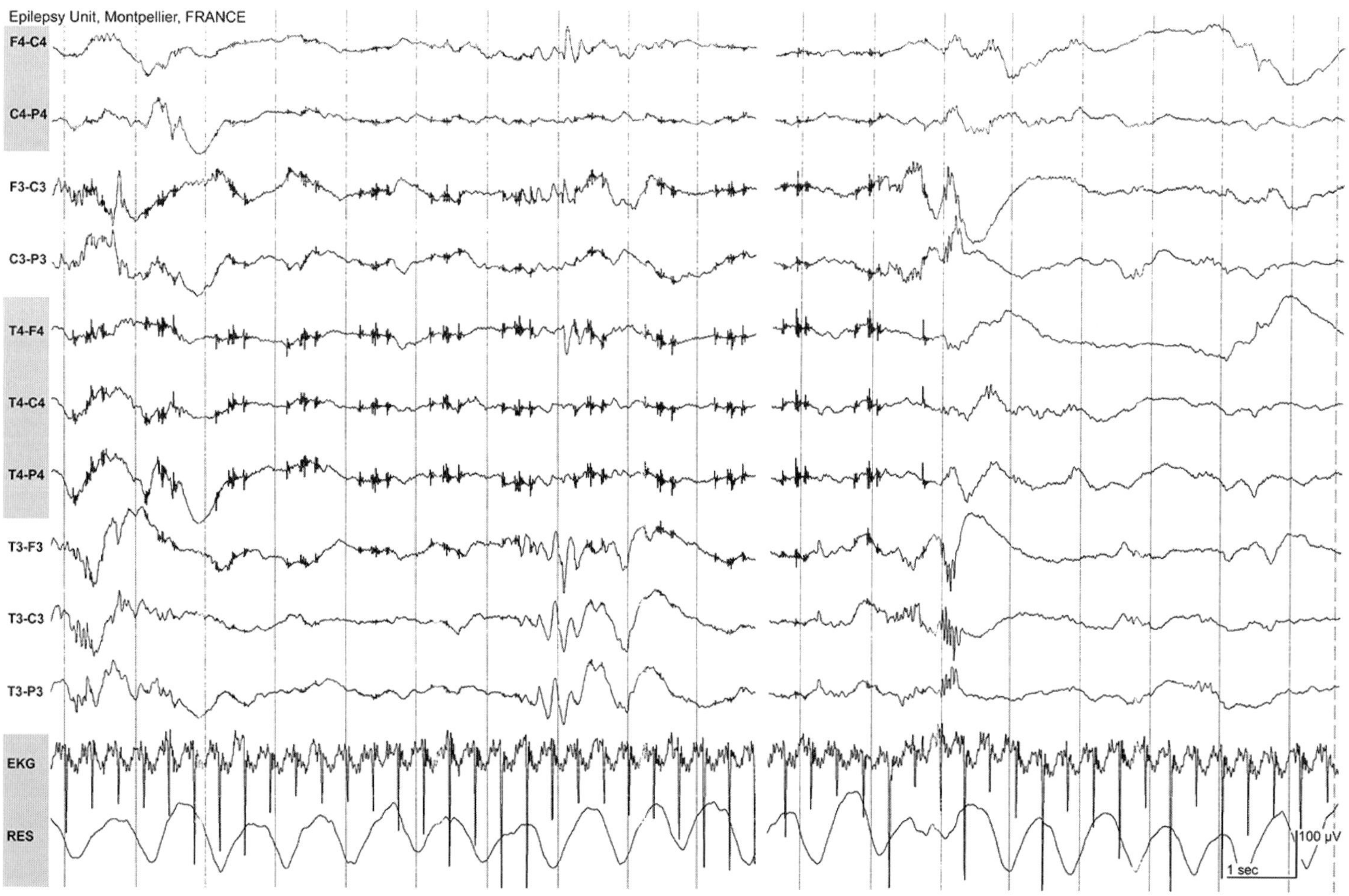

Figure a / Recording at 15 mm/s.

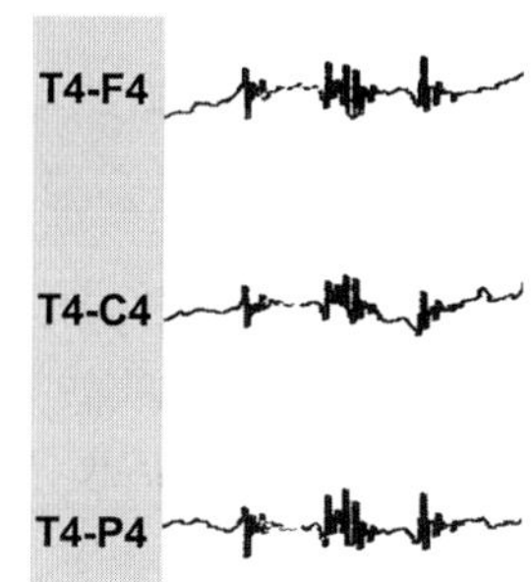

Figure b / Bursts of fast activities.

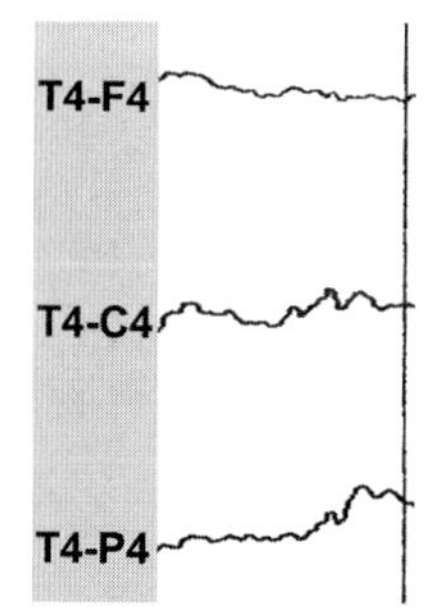

Figure c / The bursts cease when the incubator is turned off.

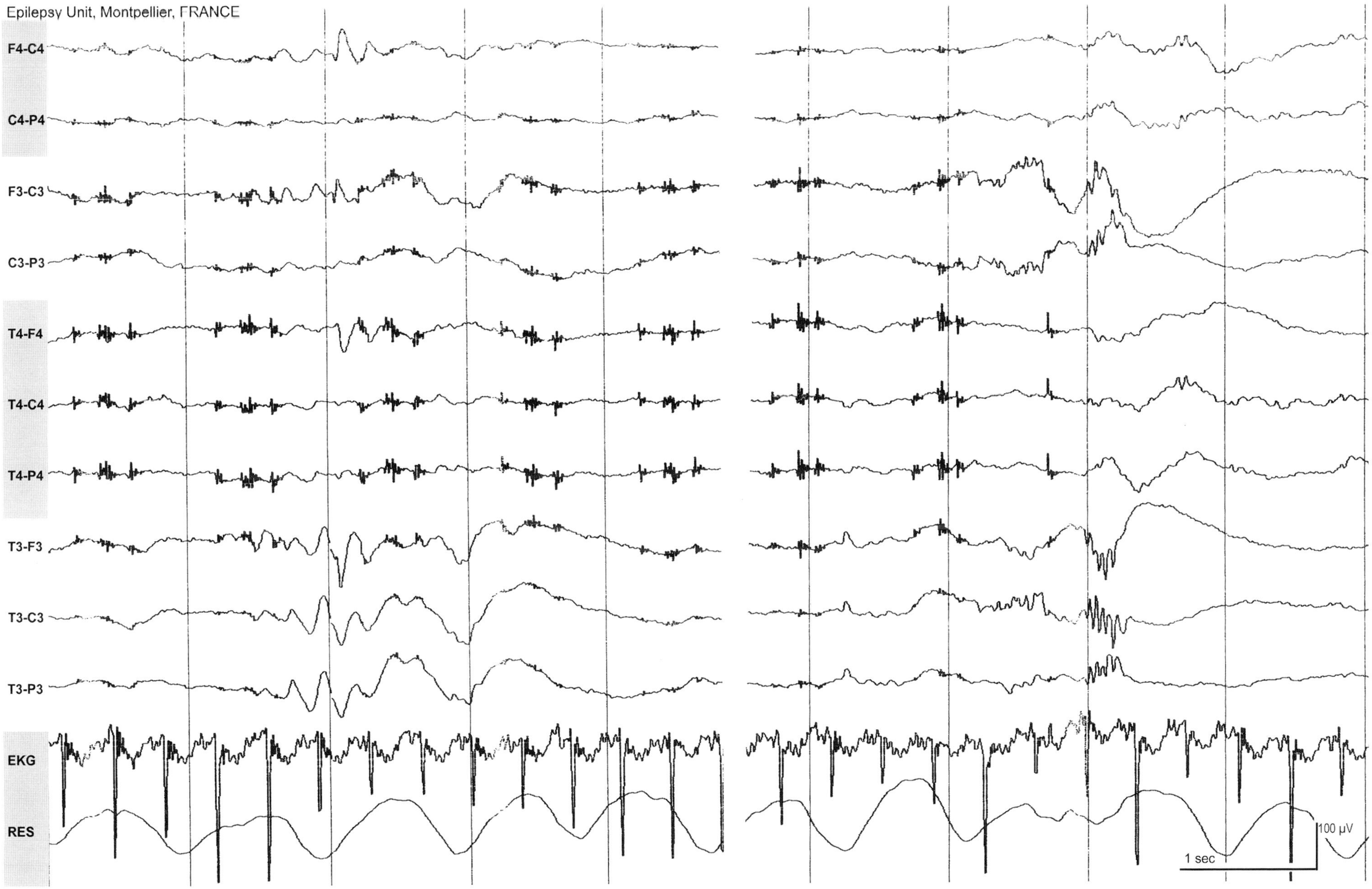

Epilepsy Unit, Montpellier, FRANCE
F4-C4
C4-P4
F3-C3
C3-P3
T4-F4
T4-C4
T4-P4
T3-F3
T3-C3
T3-P3
EKG
RES
100 µV
1 sec

IV • 27 Chewing movements (1)

Context

16-year-old woman with idiopathic generalized epilepsy.

What to note

Awake, eating lunch. Bursts of muscle potentials are predominant over the temporal regions. This muscle activity creates the false impression of a polyspike-wave discharge.

What to do and comment

Make minute notes of patient's activities does. Check the video when reading the EEG. It is important when first analyzing an EEG not to use a muscle activity filter, as filtered muscle activity can be mistaken for epileptiform activity. Likewise, when there are few electrodes, for example with ambulatory-EEG recordings, this type of activity could be mistaken for interictal or ictal epileptic activity if the patient does not indicate that he was eating.

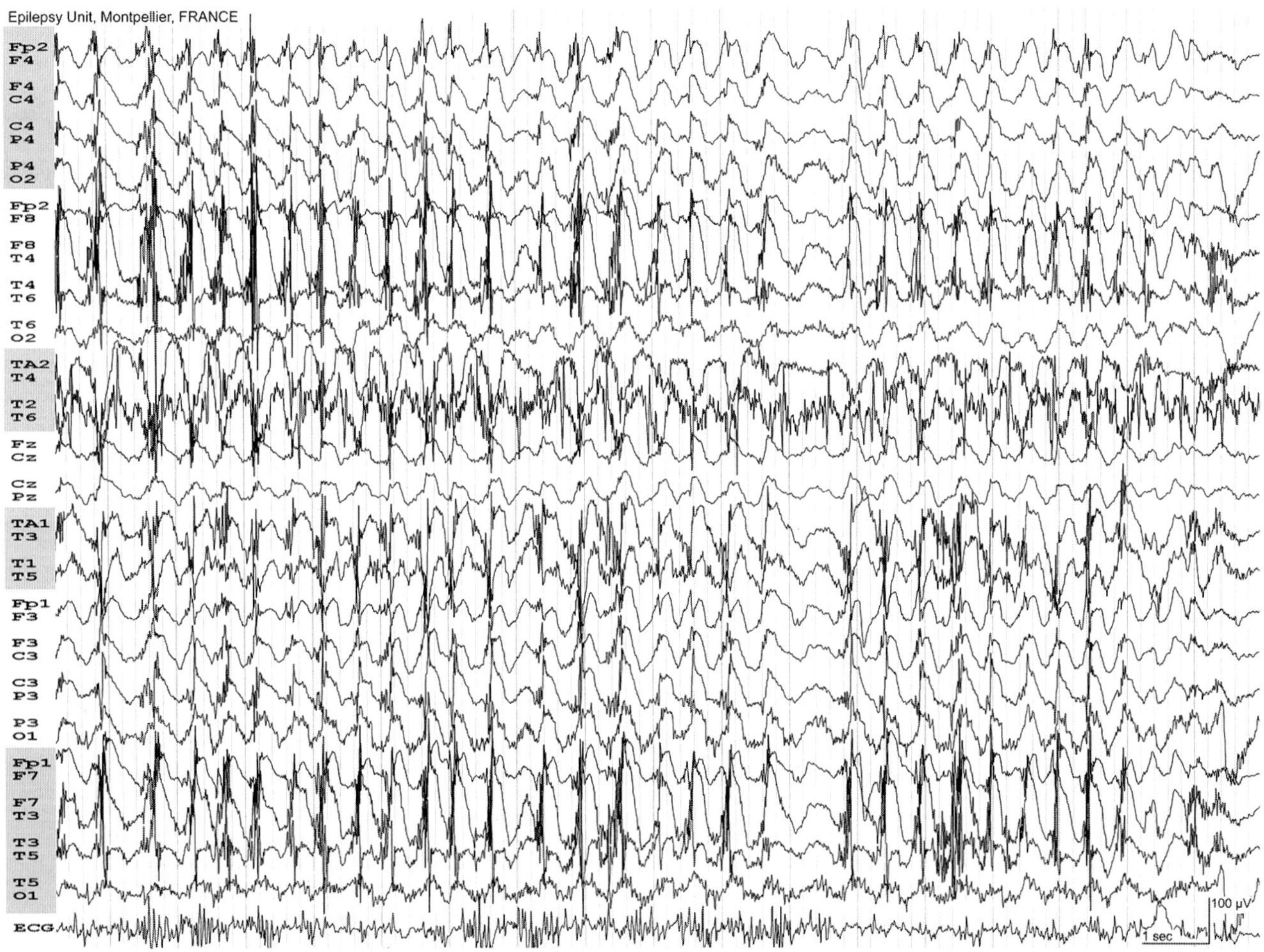

Figure a / Recording at 15 mm/s.

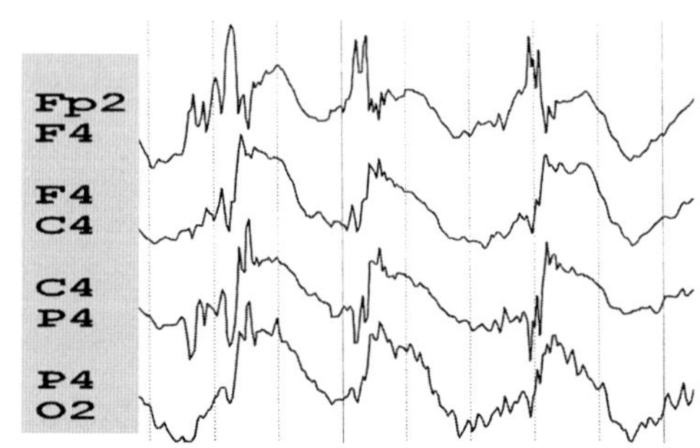

Figure b / Muscle potentials due to chewing.

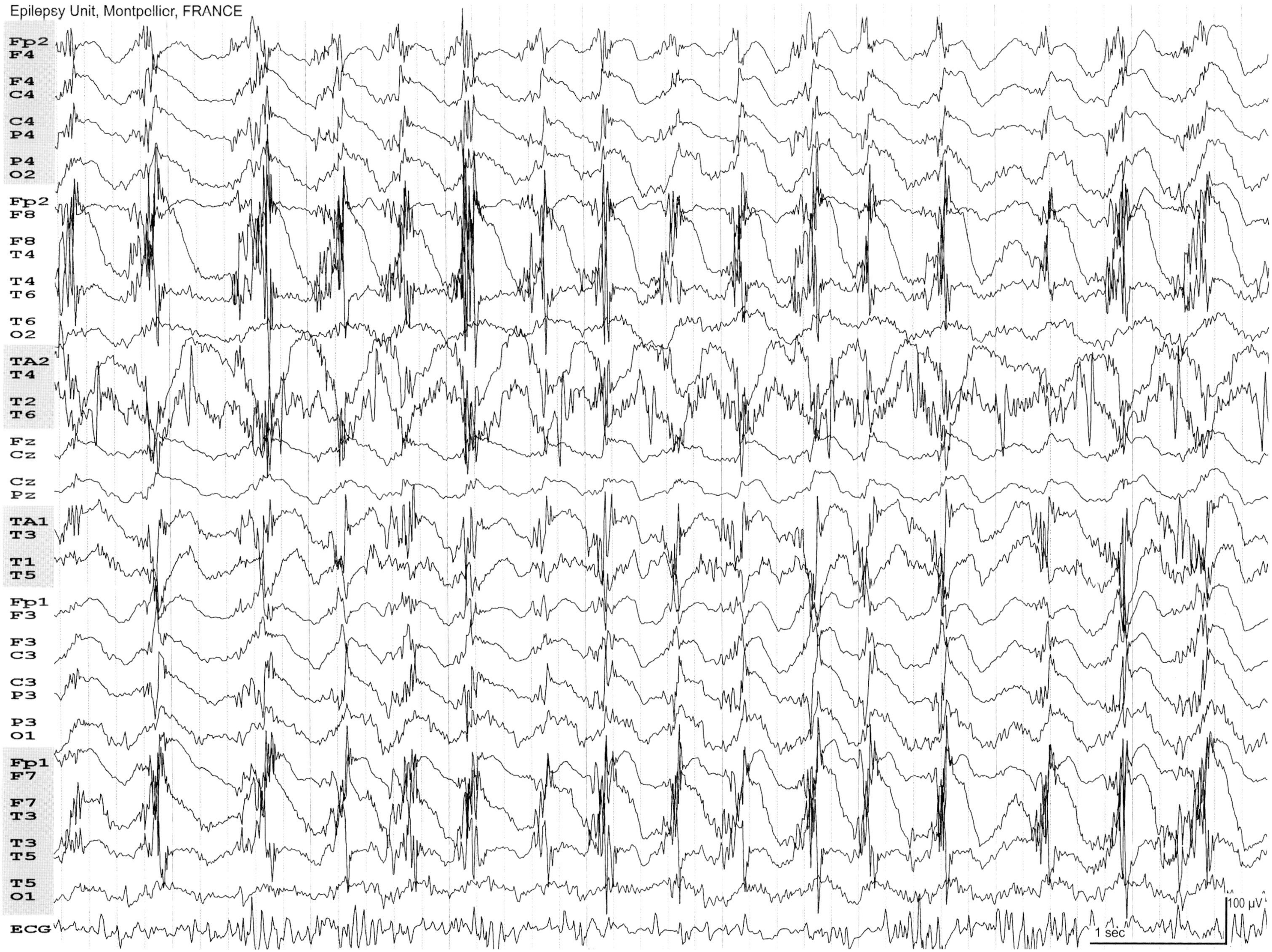
Epilepsy Unit, Montpellier, FRANCE
Fp2 F4
F4 C4
C4 P4
P4 O2
Fp2 F8
F8 T4
T4 T6
T6 O2
TA2 T4
T2 T6
Fz Cz
Cz Pz
TA1 T3
T1 T5
Fp1 F3
F3 C3
C3 P3
P3 O1
Fp1 F7
F7 T3
T3 T5
T5 O1
ECG
100 µV
1 sec

• 28 Chewing movements (2)

Context

14-old girl with juvenile myoclonic epilepsy.

What to note

Bubble-gum (should not be allowed during EEG). Bursts of muscle potentials. The bursts are generalized. Note the presence of a mu rhythm over the left central regions.

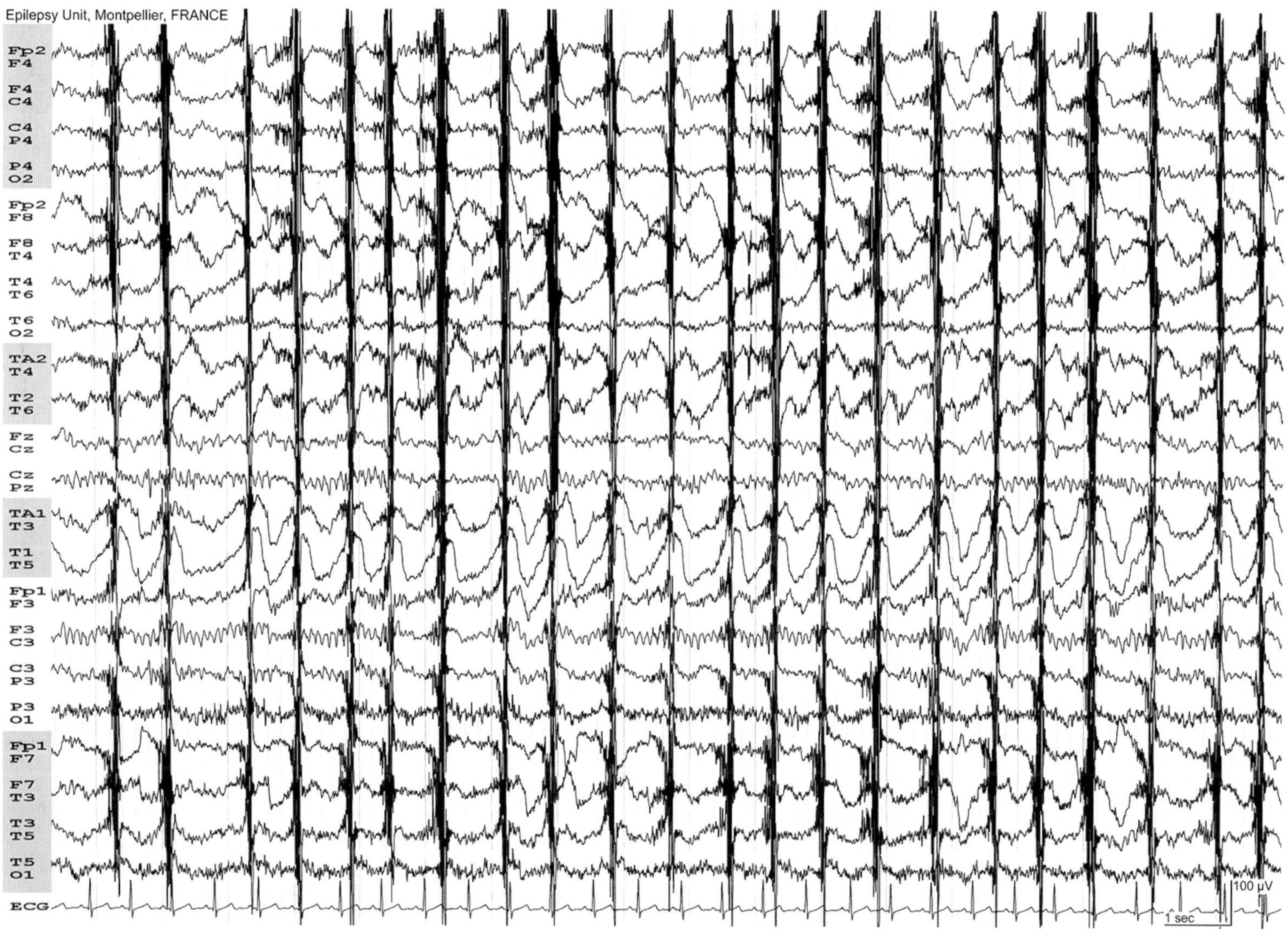

Figure a / Recording at 15 mm/s.

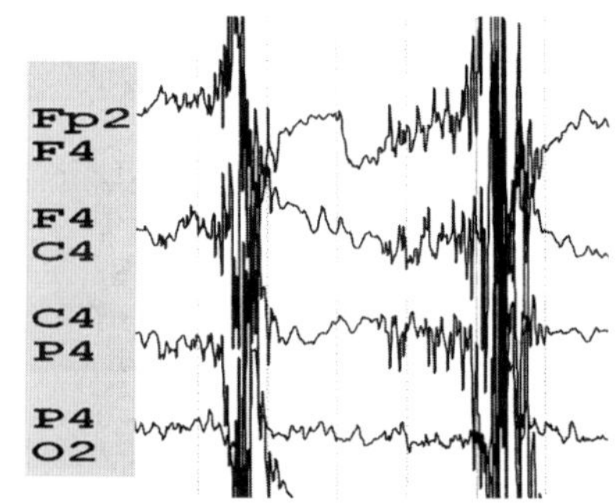

Figure b / Muscle potentials due to chewing.

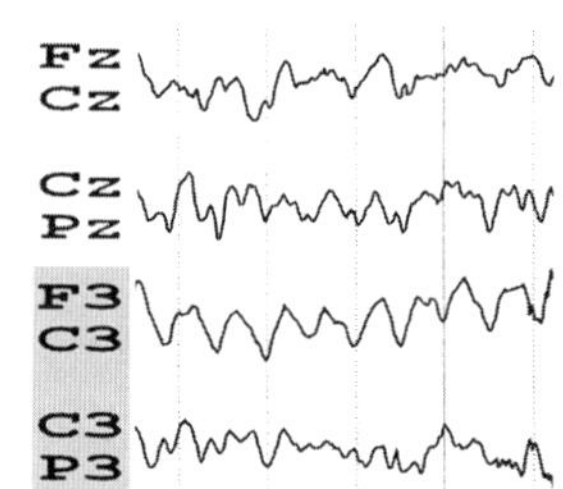

Figure c / Mu rhythm.

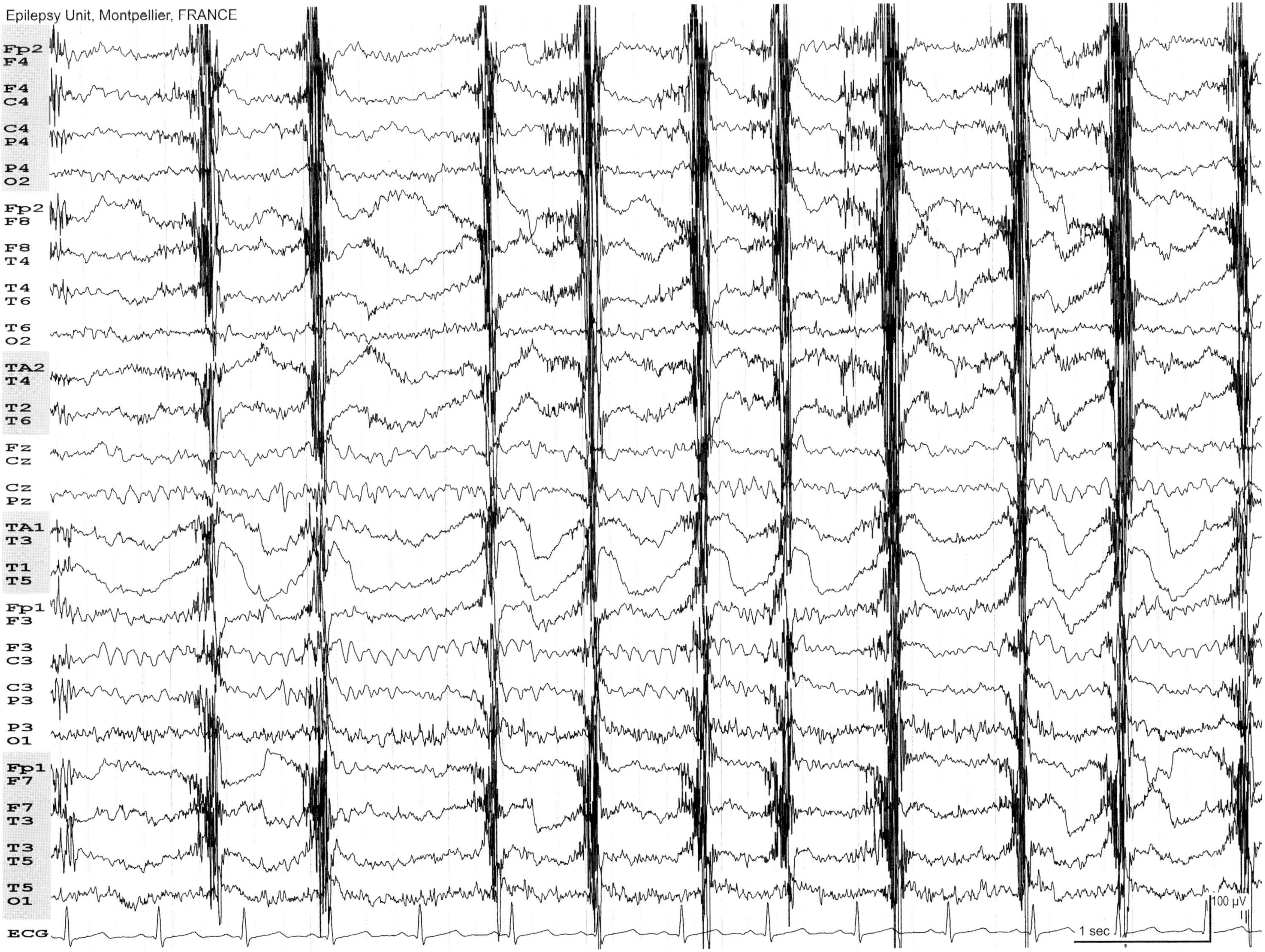
Epilepsy Unit, Montpellier, FRANCE
Fp2 F4
F4 C4
C4 P4
P4 O2
Fp2 F8
F8 T4
T4 T6
T6 O2
TA2 T4
T2 T6
Fz Cz
Cz Pz
TA1 T3
T1 T5
Fp1 F3
F3 C3
C3 P3
P3 O1
Fp1 F7
F7 T3
T3 T5
T5 O1
ECG
100 µV
1 sec

IV • 29 Glossokinetic artifact

Context

40-old man referred for episodes of loss of consciousness

What to note

Superimposed muscle activities. Bilateral delta waves at 2 Hz predominating over the anterior and temporal regions. This activity corresponds to movements of the tongue.

Comment

The artifacts produce by the tongue are in the delta range. The amplitude is greater in the temporal regions than in parasagittal regions. They may be bilateral or unilateral depending on the direction of the tongue. The artifacts may be reproduced when the patient says la-la-la.

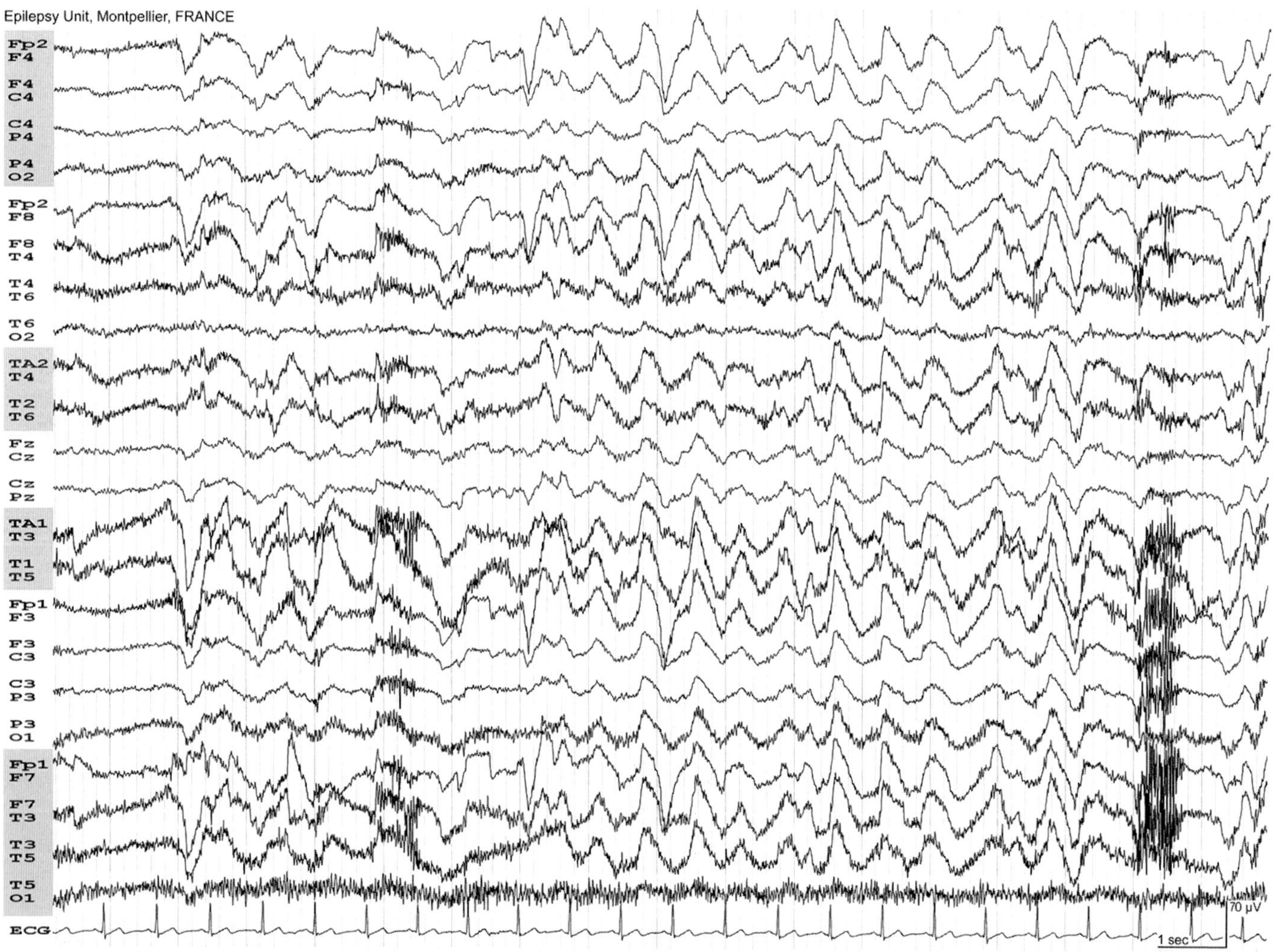

Figure a / Recording at 15 mm/s.

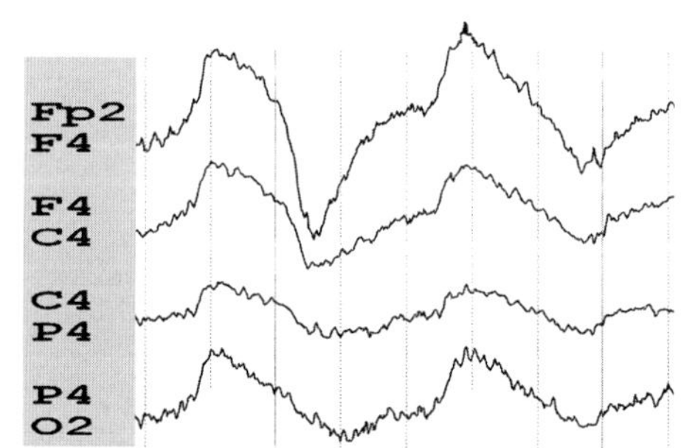

Figure b / Delta waves produced by movements of the tongue.

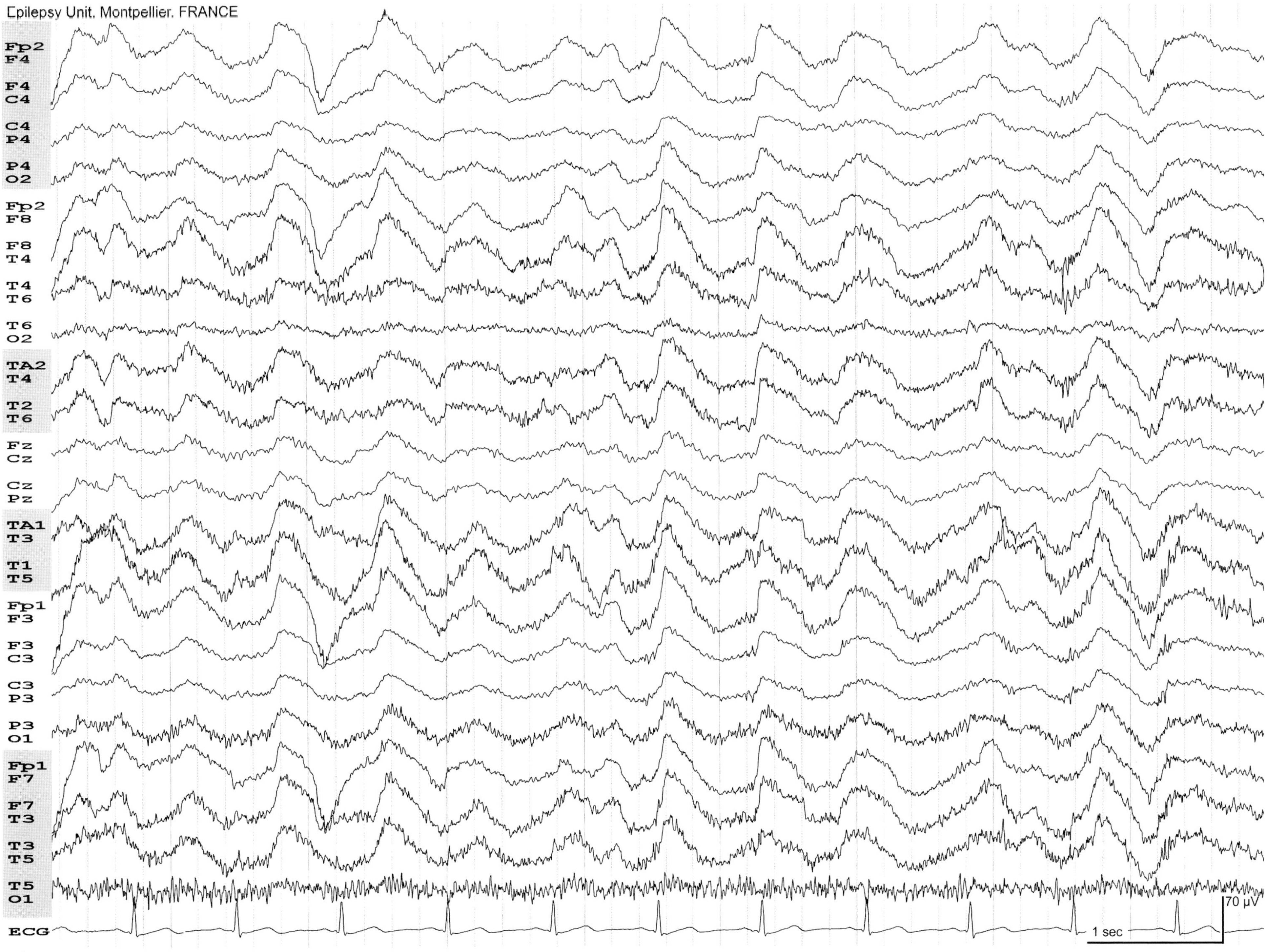
Epilepsy Unit, Montpellier, FRANCE
Fp2 F4
F4 C4
C4 P4
P4 O2
Fp2 F8
F8 T4
T4 T6
T6 O2
TA2 T4
T2 T6
Fz Cz
Cz Pz
TA1 T3
T1 T5
Fp1 F3
F3 C3
C3 P3
P3 O1
Fp1 F7
F7 T3
T3 T5
T5 O1
ECG
70 µV
1 sec

REFERENCES

Asokan G, Pareja J, Niedermeyer E. Temporal minor slow and sharp EEG activity and cerebrovascular disorder. *Clin Electroencephalogr* 1987; 18: 201-210.

Beaussart M. Benign epilepsy of children with rolandic (centro-temporal) paroxysmal foci: a clinical entity. Study of 221 cases. *Epilepsia* 1972; 13: 795-811.

Brickford RG. Activation procedures and special electrodes. *In:* Klass DW, Daly DD (eds). *Current Practice of Clinical Electroencephalography*. New York: Raven Press, 1979: 269-305.

Cavazzuti GB, Cappella L, Nalin A. Longitudinal study of epileptiform EEG patterns in normal children. *Epilepsia* 1980; 21: 43-55.

Ciganek L. Problem of rolandic "an arceau" rhythm. *Cesk Neurol* 1959; 22: 101-108.

Crespel A, Baldy-Moulinier M, Coubes P. The relationship between sleep and epilepsy in frontal and temporal lobe epilepsies: practical and physiopathologic considerations. *Epilepsia* 1998; 39: 150-7.

Crespel A, Coubes P, Baldy-Moulinier M. Sleep influence on seizures and epilepsy effects on sleep in partial frontal and temporal lobe epilepsies. *Clin Neurophysiol* 2000; 111 Suppl 2: S54-9.

Crespel A, Velizarova R, Garrigues G, Gelisse P. A new case of slow alpha variant during REM sleep. *Neurophysiol Clin* 2009; 39: 263-5.

Duntley SP, Kim AH, Silbergeld DL, Miller JW. Characterization of the mu rhythm during rapid eye movement sleep. *Clin Neurophysiol* 2001; 112: 528-31.

Dreyfus C, Curzi-Dascalova L. The EEG during the first year of life. In: Remond A (ed). *Handbook of electroencephalography and clinical neurophysiology, Vol. 6B.* Amsterdam: Elsevier, 1975: 24-30.

Eeg-Olofsson O, Petersen I. Rhythmic mid-temporal discharges in the EEG of normal children and adolescents. *Clin Electroencephalogr* 1982; 13: 40-45.

Fleming WE, Avidan A, Malow BA. Subclinical rhythmic electrographic discharge of adults (SREDA) in REM sleep. *Sleep Medicine* 2004; 5: 77-81.

Gastaut H, Terzian H, Gastaut Y. Étude d'une activité électroencéphalographique méconnue: Le rythme rolandique en arceau. *Marseille médical* 1952; 89: 296-310.

Gastaut H, Fischer-Williams M. Étude électroencéphalographique des syncopes. II. Corrélations électrocliniques chez 25 sujets enregistrés pendant leur syncope. *Rev Neurol (Paris)* 1956; 95: 542-547.

Gastaut H, Fischer-Williams M. Electro-encephalographic study of syncope; its differentiation from epilepsy. *Lancet* 1957; 273: 1018-25.

Gelisse P, Kuate C, Coubes P, Baldy-Moulinier M, Crespel A. Wicket spikes during Rapid Eye Movement Sleep. *J Clin Neurophysiol* 2003; 20: 245-350.

Gelisse P, Crespel A. Mu rhythm in the infant. *Neurophysiol Clin* 2006; 36: 261-3.

Gelisse P, Crespel A. Phantom spike-and-wave bursts during REM-sleep. *Neurophysiol Clin* 2008; 38: 249-53.

Gelisse P, Crespel A. Slow alpha variant during REM sleep. *Neurophysiol Clin* 2008; 38: 3-8.

Gelisse P, Crespel A. Mu rhythm and rhythmic midtemporal discharges in REM sleep. *Neurophysiol Clin* 2014; 44: 165-7.

Gelisse P, Serafini A, Velizarova R, Genton P, Crespel A. Temporal intermittent activity: a marker of juvenile absence epilepsy? *Seizure* 2011; 20: 38-41.

Gibbs FA, Gibbs EL, Lennox WG. Electroencephalographic response to overventilation and its relation to age. *J Pediatr* 1943; 23: 497-505.

Gibbs FA, Gibbs EL. *Atlas of Electroencephalography, vol 1.* Cambridge MA: Addison-Wesley, 1950.

Gibbs FA, Gibbs EL. *Atlas of encephalography, vol. 2.* Cambridge, MA: Addison-Wesley, 1952.

Gibbs FA, Gibbs EL. *Atlas of encephalography, 2nd ed., vol. 3* Reading, MA: Addison-Wesley Publishing Company INC, 1964.

Hughes JR. Two forms of the 6/sec spike wave complex. *Electroencephalogr Clin Neurophysiol* 1980; 48: 535-550.

Jukkarwala A, Hassan H, Nair M, Iyer RS. Extraoccipital photoparoxysmal response in a case of focal encephalitis. *Epileptic Disord* 2011; 13: 103-6.

Kasteleijn-Nolst Trenité D, Rubboli G, Hirsch E, Martins da Silva A, Seri S, Wilkins A, Parra J, Covanis A, Elia M, Capovilla G, Stephani U, Harding G. Methodology of photic stimulation revisited: updated European algorithm for visual stimulation in the EEG laboratory. *Epilepsia* 2012; 53: 16-24.

Katz RI, Horowitz GR. Sleep onset frontal rhythmic slowing in a normal geriatric population. *Electroencephalogr Clin Neurophysiol* 1983; 56: 27P.

Lairy GC, Harrison A, Leger EM. Foyers occipitaux asynchrones de pointes chez l'enfant mal voyant et aveugle d'âge scolaire. *Rev Neurol (Paris)* 1964; 111: 351-353.

Lipman IL, Hughes JR. Rhythmic mid-temporal discharges. An electroclinical study. *Electroencephalogr Clin Neurophysiol* 1969; 27: 43-47.

Naquet R, Louard C, Rhodes J, Vigouroux M. À propos de certaines décharges paroxystiques du carrefour temporo-pariéto-occipital. Leur activation par l'hypoxie. *Rev Neurol (Paris)* 1961; 105: 203-207.

Niedermeyer E, Koshino Y. Mu-Rhythmus: vorkonmmen und klinischeBedeutung. Z EEG-EMG 1975; 6: 69-78.

Niedermeyer E. Abnormal EEG patterns: epileptic and paroxysmal. In: Niedermeyer E, Lopes Da Silva F, (eds). *Elenctroencephalography: basic principles, clinical applications and related fields*, 5th edition. Philadelphia: Lippincott Williams &Wilkins; 2005: 255-280.

Okuma T, Kuba K, Matsushita T, Nakao T, Fujii S, Shimoda Y. Study on 14 and 6 per second positive spikes during nocturnal sleep. *Electroencephalogr Neurophysiol Clin* 1968; 25: 140-149.

Passouant P. EEG and sleep. Electo-clinical semeiology. In: Remond A (ed). *Handbook of electroencephalography and clinical neurophysiologie vol. 7A*. Amsterdam: Elsevier, 1975: 3-11.

Reiher J, Lebel M. Wicket spikes: clinical correlates of a previously undescribed EEG pattern. *Can J Neurol Sci* 1977; 4: 39-47.

Santoshkumar B, Chong JJ, Blume WT, McLachlan RS, Young GB, Diosy DC, Burneo JG, Mirsattari SM. Prevalence of benign epileptiform variants. *Clin Neurophysiol* 2009; 120: 856-861.

Serafini A, Crespel A, Velizarova R, Gélisse P. Activation of wicket spikes by REM sleep. *Neurophysiol Clin* 2014; 44: 245-9.

Silverman D. The anterior temporal electrode and the ten-twenty system. *Am J EEG Technol* 1965; 5: 514-515.

Stephenson JBP. *Fits and faints*. London: Mac Keith Press, 1990.

Tannier C, Bentzinger C, Feuerstein J. A case of unilateral and lesional mu rhythm-clinical and encephalographic development. *Rev Electroencephalogr Neurophysiol Clin* 1982; 12: 117-22.

Tassinari CA, Daniele O, Gambarelli F, Bureau-Paillas M, Robaglia L, Cicirata F. Quantité excessive de 7-14 positive spikes pendant la PMO chez deux jumeaux monozygotes avec retard du langage. *Rev Electroencephalogr Neurophysiol Clin* 1977; 7: 192-3.

Tsuzuki H. The 14 and 6 per sec. positive spikes during paradoxical sleep. *Folia Psychiatrica Neurologica Japonica* 1967; 21: 181-8.

Van Sweden B, Wauquier A, Niedermeyer E. Normal aging and transient cognitive disorders in the elderly. In: Niedermeyer E, Lopes Da Silva F (eds). *Elenctroencephalography: basic principles, clinical applications and related fields, 4th edition*. Baltimore: Williams & Wilkins, 1999: 340-348.

Velizarova R, Crespel A, Serafini A, Gelisse P. A new approach for the detection of the fourteen- and six-Hertz positive bursts (6-14 Hz): the lower temporal line. *Clin Neurophysiol* 2011; 122: 1272-3.

Williamson PC, Merskey H, Morrison S *et al.* Quantitative electroencephalographic correlates of cognitive decline in normal ederly subjects. *Arch neurol* 1990; 47: 1185-1188.

INDEX

IMPRIM'VERT®

Achevé d'imprimer par Corlet, Imprimeur, S.A.
14110 Condé-sur-Noireau
N° d'Imprimeur : 184450 - Dépôt légal : novembre 2016
Imprimé en France